Physical Education and the Study of Sport

Fifth Edition

We dedicate this book to all our 'A' level Physical Education and Sport Studies teachers, who have always been adaptable and enthusiastic to change. We wish them every success in their delivery of the AS/A2 programmes.

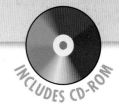

Physical Education and the Study of Sport

Fifth Edition

Bob Davis
Honorary Research Fellow, Worcester College of Higher Education
Former Principal Lecturer in Physical Education, Madeley College of Higher Education
Former Lecturer (p/t) in Sport, Health and Exercise, Staffordshire University
Chief Examiner, Reviser and Practical Moderator, A-Level Physical Education (AEB; 1986–1995)
Senior Adviser and Reviser, A-Level Physical Education (OCR; 1995–2003)

Jan Roscoe BEd(Hons) MSc
Former Teacher of A-Level Physical Education and Human Biology, Widnes Sixth Form College
Anatomy and Physiology Consultant for A-Level Physical Education (AEB; 1989–1997)
Publisher and Physical Education and Sport Resources Supplier

Dennis Roscoe
Former Head of School of Maths and Sciences, Knowsley Community College
Biomechanics Consultant (1989–1997) and Assistant Examiner and Team Leader for A-Level
Physical Education (1989–1993)
Publisher and Physical Education and Sport Resources Supplier

Ros Bull BEd(Hons) MSc
Former Principal Lecturer in Physical Education, Liverpool John Moores University
Former Chief Moderator, A-Level Physical Education and Sports Studies (AEB; 1988–1993)

Illustrations by Richard Tibbitts and Evi Antoniou-Tibbitts

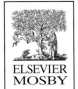

ELSEVIER MOSBY

EDINBURGH LONDON NEW YORK OXFORD PHILADELPHIA ST LOUIS SYDNEY TORONTO 2005

ELSEVIER
MOSBY

First edition published 1991 by Wolfe Publishing Ltd; reprinted 1992
Second edition published 1994; reprinted 1995, 1996
Third edition published 1997; reprinted 1998
Fourth edition published 2000, reprinted 2001, 2003

ISBN 0 7234 3375 5

Teachers' guides for Parts One and Two are available from Jan Roscoe Publications, 'Holyrood', 23 Stockswell Road, Widnes, Cheshire WA8 4PJ, UK. Teachers' guides for Part Three are available from Bob Davis, 102 High Street, Pershore, Worcestershire, WR10 1EA.

Videos © Jan Roscoe Publications 2000

British Library Cataloguing in Publication Data
A catalogue record for this book is available from the British Library

Library of Congress Cataloging in Publication Data
A catalog record for this book is available from the Library of Congress

Note
Knowledge and best practice in this field are constantly changing. As new research and experience broaden our knowledge, changes in practice, treatment and drug therapy may become necessary or appropriate. Readers are advised to check the most current information provided (i) on procedures featured or (ii) by the manufacturer of each product to be administered, to verify the recommended dose or formula, the method and duration of administration, and contraindications. It is the responsibility of the practitioner, relying on their own experience and knowledge of the patient, to make diagnoses, to determine dosages and the best treatment for each individual patient, and to take all appropriate safety precautions. To the fullest extent of the law, neither the publisher nor the authors assume any liability for any injury and/or damage.

your source for books,
journals and multimedia
in the health sciences
www.elsevierhealth.com

The publisher's policy is to use paper manufactured from sustainable forests

Printed in China

Contents

Preface   ix
Acknowledgments   x

Part 1 The performer in action   1

1 The anatomy of physical performance   **3**
  1.1 The human skeleton in action   3
  1.2 Joints in action   12
  1.3 Muscles in action   20
  1.4 Types of muscular contraction   26
  1.5 How coordinated movement is produced   31
  1.6 Skeletal muscle structure and fibre types   38

2 Cardiovascular-respiratory systems   **47**
  2.1 The heart   47
  2.2 The vascular system   58
  2.3 Blood flow in muscles   63
  2.4 Respiratory factors in physical performance   69
  2.5 Gas exchange in the lungs   76
  2.6 Lung volumes and physical activity   82

3 Energy for exercise   **89**
  3.1 Energy and work   89
  3.2 Energy creation and release within muscle   94
  3.3 The recovery process after exercise   101
  3.4 Maximal aerobic and anaerobic capacities   107
  3.5 Nutrition for exercise   112

4 Training for physical performance   **119**
  4.1 Physical fitness and fitness testing   119
  4.2 Training   132
  4.3 Types of training   146
  4.4 Children and physical activity   168

5 Fitness for life   **173**
  5.1 Obesity   173
  5.2 Cardiovascular diseases   178
  5.3 Ageing and physical fitness   181

6 Biomechanics: linear motion   **189**
  6.1 Linear motion   189

7 The nature and application of force   **199**
  7.1 The nature of force   199
  7.2 Internal forces   227

8 Rotating systems   **243**
  8.1 Angle and angular displacement   243
  8.2 Moment of inertia   247

  Synoptic investigation   258
  Glossary of terms   264

Part 2 The performer as a person

277

9 The nature and classification of skill   **279**
  9.1 Skill defined   279
  9.2 Skill classified   281
  9.3 Skill and ability   286

10 Information processing in perceptual-motor performance   **295**
  10.1 Introduction to information processing   295
  10.2 Sensory input: the receptor mechanism   299
  10.3 Perception: the DCR process   301
  10.4 Perception: selective attention and memory 303
  10.5 Decision making   308
  10.6 Motor output and feedback   315

11 Principles of learning and teaching   **325**
  11.1 Introduction: learning, performance and learning curves   325
  11.2 Learning: principles and theories   328
  11.3 Motivation and feedback   335
  11.4 Transfer of learning   340
  11.5 Teaching   343

12 Psychology of sport performance: individual differences and performance enhancement   **353**

12.1 The nature of sport psychology   353
12.2 A brief history of sport psychology   354
12.3 Personality   356
12.4 Attitudes in sport   369
12.5 Aggression in sport   374
12.6 Motivation   379

13 Psychology of sport: social influences on performance and mental preparation   **397**

13.1 Social learning   397
13.2 Groups and teams   399
13.3 Leadership   405
13.4 Competition effects on sport performance: social facilitation   409
13.5 Mental preparation for sports performance   413

Glossary of terms   431

Part 3 The performer in a social setting   **435**

14 Important concepts in physical educational and sport   **437**

14.1 Introduction   437
14.2 Towards a concept of leisure   441
14.3 Towards a concept of play   447
14.4 Towards a concept of recreation   450
14.5 What do we mean by physical recreation?   450
14.6 Towards a concept of sport   454
14.7 What is physical education?   462

15 Physical education and sport in the United Kingdom   **469**

15.1 The social setting   469
15.2 Administration of physical education   474
15.3 Administration of sport   483
15.4 Organisation of outdoor recreation and outdoor education   486

16 Sociological considerations of physical education and sport   **491**

16.1 Towards an understanding of sports sociology   491
16.2 Society, culture and sport   494
16.3 Group dynamics in sporting situations   508
16.4 Roles in sport and physical education   515

17 Some contemporary issues in physical education and sport   **521**
17.1 Societal: excellence in sport   522
17.2 Institutional: outdoor education   530
17.3 Sub-cultural: women in sport   534

Glossary of terms   543

18 Physical education and sport on the continent of Europe with particular reference to France   **545**
18.1 The social setting of physical education and sport in France   545
18.2 The administration of physical education in France   549
18.3 The administration of sport in France   553
18.4 The organisation of outdoor recreation and outdoor education in France   555

19 Physical education and sport in Commonwealth countries with particular reference to Australia   **559**
19.1 The social setting of physical education and sport in Australia   559
19.2 The administration of physical education in Australia   566
19.3 The administration of sport in Australia   571
19.4 The organisation of outdoor recreation and outdoor education in Australia   577

20 Physical education and sport in North America with particular reference to the United States   **583**
20.1 The social setting of physical education and sport in the United States of America   583
20.2 The administration of physical education in the United States   589
20.3 The administration of sport in the United States   594
20.4 The organisation of outdoor recreation and outdoor education in the United States   598

21 Physical education and sport in Communist and post-Communist countries with particular reference to the Soviet Union (Russia)   **603**
21.1 The social setting of physical education and sport in the Soviet Union and post-reform Russia   603
21.2 The administration of physical education in the USSR (Russia)   610
21.3 The administration of sport in the USSR (Russia)   614
21.4 Tourism in the Soviet Union and post-reform Russia   618
21.5 Cross-cultural review and exam-style questions   621

Glossary of terms   625

22 Historical perspectives and popular recreation   **627**
22.1 Historical perspectives   627
22.2 Factors underlying the origins of sport   630
22.3 The pattern of popular recreation in Great Britain   630

23 Athleticism in 19th-century English public schools   **651**
   23.1 Background to public school development   651
   23.2 The structural basis of the English public school system   652
   23.3 The technical development of sports in the public schools   654
   23.4 Athleticism and character development   661
   23.5 The influence of public school athleticism on sport in society   663

24 The pattern of rational recreation in 19th-century Britain   **667**
   24.1 Social factors influencing the development of rational recreation in Britain   667
   24.2 The rational development of activities and games   671

25 Transitions in English elementary schools   **681**
   25.1 19th-century drill and gymnastics   681
   25.2 The 1902 model course   682
   25.3 Early syllabuses of physical training   684
   25.4 The effects of the Second World War (1939–1945)   687
   25.5 Summary of cultural influences in the 20th century   689

   Glossary of terms   693

Index   697

Preface

The first edition of *Physical Education and the Study of Sport* was designed as a necessary text for new A-level candidates in Physical Education and Sport Studies. Written by a team of teachers engaged in producing and teaching the syllabuses, the book set out to give teachers and candidates the necessary knowledge and understanding for this level of study, while adopting a user-friendly style and practical approach.

The second, third and fourth editions of the book evolved to meet the needs of changing exam syllabuses and boards, and the changing nature of A-level as it became more closely defined as AS and A2. As with most subjects at these levels, Physical Education and Sport Studies courses became modular, with modules 1, 2 and 3 being taken at AS-level in the first year of a two-year programme, or as a stand alone AS after one year. The second year (labelled A2) incorporated modules 4, 5 and 6, and the final A-level result consisted of a combination of results from all 6 modules.

This fifth edition attempts to meet the needs of AQA, Edexcel and OCR syllabuses at AS and A2. The sections and chapters of the book retain their original structure, and the syllabus contents will need to be sought by the student from these chapter headings.

As with the fourth edition, this edition includes a CD-ROM which adds an interactive element to the use of the book and CD-ROM combined as a package.

The book appears again on the CD-ROM (for those who prefer to browse from the computer screen) with the added feature that it is possible to select your syllabus and module of study and have only relevant material appear on-screen. This should help with the confusion over whether certain parts of the subject matter (in the book) should be studied or not.

Also, the CD-ROM includes sections on:

- the synoptic assessment element (with examples of questions and sample answers for each board)
- the project element (as relevant to your course), with examples
- the PPP/IPP/PEP element with sample folios or PEPs from each syllabus
- sample exam papers from each board.

Hopefully this fifth edition package will add a cognitive element to people who love sport and want to study how it operates, and help people understand how sports performance can be enhanced by looking at theoretical aspects of sport studies. This will raise the standard of sports performance at the base of the performance pyramid and hopefully encourage an elite to establish sporting excellence in this country.

July 2004   Dennis Roscoe

Acknowledgements

We would like thank and acknowledge Richard Tibbitts and Evi Antoniou-Tibbitts who have developed and enhanced the artwork and photographs created by Shirley Doolan, John Helms, Peter Cullen, Rosemary White and Ken Travis from previous editions. We wish to thank Alan Edwards and Helen Roscoe who have prepared photographs for this new edition, in addition to photographs supplied by ActionPlus Sports Images. We wish to thank James Watkins for the use of his diagrammatic themes within the Biomechanics section.

We wish to acknowledge the tireless work of teams from OCR, AQA, Edexcel and Welsh Boards who have created AS/A2 level Sport and Physical Education syllabuses in line with the Dearing Report and for the use of their exemplar projects, personal performance profiles and examination papers within the CD-ROM.

We have a special thanks to Sarena Wolfaard, from Elsevier, who has brought together a team of specialist editors who have chased us and kept us working to fulfil those important deadlines, and to Wendy Gardiner, Gail Wright, and Colin McEwan who have co-jointly produced the book and CD-Rom. We know that users will be delighted with the enclosed exam-board specific text for AQA/OCR and Edexcel syllabuses on the first section of the CD-ROM. We wish to thank Elsevier for agreeing to allow PE staff to use this CD-ROM for classroom Powerpoint Presentations. This facility will enhance the quality of delivery in all schools and colleges.

Once again it has been a pleasure to work with Nora Naughton, our project manager and her in-house team Kathy Syplywczak, Sarah Abel and Sam Gear from Naughton Project Management. We wish to acknowledge and also express our appreciation for the important role Nora has played – for the many hours we have spent on the phone, for the prompt exchange of written sections of the manuscript and for her patience in dealing with last-minute alterations.

We wish to thank Holly Regan-Jones, who copy-edited the text, checked grammar and coding of figures and diagrams, and Debra Barrie who copy-edited the text of the CD-Rom. Stewart Larking, who designed the very colourful contemporary cover, based on an initial concept by Helen Roscoe, Judith Wright who has been responsible for the design direction of the project, and to Sharine Yap, RDC China who has been responsible for the page layouts and corrections.

A further acknowledgement is due to the MacMillan Company of Australia for their permission to use material from *Physical Education: Theory and Practice* by Davis et al in Part Two.

Part 1

The performer in action

Jan and Dennis Roscoe

1. The anatomy of physical performance
2. Cardiovascular-respiratory systems
3. Energy for exercise
4. Training for physical performance
5. Fitness for life
6. Biomechanics: linear motion
7. The nature and application of force
8. Rotating systems

Synoptic movement analysis investigation

Glossary of terms

If we are to understand the performer in action we need to know how the body is put together, how it functions, how it moves and how it applies forces to itself and other bodies with which it comes into contact.

Two main sections have been combined within Part 1. These are the application of human anatomy and physiology (Chapters 1–5) and biomechanics (Chapters 6–8) to the study of physical education and sport.

The aim of *The performer in action* is to develop, very simply and by no means completely, some of the concepts in these areas of study in the mind of the student, in as relevant and as practical a manner as possible. It will therefore be essential for the student to look at other texts on intermediate-level human anatomy, physiology, biomechanics and physics to search out more detail than is provided here or to progress the concepts further as interest takes him or her.

The results tables included in this text are available for students to copy and use.

A short bibliography of texts and reading lists, the reading of which would extend understanding and knowledge of relevant concepts, is to be found at the end of all chapters.

For the teacher, *The performer in action* provides a series of practical activities that should help the non-scientific student to understand the essentials of anatomical, physiological and biomechanical concepts without the need for a detailed programme of specialist lessons.

The anatomy of physical performance

Athletic activity in all its forms of movement is made possible by the arrangement and functioning of bodily systems. The aim of this section is to discover how we move.

1.1 The human skeleton in action

Learning objectives

On completion of this section, you will be able to:
1. Classify and identify skeletal bones in the axial and appendicular skeletons.
2. Classify and recognise the specific functions of bones according to their shape.
3. Recognise bony features and understand their functioning within the human body.
4. Appreciate variations of bone thickness, density and length in relation to sporting activities.
5. Identify the two types of skeletal tissue and be able to write briefly about their structure and function within the human body.
6. Describe the process of ossification in the different types of bones.
7. Understand the influence of exercise on the developing skeleton.

Keywords

- appendicular skeleton
- articular
- axial skeleton
- bony features
- cancellous bone
- cartilage
- compact bone
- depressions
- diaphysis
- endochondral ossification
- epiphyseal plate
- epiphysis
- flat bone
- Haversian system
- hyaline or articular cartilage
- intramembranous ossification
- irregular bone
- long bone
- osteoblast
- osteoclast
- osteocyte
- protrusions
- short bone
- skeleton
- white fibrocartilage
- yellow elastic cartilage

The human skeleton consists of 206 bones (Figure 1.1), many of which move or hinge at joints and which, in combination with over 600 skeletal muscles, enable the human body to achieve a variety of actions, such as running, throwing, striking, jumping, pulling and pushing.

Joints are covered with compressible **articular** (articular is a word that describes surfaces which move or hinge) or **hyaline cartilage**, which serves to cushion the impact of large forces on bone ends. Joint movements are varied and complex. For example, the

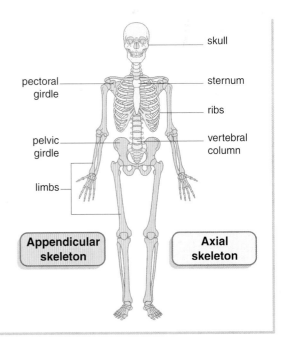

Fig. 1.1 The 206 bones are divided into the appendicular and axial skeletons.

skull
sternum
ribs
vertebral column

pectoral girdle
pelvic girdle
limbs

Appendicular skeleton
Axial skeleton

shoulder joint is constructed to permit swinging, throwing, striking and supporting movements. The **foot** is designed to support the body weight, to act as a shock absorber and to provide great flexibility of movement. All these skeletal bones and joints enable the body to carry out a vast range of complex movements demanded by a variety of differing physical and sporting situations. This section will help you to identify skeletal bones, skeletal connective tissues and their functions, to understand bone development in relation to a variety of physical activities and the influence of exercise on the developing skeleton.

The **human skeleton** has been created by evolution to perform the following functions.

1. To provide a lever system against which muscles can pull.
2. To provide a large surface area for the attachment of muscles.
3. To protect delicate organs (for example, the cranium protects the brain).
4. To give shape to the body.
5. To give support to the body (for example, the firm construction of the thorax, which permits breathing).
6. To manufacture red blood cells and to store fat, calcium and phosphate.

Investigation 1.1 Types of skeleton

Using the information in this section, work out the functions specific to the **appendicular** and **axial** skeletons.

Types of bones

The shape and size of bones are designed according to their specific functions. They can be **long, short, flat** or **irregular** (see Figure 1.2).

A long bone

A long bone consists of a hollow cylindrical shaft formed of compact bone with cancellous bone located at the knobbly ends of the shaft (see Figures 1.7 and 1.8). The **tibia** is an example of a long bone.

A short bone

A short bone is a small roughly cubed-shaped bone consisting of entirely cancellous bone surrounded by a thin layer of compact bone. The **carpals** in the wrist are examples of short bones.

Flat and irregular bones

Flat and irregular bones consist of two outer layers of compact bone with cancellous bone between them. A flat bone is smooth, flattened and usually slightly curved. The **cranium** is an example of a flat bone. Examples of irregular bones include **vertebrae, the patella** or **sesamoid** bone (sited in the patella knee tendon) and wormian bones, which are small irregular bones sometimes formed in cranial sutures.

Irregular bones have no definite shape. The **vertebral column**, which is part of the axial skeleton, is composed of 24 unfused vertebrae – five fused sacral vertebrae attached to four fused coccygeal vertebrae – making a total of 26 bones.

Investigation 1.2

Identification of skeletal bones
Materials: skeleton. Figure 1.2, posters.

Task 1
Refer to the skeleton drawing (Figure 1.2A) and identify the bones numbered 1–25.

Task 2
Define the axial and appendicular skeletons. Using a skeletal model and Figures 1.1 and 1.2A, identify the major bones that make up the axial and appendicular skeletons.

Investigation 1.3

Identification of skeletal bones

Task 1 (use the information in Figure 1.3 on p. 6)
1. Identify those structural features common to all unfused vertebrae.
2. Identify the five main regions of the vertebral column, numbered 7–11.
3. How is the basic plan of vertebrae modified in different regions of the vertebral column to perform different skeletal functions?
4. Identify the **axis** and **atlas** vertebrae. State the principal function for both vertebrae.
5. Which part of the nervous system does the vertebral column protect?

Task 2
Using the information in Figure 1.2, identify the labelled sesamoid bone. What is its function in relation to physical activity?

Task 3
Complete the adjacent exercise in which you are asked to match the bone type to an example in the body and specific function. That is, join the linked types, examples and functions as shown for the femur. ▶

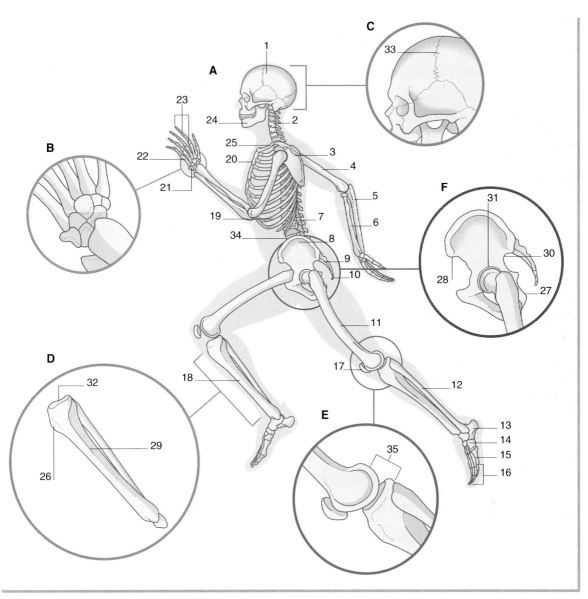

Fig. 1.2 Human skeleton in action. A. The human skeleton.
Examples and types of bones: **B.** Short. **C.** Flat. **D.** Long. **E.** Irregular. **F.** Flat.
Some examples of bony features: **26.** Tuberosity. **27.** Tubercle. **28.** Spine. **29.** Ridge. **30.** Notch. **31.** Fossa. **32.** Condyle.
Types of joint: **33.** Fibrous joint – suture. **34.** Cartilaginous joint – intervertebral disc. **35.** Synovial joint – knee.

▶ **Task 4**
Using a skeletal model and Figure 1.2, classify other examples for each of these four types of bones.

Task 5
Bend down and touch your toes. Explain what joints and bones are involved and what movement is brought about.

Bone type	Example in the body	Specific function
flat	femur	gives strength
long bone	tarsal	protective
short	axis	acts as a lever
irregular	sternum	large surface area for muscle attachment

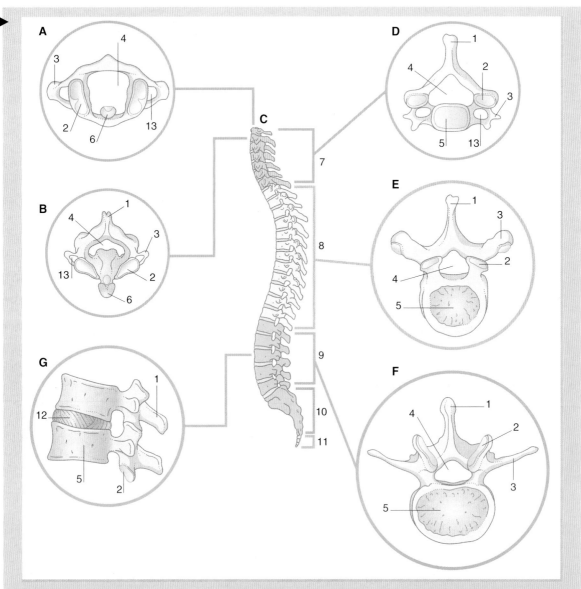

Fig. 1.3 Vertebral column. A. Atlas, superior view. **B.** Axis, superior view. **C.** Vertebral column, lateral view. **D.** Cervical vertebra, superior view. **E.** Thoracic vertebra, superior view. **F.** Lumbar vertebra, superior view. **G.** Two lumbar vertebrae.
1. Spinal process for attachment of back muscles. **2.** Articulating surface connection for ribs and other vertebrae.
3. Transverse processes provide attachment for muscles and ligaments. **4.** Spinal canal through which spinal cord runs.
5. Centrum or body of the vertebra, which bears the body weight. **6.** Odontoid process of axis. **7.** Cervical vertebrae (7).
8. Thoracic vertebrae (12). **9.** Lumbar vertebrae (5). **10.** Sacrum (fused). **11.** Coccyx. **12.** Intervertebral disc (cartilaginous joint). **13.** Foramen for vertebral artery.

Investigation 1.4   The identification of bony features

Materials: Figure 1.2 and skeletal bones.

Your task is to identify various bony features from the collection of bones supplied for this investigation and from diagrams of the skeletal bones in this text or elsewhere.

Task 1
Run your fingers along different types of long, short, flat and irregular bones. Feel for bumps and dents on the surface of these bones. These bony features are called **protrusions** and **depressions**, respectively. Identify the following types of **depressions**.

1. A **fossa**, which is a rounded depression, e.g. the acetabular fossa.

2. A **groove**, e.g. the deep bicipital groove near to the head of the humerus, which is occupied by one of the tendons of the biceps muscle.

3. A **notch**, e.g. the sciatic notch.

Protrusions are classified into the following types.

1. A **tuberosity**, which is a broad, rough, uneven bump, e.g. the tibial tuberosity.

2. A **tubercle** is a smaller version of a tuberosity, e.g. the tubercle of the iliac crest.

3. A **spine**, which is a sharp pointed feature, e.g. the iliac spine.

4. A **ridge, crest** or **line** runs along the shaft of a bone, e.g. along the tibial crest.

Protrusions that form part of a joint are called **condyles** and **epicondyles**. For example, the rounded condyles and the adjacent epicondyles of the femur form part of the knee joint.

Task 2
Identify other examples of protrusions and depressions on a skeleton.

Task 3
What do you think are the functions of the protrusions and depressions you have found?

Investigation 1.5   A comparison of bone measurements

Materials: tape measures, skeleton poster.

Task 1
Using a tape measure, on a partner or yourself, measure the circumference of bones at the wrist, elbow, ankle and knee.

1. Make a results table in which it is possible to compare measurements between males and females in the class or group.

2. Is the circumference (which is directly related to thickness) of bone an indication of the maturity and strength of bones?

Task 2
Bones of males are denser than those of females and the bones of an Afro-Caribbean skeleton are denser than those of the Caucasian skeleton. What effect would this information have when planning physical activity programmes?

Task 3
1. Identify the positions of the bones of the elbow joint (**humerus, radius, ulna**) and shoulder joint (**scapula, humerus**) on a partner and relate the positioning of these bones to a skeletal chart and/or Figure 1.2A.

2. Discuss and list the joint types and ranges of movement of the elbow and shoulder joints (see Table 1.1 (p.15) for details on joint types and movement patterns).

Task 4
1. Identify the **acromion** process of the scapula, **olecranon** process at the elbow end of the ulna and styloid **process** at the wrist end of the ulna.

2. Using a tape measure, measure the distance from the:
   a. acromion process to the styloid process
   b. acromion process to olecranon process
   c. olecranon process to the styloid process.

3. Identify the **head** of the **femur, femoral condyle** of the knee joint and **lateral malleolus** of the fibula.

4. Measure the distance from the:
   a. head of femur to the femoral condyle
   b. femoral condyle to the lateral malleolus.

5. Record the results in a table for each individual. Include gender, skeletal height, bone measurement data from above and major sporting activity.

6. Collect data from males and females and record on bar charts the distribution of measurements from all individuals for each category of measurement.

7. Discuss and comment on the distribution of results obtained from different sporting groups, and from males as opposed to females.

Task 5
Eight new events (handball, basketball and six rowing events) were introduced for women in the Olympic Games at Montreal in 1976. The data on heights of 186 medallists from these newly introduced events are shown (Figure 1.4) superimposed on the height distribution of women aged 18–24 in the United States, who were used as a reference population. (Volleyball statistics have been included to give a complete set of women's team games in these Olympic Games. Reference source data adapted from Khosla 1983.[1]

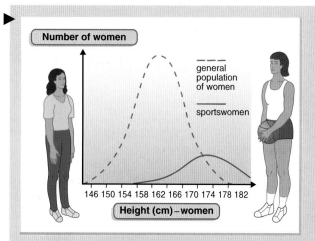

Fig. 1.4 Height distribution of female Olympic medallists compared with those of women aged 18–24 in the United States (adapted from reference[1]).

Note from Figure 1.4 that the mean height for the general population is 162 cm and for the medallists is 174 cm.

1. Using the information in Figure 1.4, discuss the proposition that there is an overwhelming bias in favour of the very tall in many team contests.

2. From the graph, work out the approximate proportion of the general population with height above 174 cm. What are the implications of this for selection of national squads from groups of ordinary sportspeople?

3. Give other examples of sports where tallness, specific limb dimensions and shortness would be beneficial to performance.

Types of skeletal connective tissue

There are two types of skeletal connective tissue: **cartilage** and **bone**.

Cartilage

Cartilage is a firm, smooth, resilient, non-vascular connective tissue. It consists of a matrix of **chondrin** (a gelatinous protein) that is secreted by specialised cells called **chondrocytes**. These cells position themselves in tiny cavities called **lacunae** and are nourished by nutrients that diffuse across from the capillary network outside the cartilaginous tissue. There are **three** types of cartilage found in the human body.

1. **Yellow elastic cartilage** (Figure 1.5A), consists of yellow elastic fibres running through a solid matrix, with cells lying between the fibres. The pinna or ear lobe and epiglottis are examples of this tissue.

2. **Hyaline** or **articular cartilage** (Figure 1.5B), appears as a smooth bluish-white matrix tissue. The matrix is solid, smooth, firm and yet resilient. The cells are grouped together to form a cell nest. This type of cartilage is located on the surfaces of bones that form joints. It forms the costal cartilages, which attach the ribs to the sternum, and is also found in the larynx, trachea and bronchi.

3. **White fibrocartilage** (Figure 1.5c) consists of a dense mass of white fibres in a solid matrix, with the cells spread thinly among the fibres. It is a tough, slightly flexible tissue that is found between the bodies of the vertebrae (called

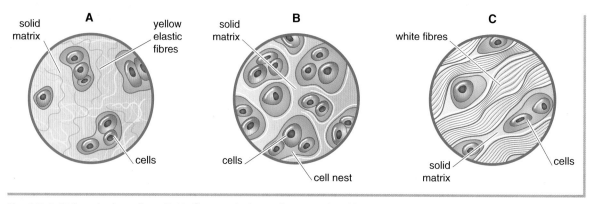

Fig. 1.5 A. Yellow elastic cartilage. **B.** Hyaline or articular cartilage. **C.** White fibrocartilage.

intervertebral discs, refer to Figure 1.3G, item 12), in semilunar cartilages in the knee joint and it surrounds the rim of the bony sockets of the hip and shoulder joints.

Bone

Bone is classified as either **hard** (or **compact**) or **spongy** (or **cancellous**). It is the hardest connective tissue in the human body and is composed of water, organic material (mainly **collagen**, a structural fibrous protein that supports many body tissues) and inorganic salts, namely calcium phosphate, calcium carbonate and fluoride salts.

Compact bone

Compact bone consists of thousands of collagen-based structures called **Haversian systems** (0.5 mm in diameter). Each Haversian system has a central canal surrounded by concentric ring-shaped calcium-based plates called **lamellae**. Figure 1.6 shows the microscopic detail of a compact bone.

Spongy or cancellous bone (Figures 1.6, 1.7, 1.8)

Spongy or **cancellous** bone has a honeycomb appearance and consists of a thin criss-cross matrix of bone tissue called **trabeculae** (a general term describing connective tissue that supports other tissues), with red bone marrow filling the tiny spaces. This criss-cross matrix acts as a scaffolding to provide greater strength and support without the greater weight of solid bone.

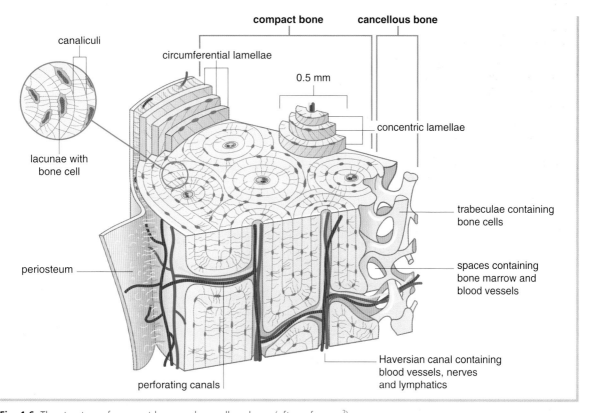

Fig. 1.6 The structure of compact bone and cancellous bone (after reference[2]).

Investigation 1.7 To examine the structure of bone

Task 1

Consider the labelled structures in Figure 1.6 and/or projector slides (if available) and relate these structures to the following description.

*Bone cells are located in spaces called **lacunae** (which contain lymph) and they are arranged concentrically around a canal containing blood vessels, nerves and lymphatics (the Haversian canal). These bone cells run into a system of fine channels or **canaliculi**. It is the lymph in these channels that is responsible for carrying food and oxygen to the bone and for removing waste products.*

Compact bone is surrounded by a tough, vascular tissue (blood vessels containing blood) called the **periosteum**.

Task 2

If you cut a long bone in half down the middle, you would be able to observe the structures shown in Figure 1.8. Using the information in Figures 1.7 and 1.8 and from specialist human biology texts, answer the following questions.

1. Where in a long bone is spongy bone located?

2. Why do you think red bone marrow is present in spongy bone?

3. Suggest reasons why long bones are hollow.

4. What is the function of the **yellow bone marrow** located in the diaphysis?

5. The surface of bones, except for articular surfaces, is covered by the **periosteum**, which attaches itself to the bone via tiny roots.

What do you think are the principal functions of the periosteum?

6. Why is it important for the ends of bones to be reinforced with a criss-cross matrix of bone tissue, as shown in Figure 1.7?

7. Observe and comment on the positioning of the compact bone in Figure 1.7.

8. Observe and comment on the positioning of the articular cartilage.

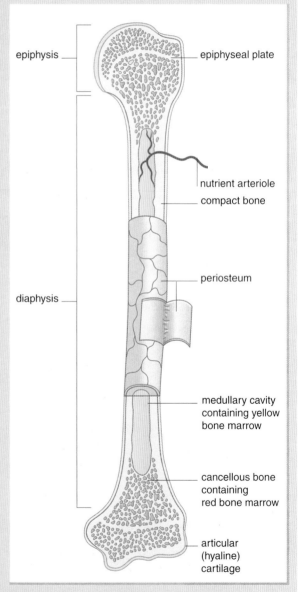

Fig. 1.8 Longitudinal section of a typical long bone.

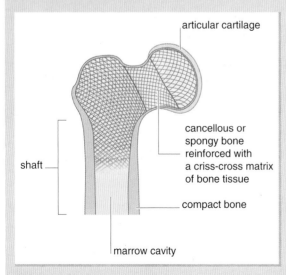

Fig. 1.7 Head of the femur.

The development of bones

Ossification is the process of bone formation or the conversion of fibrous tissue or cartilage into bone.

Within the developing foetus the short and long bones are formed as a result of **indirect ossification**, since the foetal cartilage is replaced by bone. This process is called **endochondral ossification**, as illustrated in Figure 1.9.

Throughout the development of a long bone, parts of the bone are reabsorbed so that unnecessary calcium phosphate is removed and structures such as the **medullary cavity** are created. Specialised cells called **osteoclasts** carry out this job. Remodelling is the ongoing replacement of old bone tissue by new bone tissue and redistribution of bone tissue along lines of mechanical stress.

In addition, the bone becomes wider as a result of the **osteoblasts** laying down new layers of bone tissue within the deeper layers of the periosteum.

The process of ossification in a short bone takes place from the centre of the bone and radiates outwards.

Flat and irregular bones are developed in one stage directly from connective tissue. This process is called **intramembranous ossification** and it takes place at ossification centres within the membrane. Osteoblasts

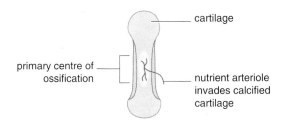

A. Bone-forming cells called **osteoblasts** (*os* means bone and *blast* means immature cell) first appear in the centre of the **diaphysis** (the primary centre of ossification) and surround themselves with calcium and phosphate ions supplied by the blood. Blood vessels invade the calcified cartilage and a cavity begins to form once the cartilage is replaced by bone. When the osteoblast becomes embedded in the lacuna of the bone matrix, it becomes an **osteocyte**.

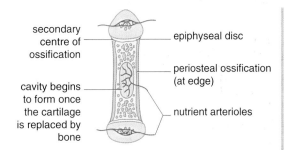

B. At birth most of the diaphysis consists of bone, and bone has started to appear in the **epiphysis** (the secondary centre of ossification). On the exterior, **periosteal ossification** continues.

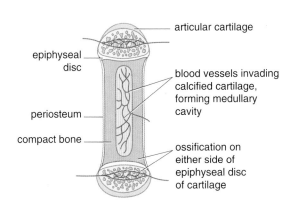

C. A disc of cartilage separates the bone at the diaphysis from the bone at the epiphysis. This disc is called the **epiphyseal disc** or growth disc because it is the only place where an increase in the length of the bone can take place. As the young child grows, increase in length of the long bone can occur only at the epiphyseal discs. On the exterior, periosteal ossification continues.

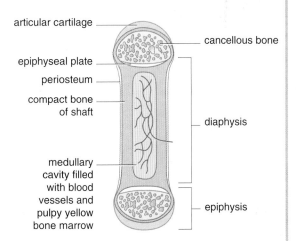

D. When the growth ceases, the bony diaphysis is united with the epiphysis and the line of fusion is marked by a dense layer of bone called the **epiphyseal plate**. The age at which this fusion occurs varies, but long bones normally cease growing in late adolescence.

Fig. 1.9 Endochondral ossification in a long bone (after reference[2]).

produce bone tissue along the membrane fibres to form cancellous bone. Beneath the periosteum, osteoblasts lay down compact bone to form the outer surface of the bone. The sutures of the skull gradually ossify during the development of a young child into adulthood, as do the clavicle, scapula and pelvis.

As a result of ossification, the two types of bone tissue described earlier are formed (Figure 1.6), namely **cancellous** and **compact bone**. It is only at the joint sites that cartilage remains to form the edges where bones meet.

Review questions

1. Draw a diagram to represent a longitudinal section of a long bone. Label your diagram to show the main structural features and the progress of ossification.
2. Describe the process by which a long bone is lengthened.
3. Distinguish between cancellous and compact bone in terms of microscopic appearance, location and function.
4. Make a list of the activities that you are involved in which may help to promote bone growth. Explain your answer.

Exam-style questions

1. What considerations, with respect to skeletal development, must a coach make in the planning of a training programme for a growing adolescent? (*6 marks*)

2. Exercise, along with an adequate diet, is essential for proper bone growth. Discuss. (*8 marks*)

1.2 Joints in action

Learning objectives

On completion of this section, you will be able to:

1. Classify joints into fibrous, cartilaginous and synovial.

2. Identify and describe the features of the different types of synovial joint.

3. Appreciate how joint structure allows for a variety of different skeletal movements.

4. Classify movement in relation to the major body planes and axes.

5. Describe briefly some of the common joint injuries and methods of prevention.

6. Appreciate what is meant by good posture and identify some of the causes and rehabilitation methods used for postural defects.

Keywords

➤ posture

Joint feature
➤ bursae
➤ joint capsule
➤ cartilaginous joint
➤ fibrous joint
➤ ligaments
➤ menisci
➤ pads of fat
➤ synovial fluid
➤ synovial joint
➤ synovial membrane

Movement patterns
➤ abduction
➤ adduction
➤ circumduction
➤ depression
➤ dorsiflexion
➤ elevation
➤ eversion
➤ extension
➤ external rotation

➤ flexion
➤ internal rotation
➤ inversion
➤ planter flexion
➤ pronation
➤ rotation
➤ supination

Synovial joints
➤ ball and socket
➤ condyloid
➤ gliding
➤ hinge
➤ pivot
➤ saddle

Cardinal planes
➤ frontal
➤ sagittal
➤ transverse

Axes of movement
➤ saggital
➤ frontal
➤ vertical

So far our investigation into how we move has been concerned with an understanding and identification of the main bones and bony tissues in the human body. This next section will help you to understand how bones are connected to each other in order to achieve movement.

A **joint** is a site in the body where two or more bones come together and joints are classified according to the amount of movement there is between the articulating surfaces.

Types of joint

Fibrous or fixed joint

A **fibrous** or a fixed joint has no movement at all. Tough fibrous tissue lies between the ends of the bone, which are dovetailed together. Examples in the human body are the sutures in the skull, as illustrated in Figure 1.10 (also refer to Figure 1.2c).

Cartilaginous joint

A **cartilaginous** joint allows some slight movement. The ends of bones are covered in articular or hyaline cartilage, separated by pads of white fibrocartilage. Slight movement is made possible only because the pads of cartilage compress. In addition, the pads of cartilage act as shock absorbers. The intervertebral discs are examples of this type of joint, as illustrated in Figures 1.11 and 1.3G.

Synovial joint

A **synovial** joint (Figure 1.12) is a freely moving joint and is characterised by the presence of a joint capsule and cavity. This type of joint is subdivided according to movement possibilities, which are dictated by the bony surfaces that actually form the joint (the knee joint is an example of this type of joint, as is illustrated in Figure 1.13).

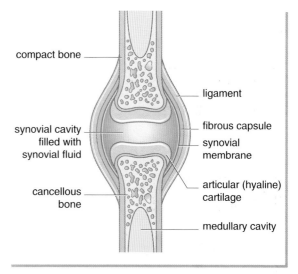

Fig. 1.12 Synovial joint.

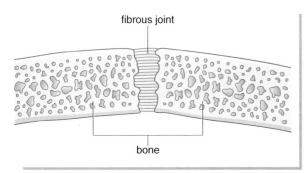

Fig. 1.10 Fibrous joint.

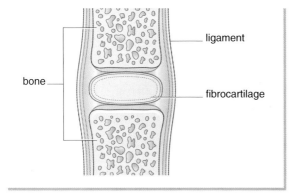

Fig. 1.11 Cartilaginous joint.

Investigation 1.8

To consider the structure and function of the main types of joints

Materials: Human skeleton, skeleton and/or joint posters.

Task 1
Identify the three types of joints classified so far. Locate the positioning of examples for each of these three types of joint on your own body.

Task 2
1. Jump off a box.
2. Run and bound.
3. Rotate your upper trunk against your lower body.

Explain the role of cartilaginous joints in these movements.

Task 1

Using the synovial joint illustrated in Figure 1.13, match each letter to one of the structures listed below and explain the function of each structure by using appropriate reference books.[2, 3] For example:

Structure:

1. **Articular or hyaline cartilage** – a smooth, shiny cartilage that covers the ends of bones and absorbs synovial fluid.

 Answer: F.

Function: to prevent friction between bones; it is thought that when the joint is exercised, synovial fluid is squeezed out of the articular cartilage at the point of contact (McCutchen's weeping lubrication theory).

2. **Joint capsule** – a sleeve of fibrous tissue surrounding the joint.

3. **Ligament** – a sleeve of tough, fibrous connective tissue, which is an extension of the joint capsule.

4. **Synovial membrane** – a sheet of epithelial cells inside the joint capsule.

5. **Synovial fluid** – the fluid enclosed in a joint, some of which is absorbed by hyaline cartilage during exercise.

6. **Pad of fat** – pads of fat that occupy gaps in and around the joint.

Task 2

Two other features, **bursae** and **menisci**, appear in synovial joints. **Bursae** are little sacs of synovial fluid and **menisci** are extra layers of fibrocartilage located at the articulating surfaces of joints. Suggest functions for these specialised joint features and give examples from the human body.

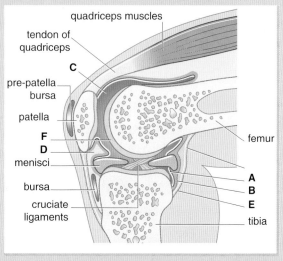

Fig. 1.13 Synovial joint: the knee.

Task 3

Identify the intracapsular ligaments.

Task 4

Sketch a diagram of a named **ball** and **socket** type of joint, labelling all the structures that provide joint strength and mobility.

Task 5

The effect of long-term training on hyaline cartilage is to cause a permanent cartilaginous thickening as a result of the laying down of additional cartilaginous cells. Suggest reasons why you think an increase in hyaline cartilage thickness would be beneficial to an athlete.

Types of synovial joints and their movement range

As the title suggests, all synovial joints are characterised by the presence of synovial fluid.

The possible ranges of movements within a synovial joint vary according to the shape of the articulating surfaces and therefore according to the joint type (this information is contained in Table 1.1). In addition, specific movement patterns are briefly described and illustrated in Figure 1.14.

A full-page illustration of these different types of synovial joint and the type of movement allowed by them can be found on pp. 7–8, Figures 1.12–1.17, of Wirhed.[3]

In Table 1.1 the movement ranges of synovial joints are classified according to their axes of movement, i.e. joints that allow only one plane of movement are identified as a one-axis joint, a two-axes joint has movement within any two planes, whereas a three-axes joint has movement in all three planes.

For a more detailed account of planes and axes of motion, refer to Wirhed[3] and Bartlett.[4]

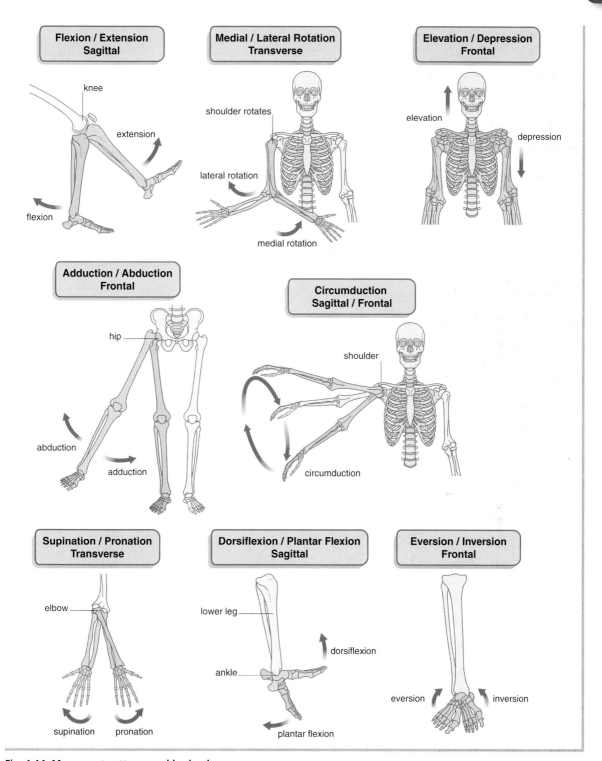

Fig. 1.14 Movement patterns and body planes.

Movement in relation to lever systems

When muscles act on joints to produce the movement patterns identified in Table 1.1, bones act as levers. A full description and application of the three lever systems is found in Section 7.2.

Table 1.1 Types of synovial joint

Joint type	Shape of joint	Movement range	Example in the body
Ball and socket	Ball-shaped bone fits into a cup-shaped socket	Three axes – flexion and extension, abduction and adduction, rotation, circumduction	Hip
Hinge	Convex and concave surfaces fitting together	One axis – flexion and extension	Distal joints of phalanges
Pivot	Ring-shaped, surrounding a cone	One axis – rotation	Radio-ulnar joint below elbow
Condyloid	A modified ball and socket	Two axes – flexion and extension, abduction and adduction, giving circumduction	Metacarpophalangeal joints of fingers
Saddle	Shaped like a saddle	Two axes – flexion and extension, abduction and adduction, giving circumduction	Carpometacarpal joint of the thumb
Gliding	Two flat gliding surfaces	A little movement in all directions	Joint between the clavicle and sternum

Movement in relation to major body planes and their axes

Planes of movement

Body planes are points of reference used to assist in the understanding of movement of body segments with respect to one another, as illustrated in Figure 1.15. Within each plane an axis can be identified in association with a particular joint about which the movement takes place. There are **three** imaginary planes of reference (known collectively as the **cardinal planes**), which pass through the centre of gravity of the body.

1. The **frontal** or lateral plane is a vertical plane that divides the body into front (anterior) and back (posterior) sections. **Abduction and adduction** movement patterns (such as those occurring in a cartwheel) and **spinal lateral flexion** (side flexion trunk bends) occur within this plane.
2. The **sagittal** plane is another vertical plane (at right angles to the frontal plane) that divides the body into right and left sections. The midline of the body is a vertical line where the sagittal and frontal planes meet. Medial points are said to be close to this midline and lateral points away to one side (left or right) of the midline. **Flexion** and **extension** movement patterns, such as in somersaulting, sit-ups and biceps curl, occur within this plane.
3. The **transverse** or horizontal plane divides the body into upper and lower sections. Within the transverse plane, **superior** means towards the top of the body and **inferior** means towards the bottom of the body. Rotational movement patterns such as **pronation**, **supination** and **spinal rotation**

occur within this plane. Spinning activities, such as in hammer throwing and the spinning skater, are examples of rotational movements within the transverse plane.

Figure 1.15 gives a diagrammatic representation of the primary cardinal reference planes.

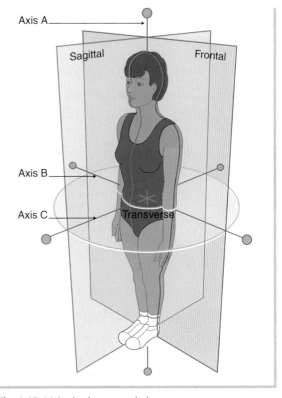

Fig. 1.15 Major body axes and planes.

Axes of movement

When movement occurs within a plane, it must rotate around an axis. There are three axes, labelled A, B and C in Figure 1.15.

The **sagittal** or transverse axis passes horizontally from back (posterior) to front (anterior), at right angles to the frontal plane. Movements in the frontal plane about the sagittal axis include abduction, adduction and spinal lateral flexion.

The **frontal** axis runs from side to side at right angles to the sagittal plane. Movements within the sagittal plane about the frontal axis are flexion, extension, hyperextension, dorisflexion and plantarflexion.

The **vertical** or longitudinal axis runs straight down through the top of the head at right angles to the transverse plane. Movements in the transverse plane about the vertical axis are rotational movements.

In Table 1.1 the movement ranges of synovial joints are classified according to their axes of movement, i.e. joints that allow only one plane of movement are identified as a one-axis joint, a two-axes joint has movement within any two planes, whereas a three-axes joint has movement in all three planes.

For a more detailed account of planes and axes of motion, refer to Wirhed[3] and Bartlett.[4]

Investigation 1.10   To associate movement patterns of synovial joints with the primary cardinal reference planes and their axes

Task 1
Table 1.1 gives examples for each synovial joint type. Identify other examples of synovial joints located in the human body.

Task 2
Using the specific terms that describe the basic movement range, identify the possible movement patterns for your selected joints.

Task 3
In Figure 1.15 the axes of motion have been labelled A, B and C. Identify each of these axes.

Task 4
Classify the movement patterns, listed from task 2 above, according to the three major body planes and axes.

Investigation 1.11   Joints in action (see Table 1.2)

Task 1
During most physical activity, the knee joint plays a vital role in movement.

1. Describe how the anatomical structures of the knee joint protect and stabilise the joint.
2. Describe how the anatomical structures of the knee joint make movement possible.
3. In many sports, the knee joint is often injured as a result of impacts (with other sportspeople or objects) or excessive forces (as in weightlifting, throwing or jumping) or overuse. Make a list of the common injuries that occur in the knee joint. (You may wish to extend this line of investigation to other joint sites.)
4. Describe some of the ways in which you could prevent such injuries from occurring.

A good reference book for questions 3 and 4 is Bird et al.[5]

Task 2
Working with a partner, locate the joints identified in Table 1.2 and identify the joint type. Place a tick in the appropriate boxes relevant to the movement patterns for each of the joints listed.

Task 3
Define circumduction and, using the information in Table 1.2, list the joints where this can occur.

Task 4
Observe the action pictures in Figure 1.16. Name the types of synovial joint located at the knee and hip of the swimmer and basketball player. Analyse the movement patterns happening at these joints. You may wish to select your own action pictures and answer the same questions.

Task 5
Identify the plane and axis of rotation during the preparatory leg action of the basketball shot shown in Figure 1.16B.

Task 6
Choose a selection of flexibility exercises that are part of your normal warm-up (refer to pp. 157–158 onwards for ideas). Within small groups, compare the ranges of flexibility at selected joint sites. You may wish to use the mobility assessment test described in Chapter 4.

▶

Table 1.2 Joint analysis

Joint	Joint type	Flexion	Extension	Abduction	Adduction	Rotation	Supination	Pronation
Wrist								
Radio-ulnar								
Elbow								
Shoulder								
Shoulder girdle								
Spine								
Hip								
Knee								
Ankle								

Joint	Elevation	Depression	Plantarflexion	Dorsiflexion	Inversion	Eversion
Wrist						
Radio-ulnar						
Elbow						
Shoulder						
Shoulder girdle						
Spine						
Hip						
Knee						
Ankle						

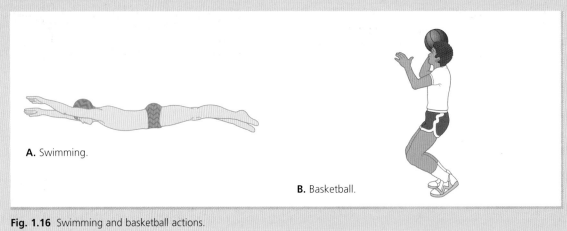

A. Swimming.

B. Basketball.

Fig. 1.16 Swimming and basketball actions.

Investigation 1.12   Postural factors and physical activity

Figure 1.17A is thought to be the most efficient way of standing to minimise joint and skeletal stress, whilst maximising muscular function.

1. In what ways does the inefficient postural stance in Figure 1.17B differ from that of Figure 1.17A?

2. Using a specialist sports injury text (such as Bird et al[5]), identify some of the factors that result in the development of poor posture.

3. In many sports there is a natural tendency to kick more frequently with one foot, play tennis or throw an implement either right handed or left handed. This often results in the dominant side becoming bigger, stronger, better controlled and better coordinated. By referring to Sections 1.4, 4.1 and specialist sports injuries texts,[5] identify the way in which the weakness of a muscle group could be assessed and treated in the rehabilitation of muscular imbalance.

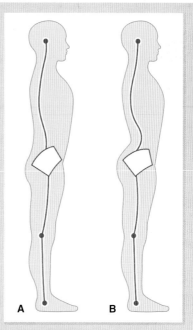

Fig. 1.17
A. Anatomically efficient posture.
B. Inefficient posture.

A   B

Review questions

1. Define articulation. What factors determine the degree of movement at joints?

2. List the bones that articulate in the following joints:
   a. knee
   b. elbow
   c. shoulder
   d. thoracic vertebrae
   e. hip.

3. Explain how the articulating bones in a synovial joint are held together.

4. What differences in their joints produce the differences in mobility between the hip joint and the elbow joint?

5. Identify and categorise **four** joints involved in the arm action of the tennis serve.

6. Identify the movement patterns performed at the joint sites listed for the following physical activities:

   a. pushing hockey ball: knees, elbows, wrists

   b. sit and reach test (task 5 described in Investigation 4.1): trunk, hip

   c. step up onto a bench (task 3 described in Investigation 4.1): knees, hip

   d. basketball shooting: wrists, elbow, shoulders

   e. vertical jump (task 1(2) described in Investigation 4.1): ankles, knees, hip.

Exam-style questions

1. a. Figure 1.18 shows a gymnast in the crucifix position on the rings. Identify the **three** planes and the **three** axes of motion indicated in the diagram. (*3 marks*)

  b. In which plane does each of the following movements take place:
-   **i.** cartwheel?
-   **ii.** forwards somersault?
-   **iii.** ice skating spin with legs together and arms overhead? (*3 marks*)

  c. Identify the main axis of rotation for each of the sports movements shown in Figures 1.19A–C. (*3 marks*)

(Total 9 Marks)

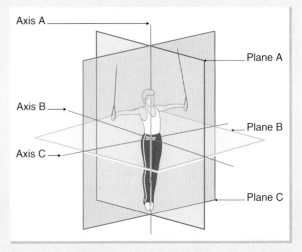

Fig. 1.18 Crucifix position on the rings.

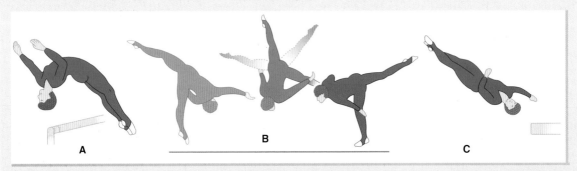

Fig. 1.19 Identify axes of rotation for **A.** rear layout dismount, **B.** aerial walkover and **C.** twisting dismount..

1.3   Muscles in action

Learning objectives

On completion of this section, you will be able to:

1. Classify and identify skeletal muscle according to its shape and group.

2. Locate, name and appreciate the movement patterns of major muscles.

3. Discuss the relationship between muscle size and performance.

4. Understand the role of musculo-skeletal attachments in limb movement.

5. Analyse movements in terms of muscle action.

6. Understand what is meant by origin, insertion and antagonistic muscle action.

Keywords

- ➤ agonist
- ➤ antagonist
- ➤ antagonistic muscle action
- ➤ aponeuroses
- ➤ fascia
- ➤ fixator
- ➤ fusiform
- ➤ insertion
- ➤ ligaments
- ➤ muscle group
- ➤ origin
- ➤ pennate
- ➤ periosteum
- ➤ skeletal muscle
- ➤ synergist
- ➤ tendon

One of the important functions of the human skeleton is to enable movement. Physical activity is achieved as a result of the action of over 600 muscles that contract or shorten, thereby facilitating the movement of the skeleton across its joints.

Muscles are the converters of energy, since they change chemical energy into mechanical energy. This is achieved as a result of the contraction of hundreds of muscle fibres within the connective tissue of each muscle.

During muscular contraction a muscle tightens to produce a state of tension that is adequate to meet the demands of the activity. The effect of regular physical activity is to develop and sustain local muscle strength and endurance. Some skeletal muscles, for example the soleus muscle, are very fatigue resistant (this is because they consist of a high proportion of **slow-twitch** fibres). Other muscles, for example the biceps and gastrocnemius muscles, fatigue more quickly because they are essentially **fast twitch** (the details of slow- and fast-twitch muscle fibres are described in Section 1.6). The effects of training in adapting muscle tissue to stress demands are discussed in Chapter 4. However, all muscles will contract *only* when stimulated by nerve impulses.

Shapes of muscles (Figures 1.21B–E)

Skeletal muscles vary in shape and function. Each muscle shape, its origins, insertions and positioning, have evolved specifically to deal with its unique functioning.

Fusiform

Fusiform means **spindle shaped**, since the muscle fibres run the length of the muscle belly to converge at each end. This strap-like, round shape enables the muscle to perform a large range of movement.

Pennate

Pennate means **featherlike**. A pennate muscle is a flat muscle in which fibres are arranged around a central tendon, like the barbs of a feather.

The major types of pennate muscles are grouped according to the way in which the fibres are arranged around the central tendon (Figure 1.20). Pennate muscles have a very limited range of movement, but are very strong.

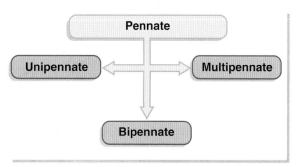

Fig. 1.20 Pennate muscle types.

Investigation 1.13

Identification of muscle shapes and the relationship of muscle shape to its function

1. Give an example for each type of fusiform and pennate muscle shape illustrated in Figures 1.20 and 1.21.

2. Describe how the three types of pennate muscle shape are designed for efficient functioning within the human body.

The above investigation could be extended to consider the relationship between muscle shape and muscle force.[3]

Investigation 1.14

Identification of muscles and their movement patterns

Materials: Figure 1.21 and muscle chart and/or slides.

Task 1
Identify and label the muscles numbered 1–34 in Figure 1.21.

Task 2
Using the labelled muscles from Figure 1.21 and other reference material,[3,6,7] identify groups of muscles of the upper leg, their origins and insertions and classify them into functional categories: that is, flexors, extensors, adductors, abductors and rotators (for an example, see Table 1.3).

Task 3
Identify the groups of muscles of the shoulder and upper arm according to functional categories.

Task 4
Identify the groups of muscles of the trunk according to functional categories.
You may wish to extend this investigation by identifying the origins and insertions of other major muscles on skeletal bones.

▶

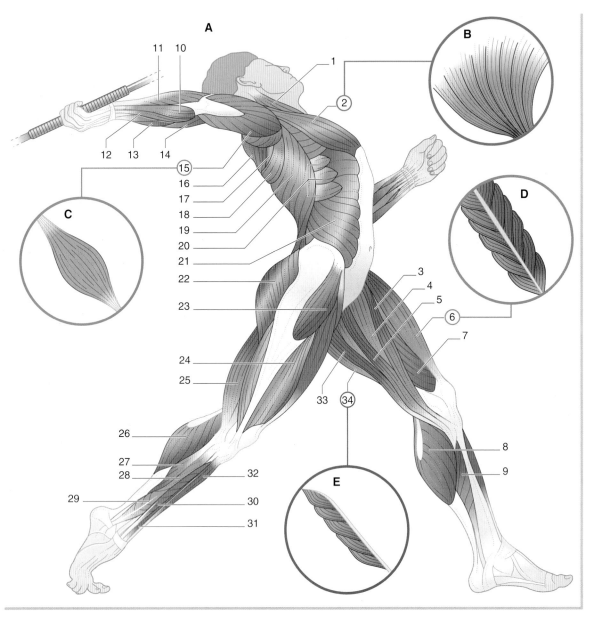

Fig. 1.21 Muscles in action. A. Superficial muscles of the human body (1–34).
Muscle shapes: **B.** Multipennate. **C.** Fusiform. **D.** Bipennate. **E.** Unipennate.

Table 1.3 Flexors – bending of the knee		
Muscle group	Origin	Insertion
Hamstrings Biceps femoris	**Long head** – ischial tuberosity **Short head** – linea aspera of femur	Head of fibula and lateral condyle of tibia
Semimembranosus	Ischial tuberosity	Medial condyle of tibia
Semitendinosus	Ischial tuberosity	Below medial condyle of tibia

Investigation 1.15   To identify muscles in relation to simple motor tasks and to relate muscle size to performance

Materials: tape measures, muscle chart.

Task 1
Perform a standing long jump (Figure 1.22) and measure the distance covered from the start line to the nearest point of landing. Record the best of three trials.

Task 2
By appropriate use of the muscle chart and by palpation, identify the muscles on the front of the thigh.

1. What is this group of muscles commonly called?
2. Name each main muscle located within this group.

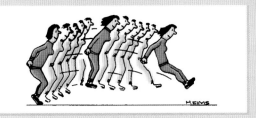

Fig. 1.22 A standing long jump.

Task 3
Stand normally, feet slightly apart. Using the tape, your partner measures (in cm) the circumference of your contracted thigh at its maximum girth or mid-distance from the hip to the knee joint, for both left and right legs. Record these measurements in Table 1.4.

Task 4
1. Compare within small groups the relationship between standing long jump and maximum thigh girths. Plot a graph of performances from the standing long jump (*x*-axis) against the maximum thigh girths (*y*-axis) of as many of your colleagues as possible. What does your graph show?

2. Are there differences in left and right thigh girths? Give possible reasons for any differences.

3. Identify any errors that may have affected your results.

You may wish to extend this investigation by using other muscle groups such as those of the trunk and shoulder regions of the body.

Table 1.4 Results table – the relationship of muscle size to performance					
	Performance and measurements of class members				
	Self	1	2	3	4
Standing long jump					
Distance in metres					
Thigh girths					
left thighs in cm					
right thighs in cm					

How skeletal muscle works

Muscles and bones have specialised skeletal structures, such as **tendons** and the **periosteum** (*peri* around, *oste* bone) of a bone, which generally transmit muscular forces to bones or, in the case of ligaments, attach bone to bone (**ligaments** limit the range of movement of joints). These structures are commonly known as **musculo-skeletal attachments**.

Tendons
Muscles are attached to bones by tendons, which pass over joints. Tendons are strong, mainly inelastic and

vary in length and structure. Small tendons, such as those to the muscles that control eye movement, have no nerve and blood supply whereas large tendons, such as the Achilles tendon, are connected to the **central nervous system** and the **circulatory system**. Therefore, these larger tendons have nerves and blood supply, both of which are substantially less prolific and effective than in the actual muscles. In some cases the tendinous attachment to bone is a more flattened or ribbon-shaped connection, called an **aponeurosis**. This type of tendon is without nerves. An example is the aponeurosis of the internal oblique muscles (which tilt and rotate the trunk relative to the hip girdle).

Tendons are rigidly cemented to the periosteum, as illustrated in Figure 1.23. Where the tendon fastens on to the periosteum, structures called **Sharpey's fibres** firmly attach tendon tissue on to periosteal bone tissue. The **periosteum** is tough connective tissue whose function is to attach muscle tendons to bone and to assist bone growth.

Other connective tissue

Fascia is a general form of connective tissue that overlays or underlines many body structures. A specialist example of this is the **epimysium**, which is the name for the sheath or outermost layer of connective tissue that surrounds the whole muscle (shown in Figure 1.23 and discussed in more detail later in this chapter). **Superficial fascia** underlies the skin and forms the connective link between the skin and **deep fascia** of muscle.

The origin and insertion of muscles

The tendon at the static end of the muscle is called the **origin** and the tendon at the end of the muscle closest to the joint that moves is called the **insertion** of that muscle.

The arrangement of muscles

Muscles that cause joints to bend are called **flexors**, while those that straighten a joint are called **extensors**. Skeletal muscles are normally arranged in pairs, so that as one muscle is contracting the opposing muscle is relaxing, thus producing coordinated movement.

The muscle that actually shortens, to move the joint, is called the **prime mover** or **agonist**, whereas the muscle that relaxes in opposition to the agonist is called the **antagonist**. Muscles that are prime movers for one movement act as antagonists for the opposite movement. For example, the **biceps** (agonist) contracts while the **triceps** (antagonist) relaxes (Figure 1.24A). This combined action causes the elbow to flex. When the elbow straightens the reverse occurs: the **triceps** (agonist) contracts while the **biceps** (antagonist) relaxes (Figure 1.24B). The action of muscles working in pairs is called **antagonistic muscle action**. Antagonistic muscle action limits and controls movements, especially when there are groups of muscles acting together.

In addition, there are muscles that stabilise the origin to the prime mover so that only the bone into which it is inserted will move. These are called **fixators** and **synergists**.

Fixator muscles hold joints in position and are sited so that the origin and insertion are on opposite sides of a stabilised joint. **Synergists** are muscles that work together to enable the agonist muscle to operate (*syn* together, *ergon* work). Note that the terms 'fixator' and 'synergist' could be applied to the same muscle.

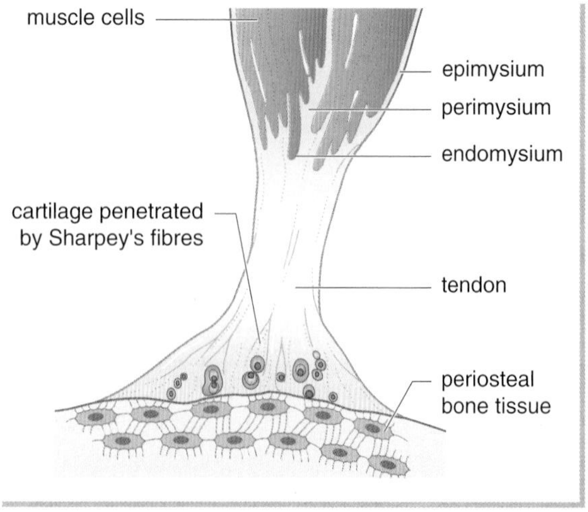

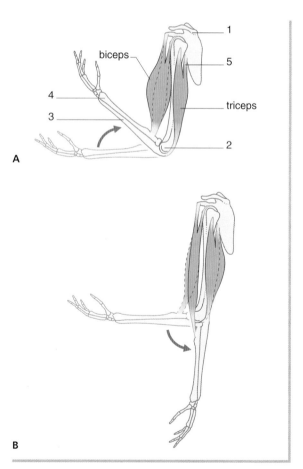

Fig. 1.23 How a tendon connects muscle to bone (after Solomon[8]).

Fig. 1.24 A. Flexion of the elbow. **B.** Extension of the elbow.

Investigation 1.16   An analysis of limb movement

Materials: bar with secured discs, Figures 1.24 and 1.25.

Task 1

1. Perform a curl with a light bar (see Figure 1.25: make sure that your teacher shows you the correct technique).
2. Identify the bones numbered 1–4 in Figure 1.24A.
3. Identify the structure numbered 5 in Figure 1.24A.
4. Using an example from one of the muscles shown in Figure 1.24A, explain what is meant by 'origin' and 'insertion'.
5. Identify and classify the muscles that are used in the action of curling a bar into the functional categories of agonist (or prime mover) and antagonist.
6. Using your own musculature and Figure 1.21, identify those muscles that act as fixators and synergists in the action of curling a bar.

Task 2

1. List the main agonists active in:
   a. legs whilst cycling
   b. leg action of a swimmer during breast stroke
   c. shoulder, arm and forearm whilst performing a push-up.

2. Work out the muscles that are relaxing in opposition to the agonist muscles in a, b and c.

Further practical work, which identifies specific exercises to increase strength and flexibility of muscles, is located in Section 4.3.

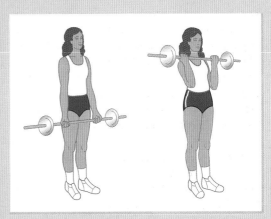

Fig. 1.25 Performing a curl with a light bar.

Review questions

1. What is the function of tendons?
2. What is the function of ligaments?
3. What are the functions of periosteal layers?
4. Identify the agonists that are active in:
   a. elevating the shoulders
   b. hyper-extending the back
   c. abducting the hip
   d. dorsiflexing the ankle
   e. flexing the knee.

5. Work out the muscles which are relaxing in opposition to the agonist muscles of 4a–e.

6. Identify the agonist muscles that are active in:
   a. a pull-up
   b. hitting a stationary hockey ball
   c. a sit-up
   d. a vertical jump
   e. shooting in basketball.

Exam-style questions

1. A backward roll, as illustrated in Figure 1.26, involves a series of coordinated muscle actions.

   a. Describe the movement patterns created at the hip and knee joints during the whole of the backward roll. (*4 marks*)

   b. Identify **two** agonist muscles acting on the shoulder joint during the push-off phase from the mat. (*2 marks*)

   c. Distinguish between hip flexion and trunk flexion. (*4 marks*)

   (*Total 10 marks*)

2. Figures 1.27A and B show a shot putter during the delivery phase of the technique.

   a. List the bones that articulate in the shoulder and knee joints. (*4 marks*)

b. Briefly explain the movement sequence of the right arm during the delivery phase of the shot put. (*3 marks*)

c. With reference to Figures 1.27A and B, name the main contracting muscles involved in the extension of the right elbow, knee and hip joints. (*6 marks*)

d. Using an example from either Figure 1.27A or B, explain what is meant by a fixator muscle. (*2 marks*)

e. Identify and describe an exercise that would improve the strength of the shoulder musculature of a shot putter. (*3 marks*)

f. Why is important to warm-up muscle tissue prior to vigorous activity such as shot putting? (*2 marks*)

(*Total 20 marks*)

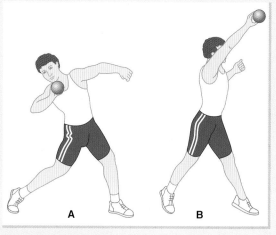

Fig. 1.27 Shot put action.

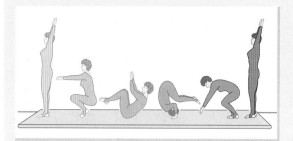

Fig. 1.26 Backward roll.

1.4 Types of muscular contraction

Learning objectives

On completion of this section, you will be able to:

1. Understand the concepts and the advantages and disadvantages of dynamic (isotonic and isokinetic) and static (isometric) contractions.

2. Understand the concepts of concentric and eccentric contractions.

3. Identify types of muscle contraction in relation to practical situations, co-jointly with agonist muscle identification.

Keywords

➤ concentric contraction
➤ dynamic contraction
➤ eccentric contraction
➤ isokinetic muscle contraction (mc)
➤ isometric mc
➤ isotonic mc
➤ muscular contraction
➤ plyometrics
➤ static contraction

In Investigation 1.16 you flexed or contracted the biceps muscle in your upper arm. This action was brought about by a changing state of contraction within the muscle tissue.

Muscular contractions can vary in speed, force and duration. For example, in cycling the action is cyclical and rhythmical, involving the interplay of agonist and antagonist. Whereas the action of a boxer throwing a punch is ballistic in nature, since the arm is moved fluidly by a short, fast contraction of the agonist and the movement is stopped as a result of the antagonist brake action.

During muscular contraction, a muscle may shorten, lengthen or stay the same. Where a muscle changes length, the contraction is classified as

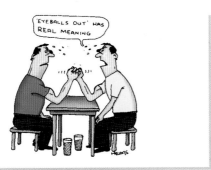

Fig. 1.28

dynamic. When a muscle remains the same length, a **static** contraction occurs.

Static contractions – isometric muscle contraction

Another name for a static muscular contraction is an **isometric** contraction (*iso* means same and *metric* means length, hence same length). This concept can be expressed as in Figure 1.28 or as:

Force of muscle contraction = Force expressed by resistance

The result is that the muscle length and tension in the arm-wrestling contest remain static. It is found that pushing or pulling **without moving** can produce a strength gain in the muscles used. In a training situation this is done by exerting the maximum possible force in a fixed position for sets of 10 seconds, with 60 seconds recovery interval. Its advantage is that a large amount of strength training can be done in a short time. Another advantage of **isometric training** is that it needs no special place or equipment and it can be done at any time throughout the day. However, it does little for cardiovascular fitness.

Concentric contractions – isotonic and isokinetic muscle contraction

The sort of exercise in which muscles are used in a normal **dynamic** way and in which muscles contract at a speed controlled by the sportsperson is called **isotonic**. In this case, the work is labelled **concentric** or positive because the resulting tension causes the muscle to create movement by shortening its length. The advantage of this type of exercise is that it stimulates real sporting use of the musculature. One of the adaptations produced by this type of training or exer-

cise is to increase the capillarisation of both skeletal and cardiac muscle and to enable these muscles to become more resistant to the onset of fatigue. Therefore, it is most likely to lead to improvement in sporting performance.

In **isokinetic** exercise, the point at which force acts moves at constant speed. For example, in a squat the shoulders move upward at a constant speed regardless of the effort put into the exercise. Special machines are needed for isokinetic work (the nearest usually available is a hydraulic exercise machine). Isokinetic exercises (concentric and eccentric) are used in special strength-training programmes and human movement research.

The advantage of isokinetic training is that it removes from the exercise the differences between forces exerted at different angles of limbs at a joint (refer to Investigation 7.5, task 7 for a discussion on the effect of joint angle on forces applied by muscle systems). Like isotonic exercise, isokinetic training improves muscle strength and endurance, as well as cardiovascular fitness.

Eccentric contractions

It is found that if maximum effort is put into an exercise **while a muscle group is lengthening**, then the muscle exerts a bigger force than in any of the other types of exercise mentioned above. In this case the work is labelled **eccentric** or negative, as, for example, in the controlled lowering of a weight.

This is the effect of the stimulus trying to prevent muscle lengthening and it produces the biggest overload possible in a muscle, thereby enhancing its development as far as strength is concerned. Eccentric contractions can be produced isotonically and isokinetically.

The chief practical use of eccentric contractions is in **plyometric work**. Plyometric work is also referred to as **elastic/explosive strength work**. Examples of plyometric work are illustrated in Figure 1.29. In Figures 1.29A and B a sportsperson is bounding over a series of hurdles and jumping on and off low boxes respectively. The effect of dropping from a height is to place an eccentric load on the calf muscles and Achilles tendon, thus creating a loaded stretch on this muscle–tendon unit. The explosive muscular, concentric take-off power results from a combination of motor unit recruitment and stored energy within the working muscles. In Figure 1.29C eccentric work on the shoulder girdle is performed as a result of a

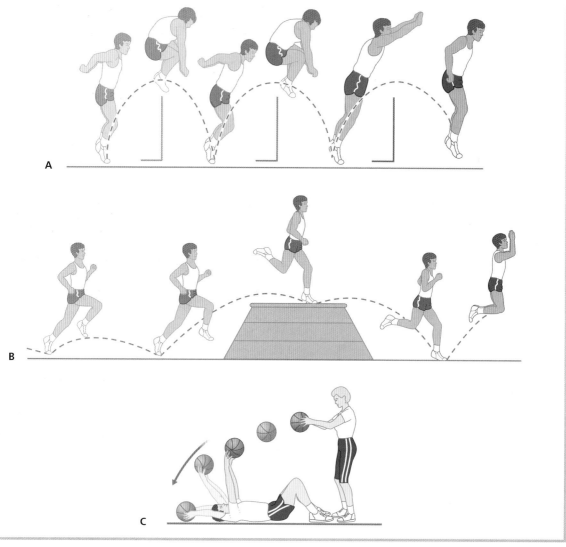

Fig. 1.29 Examples of eccentric exercises. **A.** Plyometric bounds over hurdles. **B.** Plyometric jumps on and off a box top. **C.** Pull-over catch.

medicine ball being fed to the athlete lying on the floor, who catches the ball with extended arms to pass back to a partner. Again, a stretch reflex is initiated as the shoulder girdle is overloaded. You may wish to try some of these examples! (For a detailed discussion on the adaptations produced by training, refer to Chapter 4 and for further insight into plyometic work see references[9, 10].)

Investigation 1.17 Types of muscular contraction in relation to physical activity

Materials: chinning bar.

Task 1
1. Hang from a bar, as shown in Figure 1.30A, holding a 90° angle in the elbow joint.

2. From the bent arm position, pull yourself up, as shown in Figure 1.30B.

3. When you have completed the chin-up, lower yourself slowly down to an arms-extended position, as shown in Figure 1.30C.

▶

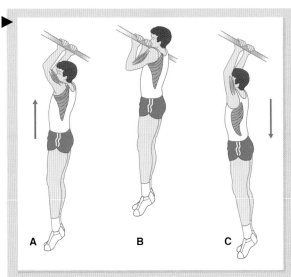

Fig. 1.30 Chinning bar.

Task 2
With the aid of the diagrams, work out the agonist muscles used for each exercise, their origins and insertions and the type of muscular contraction being used. Write your answers in Table 1.5.

Task 3
1. In which part of the movement sequence is eccentric work being done?

2. Identify the muscle that is exerting force while lengthening.

Task 4
Figure 1.31 shows four different actions from different sports. The muscles drawn in these action figures are the active ones used in the position or movements.

Make a table similar to Table 1.5 and complete the task of identifying the active muscles, their origins and insertions and the type of muscle contraction. (Adapted from Klausen.[11])

Table 1.5 Results

	Agonist muscles	Origin	Insertion	Type of contraction
A.				
B.				
C.				

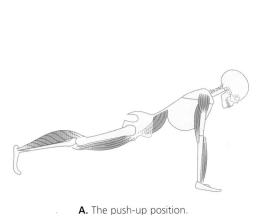

A. The push-up position.

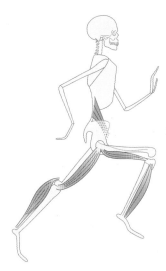

B. Sprinting.

Fig. 1.31

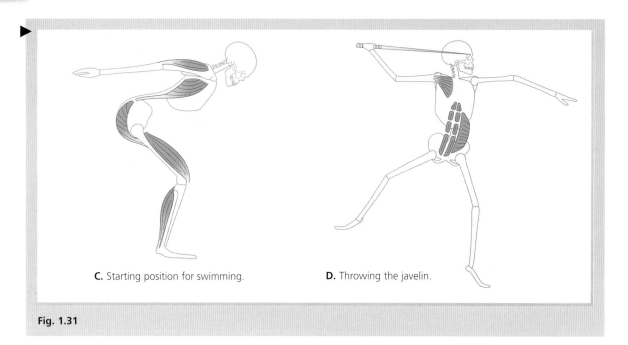

C. Starting position for swimming.

D. Throwing the javelin.

Fig. 1.31

Synoptic movement analysis

A practical analysis and review of limb movement, that includes all topics taught up to this point in time alongside biomechanical applications, is located at the end of Chapter 8 on pp. 264–267. This synoptic investigation for part 1 is intended to summarise and establish connections between these subject areas.

Exam-style questions

Figure 1.32 shows the relationship between eccentric, isometric and concentric work.

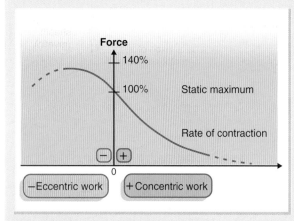

Fig. 1.32 The relationships between eccentric, static and concentric work.

1. a. Compare and account for muscle forces made at maximum eccentric work with their static maximum. (*4 marks*)

   b. Explain why an eccentric contraction is called negative work and a concentric contraction is called positive work. (*2 marks*)

   c. Identify and describe a physical activity that would produce results similar to those shown in Figure 1.32. Identify the movement sequence in relation to concentric, static and eccentric work. (*6 marks*)

   (*Total 12 marks*)

2. Describe two training exercises that could be included in a plyometric session for a basketball player. (*4 marks*)

3. Research suggests that delayed muscle soreness is greatest following eccentric contractions. Suggest why this is so. (*4 marks*)

1.5 How coordinated movement is produced

Learning objectives

On completion of this section, you will be able to:

1. Have a brief understanding of the structures and functions of the nervous system necessary for the production of coordinated movements in the human body.

2. Describe how an action potential is propagated along a cell's membrane.

3. Describe how co-ordinated movement is produced in relation to strength of stimulus, gradation of contraction, spatial summation and wave summation.

4. Understand the origins of voluntary and involuntary movements and describe the reflex arc.

Keywords

- acetylcholine
- action potential
- all-or-none law
- central nervous system
- cerebellum
- depolarisation
- Golgi tendon organ
- gradation of contraction
- hyperpolarisation
- inhibition
- motor end-plate
- motor neurone
- motor neurone pool
- motor unit
- muscle spindle apparatus
- muscle twitch
- peripheral nervous system
- potassium/sodium exchange pump
- reflexive movement
- repolarisation
- saltatory conduction
- sensory neurone
- single muscle fibre block
- spatial summation
- synapse
- tetanic contraction
- voluntary movement
- wave summation

Muscle can contract only when a nerve ending is stimulated by outgoing impulses from the **central nervous system** (CNS), which consists of the brain and spinal cord. The contractile system for muscles is organised into a number of distinct parts, each of which is controlled by a single **motor neurone** (Figure 1.33B), and each motor neurone controls a large number of muscle fibres. A group of fibres (referred to in this text as a **single muscle fibre block**) and its neurone is called a **motor unit** (Figure 1.33A).

A **motor neurone** (Figure 1.33B) consists of three major parts including **a cell body** containing the nucleus, mitochondria and other organelles, cellular extensions called **dendrites** and an **axon**. **Dendrites** are highly branched extensions of the cytoplasm that project from the cell body within the grey matter of the spinal cord. Following sensory stimulation, a relay neurone transmits neural impulses to the dendrites of the motor neurone; they are specialised to receive and conduct these electrical impulses towards the cell body. The **axon** arises from the thickened area of the cell body and emerges out of the ventral root of the spinal cord. Its function is to transmit neural impulses away from the cell body towards muscle tissue or a gland. The surrounding **myelin sheath** acts as an insulator to speed up the transmission of the impulse. A typical motor neurone divides into several branches as it reaches the muscle bed. These branches connect the motor neurone to the muscle fibres by specialised structures known as **motor end-plates** (Figure 1.33).

Control by the brain is possible because of the ascending and descending fibres to the motor cortex.

The transmission of neural messages along a neurone is an electrochemical process. When a neurone is not conducting an impulse it has a **resting**

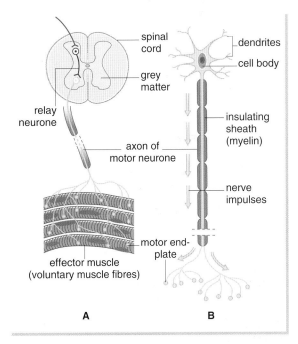

Fig. 1.33 A. A motor unit. **B.** A motor neurone.

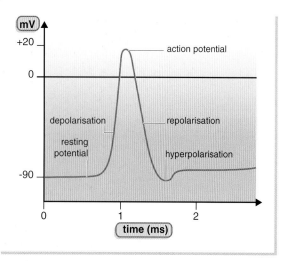

Fig. 1.34 An action potential.

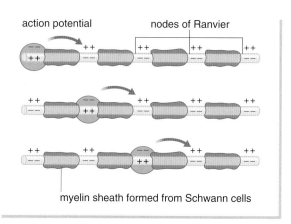

Fig. 1.35 Conduction of an action potential along a myelinated axon.

potential brought about by the outward diffusion of potassium ions (K^+) along a concentration gradient and a negatively charged inside cell membrane when compared with the outside of the cell membrane.

An **action potential** (Figure 1.34) occurs at the point along the axon where the neural impulse is being propagated. It is initiated when sufficient numbers of sodium ions (Na^+) are allowed to diffuse into the neurone. This **depolarises** the axon to a critical threshold level. Action potentials occur in an **all-or-none** fashion. If an action potential occurs at all, it is of the same magnitude and duration no matter how strong the stimulus.

Repolarisation is the return of the membrane potential towards the resting membrane potential because of K^+ movement out of the cell and because Na^+ movement into the cell slows to resting levels. The **after potential** is a short period of **hyperpolarisation**. The **resting potential** is restored by the sodium/potassium exchange pump, which returns ion concentrations to their resting values.

An action potential initiated in one part of the cell membrane stimulates action potentials in adjacent parts of the membrane and so on (Figure 1.35). The speed of propagation along neurones varies greatly from cell to cell. Neurones that have large-diameter myelinated axons conduct action potentials faster than small-diameter unmyelinated axons. A myelin sheath (see Figure 1.35) offers increased conduction velocity as a result of the action potential jumping from node to node. This process is called **saltatory conduction** and is less costly in terms of ion 'run down' since ion exchange occurs only at the **nodes of Ranvier**.

Transmission of an impulse between sensory and relay, and relay and motor neurones occurs at specialised junctions called **synapses** (Figure 1.36). The wave of depolarisation is unable to jump across the synaptic cleft; however, the problem is solved by the release of transmitter substances, such as **acetylcholine**, from the synaptic knobs. This transmitter substance diffuses across the synaptic cleft to bind with postsynaptic receptors. The sodium gates in the membrane open, allowing sodium to enter the axon and initiate the action potential. The electrical impulse can now pass directly from one cell to another. Once the action potential is completed, the enzyme **acetylcholinesterase**

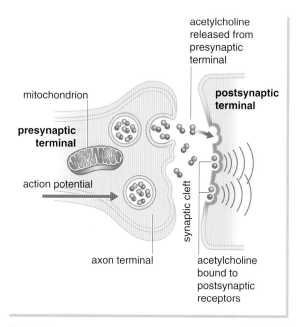

Fig. 1.36 A synapse.

breaks down the acetylcholine, thus clearing the gap in readiness for the arrival of the next impulse.

Transmission of an impulse at the motor end-plate works in a similar way to a synapse, as illustrated in Figure 1.37 stages 1–8. The electrical impulse travels down the spinal cord and motor neurone to the **effector** or active muscle in the way described above. The function of the motor end-plates is to transfer impulses from the small, branching motor neurones to large muscle fibres (in all directions). This is achieved when the **nerve action potential** is followed by a **muscle action potential**. There is a delay of 0.5 milliseconds (ms) which is the time needed for the release of acetylcholine from the synaptic knobs. An area of depolarisation travels down the muscle cell, passing the entrances to the 'T' vesicles, which secrete Ca^{++} needed to initiate muscle contraction (see p. 42 for the subsequent reactions within the muscle cell). Each different fibre type is innervated by a different kind of motor neurone. When an electrical impulse reaches the muscle fibres (i.e. single muscle fibre block) of a single motor unit, the muscle cells contract simultaneously since they receive the same impulse from a single cell body of a motor neurone.

Each whole muscle consists of a large number of motor units. In muscles such as those in a leg or arm, there are about a thousand muscle fibres serviced by one motor unit; whereas, on smaller, more sensitive muscles such as those in fingers, there are fewer fibres per motor unit. The nerve cell bodies of all motor units are, for a given muscle, bound together at an appropriate level in the spinal cord to give the nearest access point to that specific muscle and leave as a concentrated bundle from the ventral root of the spinal cord. These concentrated bundles or patches are called **motor neurone pools** and there is a motor neurone pool for each muscle in the body.

The nature of the stimuli received at the muscle bed will determine the type of muscular response.

Motor-neural firing patterns

A muscle twitch (see Figure 1.38)

Stimuli received by the motor neurone pools are transmitted to the different motor units, which do not necessarily work in unison. The strength of the stimulus must be sufficient to activate at least one motor unit to produce any contraction at all. Once activated, **all** the muscle fibres (within a single muscle fibre block) in that motor unit will contract maximally to produce a muscle twitch that lasts a fraction of a second. This is known as the **ALL-OR-NONE LAW** as neurones and muscle fibres either respond completely (all) or not at all (none) to a stimulus.

The contractile time of fast-twitch fibres is much quicker than that in slow-twitch fibres. Therefore, fast-twitch fibres produce greater contractile forces sooner (see Table 1.6, p. 43).

Region A (of Figure 1.38) shows the approximate time scale for a single motor unit muscle twitch.

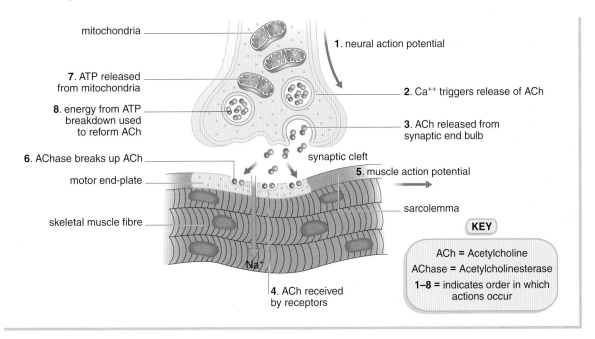

mitochondria

1. neural action potential

7. ATP released from mitochondria

2. Ca^{++} triggers release of ACh

8. energy from ATP breakdown used to reform ACh

3. ACh released from synaptic end bulb

6. AChase breaks up ACh

motor end-plate

synaptic cleft

5. muscle action potential

skeletal muscle fibre

sarcolemma

Na^+

KEY

ACh = Acetylcholine
AChase = Acetylcholinesterase
1–8 = indicates order in which actions occur

4. ACh received by receptors

Fig. 1.37 Impulse transmission at a neuromuscular junction.

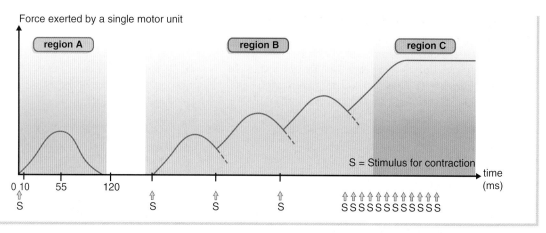

Fig. 1.38 Motor-neural firing patterns.

Wave summation

The strength of a single muscle fibre block (within a motor unit) can be increased in another way when a second stimulus, at the motor neurone pool, is received very quickly after the first stimulus. Hence the time interval between stimuli (marked in Figure 1.38 as 'S' in region B) is not long enough for relaxation of the muscle fibre block to occur. Hence the tension in the muscle block rises. This adding on of contractions to produce a stronger effect, due to an increase in the rate of stimulation, is known as **wave summation**.

Tetanic contraction

When impulses fire off so fast that there is no time for any relaxation at all, a state of absolute contraction is produced, called a **tetanic contraction**. Region C of Figure 1.38 shows this effect.

Gradation of contraction

Gradation of contraction refers to ability of muscles to produce forces varying from very light to maximal force or tension. This is achieved in two ways.

1. By varying the frequency of the stimulus (the number per unit time), contractions of different strengths can be produced i.e. low frequencies produce relatively weak contractions, whereas high frequencies produce more powerful contractions (refer to wave summation).
2. By varying the number of motor units recruited for the activity (different motor units will be

involved, not necessarily the same ones in succession).

This combined effect enables a muscle to exert forces of graded strengths, whose efforts range from fine, delicate, precision-controlled movements to strong, dynamic, powerful movements. This is called **gradation of contraction**.

Spatial summation (see Figure 1.39)

The term **spatial summation** refers to that fact that any given stimulus will cause motor units to be successively activated over the volume of muscle, i.e. different motor units are involved throughout the muscle. The

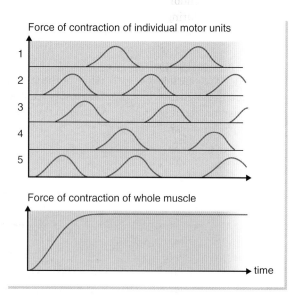

Fig. 1.39 Spatial summation.

advantage of different muscle fibre blocks being activated throughout a muscle is that ATP consumption (the energy-producing reaction) is shared throughout the muscle instead of being confined to single motor units and therefore fatigue is spread throughout the muscle instead of being confined to small groups of fibres.

Spatial summation is shown in Figure 1.39 in which the effects of five different motor units add up to produce a resultant whole muscle contraction.

This slight **out-of-step** action of motor units is a very important factor in maintaining sustained contraction at any strength. If some motor units are contracting whilst others are relaxing and if this is staggered throughout the muscle, quite long periods of sustained contraction can be achieved, depending on the load being moved or, in the case of **isometric contraction**, the tension being produced. All muscular action has to develop sufficient isometric tension in order to apply sufficient force to begin movement.

All the above ways of varying the strength of contraction depend on the size of stimulus and normally they are used together to produce coordinated movement patterns that may vary from finely graded strengths to maximal contractions.

In addition to the action of motor units, coordinated movements are adjusted by **sensory feedback**. Within physical performance, the sportsperson is aware of pressure, pain, joint angles, muscle tension and speed of actions as a result of specialised proprioceptors such as **Golgi tendon organs** and **muscle spindle apparatuses**.

The **Golgi tendon organs** continuously monitor **tendon tension** during a contraction or passive stretch. The organs are held within a small capsule through which a small bundle of tendon fibres pass and which lie close to the tendon fibres' attachment to a muscle fibre. They are sensitive to the tension in the muscle and tendon combination and provide sensory feedback of information about the tendon tension to the spinal cord. During **excessive** tension (created by a muscle when it is undergoing either a concentric or eccentric contraction) or during **excessive** passive stretching (during PNF mobility training, for example, refer to p. 157), the Golgi receptors conduct their signals rapidly to the spinal cord. This then triggers the motor or efferent nerves to relay electrical impulses back to the muscle bed to bring about a reflex **inhibition** of the **agonist** muscles (to which the tendon is attached) and excite contraction of the **antagonist** muscles involved. This protects muscle tissue from potential injury by **inhibiting** contraction of the agonist muscle

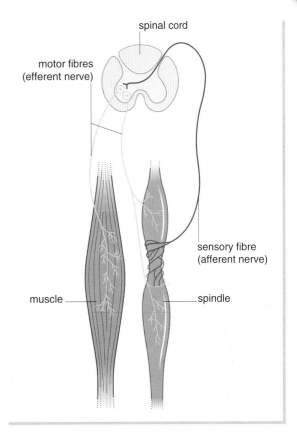

Fig. 1.40 Muscle spindle apparatus.

and **exciting** contraction of the antagonist muscle if the tendon is overstretched. Certain types of strength training can reduce the influence of the Golgi tendon organs (in inhibiting muscle contraction), thereby increasing the forces that can be applied by a muscle.

The muscle spindle apparatus detects and monitors muscle activity (Figure 1.40). When muscle fibres contract, ends of the muscle spindle come closer together, stimulating the sensory or afferent nerves which relay electrical impulses to the spindle cord. Motor or efferent nerves then relay electrical impulses to the muscle bed, followed by an adjustment in the state of muscle tension required for the execution of the physical task. This involuntary stretch reflex provides information such as state of muscle tension, length, position and rate of change of muscle length. Muscle spindles are important in the control and tone of postural muscles. Information from such proprioceptors is used as a basis for **decision making**. This sensory aspect of physical activity is included in the area 'The Performer as a Person' and provides the initial source of information that enables the muscle system to operate **stretch reflexes**.

The role of reflexes in coordinated movement

Reflexes play an important role in all forms of movement. The two types of reflex that originate from the CNS are:

1. **voluntary reflexes**, where impulses originate in the voluntary motor cortex
2. **involuntary reflexes**, which originate from the stimulation of sense organs, to produce electrical impulses in sensory neurones.

The **reflex arc** is the pathway along which unlearned and automatic learned responses travel.

How reflexes work

Figure 1.41 shows the unlearned reflex of the knee jerk reflex. The hammer strikes the knee and the impulse travels up the sensory neurone into the spinal cord to the motor neurone, which transmits the impulse to motor units of quadriceps femoris, stimulating it to contract, thus causing the lower leg to jerk outwards. This is a **monosynaptic** reflex because a chain of only two neurones (one synapse) is necessary.

Modification of movements

The self-regulation of rhythmical movements between one muscle group and its antagonist is called **reciprocal innervation** or reciprocal inhibition. This concept explains how the flow of sensory information (from the muscle to the spinal cord) is linked within the grey matter of the spinal cord to the motor neurone of the antagonistic muscle. For example, reciprocal innervation is involved in the knee jerk reflex, illustrated in Figure 1.41. As the knee flexors become inhibited, the leg extensors are stimulated and relax as a result of the reflex action. Hence reciprocal innervation provides the necessary feedback for the continual adjustments of tension between muscle groups.

Modification of all muscular actions is under the control of the **cerebellum** of the brain. The cerebellum

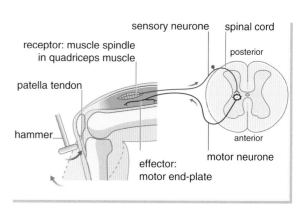

Fig. 1.41 Mechanism of knee jerk reflex.

is rather like a final sorting section of a computer being fed continuously with information from all the sense organs, giving position of limbs, state of muscles (whether contracting or relaxing) and so on. It helps to create fine coordination and ensures that physical activity is carried out smoothly.

Investigation 1.18 The reflex arc

Task 1
Work in pairs. One of you sits with legs crossed in a relaxed position. Your partner firmly taps your patella tendon using a patella hammer or ruler (the patella is positioned just below the knee cap). Describe and record the response of the knee to the tap. How can you tell that this response was a reflex action?

Task 2
Give an example of a skill you have learned that has become an automatic response to a stimulus.

Task 3
Distinguish between automatic (reflex response) and fast reactions. Use examples from sporting situations to illustrate your answer.

For a fuller account of nervous control of muscular movement, see references [2,12–17].

Exam-style questions

1. Name the different regions of a motor neurone. (*3 marks*)

2. Figure 1.42 has been created from a slide of skeletal tissue as seen with a light microscope at a magnification of 800 times. It shows part of two motor units.

   a. Use evidence from the drawing to suggest:

   i. a meaning for the term 'motor unit' (*2 marks*)

   ii. why all the muscle fibres shown will not necessarily contract at the same time. (*3 marks*)

   ▶

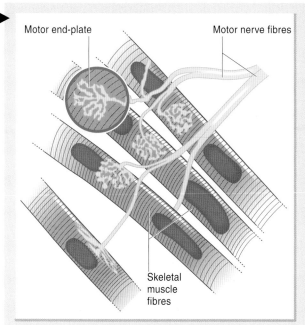

Fig. 1.42 Two motor units in skeletal tissue.

b. Briefly describe the sequence of events at the muscle end-plate that leads to an action potential passing along the muscle fibre. *(4 marks)*

c. Describe some of the factors that determine muscle speed and tension characteristics. *(4 marks)*

d. Explain the role of motor units in controlling the strength of muscular contractions in sports movements. *(10 marks)*

(Total 26 marks)

3. Figure 1.43 shows the pathways of transmission of impulses through the central nervous system during the knee jerk reflex.

a. Give the names of the **five** structures lettered P–T on Figure 1.43. *(3 marks)*

b. With reference to the diagram, briefly describe the sequence of events in a knee jerk. *(3 marks)*

c. Briefly describe the structure and function of a synapse. *(3 marks)*

d. Explain the difference between this reflex action and a similar movement carried out under voluntary control. *(4 marks)*

e. A sports commentator might say a 'games player' has **lightning reflexes**, when referring to a good interception made by him or her. Discuss whether or not reflex is the correct term for such an interception. *(5 marks)*

(Total 18 marks)

4. The trace in Figure 1.44 shows an intracellular recording of the potential within a nerve cell and the changes resulting from its excitation by other nerves that synapse with it.

a. Explain the following terms:
   i. resting membrane potential *(3 marks)*
   ii. action potential. *(2 marks)*

b. Explain why, individually, the excitatory impulses did not generate an action potential but collectively they did. *(3 marks)*

c. Explain briefly how the myelin sheath influences the speed of contraction of a nerve impulse. *(3 marks)*

d. Explain why the release of a transmitter substance, such as acetylcholine, into a neuromuscular junction does not stimulate the muscle to go into prolonged contraction. *(3 marks)*

(Total 14 marks)

5. a. Identify the three components of a stretch reflex (refer to Figure 1.40). *(3 marks)*

b. Under what conditions would the Golgi tendon organ function to protect voluntary muscle. *(2 marks)*

c. Explain the role of the muscle spindle apparatus when performing a triple jump. *(4 marks)*

(Total 9 marks)

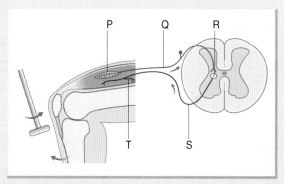

Fig. 1.43 Knee jerk reflex.

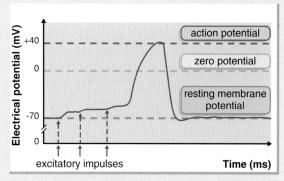

Fig. 1.44 Electrical potential across the membrane of a motor neurone during the propagation of a nerve impulse.

1.6 Skeletal muscle structure and fibre types

Learning objectives

On completion of this section, you will be able to:
1. Describe the gross and microscopic structural detail of striated muscle cells.
2. Understand the mechanisms involved in striated muscle contraction.
3. Relate tension to types of exercise and muscular contraction.
4. Understand the role of fibre types with respect to sporting situations.

Keywords

- cross-bridge
- endomysium
- epimysium
- filaments – actin and myosin
- Huxley's sliding filament theory of muscle contraction
- muscle fibre
- myofibril
- myoglobin
- nervous impulse
- perimysium
- ratchet mechanism
- red muscle
- sarcolemma
- sarcomere
- sarcoplasm
- striated muscle
- triad or 'T' vesicle
- troponin
- tropomyosin
- white muscle

Fibre type
- type I
- type IIa (FOG)
- type IIb (FG)
- type IIc

To understand how a muscle converts chemical energy into mechanical energy, we need to understand the structural detail of voluntary muscle and what makes it contract.

Voluntary muscle is often referred to as **skeletal** muscle because it normally moves bones. Other descriptions include **striped** or **striated**, which derive their names from the striped microscopic appearance of the muscle cells.

A typical muscle is the gastrocnemius or calf muscle, which has its origin on the lateral and medial condyles of the femur and its insertion through the Achilles tendon on the calcaneum or heel bone (Figure 1.45B).

Figure 1.45C shows the entire muscle surrounded by a layer of connective tissue called the **epimysium**, which consists mainly of collagen fibres. The function of the epimysium is to provide a smooth surface against which other muscles can glide and to give the muscle its form. The epimysium is the total envelope surrounding the muscle and connects muscle tissue to outer **fascia**.

Within the muscle are large bundles of muscle fibres or **fasciculi**, which are surrounded by the **perimysium** (middle layer) consisting of collagen and elastic fibres. These structures are shown in Figures 1.45C and D.

Within each bundle or fasciculus are **muscle cells** or **fibres**, each individually wrapped by a very thin layer of connective tissue or **endomysium** (*endo* final, *mysium* muscle; see Figure 1.45D).

All three connective tissue layers (epimysium, perimysium and endomysium) are connected to each other so that when the muscle fibres contract, they are ultimately linked to a tendon attached to a bone across a joint, thus creating voluntary movement.

The muscle cell (see Figure 1.45E)

Each cell consists of a multinucleate (containing many nuclei) fibre and is highly specialised for contraction. Although the diameter of the muscle cell is very small (10–100 µm (microns)), its length can be extremely long (up to 0.5 m), depending on the length of the whole muscle. Therefore, it is important that the muscle cell can transmit its nerve impulses throughout the entire length of the fibre. As a consequence, skeletal muscle is a good conductor of electricity. The cell membrane or **sarcolemma** is very thin to enable efficient diffusion of oxygen and glucose into the cell and carbon dioxide out of the cell. Positioned just inside the sarcolemma are numerous nuclei, hence the term 'multinucleate'. (The **nucleus** is the control centre of a cell.)

The sarcoplasm inside the cell is a specialised cytoplasm containing sarcoplasmic reticulum, 'T' (triad) vesicles, enzymes and mitochondria.

The sarcoplasmic reticulum is a network of internal membranes that run throughout the sarcoplasm and is responsible for the transportation of materials within the cell. A 'T' vesicle is a sac that contains cellular secretions, such as calcium ions, needed to initiate muscle contraction. Enzymes are the organic catalysts that regulate all chemical reactions within the cell (for example, ATPase is needed to activate adenosine triphosphate (ATP), which provides the energy needed for muscular contraction). Mitochondria

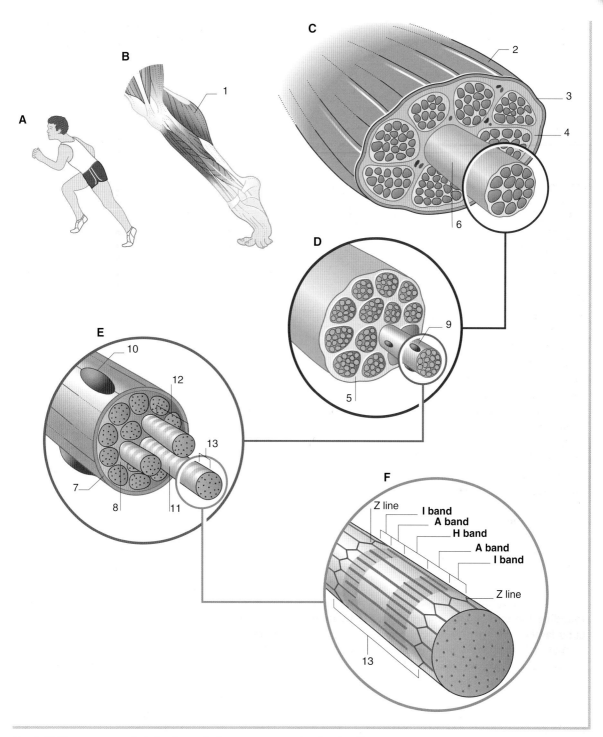

Fig. 1.45 The structure of skeletal muscle from gross to molecular detail.
A. Sprinter in action. **B.** Lower part of leg showing positioning of the gastrocnemius muscle. **C.** Cross-section through the gastrocnemius muscle. **C, D.** Sections of the fasciculi. **E.** Muscle cell. **F.** Myofibril.

1. Gastrocnemius muscle. **2.** Belly of muscle. **3.** Epimysium. **4.** Perimysium. **5.** Endomysium. **6.** Muscle bundle or fasciculus. **7.** Sarcolemma. **8.** Sarcoplasm. **9.** Muscle cell. **10.** Nucleus. **11.** Myofibril. **12.** Banding pattern of myofibril. **13.** Sarcomere with labelled banding pattern.

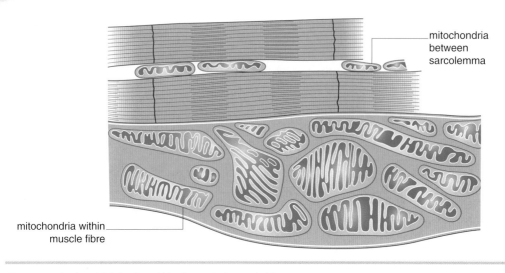

mitochondria
between
sarcolemma

mitochondria within
muscle fibre

Fig. 1.46 Mitochondrial density within slow-twitch muscle fibres.

are often referred to as the power plants of the cell, because most of the reactions of cellular respiration, and hence energy release, take place within them.

Figure 1.46 shows the distribution of mitochondria within slow-twitch, type I muscle fibres (refer to Table 1.6 for details on slow-twitch fibres). Those mitochondria positioned beneath the sarcolemma provide energy for the transport of ions and metabolites across the sarcolemma. Those mitochondria positioned deep within the muscle fibres provide energy for muscle contraction via ATP regeneration (refer to p. 98 for additional information on the role of mitochondria within skeletal muscle tissue).

Some muscle fibres contain more sarcoplasm than others; these appear darker due to the presence of **myoglobin** (a form of haemoglobin that occurs in muscle cells). This type of muscle is called **red muscle** and is best suited for long-term powerful contractions, as in the postural extensor muscles (such as the rectus abdominis or erector spinae muscles, which hold the body upright). **White muscle** contains less sarcoplasm and myoglobin but more ATPase (the enzyme needed to assist release of energy from ATP; see Chapter 3.2 for a discussion on energy generation and ATP). Therefore white muscle is best suited for speed. Flexor muscles, such as vastus medialis or biceps muscles, which can move limbs quickly, are examples of white muscle. Red and white muscles are also described as slow- and fast-twitch muscles, respectively. The properties of these different types of muscle cells or fibres are discussed in detail in the section on types of muscle fibre (Table 1.6, p. 43).

Muscle myoglobin

Muscle myoglobin (a molecule similar to haemoglobin) has a temporary but **greater** affinity for oxygen than does haemoglobin. Therefore, muscle myoglobin captures oxygen from saturated haemoglobin, thereby transferring oxygen into the muscle cell structure. Since myoglobin is present throughout the cell, oxygen is transferred from myoglobin molecule to myoglobin molecule until it reaches the mitochondria (where it is needed for energy-producing reactions). This process is in addition to the diffusion of oxygen (carried by haemoglobin in red blood cells) from capillaries into muscle cells, caused by the larger concentration (or partial pressure) of oxygen in haemoglobin than in muscle cells (see pp. 77–78 for a discussion about gas diffusion into muscle cells).

Muscle cell structure (see Figure 1.45E and F)

Running longitudinally within the sarcoplasm are long, slender, light and dark structures called **myofibrils** (3 µm in diameter), which therefore create a striated appearance. Each myofibril consists of numerous units called **sarcomeres**.

The sarcomere (see Figures 1.45F and 1.47)

Each sarcomere is the functional basic unit of a myofibril and thousands of sarcomeres form a long chain within each myofibril. The **Z** membrane indicates the boundary between one sarcomere and the next.

The reason for this light and dark striated banding pattern (hence the name **striped muscle**) is that it is composed of two types of longitudinal protein filaments:

1. **Thick filaments of myosin** – confined to the dark **A** band and **H** zone in the middle, which has only thick myosin filaments.
2. **Thin filaments of actin** – which are found in the light **I** band and between myosin at the ends of the dark **A** band. An actin filament is composed of molecules of **actin, tropomyosin and troponin**.

The **A** bands are positioned in the central section of the sarcomere and consist of thick and thin filaments separated by an **H** zone that has only thick filaments. The **I** band is positioned at both ends of the sarcomere and consists exclusively of thin filaments.

The thin filaments connect the **Z** membrane and the inner edge of the nearer **A** band at each end of the sarcomere. The thick filaments join the outer edges of both **A** bands and therefore overlap the thin filaments located within the **A** band. This arrangement is illustrated in Figure 1.47A.

What happens when the muscle contracts?

The theory of muscle contraction is based on Huxley's sliding filament theory of muscle contraction.[18] In relaxed muscle all the bands are visible, whereas in contracted muscle the light **I** band narrows and then disappears, since the thin actin filaments are being drawn further in between the thick myosin filaments (refer to Figure 1.47 to observe these differences between relaxed and contracted muscle).

How do the two sets of filaments move between each other?

The key to the process of muscle contraction lies in the **overlapping** of the thick myosin and thin actin filaments, as seen in Figure 1.47. The thin actin filaments are made up of two chains of globular proteins, called **tropomyosin** and **troponin**. Tropomyosin strands are

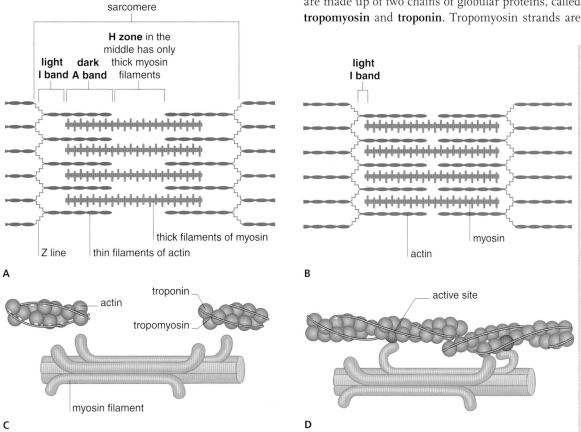

Fig. 1.47 Diagrammatic detail of sarcomere (after Huxley[18]). **A, C.** Relaxed muscle. **B, D.** Contracted muscle. During muscle contraction the light I band narrows, then disappears, as actin filaments are drawn further and further between filaments of myosin.

wound about the thin actin filaments and troponin is attached to the tropomyosin at regular intervals. At rest troponin holds the tropomyosin in position to block the myosin-binding sites on actin filaments (Figure 1.47c).

In Section 1.5 the transmission of a neural impulse at a neuromuscular junction is described in Figure 1.37. At stage 5, a neural action potential is converted to a muscle action potential. As the nervous impulse reaches the muscle cell it initiates the release of calcium ions (Ca^{++}) from special storage 'T' vesicles in the sarcoplasmic reticulum. Troponin has a high affinity for calcium ions and, as the Ca^{++} bind to the troponin, the shape of the troponin–tropomyosin complex changes to expose the **active sites** on the actin filaments. The calcium ions stimulate the contraction of the muscle by exposing the active sites on the actin filaments, as observed in Figure 1.47D.

At the same time the heads of the myosin filaments become activated by ATP which, when broken down into ADP and free phosphate (P_i), releases large amounts of energy. The myosin heads attach themselves to selected sites on nearby actin filaments to form **actin–myosin** bonds, usually called **cross-bridges**. This process is illustrated in Figures 1.47D and 1.48. This is immediately followed by the detachment of cross-bridges and the reattachment of the myosin heads to the next actin sites and so on. The whole effect is to pull the actin filaments past the myosin filaments so that they form a bigger overlap (than in the resting state) and therefore shorten the sarcomere. The attachment, detachment and reattachment of cross-bridges are referred to as the **ratchet mechanism**.

With many thousands of thin filaments pulling past thick filaments within a single cell and many thousands of muscle cells contracting in this way, skeletal muscle can quickly respond to the demands of ballistic activity, such as in a flat-out 100 m swim or sprint. The strength of the muscular contraction is proportional to the number of cross-bridges in harness; with the result that a muscle, in a full state of contraction, has a greater region (within each cell) of actin–myosin overlap and hence a greater number of cross-bridges in harness. There is no slippage within the cross-bridges because of the non-aligned or offset attachments of the actin–myosin bonds (see Figure 1.48).

When the calcium is reabsorbed and the nervous stimulation withdrawn, the troponin–tropomyosin system resumes the blocking of cross-bridge connections, contraction stops and the muscle relaxes (see Figures 1.47A and 1.47C).

Types of muscular contraction (see Section 1.4)

When the muscle fibre is held at a certain point of stretching simultaneous with the actin–myosin bonding occurring, the result will be an isometric contraction (although what happens in this sort of contraction is that different muscle fibre blocks alternate in contraction; spatial summation on p. 34).

When the muscle fibre is stretched outwards at the same time as the occurrence of actin–myosin bonding, an eccentric contraction will take place. The contraction becomes concentric when the actin filaments slide in between the myosin filaments.

Energy used for muscular contraction is derived from glucose and free fatty acids, which are converted in the mitochondria into ATP which is then delivered to the contractile filaments.

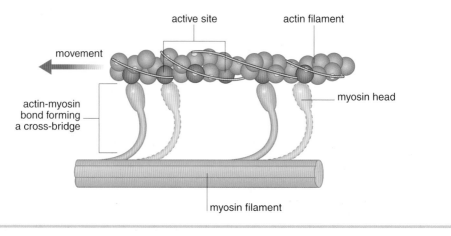

Fig. 1.48 Sliding filament theory: actin–myosin bonds.

Types of muscle fibre

The muscle fibres within a given motor unit may be either **slow-twitch fibres** (or **type I**) or **fast-twitch fibres** (or **type II**). Within an individual there are different proportions of these fibre types found in different muscles and evidence supports the view that fibre type distribution is inherited.

All muscle contains a mixture of **slow-** and **fast-twitch fibres**. The major differences between the two types are related to:

- **speed of contraction** – slow-twitch muscle fibres contract at a rate of about 20% when compared with fast-twitch muscle fibres
- **muscle fibre force** – fast-twitch fibres are bigger in size than slow-twitch fibres, have larger motor neurones and therefore can generate high force rapidly

- **muscle endurance** – slow-twitch fibres are capable of resisting fatigue whereas fast-twitch fibres are easily fatigued.

Type I fibres have the highest aerobic capacity. Type II fibres are subdivided into type IIa, type IIb and type IIc.

Type IIa fibres, otherwise known as FOG (**F**ast-**O**xidative-**G**lycolytic), have a greater resistance to fatigue compared with type IIb fibres (**F**ast-**G**lycolytic – FG) that have only a high capacity for anaerobic, glycolytic metabolism. The fatigue-resistant nature of type IIa is thought to be due to muscle adaptation in response to endurance training. Although little is known about **fast-twitch type c** fibres, it is thought that this recently discovered category operates at the far end of the anaerobic metabolic continuum.

A summary of comparisons of these three types of muscle fibres is listed in Table 1.6.

Table 1.6 Structural and functional characteristics of type I and type II (IIa and IIb) muscle fibres

	Slow-twitch	Fast-twitch	
Characteristic	type I	type IIa (FOG)	type IIb (FG)
Structural aspects			
Colour	Red	Red-pink	White
Fibre diameter	Small	Medium	Large
Fibres per motor unit	10–180	300–800	300–800
Capillary density	High	Medium	Low
Myoglobin content	High	Medium	Low
Mitochondrial density	High	High	Low
Sarcoplasmic reticulum development	Low	High	High
Triglyceride stores	High	Medium	Low
Glycogen stores	Low	High	High
Phosphocreatine content	Low	High	High
Functional aspects			
Myosin-ATPase activity	Low	High	High
Glycolytic enzyme activity	Low	High	High
Oxidative enzyme activity	High	Midway	Low
Ability to generate ATP	High	Midway	Low
Energy pathway used	Aerobic	Aerobic/anaerobic	Anaerobic
Fatigue level	Low	Midway	High
Recruitment order	First	Second	Third
Twitch (contractile time) ms	Slow	Fast	Fast
Relaxation time	Slow	Fast	Fast
Primary function	Maintaining posture/ endurance-based activities	Running/sprinting	High-intensity rapid activity

Some of the terms used to describe the characteristics of fibre types may be unfamiliar but you should be able to understand them once you have referred to relevant sections within this text.

Investigation 1.19 To consider some of the characteristics of fibre types

Task 1
1. It can be deduced from the information summarised in Table 1.6 that slow-twitch fibres are best suited to **aerobic** (performed with a full and adequate supply of oxygen) types of exercise. On the other hand, fast-twitch fibres are specifically adapted for high-intensity and mainly **anaerobic** (performed without sufficient oxygen to cope with the energy demand) types of exercise. Describe some of the characteristics that support this deduction.

2. The effects of specialised training can alter the metabolic functioning of fast-twitch type IIb fibres so that they take on some of the characteristics of type I fibres to become type IIa fibres. Describe the ways in which metabolic functioning of type IIa fibres changes as a result of specialist aerobic training.

3. In which sporting activities would the adaptation of fast-twitch (type IIb) fibres to type IIa fibres be relevant to a sportsperson?

4. What types of training would cause the adaptation of fast-twitch fibres to type IIa fibres?

5. Give examples of types of training that would stress slow-twitch fibres and fast-twitch glycolytic fibres.

Task 2

Using the information in Figure 1.49, describe the order in which fibre types are recruited as the number of motor units increase.

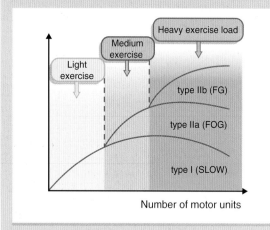

Fig. 1.49 Recruitment of fibre types (after reference[3]).

Task 3

Another interesting study is the relationship between distribution of fibre type and different sporting activities, as illustrated in Table 1.7. Basically, the more explosive and intense the demands of the sport, the more likely it is that successful sportspeople will have a higher proportion of fast-twitch muscle fibres in their muscles.

1. Using the information in Table 1.7, comment on the distribution of fibre type with respect to different sporting activities.

2. Compare and account for differences in percentage fibre distribution with respect to males and females.

3. Compare and account for differences in percentage fibre distribution between untrained and trained performers.

4. Discuss the role of genetics in determining the proportions of muscle fibre types and the potential for success in selected activities.

5. What is the pattern of muscle fibre recruitment during:

   a. a high jump?

   b. a 5 km race?

   c. a 400 m race?

6. Using the information contained within Table 1.6, give two pieces of evidence that:

   a. suggest that fast-twitch fibres may easily build up an oxygen debt

   b. might account for the difference in speed of contraction of the two types of fibre.

7. Suggest why muscles concerned with maintaining body posture might be expected to have a large proportion of slow-twitch fibres.

Table 1.7 Percentages of slow-twitch (type I) and fast-twitch (type II) fibres in males and females (found in leg muscles) compared to sporting activity (based on references[19–22])

	% Type I		% Type II	
Event	Males	Females	Males	Females
Distance runners	79	69	21	31
Cross-country skiers	64	59	36	41
Cyclists	60	52	40	48
800 m runners	48	61	52	39
Javelin throwers	50	43	50	57
Shot putters	38	50	62	50
Sprinters	24	29	76	71
Untrained	45	55	55	45

Review questions

1. Define sarcolemma, sarcoplasm, myofibril and sarcomere.

2. List the proteins involved in muscular contraction and describe the role of each one.

3. Explain how the arrangement of actin filaments and myosin filaments produces **I** bands, **A** bands and **H** zones.

4. With the aid of diagrams, compare the structure of relaxed skeletal muscle with that of contracted skeletal muscle.

5. Comment on the number and distribution of mitochondria with respect to muscle fibre types.

Exam-style questions

Table 1.8 shows the percentage composition of slow-twitch fibres found in leg muscles of male athletes specialising at different running distances.

1. a. Briefly discuss the relationship between the percentage of slow-twitch fibres and race distance, as suggested by the data in Table 1.8. *(3 marks)*

   b. Which group of athletes is the most specialised in terms of slow-twitch muscle composition? Explain your choice by reference to Table 1.8. *(2 marks)*

   c. Arrange the group of runners in rank order according to how close their slow-twitch muscle fibre composition matches the 'ideal' for their distance. *(6 marks)*

   d. List **three** features of slow-twitch fibres that contribute to their greater aerobic capacity. *(3 marks)*

   e. In terms of muscle fibre types, explain why it is sometimes said that 'endurance kills speed'. *(3 marks)*

   f. Why is it more accurate to refer to slow-twitch motor *units* rather than slow-twitch muscle fibres? *(3 marks)*

   (Total 20 marks)

Table 1.8 Percentage composition of slow-twitch fibres in male leg muscles		
Event	*Mean % slow-twitch fibres*	*Range of % slow-twitch fibres*
Marathon runners	85	50–95
800m runners	55	50–80
100/200m sprinters	35	20–55

2. a. Explain, in terms of the sliding filament mechanism, why a fully extended muscle cannot exert its maximum force. *(4 marks)*

   b. Explain why muscles can only contract actively and how a contracted muscle is subsequently restretched when relaxed. *(4 marks)*

   c. An understanding of the functional structure of muscle cells is an important basis for an understanding of physical activity. Discuss this statement. *(12 marks)*

   (Total 20 marks)

For further development of muscle functioning, refer to Section 4.1 which illustrates aspects of fitness such as strength, speed, local muscle endurance and Section 4.2 on p. 145 which considers the effect of warm-up on skeletal muscle tissue.

For a fuller account of the structure and function of muscle tissue, refer to references[2, 3, 11–17].

References

1. Khosla T 1983 *Sport for tall*. British Medical Journal 287:736–738

2. Seeley R R, Stephens T D, Tate P 2003 *Anatomy and physiology*, 6th edn. McGraw Hill, New York

3. Wirhed R 1997 *Athletic ability and the anatomy of motion*, 2nd edn. Mosby, London

4. Bartlett R 1997 *Introduction to sports biomechanics*. Spon/Routledge, London

5. Bird S, Black N, Newton P 1997 *Sports injuries*. Stanley Thornes, Cheltenham
6. Blakey P 1992 *The muscle book*. Bibliotek Books, Stafford
7. Thompson C W 2003 *Manual of structural kinesiology*, 15th edn. McGraw Hill, New York
8. Solomon E P, Davies P W 1983 *Human anatomy and physiology*. CBS College Publishing, Philadelphia
9. Chu D A 1998 *Jumping into plyometrics*, 2nd edn. Human Kinetics, Champaign, Illinois
10. Chu D A 1993 *Jumping into plyometrics video*. Human Kinetics, Champaign, Illinois
11. Klausen K, Hemmingsen I, Rasmussen B 1982 *Basic sport science*. McNaughton and Gunn
12. Foss M L, Keteyian S J 1998 *Fox's physiological basis for exercise and sport*, 6th edn. McGraw Hill, New York
13. Tortora G 2003 *Principles of anatomy and physiology*, 10th edn. John Wiley, New York
14. McKenna B R, Callendar R 1996 *Illustrated physiology*, 6th edn. Churchill Livingstone, Edinburgh
15. Bastian G F 1993 *An illustrated review of anatomy and physiology: the skeletal/muscular systems*. HarperCollins, New York
16. Clegg C 1995 *Exercise physiology*. Feltham Press, New Milton
17. Wilmore J H 2004 *Physiology of sport and exercise*, 3rd edn. Human Kinetics, Champaign, Illinois
18. Huxley H 1969 *The mechanism of muscular contraction*. Science 164(3886):1356–1366
19. Burke F, Cerny F, Costill D, Fink W 1977 *Characteristics of skeletal muscle in competitive cyclists*. Medical Science in Sports and Exercise 9:109–112
20. Costill D, Daniels J, Evans W, Fink W, Krahenbuhl G, Saltin B 1976 *Skeletal muscle enzymes and fibre composition in male and female track athletes*. Journal of Applied Physiology 40:149–154
21. Gollnick P R, Armstrong R, Saubert C, Piehl K, Saltin B 1973 *Enzyme activity and fibre composition in skeletal muscle of untrained and trained men*. Journal of Applied Physiology 33(3):312–319
22. Thorstennsson A, Larsson L, Tesch P, Karlsson J 1977 *Muscle strength and fibre composition in athletes and sedentary men*. Acta Physiologica Scandinavica 98:318–322

Further reading

Delavier F 2001 *Strength training anatomy*. Human Kinetics, Champaign, Illinois
James R, Thompson G, Wiggins-James N 2003 *Complete A–Z physical education handbook*, 2nd edn. Hodder and Stoughton, London
Jarmey C 2003 *The concise book of muscles*. Lotus Publishing, Chichester
McMinn R M H *et al.* 1987 *The human skeleton*. Wolfe, London
Roscoe D A, Roscoe J V, Honeybourne J, Davis R J, Galligan F 2003 *Physical education and sports studies AS/A2 level student revision guide,* 3rd edn. Jan Roscoe Publications, Widnes
St John Ambulance 1998 *Young people's first aid*, 2nd edn. Mosby, London

Multimedia

Video

Functional Anatomy – The Sports Science Series, The University of Western Australia. UK supplier Boulton and Hawker Films Ltd, 1988

CD-ROMs

Adams *Interactive Physiology – Muscular System*. Benjamin/Cummings, California, 2004
Roscoe D A, Roscoe J V 2002 *OCR/AQUA/Edexcel Science and Sport Psychology Powerpoint Classroom Presentation CD-ROM*. Jan Roscoe Publications, Widnes
Roscoe D A, Roscoe J V, Honeybourne J, Davis R J, Galligan F 2003 *Physical Education and Sports Studies AS/A2 Level Student Revision Guide, CD-ROM,* 3rd edn. Jan Roscoe Publications, Widnes
Roscoe D A 2004 *Teacher's guide to physical education and the study of sport, part I, the performer in action, anatomy and physiology CD-ROM, 5th edn.* Jan Roscoe Publications, Widnes

Cardiovascular-respiratory systems

Athletic activity in events such as hockey, tennis, middle- and long-distance running and cross-country skiing requires the body to be able to endure tremendous physical and physiological stress.

This ability is commonly known as **staying power** or **endurance** and is limited by the capacity of the **cardiovascular system**. This comprises the **heart** (whose job is to pump blood around the body), the **vascular system** (consisting of **blood** and **circulatory vessels**) and the **lungs** (where the exchange of oxygen and carbon dioxide takes place). The function of the **vascular system** is to transport nutrients, waste products, hormones and other essential chemical compounds throughout the body and to link all other systems within the body.

The cardiovascular system works to ensure that adequate amounts of oxygen are delivered to muscles and other tissue cells to meet the demands of exercise.

The capacity at which the **cardiovascular-respiratory systems** operate will depend on the intensity, duration and type of muscular contraction being performed. For example, the longer and lighter the activity, the more the body will be limited by the capacity of the **aerobic energy system**. The shorter and higher the intensity of exercise, the more the body will be limited by the capacity of the **anaerobic energy systems**. (See Section 3.2 for a detailed explanation on these energy systems.)

Exercise, particularly aerobic endurance training, has the effect of improving cardiovascular-respiratory functioning, especially that of the heart. (Cardiac functioning is used as a criterion to assess **physical fitness** levels.)

This chapter will help you to understand the structure, actions and adaptations of the **cardiovascular-respiratory** systems in response to physical activity and exercise stress.

2.1 The heart

Learning objectives

On completion of this section, you will be able to:

1. Be familiar with the functions of the coronary arteries and veins.

2. Identify and understand the structure of heart tissue in relation to its functioning.

3. Understand the concepts of cardiac impulse, cardiac cycle, cardiac output, Starling's Law of the Heart and pulse rate, and be able to describe the events of the cardiac cycle.

4. Appreciate that the heart is myogenic, since it initiates its own electrical impulse.

5. Interpret an ECG trace of electrical activity of heart muscle.

6. Understand that the changing rate of heartbeat is controlled by two sets of nerves – the sympathetic and parasympathetic nerves – and that factors such as hormones, temperature, venous return and electrolyte balance affect heart rate.

7. By using investigational methods, describe the effects of changing the body position on resting heart rate.

8. Identify factors that affect stroke volume and understand heart rate response to varying workloads.

9. Interpret data on cardiac dynamics.

Keywords

- adrenaline
- aorta
- atrioventricular node (AV node)
- atrioventricular valve
- atrium
- bundle of His
- cardiac
- cardiac cycle
- cardiac impulse
- cardiac output ($\dot{Q}$)
- carotid artery
- diastole
- electrocardiogram (ECG)
- endocardium
- heart rate (HR)
- heart sounds
- mitral valve
- myocardium or striped cardiac tissue
- myogenic
- parasympathetic nervous system
- pericardium
- pulmonary arteries
- pulmonary veins
- pulse
- Purkinje fibres
- radial artery
- semilunar valves
- sinoatrial node (SA node) or pacemaker
- Starling's Law of the Heart
- stroke volume (SV)
- sympathetic nervous system
- systole
- tricuspid valve
- venae cavae
- ventricle

The **heart** is a pear-shaped organ located in the thoracic (chest) cavity. It lies just underneath the sternum between the lungs, with its apex positioned slightly to the left of centre of the body.

The heart consists of three layers.

a) The **pericardium** is an outer, double-layered bag or **serous membrane** containing a thin film of fluid called the **pericardial fluid** (serum is a watery liquid, consisting of plasma minus fibrinogen – a blood protein used in the clotting mechanism). The functions of the pericardium are to reduce friction (with the other contents of the thoracic cavity and the cavity wall itself) and maintain heart shape.

b) The **myocardium** (Figure 2.1E and F) or **cardiac striped muscle tissue** forms the largest part of the heart wall. Cardiac muscle contracts in the same way as skeletal muscle. Each cell, with one nucleus positioned towards the cell centre, branches to unite with other cells. It is separated from adjacent cells by an **intercalated disc**, which offers very little resistance to the neural impulse. Therefore, the cardiac impulse is transmitted throughout the myocardium. The whole effect is to create a united sheet of muscle.

The heart has a **pacemaker** (see Figure 2.2), which initiates and sends impulses throughout the myocardium. The pacemaker is independent of the **central nervous system (CNS)** (since the heart generates its own impulses it is said to be **myogenic**). Because of its united structure, all cells forming the entire myocardium muscle sheet contract together to produce a heartbeat. This is an application of the **all-or-none law**.

c) The **endocardium** is a smooth, glistening, **inner serous membrane** consisting of flattened epithelium that lines the heart cavities. Its function is to prevent friction between the heart muscle and flowing blood.

Investigation 2.1 To examine the structure of the heart

Materials: heart model, heart and circulatory posters, fresh hearts (pig or sheep), dissection materials, disposable gloves.

The following tasks assume the availability of animal hearts for dissection. If none are available, then these can be replaced by the appropriate use of models and charts. Not all the practical tasks within this investigation may be possible, since they rely on an 'intact' heart.

Task 1 – external features

1. Work out the ventral (the front surface) and dorsal (the rear surface) sides of the heart.

2. Identify the external features of the heart that are labelled in Figure 2.1B.

3. Observe and identify the narrow vessels branching over the surface of the ventricles. These blood vessels supply the heart with food and oxygen and transport carbon dioxide and other waste products away from the heart.

4. What happens if one of the main arteries to the myocardium becomes blocked with fatty lesions or a blood clot?

Task 2 – heart valves (Figure 2.1C and D)

1. Cut a small opening in the right atrium and look down into the atrioventricular opening (this opening is between the top and bottom chambers of the heart). Pour a small amount of water into the atrium and observe the action of the valve as the bottom chamber fills. Write down your observations.

2. Now squeeze the bottom chamber containing the water. Observe and identify the vessel from which the water emerges.

▶

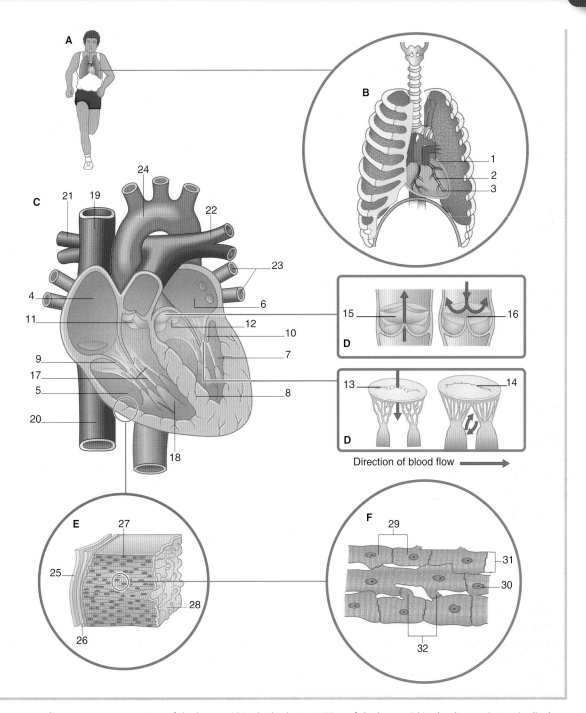

Fig. 2.1 Cardiac anatomy. A. Position of the heart within the body. **B.** Position of the heart within the thorax. **C.** Longitudinal section of the heart. **D.** Heart valves. **E.** Heart wall. **F.** Microscopic detail of myocardium.

1. Pericardium. **2.** Coronary artery. **3.** Coronary vein. **4.** Right atrium. **5.** Right ventricle. **6.** Left atrium. **7.** Left ventricle. **8.** Septum.

Atrioventricular valves: **9.** Tricuspid valve. **10.** Mitral valve or bicuspid valve.

Semi-lunar valves: **11.** Pulmonary valve. **12.** Aortic valve.

13. Mitral valve open. **14.** Mitral valve closed. **15.** Semi-lunar valve open. **16.** Semi-lunar valve closed by cusps. **17.** Chordae tendinae. **18.** Papillary muscle. **19.** Superior vena cava. **20.** Inferior vena cava. **21.** Right pulmonary artery. **22.** Left pulmonary artery. **23.** Left pulmonary veins. **24.** Aortic arch. **25.** Parietal pericardium. **26.** Visceral pericardium. **27.** Myocardium. **28.** Endocardium. **29.** Striations made up of myofibrils. **30.** Nucleus. **31.** Step-like intercalated discs. **32.** Connecting branches.

3. Repeat this task on the left side of the heart.
4. Identify the valves located between the top and bottom chambers on both sides of the heart.
5. How are these valves supported?
6. Identify the heart valves sited in the vessels leaving the bottom chambers.
7. What is the function of heart valves?

Task 3 – heart muscle (Figure 2.1C–F)
1. Cut off a small part of the apex of the heart. Observe the myocardial tissue and small openings to the ventricles. Observe the very thick section of the myocardial tissue and place a seeker into this small opening. The seeker should emerge out of the aorta. Now repeat this process on the right side of the heart. Which vessel does the seeker emerge from on this side?
2. Cut the heart open longitudinally into two equal halves. Observe that the heart is divided into a four-chambered muscular bag.

3. Identify and name the structure that separates the left and right sides.
4. Name the top and bottom chambers.
5. Describe how the top chambers differ in their shape and thickness when compared with the bottom chambers. Suggest reasons for the functional significance of these differences.
6. Observe the walls of both bottom chambers. What type of tissue are these walls made of?
7. In Figure 2.1F each cardiac muscle fibre is connected by a specialised junction called an **intercalated disc**. What is the function of this specialised junction?
8. The left bottom chamber has a thicker wall than the right bottom chamber. What is the functional significance of this difference?

Task 4 – vessels attached to the heart
Observe and identify the large vessels attached to the heart.

Review questions

1. The pathway of blood through the heart may be traced from the superior and inferior venae cavae, which empty deoxygenated blood into the right atrium. With the aid of Figures 2.1C, 2.3A–D and 2.16B, trace the pathway of blood from these large veins until it reaches the aorta. In your account briefly mention the structure and function of the heart chambers, valves and blood vessels through which the blood flows.

2. How is the heart's structure suited to its function as a dual-action pump?

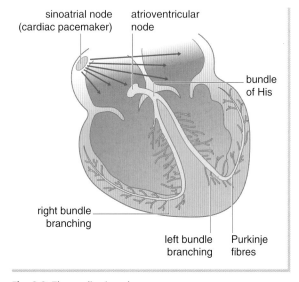

Fig. 2.2 The cardiac impulse.

How the heart works

The dynamic action of the heart is that of a dual-action pump in that both sides of the heart contract simultaneously, even though the functions of the two sides are entirely different.

The cardiac impulse (see Figure 2.2)
Cardiac contractions are initiated by an electrical impulse (the **cardiac impulse**) that originates from the **pacemaker** or **sinoatrial node** (SA node). The electrical impulse (also known as an action potential) travels down the atrial myocardium until it reaches the **atrioventricular node** (AV node) situated in the wall of the atrial septum. There is a slight delay before **atrial systole** (described below) is completed. The impulse then spreads into a specialised tissue, known as the **bundle of His**, which connects the AV node to a branched network of **Purkinje fibres**, located within the septum and the ventricle walls. The Purkinje fibres are connected to ordinary cardiac muscle fibres. As a result of this branching network, the impulse spreads throughout the ventricular walls, causing the ventricles to contract. This contraction is called **ventricular systole** as described below.

The heart's conducting system regulates the sequence of events that make up the **cardiac cycle**.

The cardiac cycle (see Figure 2.3)

The cardiac cycle is a sequence of events that make up one heartbeat and lasts for about 0.8 seconds, thus occurring about 72 times per minute, depending on one's state of fitness. **Heart rate** is defined as the number of heart contractions per minute.

The cardiac cycle consists of a period of relaxation of the heart muscle, known as **diastole** (0.5 seconds) followed by a period of contraction of the heart muscle, known as **systole** (0.3 seconds), during which time the electrical impulse from the SA node is initiated in a set timed sequence.

Cardiac diastole

In **cardiac diastole** the heart relaxes for 0.5 seconds, during which time the sequence of events shown in Figures 2.3A and B occurs.

Cardiac systole

During the 0.3 second contraction called systole, atrial systole is followed by ventricular systole and then the cycle begins again.

Atrial systole (Figure 2.3c)

First, the SA node initiates an electrical impulse that travels across the atrial walls (as described above). This is followed by a wave-like contraction across the myocardium of each atrium. The effect of atrial systole is to force **all** remaining blood past the atrioventricular valves into the lower chambers. The semi-lunar valves (pulmonary and aortic valves) are closed during this activity.

Ventricular systole (Figure 2.3d)

The electrical impulse passes from the AV node to the Purkinje fibres (as described above). Once ventricular myocardium is stimulated, a second wave-like contraction spreads across the ventricular walls, whilst the **atrioventricular valves** remain **closed** (these are the tricuspid and mitral (bicuspid) valves). Pressure inside the ventricles continues to rise. The ventricles continue to contract, until the continued increase in pressure pushes open the semi-lunar valves (pulmonary valve on the right side of the heart and aortic valve on the left side of the heart). The result is that blood flows into

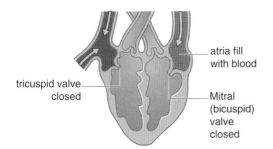

A. The atria fill with blood while the atrioventricular (mitral and tricuspid) valves are closed.

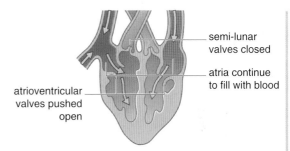

B. The atrioventricular valves are pushed open by rising atrial pressure and the ventricles start to fill with blood. During this time the semi-lunar (aortic and pulmonary) valves are closed.

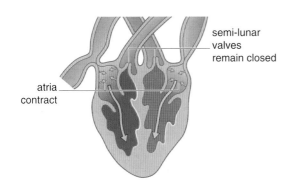

C. The atria contract, forcing remaining blood down into the ventricles.

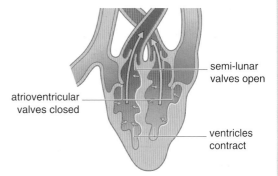

D. The ventricles contract and atrioventricular valves close. Ventricular contraction forces open the semi-lunar valves, so that blood is ejected into pulmonary artery and aorta.

Fig. 2.3 The cardiac cycle.

the pulmonary (lungs) and systemic (around the body) circulatory systems, respectively.

Heart sounds

Heart sounds heard through the stethoscope are described as **'lub-dub'** and are produced each time the heart valves close. The 'lub' sound is heard at the beginning of ventricular systole and is caused by the closure of the mitral and tricuspid valves. The 'dub' sound is heard at the beginning of ventricular diastole and is caused by the closure of the semi-lunar valves.

Cardiac output

When the ventricles contract, about 70–90 cm^3 of blood is ejected into the pulmonary and aortic arteries. This volume is called the **stroke volume**. Stroke volume is regulated by venous return and neural control (refer to Regulation of heart rate, p. 53).

Cardiac output ($\dot{Q}$) is defined as the volume of blood pumped by each ventricle in one minute. At rest this is approximately 5 dm^3 or l min^{-1}. During vigorous exercise cardiac output may increase up to 30 dm^3 or l min^{-1}.

The following formula links cardiac output to stroke volume and heart rate:

$$\text{cardiac output} = \text{stroke volume} \times \text{heart rate}$$

or $$\dot{Q} = SV \times HR$$

For example, if a person has a stroke volume of 75 cm^3 and a heart rate of 70 beats per minute (bpm), the cardiac output would be:

$$\dot{Q} = 75 \times 70$$
$$= 5250 \text{ cm}^3$$
$$= 5.25 \text{ dm}^3 \text{ or l min}^{-1}$$

Starling's Law of the Heart

Cardiac output is dependent on the amount of venous blood returning to the right side of the heart, otherwise known as **venous return**. During exercise, venous return increases and therefore cardiac output increases. This is caused by the myocardium being stretched, resulting in the myocardium contracting with greater force. Therefore, the stimulus that causes the greater force of contraction is the stretching of the muscle fibres themselves. This relationship is known as **Starling's Law of the Heart**. **Intrinsic factors** such as Starling's Law of the Heart, changes in electrolyte balance (sodium and potassium) in the heart muscle and increased myocardial temperature, result in changes in heart rate.

The pulse

The **pulse** is a peristaltic wave produced in an artery. It is due to the contraction of the left ventricle forcing out 70–90 cm^3 of blood (stroke volume) into an already full aorta. The frequency of waves represents the number of heartbeats per minute.

Electrical activity of the heart

Heart rate can be measured by **palpation, heart rate telemetry** or by using an **electrocardiogram (ECG)**. As the cardiac impulse travels across the atria and ventricular walls its electrical activity produces a recorded trace (ECG), as in Figure 2.4 which shows the three components of an ECG:

1. the **P** wave
2. the **QRS** complex
3. the **T** wave.

The **P** wave represents the excitation of both atria, known as **atrial depolarisation** (this concept is explained on p. 32). It occurs when the electrical impulse travels from the SA node across the atrial walls to the AV node. The **QRS** complex of waves represents excitation of both ventricles, known as **ventricular depolarisation**. It occurs when the electrical impulse travels from the AV node via the bundle of His to the Purkinje fibres (refer to Figure 2.2). The **T** wave indicates the **repolarisation** of both ventricles as they relax. You can see from this diagram that the heart spends more time in its resting state than in the working phase. For further information, refer to a specialist physiology text, such as references[1,2]. Heart rate taken during or immediately after exercise can be used to indicate cardiovascular-respiratory or **aerobic fitness**.

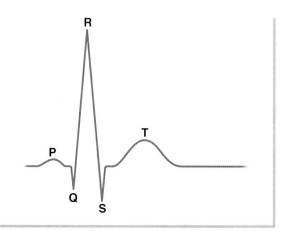

Fig. 2.4 ECG trace showing electrical activity of the heart.

Regulation of heart rate

The continual adjustment of heart rate is controlled by the **sympathetic** and **parasympathetic nervous systems**, as illustrated in Figure 2.5.

These two nervous systems originate in the **cardiac centre** of the **medulla oblongata** and they work antagonistically. The effect of exercise is to speed up heart rate. This is achieved by the sympathetic nerves transmitting impulses (initiated in the cardiac accelerator centre) and releasing **noradrenaline** onto the SA node. (Noradrenaline is produced by the adrenal medulla that forms part of the inner section of the adrenal glands.)

On the other hand, circulatory messages initiated by **baroreceptors** (located in the aorta and carotid artery) respond to high blood pressure and are received by the cardiac inhibitory centre. Impulses from the cardiac inhibitory centre are transmitted, via the **vagus nerve** (parasympathetic nerve), to the SA node to slow down heart rate. This is an example of **negative feedback control**, important in maintaining homeostasis within the body (a term described in Chapter 4 in the section looking at control of body temperature).

Other factors, such as elevated temperature, and other hormones, such as adrenaline, increase heart rate. For example, just before a competitive situation, the hormone **adrenaline** (released from the adrenal medulla) prepares the body for action. This hormone targets the heart, blood vessels, liver and fat cells. The release of adrenaline stimulates glycogenolysis (the process of breaking down glycogen to liberate glucose), intracellular metabolism of glucose in skeletal muscle cells and the breakdown of fats and proteins to form glucose.

The release of adrenaline results in reduced blood flow and reduced cellular activity to organs such as the gut, skin and kidneys that are not essential for physical activity. It increases blood flow to physically active organs such as skeletal muscle, lungs and cardiac muscle (fight or flight) (refer to Figure 2.21, p. 66). The effect of adrenaline lasts but a few minutes because it is rapidly metabolised, excreted or taken up by other tissues.

On the other hand, excessive potassium intake can slow down heart rate. In addition, gender and age also influence heart rate. It is found that females tend to have slightly higher heart rates than males and that heart rate generally slows down with age.

Ultimately, heart rate is dependent on a fine balance between the sympathetic and parasympathetic nerves, which continually adjust to changing conditions.

Other references that expand this section on cardiac structure and dynamics are [1-6].

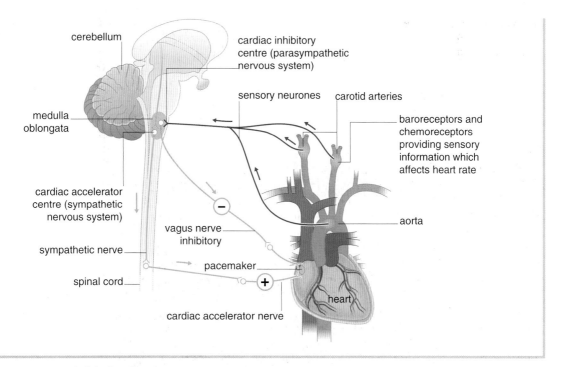

Fig. 2.5 Nervous control of the heartbeat.

Investigation 2.2   Measuring heart rate

Materials: stopwatch or stopclocks, heart and circulatory chart.

It is suggested that you work in mixed groups of five or six people.

Task 1

1. Monitor your resting heart rate by palpation at the carotid artery and radial artery (the pulse can be located by pressing softly at the carotid artery, alongside the trachea in the neck and across the wrist, the radial artery, when the arm is in a supine position). Count for 6 seconds, remembering that the count starts at zero. Then calculate your resting heart rate in beats per minute.

2. Repeat at each site using 10-second and 15-second counting periods. Do these counts in three positions:
   a. sitting
   b. lying down
   c. standing.

Task 2
Collate your group results using a table like Table 2.1.

Task 3

1. Are there any differences between heart rate taken at the radial and carotid arteries? Suggest reasons for your answer.

2. Many factors affect resting heart rate. Consider the differences in heart rate within your group and give reasons for these differences.

3. How does body position affect resting heart rate? Suggest reasons for variation of resting heart rate in the sitting, lying and standing positions.

4. What is being measured when you measure heart rate?

(Allow 2 minutes adjustment time for each of these positions prior to counting heart rate.)

Table 2.1 Results table – sitting

	Heartbeats/min, radial artery			Heartbeats/min, carotid artery		
Name	6	10	15	6	10	15
Self						

Investigation 2.3   To listen to the heart rate using a stethoscope

Materials: stethoscope.

1. Place the stethoscope upon the chest wall in the centre of the chest at the 5th intercostal space, as illustrated in Figure 2.6.
2. Describe what you can hear and which parts and actions of the heart are causing these sounds.

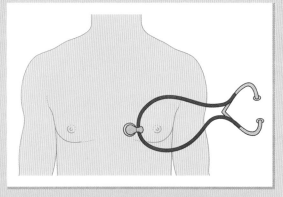

Fig. 2.6 Listening to heart sounds using a stethoscope.

Investigation 2.4 To measure heart rate response to varying intensities of workload

Materials: select EITHER the step test OR cycle ergometer test described below for this investigation. Stopwatch or stopclock. (Work in a mixed group so that you can compare your results.)

Task 1
This investigation is best achieved with a heart-rate monitor. If one is not available, work in pairs and get the passive partner to take and record heart rate values. Convert all 10-second counts to beats per minute (bpm).

1. Note your heart rate at the beginning of the lesson for a 10-second count.

2. Record your heart rate immediately before the exercise commences for a 10-second count.

3. Commence exercising by either riding the bike or stepping on and off a bench at a low-intensity (HR 120–130 bpm) work rate, for a period of 3 minutes. (For the cycle ergometer test this could be achieved without resistance and in the case of the step test with the aid of a metronome, which establishes a low fixed rate of stepping.)

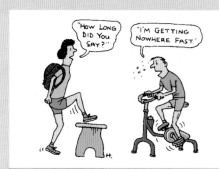

Fig. 2.7

4. Take heart-rate values for a 10-second pulse count:
   a. 1 minute after the start of the exercise
   b. 2 minutes after the start of the exercise
   c. at the end of the 3 minutes of exercise.
   d. Repeat the pulse count measurements every minute during the recovery phase until your heart rate has returned to its resting value prior to exercise.

5. Once your heart rate has returned to its resting value, repeat the same investigation but increase the workload (aim to achieve a heart rate of between 150 and 160 bpm). This can be achieved by increasing the frequency or resistance. (A weighted rucksack would be one way of increasing the resistance for the step test or, alternatively, one could increase the rate of stepping, which equates to an increase in the frequency of muscle contraction. Resistance or frequency could also be increased for the cycle ergometer investigation.)

6. Repeat this investigation once more at a workload just under maximal effort (in excess of 180 bpm), again by increasing the workload or frequency of exercise.

Task 2
1. Collate your results in table form (Table 2.2).

2. Convert heart-rate values into beats per minute. Draw a graph of your own results, with time in minutes on the x-axis (from heart rate prior to exercise to full recovery period) and heart rate in beats per minute on the y-axis, for the three different workloads.

Task 3
1. Account for any differences between your heart-rate counts at the start of the lesson and just prior to exercise.

Table 2.2 Results table – heart rate

Intensity of workload	HR at start of class (bpm)	HR prior to exercise (bpm)	HR 1 min after start of exercise (bpm)	HR 2 min after start of exercise (bpm)	HR at end of exercise (3 min) (bpm)	HR during recovery (min) 1, 2, 3, 4, etc. (bpm)
Low						
Medium						
High						

2. Using your own results, describe the relationship between heart rate and low-, medium- and high-intensity workloads.

3. Suggest physiological reasons for increased heart-rate values as workload intensifies.

4. Suggest physiological reasons for the differing patterns of recovery from the stress of the exercise.

5. A low heart rate during exercise and a small increase in heart rate as the intensity of the work increases generally reflect a high level of cardiovascular fitness. Compare your own results with those of your group members. Discuss your results in relation to gender, size, weight and levels of fitness.

6. Heart rate is increased and decreased as a result of the sympathetic and parasympathetic nervous systems, respectively. Using the information in the text, describe some of the factors that can influence heart rate.

Task 4
1. How reliable are the results of your investigation?

2. Does your investigation test what you set out to test?

3. Does your investigation produce a consistent pattern of results?

The answers to these questions will outline the concepts of **reliability** and **validity** in scientific investigations.

Review questions

1. Describe the relationship between stroke volume and submaximal and maximal exercise illustrated in Figure 2.8. Suggest reasons why maximal values for stroke volume are reached very early on in submaximal exercise.

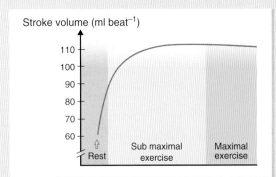

Fig. 2.8 Stroke volume and exercise.

2. Compare and suggest reasons for the trends shown in Figure 2.9, between cardiac output (bottom), stroke volume (top) and heart rate (middle) during rest, exercise and recovery.

3. When you are running, contraction of skeletal muscles in the legs helps blood return to the heart more rapidly. Would this effect increase or decrease stroke volume? Explain your answer.

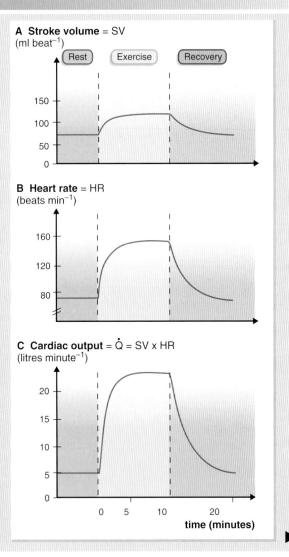

Fig. 2.9 A. Stroke volume, **B.** heart rate and **C.** cardiac output during rest, exercise and recovery (after reference [4]).

4. Trained athletes often have resting heart rates of less than 60 bpm. This condition is known as **bradycardia** (*brady* meaning slow). Using the information in Figure 2.10, compare and contrast the hearts of a trained athlete and an untrained person.

5. Give values for cardiac output at rest and during maximal exercise for: A. untrained males and females; B. trained males and females.

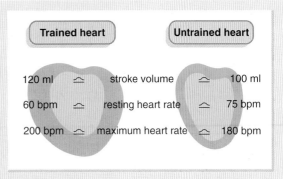

Trained heart		Untrained heart
120 ml	stroke volume	100 ml
60 bpm	resting heart rate	75 bpm
200 bpm	maximum heart rate	180 bpm

Fig. 2.10 Typical data for trained and untrained hearts.

Exam-style questions

1. One cardiac cycle includes all the events that occur between two consecutive heartbeats, as illustrated in Figure 2.11.
   a. i. Identify the **P** wave, **QRS** complex and **T** wave. *(3 marks)*
      ii. What events in the cardiac cycle do the P, QRS and T represent? *(3 marks)*
   b. Identify the cardiac phases labelled **A** and **B**. *(2 marks)*
   c. Using the information in this diagram, describe the relationship of an ECG to the cardiac cycle. *(4 marks)*
   d. Indicate on Figure 2.11 the timing of the heart sounds 'lub-dub' in relation to the cardiac cycle. *(2 marks)*

   (Total 14 marks)

2. Figure 2.12 shows a normal resting ECG (**A**) and an exercising ECG (**B**). Calculate the heart rates for both ECGs. *(2 marks)*

3. a. i. Define what is meant by a pulse and briefly describe how it is measured. *(3 marks)*
      ii. Define what is meant by the cardiac impulse. *(2 marks)*

   b. Aerobic performance is dependent upon the heart supplying blood to skeletal muscle.
      i. Describe the flow of blood through the heart during one cardiac cycle (diastole and systole). *(4 marks)*
      ii. Explain how heart valves (cuspid and semi-lunar) help control the direction of blood flow through the heart. *(4 marks)*

   (Total 13 marks)

4. A fit 18-year-old female student performs a 400 metre time trial in 1 minute.
   a. Sketch and label a graph to show a typical heart rate response. Start with the resting heart rate, then during the time trial, and then over a 20-minute recovery period. *(4 marks)*
   b. State **two** reasons for the increased heart rate during the exercise period. *(2 marks)*
   c. Explain why heart rate takes some time to return to its resting value following the exercise period. *(3 marks)*

   (Total 11 marks)

5. During and after exercise, the performer's heart rate will increase and decrease. Describe how neural control regulates these changes. *(4 marks)*

6. Training-induced changes of the heart may be considered as structural and functional. Discuss. *(10 marks)*

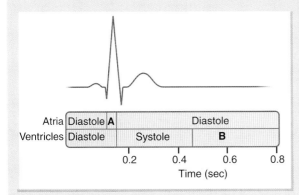

Atria	Diastole	**A**		Diastole	
Ventricles	Diastole		Systole	**B**	
	0.2	0.4	0.6	0.8	

Time (sec)

Fig. 2.11 The relationship of the ECG to the cardiac cycle.

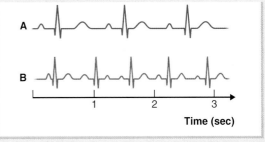

Fig. 2.12 A. Resting ECG and **B.** exercising ECG.

2.2 The vascular system

The key role of the **vascular system**, which comprises **blood** and **circulatory vessels**, is **transportation**. The effect of athletic activity is to increase the demand from body cells for both nutrients from the digestive system and oxygen from the lungs and to produce additional waste, which needs to be carried from body cells to the lungs and kidneys.

Blood is the specialised fluid tissue that carries out these functions within a closed system of vessels.

Blood

Blood is made up of 55% **plasma** and 45% **corpuscles**. In addition to the functions described above, it is involved in clotting, helps regulate body temperature and transports hormones such as adrenaline around the body.

Plasma is a straw-coloured fluid that contains approximately 90% water, 8% blood proteins, 1% salts, 0.5% food substances, 0.04% waste products, gases such as oxygen and carbon dioxide, enzymes, hormones, antibodies and antitoxins.

You may wish to find out more about each of these constituents of blood. For example, the plasma and red blood cell proportions can be determined using a technique for measurement called a haematocrit; see Green.[7] For a fuller blood profile see McKenna & Callendar.[1]

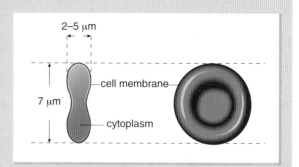

▶ **Task 2 – structure and function of white blood cells**

1. Using Figure 2.14, identify, draw and label two types of white blood cell, one granulocyte and one non-granulocyte, giving the percentage of each found in blood.

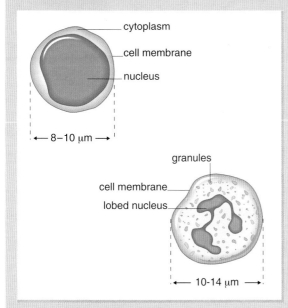

Fig. 2.14 White blood cells.

2. What are the functions of these two types of cells?

3. Where are white cells formed and how many occur per mm³ of blood?

4. Of what relevance are white blood cells to the active sportsperson?

Task 3 – structure and function of platelets

1. Using Figure 2.15, identify and draw a platelet.

2. Where are platelets formed?

3. What is their function and how many occur per mm³ of blood?

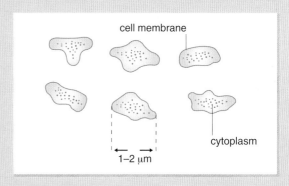

Fig. 2.15 Platelets.

Blood circulation (see Figure 2.16)

As a result of the dual pumping action of the heart, there are about 5.5 litres (5.5 dm³) of blood continually circulating throughout the body.

The closed system of vessels containing circulating blood flows within two major circulatory systems:

1. pulmonary circulatory system
2. systemic circulatory system.

These two systems are illustrated on the diagrammatic plan of Figure 2.16B.

Investigation 2.6 To consider the two circulatory systems and the principal types of blood vessels

Materials: transverse section (TS) of blood vessels, microscopes, circulatory system poster.

Task 1 – blood circulation

1. Using Figure 2.16B, describe in your own words the course of blood from the time it enters the right atrium (then passes through the heart and the two circulatory systems) until it eventually returns to the right atrium again. Describe the changes in the composition of blood during this double circulation and name the heart chambers, organs and vessels the blood flows through.

2. One of the effects of exercise is to speed up heart rate. What effect will an increased heart rate have on blood circulation?

Task 2 – blood vessels (refer to Figure 2.16 and text below)

Blood vessels vary in thickness and structural composition of their walls, diameter and overall length, according to their specific function.

1. Using the information in Figure 2.16E–G and prepared slides of blood vessels, identify an artery, a vein and a capillary network.

2. Observe the three layers of tissue that make up the walls of an artery and vein.

3. With the aid of diagrams, describe the structure of an artery, a vein and a capillary.

4. How is the structure of each of these three types of blood vessel suited to its specific function?

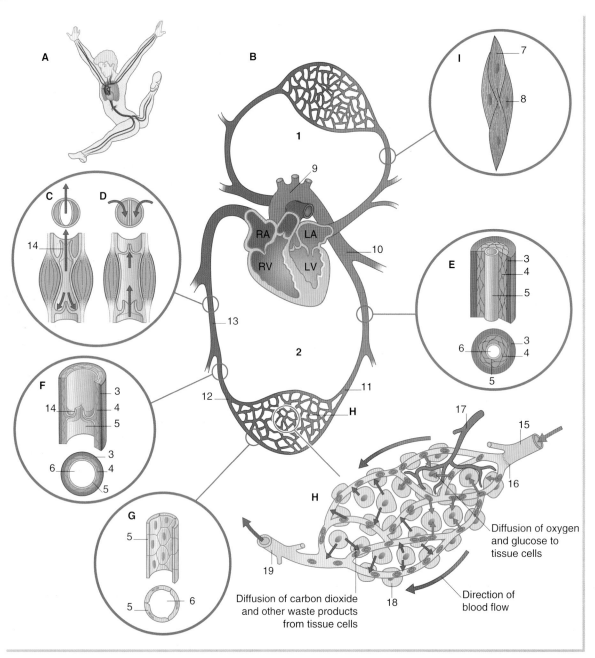

Fig. 2.16 Blood circulation. A. The human circulatory system. **B.** Diagrammatic plan of circulatory system. **C.** Skeletal muscle contracts: upper valve opened, lower valve closed. **D.** Skeletal muscle relaxes: upper valve closed, lower valve opened. **E–G. Longitudinal and transverse section through: E.** artery; **F.** vein; **G.** capillary. **H.** Capillary bed for gaseous exchange. **I.** Involuntary or smooth muscle in walls of blood vessels.

1. Pulmonary circulatory system. **2.** Systemic circulatory system. **3.** Tunica externa (fibrous collagen layer). **4.** Tunica media (smooth muscle and elastic fibrous layer). **5.** Tunica intima (endothelial layer). **6.** Lumen. **7.** Smooth muscle (spindle shaped). **8.** Centrally positioned nucleus. **9.** Aortic arch (leading to aorta). **10.** Artery. **11.** Arteriole. **12.** Venule. **13.** Vein. **14.** Pocket valve. **15.** Arteriole end of capillary bed (high pressure – oxygenated blood). **16.** Precapillary sphincter. **17.** Lymph vessel. **18.** Tissue cell. **19.** Venule end of capillary bed (low pressure – deoxygenated blood).

The general structure of arteries and veins

Blood vessels have properties that help circulation and allow blood to perform many of its functions. The walls of arteries and veins conform to a basic structural pattern as illustrated in Figures 2.16E and F. There are **three** main layers within these walls.

1. On the inside of the wall (next to the flowing blood) the **tunica intima** consists of a single layer of flat cells (endothelial layer) supported by a basement membrane and connective tissue containing collagen.
2. The **tunica media**, or middle layer of the wall, consists of circular, smooth involuntary muscle and elastic fibres. This layer varies in thickness in different vessels as described below.
   Figure 2.16I illustrates the structure of smooth muscle. Each cell consists of a spindle-shaped muscle fibre containing one centrally positioned nucleus. Unlike skeletal and cardiac muscles, smooth muscle fibres lack striations, hence the name 'smooth'. The function of smooth muscle is to control the diameter of blood vessels via **vasomotor** and **venomotor control** (refer to p. 63).
3. The fibres of the **tunica externa** or outer layer of the wall, contain collagen – a tough, relatively rigid supportive structure of blood vessel walls.

Blood vessels transporting blood away from the heart

Elastic arteries – thin walled with large diameters (Figure 2.16B)

The aorta and other large arteries are known as the 'elastic arteries' because the tunica media contains a large proportion of elastic tissue and only a small proportion of smooth muscle tissue. During ventricular systole, these arteries **extend** with a rise in left intraventricular pressure and **recoil** during ventricular diastole. These elastic arteries transport blood under **high pressure** to the muscular arteries and larger arterioles.

Muscular arteries and larger arterioles (Figures 2.16B, E and H)

These vessels are thick walled with small diameters. The tunica media consists of some elastic fibres and relatively large amounts of smooth muscle which control the shape of the lumen by contracting and hence reducing the width of the vessel (**vasoconstriction**), and relaxing and hence allowing the expansion of the vessel (**vasodilation**) known as **vasomotor control** – see p. 63. Hence these vessels are responsible for the redistribution of blood flow and alterations in blood pressure, as described in Section 2.3.

Smaller arterioles (Figure 2.16H)

Arterioles reduce in size and muscular content as they get closer to the capillary bed. The tunica media consists of smooth muscle cells and a few elastic fibres. The combined action of smooth muscle and the **precapillary sphincter** contracting and relaxing, control blood flow into the capillary bed.

Capillaries

Arterioles subdivide into **capillaries**, which are the smallest blood vessels in the body and which pass near to most muscle and other tissue cells.

The term **capillary bed** describes the total capillary structure within a muscle or other body organ. A capillary bed may contain thousands of **capillaries** for a given muscle; the number of capillaries passing through a muscle can be increased by exercise, with the result that oxygen and other nutrients can be more efficiently carried to individual muscle cells.

Also note that the large number of capillaries that eventually open out from the original artery have a much larger **total cross-sectional area** than the artery as a whole (see Figure 2.18). This means that blood slows down dramatically as it enters the capillary system and speeds up again as it leaves.

Capillary walls consist of a single layer of endothelium tissue (a simple tissue that lines all blood vessels), shown in Figure 2.16G. Their function is to be an exchange tissue, whereby dissolved materials diffuse in and out of the surrounding cells.

As blood passes through a muscle (or other) capillary system, it gradually gives up oxygen and nutrients and collects carbon dioxide and other waste products such as urea (as illustrated in Figure 2.16H and known as **gaseous exchange**). On leaving the venous end of the capillary bed, the blood enters **venules** (refer to Figure 2.16B), which transport blood to the larger veins.

Blood vessels transporting blood towards the heart – venous return

Venules (refer to Figure 2.16H)

On emerging from muscle tissue, capillaries unite to form venules, which have walls that consist of a tunica intima and tunica externa. **Venules** collect the outflow of blood from the capillary bed at **low pressure**. As they approach the veins they develop a thin tunica media coat.

Muscular veins (refer to Figures 2.16c, d and f)
These veins are supported by a thicker tunica externa, consisting mainly of collagen. They contain less smooth muscle and fewer elastic fibres than arteries of the same size and so are supported by pocket valves, which prevent backflow of blood. The tunica media is under **venomotor control** as described on p. 63.

Veins act as low-pressure reservoirs and move stored blood into general circulation during exercise in order to transport blood towards the vena cavae.

Vena cavae
These large-diameter, valveless, venous vessels have more smooth muscle in the tunica media which contracts to prevent backflow of blood and to deliver blood to the right atrium of the heart.

Investigation 2.7   Blood vessels

Task 1 – arterioles
'Dilate' means to widen and 'constrict' means to narrow. Why is it physiologically important for an arteriole to dilate and constrict and therefore allow blood to flow or prevent it from flowing?

Task 2 – capillaries
Using the information in Figure 2.16H, explain how capillaries act as exchange beds.

Task 3 – veins
1. How do pocket valves operate? (Refer to Figures 2.16C and D.)

2. Why are veins situated between muscles?

For further expansion on blood vessel structure, see references [2, 3].

Review questions

1. Figure 2.17 shows a diagrammatic representation of blood flow for both pulmonary and systemic circulation. Copy this diagram and:
   a. label the pulmonary and systemic circulation
   b. label the blood vessels leaving and entering the heart
   c. use arrows to indicate the direction of blood flow within both systems
   d. colour in the appropriate sections of each circulatory loop using blue for deoxygenated blood and red for oxygenated blood
   e. suggest a reason why the human body needs a double circulatory system.

2. Describe two important mechanisms for returning blood back to the heart, while exercising in an upright position.

3. Construct a table that lists the different types of blood vessels and their structural and functional details.

4. In some ways heart muscle is similar to skeletal and smooth muscle. In other ways these three types of tissue are different. Make a list of the similarities and differences between these three types of muscle tissue.

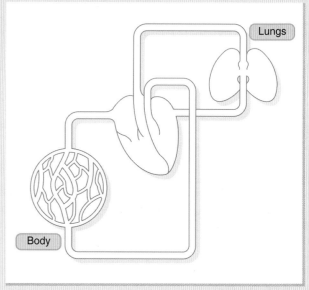

Fig. 2.17 Blood flow through pulmonary and systemic circulatory systems.

2.3 Blood flow in muscles

Learning objectives

On completion of this section, you will be able to:

1. Define blood pressure and describe the relationship between blood flow and peripheral resistance.

2. Understand what is meant by vasomotor and venomotor control.

3. Compare blood pressure in different blood vessels and describe the effects of exercise on blood pressure and blood flow.

4. Understand what is meant by the venous return mechanism and the phenomena 'muscle pump' and 'respiratory pump'.

5. Explain the significance of a lower blood pressure in the pulmonary circulatory system when compared with the blood pressure in the systemic circulatory system.

6. Explain how body temperature, water and electrolyte balance are regulated during exercise.

7. Describe how tissue fluid is formed and drained away and explain the changes in flow that occur during exercise.

8. Have a basic understanding of the importance of lymph glands in the defence of the body against infection.

Keywords

- ➤ baroreceptor
- ➤ blood flow
- ➤ blood pressure
- ➤ diastolic blood pressure
- ➤ lymph
- ➤ muscle pump
- ➤ peripheral resistance
- ➤ resistance
- ➤ respiratory pump
- ➤ sphygmomanometer
- ➤ systolic blood pressure
- ➤ tissue fluid
- ➤ vascular shunt
- ➤ vasoconstriction
- ➤ vasodilation
- ➤ vasomotor control
- ➤ venoconstriction
- ➤ venomotor control
- ➤ venous return mechanism
- ➤ viscosity

The rate at which blood circulates around the body depends on the needs of the body. During physical activity, working muscles may increase their oxygen consumption 20-fold when compared with the body's needs at rest. This section will help you to understand how and why the rate of blood flow changes as a result of physical activity.

The rate of blood flow depends on cardiac output ($\dot{Q} = SV \times HR$) and circulation. Furthermore, any changes in cardiac output will result in changes in blood pressure.

Blood pressure = Blood flow × Resistance

The **resistance** to blood flow is caused by fluid friction between blood and the walls of blood vessels. Hence as friction increases so does the resistance to flow.

Resistance to blood flow within blood vessels is called **peripheral resistance** and it depends on three factors.

1. The **viscosity** or thickness of blood (viscosity is a term that describes the resistance to flow of any fluid, in this case a steady flow of blood through the vessels). In the case of illegal blood doping techniques (refer to p. 169) as red blood cell count rises, blood viscosity increases. One of the benefits of 'warm-up' is to reduce blood viscosity and hence increase blood flow.
2. Blood vessel length since the longer the blood vessel, the greater the resistance to blood flow.
3. Blood vessel diameter, which is under the control of the **vasomotor** and **venomotor centres**.

Vasomotor and venomotor centres

Both control centres are located in the medulla oblongata (in the brain) and are regulated by the sympathetic and parasympathetic nervous systems (refer to Figure 2.5).

Vasomotor control and exercise

Changes in blood vessel diameter depend upon the metabolic needs of the body tissues. Blood pressure is monitored by **baroreceptors** (Figure 2.5) located in the aortic arch and carotid arteries. As cardiac output increases these sensory receptors are stimulated. This sensory information is received by the **vasomotor centre**, which stimulates nerves which innervate the smooth muscle walls of muscular arteries and arterioles.

1. To **increase** stimulation and hence cause **vasoconstriction** of blood vessels transporting blood to **non-active** tissue, hence **reducing** blood flow here.
2. To **decrease** stimulation and hence allow **vasodilation** of blood vessels transporting blood to **active** skeletal muscle, hence **increasing** blood flow here.

As a result of vasomotor control blood is diverted to skeletal muscle tissue where it is needed. The re-distribution of blood is otherwise known as **blood shunting** or the **vascular shunt** (refer to Figure 2.21).

The reverse of this process occurs during recovery **after** exercise to re-establish majority of blood flow to tissues as at rest (see Figure 2.21).

Venomotor control and exercise

Veins have a limited capacity to change their shape. This is the result of **venomotor tone**, whereby the vein's muscular coat receives stimulation from the sympathetic nervous system. The effect of limited vaso-constriction of veins causes a small increase in blood velocity and hence **an increase** in venous return.

Investigation 2.8   To consider blood pressure

Using the information in Figure 2.18 and Investigation 2.9, answer the following questions.

Task 1

1. Suggest reasons why systolic and diastolic blood pressure drops as the blood travels away from the left ventricle.
2. How does peripheral resistance vary from the aorta to the venae cavae?
3. As blood flows through the capillaries, there is a negligible effect of the pulse on blood flow. Compare the pressures in the arteries, capillaries and veins. Why is the pressure in veins so low?
4. The total cross-sectional area of the aorta is smaller than that of the arteries that branch from it; the cross-sectional area of the arterioles is greater than that of the arteries; the total cross-sectional area of the capillaries is greater than that of the arterioles.
   a. What will be the effect on blood flow as it travels from the aorta to arteries to arterioles to capillaries?
   b. Describe the changes in cross-sectional area from the capillaries to the venae cavae and the effect of these changes on blood flow.
5. What would be the effect of exercise on:
   a. rate of blood flow within the systemic circulatory system?
   b. blood pressure?

Task 2
Blood pressure rises and falls in relation to the cardiac cycle. Sketch a graph of the relationship of blood pressure (*y*-axis) to points of time on the cardiac cycle (*x*-axis).

Fig. 2.18 Changes in blood pressure, cross-sectional area of blood vessels and blood velocity as blood flows through the systemic system.

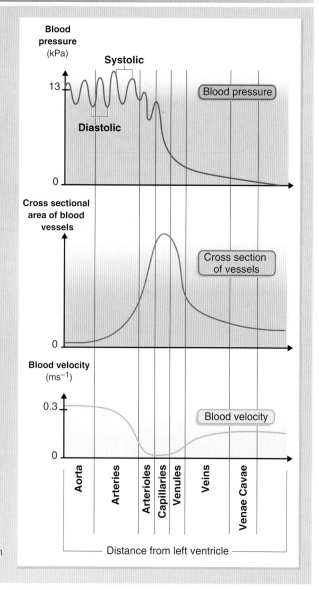

Investigation 2.9   To record blood pressure at rest

Materials: blood pressure meter
(**sphygmomanometer**). (Blood pressure meters
supplied by companies such as Griffin and George give
digitalised values.) A sphygmomanometer is used to
record blood pressure. The recording is written as:

120 mmHg	or	15.8 kPa (systolic BP)
80 mmHg		10.5 kPa (diastolic BP)

Task 1
The cuff is wrapped around the arm to cover the
brachial artery (upper arm). Air is pumped into the cuff
to **no more** than 180 mmHg (24 kPa), by which time the
cuff will feel tight around the arm and the tightness of
the cuff will compress the brachial artery so that no
pulse is recorded. The air pressure inside the cuff is
gradually released until the blood is felt spurting into
the artery. The pressure (systolic) is now read and more
air is released until the artery is completely open when
the pressure is read again (diastolic). Both these values
will be displayed on your monitor, in addition to pulse
count. The top line represents the **systolic blood
pressure**, which is the maximum pressure produced by
the left ventricle during systole. The bottom line is the
diastolic blood pressure or pressure in the artery at the
end of diastole.

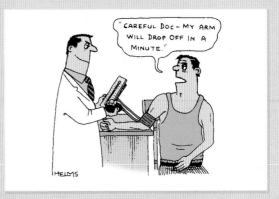

Fig. 2.19 Blood pressure cut off on arm.

It is important that you follow your teacher's
instructions carefully when using the blood pressure
meter.

Task 2
1. Measure and record your own blood pressure.
2. Compare and account for differing blood pressures
    within your class members.

Investigation 2.10   The effects of exercise on blood pressure, heart rate and blood flow

Materials: equipment for selected activity, blood
pressure and pulse meter, graph paper, strip
thermometer (a liquid crystal thermometer).

Task 1
1. Work in mixed groups and select a demanding
    physical activity that your group can manage.
    You may choose a static or dynamic type of
    exercise. Make sure that you warm up prior to
    exercising. (A warm-up could consist of 5 minutes

jogging, 5 minutes general muscle stretching, five
press-ups, five free squats and five sit-ups.)
2. Record your heart rate (HR), blood pressure (BP)
    and skin temperature (ST) prior to warm-up and
    flat-out exercise.
3. Exercise flat out for a 1-minute period, then retake
    your blood pressure, heart rate and skin
    temperature immediately after completion of the
    exercise. Make sure that you cool-down, once you
    have recorded your data.

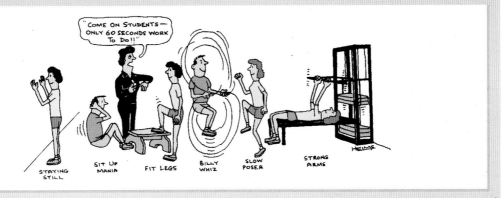

Fig. 2.20

▶ **Task 2**
Record your results in Table 2.3.

Table 2.3 Results table

SELECTED EXERCISE

	Prior to exercise	*At the end of exercise*
HR		
BP		
ST		

Task 3 – analysis of results

1. Plot your results on graph paper using the same x-axis for direct comparison.

   Graph A: arterial BP (mmHg) (y-axis) against time (min) (x-axis).

   Graph B: heart rate (bpm) (y-axis) against time (min) (x-axis).

   Graph C: skin temperature (°C) (y-axis) against time (min) (x-axis).

2. Compare the relationships between blood pressure, heart rate and skin temperature.

3. What is the effect of dynamic and/or static exercise on systolic and diastolic blood pressure?

4. A small increase in skin temperature indicates that there has been a shift of blood flow to the skin. Where has the blood come from and why does this happen?

5. Which part of the brain is responsible for detecting blood temperature?

6. Why is it advisable to 'warm-up' prior to intensive exercise and 'cool-down' at the end of an exercise period? (Refer to p. 145 for information on 'warm-up' and 'cool-down'.)

Task 4
The chart in Figure 2.21 shows how the percentage distribution of blood flow between different body systems changes from a resting state to when exercise is taken.

Note that in the example the **total** blood flow is increased by **five** times during exercise compared to blood flow when a sportsperson is resting. This means that the heart muscle, for example, takes 5% of 5 litres per minute at rest (i.e. 0.25 litres per minute), whereas it takes 4% of 25 litres per minute during exercise (i.e. 1 litre per minute), an increase of four times the actual blood flow to the heart. Total blood flow will depend on the intensity of exercise; it is possible to increase blood flow by up to 10 times the resting value. (The estimated blood flow to fatty tissue, up to 10% at rest and about 1% during exercise, is not included in the graph.)

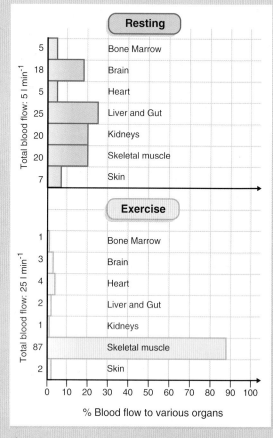

Fig. 2.21 Changes in percentage distribution of blood flow to various organs, from rest to exercise.

1. Using the information in Figure 2.21, describe the proportion of total blood flow going to different organs or body systems during rest and during exercise.

2. Suggest physiological reasons that explain how and why blood redistribution occurs during exercise.

3. With reference to Figure 2.21, explain why it is recommended that a sports person should refrain from eating for at least one hour prior to exercise.

Task 5
The effect of exercise on heart muscle is to increase blood flow to the myocardium by up to five times the resting value. Explain possible reasons for this increase.

Task 6

1. During exercise the heat generated by active muscles must be dissipated. Describe the method by which the body loses heat.

2. Describe how the body may gain heat.

3. What is meant by the term 'heat balance'?

4. How does the body minimise excessive heat loss during cold exposure?

5. What factors should be considered to provide maximum protection when exercising in the cold?

6. The body's ability to lose heat generated during exercise depends on the formation and evaporation of sweat. Water loss is accelerated during exercise. Total water loss from the body at rest in a cool environment has been estimated at approximately 95.9 ml h^{-1}, whereas during prolonged exercise it increases to values around 1325 ml h^{-1}. Identify the ways in which the body loses water and describe how most of the water loss is excreted.

7. What factors will affect the amount of sweat produced?

8. What effect does dehydration have on blood volume, heart rate and body temperature? How else can dehydration affect performance?

9. Electrolyte loss (such as sodium and chloride) during exercise occurs primarily along with water loss from sweating. How would you regulate salt and water replacement as a consequence of exercising in the heat? Identify some of the obvious benefits.

10. List the 'drinking guidelines' for athletes.

Two good references which will help you to answer the questions in Task 6 are Wilmore[8] and Foss & Keteyian.[4]

The venous return mechanism

The volume of blood leaving the heart depends directly upon the pumping action of the heart. This also results in an increase in blood flow in veins (see Figure 2.16C and D), known as the **venous return mechanism**.

At any one time veins contain three-fifths of circulating blood. This volume is significant, since venous return must be in excess of the rest of the circulating blood. Veins offer little resistance to blood flow and they can alter their shape as a result of **venomotor** control. **Venoconstriction** increases venous return by reducing the volume-capacity of veins to store blood as described above. This means that more blood is moved back towards the heart.

During exercise, skeletal muscle contracts and relaxes, squeezing sections of veins and thereby increasing venous return (see Figure 2.16C and D). This phenomenon is called the **muscle pump**.

During inhalation the pressure in the thoracic cavity is reduced, whilst the abdominal cavity pressure and pressure in other parts of the body is higher than the thoracic cavity pressure. Hence blood flowing towards the thoracic cavity will experience a force in the general direction of the heart. This phenomenon is called the **respiratory pump**. Stroke volume increases until it levels off prior to maximal effort being achieved (refer to Figure 2.8).

Blood pressure and blood flow in the pulmonary circulatory system

Venous blood leaves the right ventricle and enters the pulmonary artery at a rate of about 5 litres per minute. The pulmonary blood vessels offer little resistance to blood flow (since they contain much less smooth muscle than systemic arteries, there is less energy stored in them during systole). The whole effect is to reduce peripheral resistance to blood flow.

Once blood reaches the vast surface area of the pulmonary capillaries, it picks up oxygen by **gaseous exchange** from the alveoli. Then venules and veins stretch to accommodate the oxygenated blood and decreased blood flow as it travels to the left atrium of the heart.

Tissue fluid formation and drainage during exercise

At the arteriole end of the capillary bed, high pressure forces fluid (containing oxygen and glucose) through the capillary wall (Figure 2.22). This fluid permeates the spaces between the cells of all living tissues to become tissue fluid. Tissue cells extract the oxygen and glucose needed for tissue respiration; they excrete waste material, such as carbon dioxide and urea, at the venous end of the capillary bed, where blood pressure is low and where most of the tissue fluid returns into the capillary vessels.

Excess tissue fluid enters the surrounding lymph vessels and eventually returns to the blood via the lymphatic system. From this account it is clear that the lymphatic system plays a crucial role in maintaining the appropriate fluid levels in tissues, as well as maintaining blood volume itself.

One of the effects of exercise is to increase systolic blood pressure and hence to increase the formation of tissue fluid so that more nutrients are made available for tissue-cell respiration. During exercise, lymph is returned to the blood more quickly due to the combined

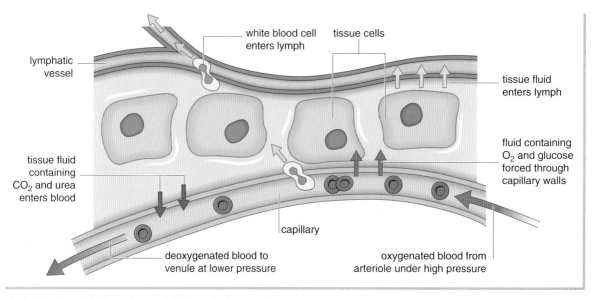

Fig. 2.22 Tissue fluid formation and drainage during exercise.

action of the muscle and respiratory pumps. These pumps contract and compress more forcibly on lymph vessels, thereby speeding up lymph flow.

Lymph nodes

The lymphatic system is not a major area of concern in the study of exercise physiology. However, whilst being a small part of the lymphatic structure as a whole, the tissues known as **lymph nodes** are relevant to our work. As lymph is transported, it passes through clusters of cells called lymph nodes (spread in groups throughout the lymphatic system), which contain cells that filter out and destroy debris such as damaged cells. Lymph nodes also contain lymphocytes that are part of the body's defence system. (You may wish to extend this area of study by referring to a specialist human biology text, such as Seeley et al.[2]) For further reading on blood flow through muscles, see references [3–5, 8].

Review questions

1. What is the specialised structure in veins that prevents excessive distension and backflow of blood?

2. What effect will an increase in stroke volume have on venous return?

3. Why is it important that pressure and flow are low in the pulmonary circulatory system when compared with the systemic circulatory system?

4. Explain how arterioles affect blood pressure.

5. Define blood pressure, blood flow and peripheral resistance. How can each be determined?

6. What factors are involved in the maintenance of blood pressure? Explain what they do.

7. a. How does venous blood manage to return to the heart, despite the fact that it is travelling against gravity?

   b. Describe two factors that affect flow of blood through the veins and back to the heart.

8. Explain which is more important in determining arterial blood pressure during rhythmical exercise: changes in vascular resistance or changes in cardiac output?

Exam-style questions

Figure 2.23 shows the variations in pressure and velocity of blood as it passes through the circulatory system while the body is at rest.

1. a. What types of blood vessels are represented by **A**, **B**, **C**, **D** and **E**? *(3 marks)*

   b. Explain the variations in velocity and pressure in vessel type **A**. *(5 marks)*

   c. Why is the velocity of the blood low in vessel type **C**? *(2 marks)*

   d. What is the physiological significance of this? *(5 marks)*

   e. What changes in Figure 2.23 would you expect during some form of rhythmic exercise? Explain your answer. *(5 marks)*

(Total 20 marks)

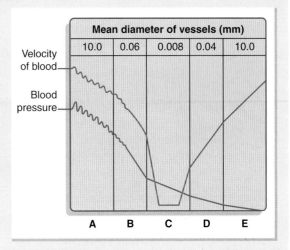

Fig. 2.23 Variations in pressure and velocity of blood in the circulatory system.

2.4 Respiratory factors in physical performance

Learning objectives

On completion of this section, you will be able to:

1. Describe the structure and function of the nasal cavity, pharynx, trachea, bronchi, bronchioles, terminal respiratory units and alveoli in the transportation of atmospheric air in and out of the lungs.

2. Understand the process by which air moves in and out of the lungs (pulmonary ventilation) and how this process is achieved by the action of muscles at rest and during exercise.

3. Understand the nervous and chemical regulation of breathing and how they affect ventilation rates.

4. Appreciate the effects of training on improving pulmonary function.

5. Consider the effects of asthma on athletic performance.

Keywords

- alveolar duct
- alveolar ventilation
- alveolus
- anaerobic threshold (AT)
- asthma
- blood acidity
- breathing
- bronchus
- bronchiole
- chemoreceptor
- epiglottis
- expiration
- glottis
- Hering–Breuer reflex
- inspiration
- intercostal nerve
- larynx

- medulla oblongata
- nasal cavity
- parietal membrane
- pharynx
- phrenic nerve
- pleural cavity
- pleural fluid
- pneumotaxic centre
- proprioceptor
- pulmonary pleura
- pulmonary ventilation
- respiratory bronchiole
- respiratory centre
- respiratory muscles
- tissue respiration
- trachea
- visceral membrane

Running fast and breathing rapidly go hand in hand. As with the increase in heart rate, there is a corresponding increase in rate and depth of breathing. This is brought about by the actions of the **breathing system**, which is the mechanism whereby the gases, oxygen and carbon dioxide are exchanged between the atmosphere and the blood vessels in the lungs during **gaseous exchange**.

This section will help you to understand the structure of the breathing system, the mechanics involved and the ventilatory responses to exercise.

Tissue respiration is the process by which cells use oxygen in order to release energy.

Pulmonary ventilation is the process of supplying fresh air to the **alveoli**, which make up the lung tissue.

Alveolar ventilation is the volume of inspired air that reaches the alveoli for gaseous exchange. It is normally expressed as volume per minute, that is:

> Alveolar ventilation = (tidal volume – anatomical dead space) × respiratory frequency.

The structure of the lungs

Figure 2.24B illustrates the anatomy of the breathing system. Each lung is covered by serous membranes called the **pulmonary pleura**. They are arranged like a double skin bag in which the outer membrane, called the **parietal membrane**, lines the chest cavity and the inner membrane, called the **visceral membrane**, lines each lung. In between the two membranes is the **pleural cavity**, which contains **pleural fluid**. The function of this lubricating fluid is to reduce friction between the two membranes during the dynamics of breathing. The pressure of this fluid is lower than the atmospheric pressure of air in the lungs. Atmospheric air pressure forces the pleural membranes against the inside of the thoracic cavity when it expands during inspiration (breathing in), thus causing the lungs to move with the chest during the breathing action.

The route by which air reaches our lungs

Air enters the breathing system through the nose (consisting of two nostrils and a nasal cavity) and mouth.

The nose is lined with a dense blood capillary network and a ciliated mucous membrane. The air is **warmed**, **filtered** and **moistened** by this lining.

Incoming air proceeds into the **pharynx** (which is involved in both respiratory and digestive systems). The incoming air is warmed and moistened as it passes through the pharynx.

Next, the air passes through the **larynx** (the voice box situated at the top of the trachea), where it is further warmed, filtered and moistened. The larynx contains a semicartilaginous flap called the epiglottis which, when closed over the **glottis**, prevents food from entering the **trachea** (breathing stops when food is swallowed). The trachea is a single airway that extends from the larynx to the two dividing bronchi.

Air then passes down the trachea which divides into two short branching **bronchi** approximately level with the fifth thoracic vertebra (one **bronchus** going to each lung). The bronchi further subdivide into smaller branches called **bronchioles**. Bronchioles consist of smooth muscle with no supporting cartilage in their walls. Hence muscle spasms can close off the airways to cause an asthma attack.[9] **Epithelium** (a general term used to describe the type of tissue lining inner body cavities) lines the trachea, bronchi and bronchioles and contains **goblet mucus cells** and **cilia** (Figure 2.24C). Cilia carry the mucus, with trapped dust and pathogens, to the back of the throat where it is swallowed.

The bronchioles further subdivide into **respiratory bronchioles**, which lead to **alveolar ducts**. Finally, the incoming air reaches millions of thin-walled air sacs, or **alveoli**, inside the lungs. **Gaseous exchange** takes place between the surface of the alveoli and the **pulmonary capillaries**, which are separated by single walls of both systems. The surface area of the delicate alveoli membrane is estimated at over 50 m^2 or the equivalent surface area of a tennis court (Figure 2.24D and E).

The alveoli contain **macrophage cells** involved in the lung's defence mechanism. These cells engulf pathogens and transport them to the bronchioles. The pathogens are subsequently dealt with by the cleaning mechanism of the lungs, as described above.

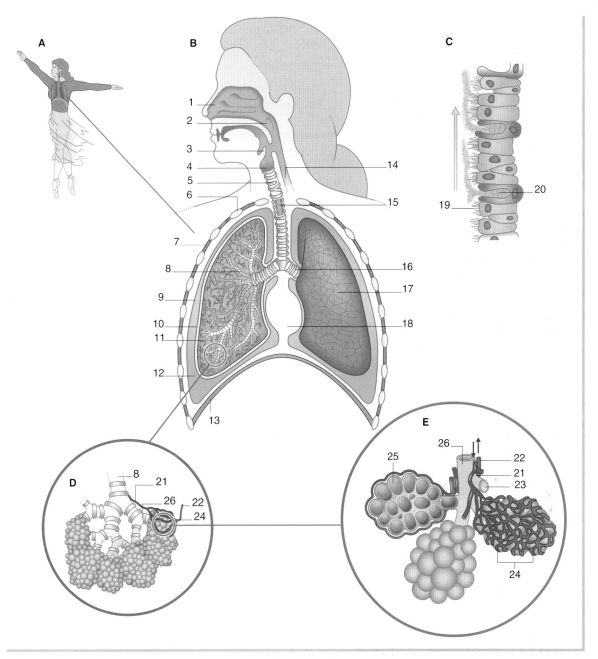

Fig. 2.24 The anatomy of the breathing system. A. The human breathing system.
B. Section of head and thorax: left lung, surface view; right lung, section.
C. Epithelial lining of cilia and goblet cells (found in structures 1, 2, 4, 8, 15 and 16).
D. Respiratory bronchioles leading to alveoli. **E.** Alveoli.

→ Flow of mucus and trapped pathogens and dust. ⇄ Direction of blood flow.

1. Nasal cavity. **2.** Pharynx. **3.** Epiglottis. **4.** Larynx. **5.** Incomplete ring of cartilage. **6.** Rib. **7.** Intercostal muscle. **8.** Bronchiole.
9. Parietal membrane. **10.** Visceral membrane. **11.** Right lung. **12.** Pleural cavity containing pleural fluid. **13.** Diaphragm.
14. Oesophagus. **15.** Trachea, section. **16.** Bronchus. **17.** Left lung. **18.** Position of heart. **19.** Cilia. **20.** Goblet mucus cell.
21. Branch of pulmonary artery (poor in O_2). **22.** Branch of pulmonary vein (rich in O_2). **23.** Alveolar duct. **24.** Alveoli surrounded by capillary network. **25.** Alveolus, section. **26.** Respiratory bronchiole.

Investigation 2.11   To understand the structure and functioning of the respiratory organs

Task 1 – to examine the structure of the trachea

Materials: transverse section (TS) slide of a trachea.

1. The trachea has walls supported by curved hoops (incomplete rings of cartilage). Feel the cartilaginous rings through the skin of your own neck just below the larynx. What is the function of these rings of cartilage?
2. Why are these rings of cartilage incomplete?
3. Make a drawing that shows the TS of the trachea. Indicate on it where you think the oesophagus is positioned.

Task 2 – to examine the structure of animal lungs

Materials: lung model, fresh animal lungs, rubber tubing and disinfectant, disposable gloves, suitable charts and diagrams. (The following task assumes the availability of fresh animal lungs – if they are not available, charts or models should be substituted.)

1. How many lobes has each lung?
2. Press the lung tissue with your fingers. Describe what it feels like.
3. Identify the larynx, trachea and bronchi.
4. Using a piece of tubing, fill the lungs with water from the tap. Alternatively, use an electrical air pump. Describe what happens to the lungs and explain your observations.
5. Empty out the water, then cut through a small section of lung tissue below one of the bronchi. Identify the smaller branching bronchioles, arterioles and venules.

Task 3 – to examine the structure of alveoli

Materials: TS slide of lung tissue, microscope.

1. Examine the prepared slide of a section of lung tissue.
2. Describe the structure of an alveolus. Figure 2.24E may assist you to observe some of the structures.
3. Why does the connective tissue below the epithelium lining the alveolus contain elastic tissue?
4. There are approximately 3 million alveoli in a pair of human lungs, varying in diameter between 70 and 300 microns (μm – a millionth of a metre or 10^{-6} m). Why is it important to have such a vast surface area of alveoli?
5. Surrounding each alveolus is a network of capillaries, as illustrated in Figure 2.24E. Why is this blood supply necessary?
6. What effect does physical activity have upon size, structure and functioning of the alveoli?

Review questions

1. Beginning with atmospheric air entering the nasal cavities, trace the pathway of an oxygen molecule until it reaches an alveolar duct and identify all the respiratory structures it passes on the way.
2. Using the information in Figure 2.24 and the text above, work through the pathway of outgoing air.

Exam-style questions

1. Distinguish between pulmonary ventilation, alveolar ventilation and tissue respiration. *(3 marks)*
2. How would breathing in cold air affect the capability to perform exercise? *(4 marks)*
3. Asthmatic attacks often occur after exercise, reaching a peak response within 5 minutes after exercise has ceased.
   a. Identify some of the causes of exercise-induced asthma. *(4 marks)*
   b. Explain how you could help a friend who is suffering from an asthma attack. *(4 marks)*

(Total 8 marks)

References[4, 9] will help you to answer question 3.

The mechanics of breathing

The actual mechanism of breathing is brought about by the changes in air pressure (intrapulmonary pressure) in the lungs, relative to atmospheric air pressure. Changes in intrapulmonary pressure are the result of the muscular actions of the **intercostal muscles** and **diaphragm**.

The respiratory muscles

The intercostal muscles (Figure 2.25)

The 11 pairs of intercostal muscles (which are arranged in two layers) occupy the spaces between the 12 pairs of ribs. The layers nearest to the lungs are called the **internal intercostal muscle fibres**. These fibres extend in a downwards and backwards direction from the lower margin of the rib above to the upper margin of the rib below, with the upper attachment being nearer to the sternum. The **external intercostal muscle fibres** lie on top of the internal intercostal muscle fibres and extend in a downwards and forwards direction, with the lower attachment nearer to the sternum, in opposition to the internal intercostal muscle fibres.

The first rib is a fixed rib and so when the external intercostal muscles contract, the other ribs are pulled

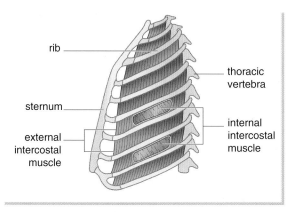

Fig. 2.25 Lateral view of rib cage to show intercostal muscles.

towards this fixed rib, resulting in an upwards and outwards movement of the thoracic cage during the process of breathing in. During quiet breathing the internal intercostal muscles remain passive.

The **intercostal nerves**, which originate from the **medulla oblongata** located in the brain, stimulate the intercostal muscles.

The diaphragm (Figure 2.26)

The **diaphragm** is a dome-shaped sheet of muscle forming the floor of the thoracic cavity. It is attached to the vertebral column, lower ribs and sternum and radiates from a central tendon. The diaphragm separates the thoracic cavity from the abdominal cavity and it is innervated by the phrenic nerves, whose nerve impulses originate from the medulla oblongata.

When the diaphragm contracts, its muscle fibres shorten and the central tendon is pulled downwards. The effect is to increase the depth of the thoracic cavity (and therefore assist in the intake of air).

The breathing mechanism at rest

During inspiration (Figure 2.26A)
The **external intercostal** muscles **contract**, whilst the **internal intercostal** muscles **relax**. This action causes the ribs and sternum to move upwards and outwards, thereby increasing the chest width from side to side and from front to back. In the meantime, pressure between the pleural membranes is reduced from −2 mmHg (−0.26 kPa) to −6 mmHg (−0.79 kPa). This negative pressure, relative to the gas pressure in the lungs, allows the pressure of air in the lungs to stretch the elastic pulmonary tissue in contact with the chest cavity. At the same time the **diaphragm contracts**, causing this dome-shaped sheet of muscle to descend by approximately 1.5 cm (the effect is to increase the depth of the thoracic cavity). Stimulation of the phrenic and intercostal nerves causes the contraction of these breathing muscles.

The combined effect of the contraction of the external intercostal muscles and of the diaphragm is to increase the volume occupied by the lungs. Therefore, the air pressure inside the lungs reduces. This results in atmospheric air being forced into the lungs via the nasal passages, trachea, bronchi and bronchioles, until air reaches the alveoli and air pressure inside the lungs is equal to the atmospheric pressure.

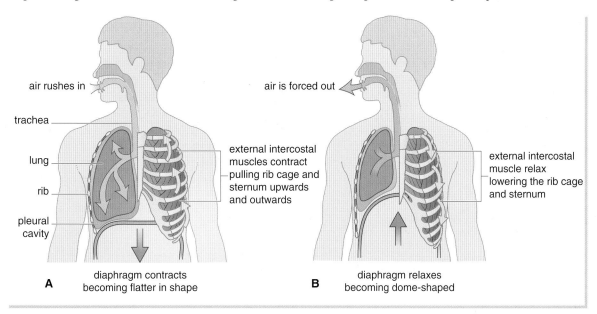

Fig. 2.26 The breathing mechanism. **A.** Breathing in. **B.** Breathing out.

During expiration (Figure 2.26B)

The **diaphragm** and **external intercostal** muscles **relax** and return to their original positions. The ribs and diaphragm press on the pleural fluid. The relative pressure between the pleural surfaces increases from −6 mmHg (or −0.79 kPa) to −2 mmHg (or −0.26 kPa). This combined effect is to reduce the lung volume, thereby increasing air pressure inside the lungs so that it is above atmospheric pressure and so air is forced out via the respiratory passages. This is aided by the elastic recoil of alveolar tissue (from the stretched state of full lung expansion) until the lungs deflate to their original volume.

The breathing mechanism during exercise

During inspiration

A much larger volume of inspired air is achieved by the contraction of accessory inspiratory muscles.

In addition to the external intercostal muscles and diaphragm muscles contracting, **scaleni** and **sterno-cleidomastoids** contract to raise the first and second ribs and sternum, respectively. During maximum efforts, the **trapezius** and **back** and **neck extensors** also contract and increase the size of the thorax even more.

During expiration

The combined contraction of the **internal intercostal** and **abdominal** muscles forces air **out** of the lungs (when the internal intercostal muscles shorten, the rib cage is actively moved downwards and the abdominal muscles force the diaphragm upwards).

Nervous and chemical regulators of the breathing mechanism

The rate of breathing is controlled subconsciously by the **medulla oblongata**, which regulates inspiration, and by the **pneumotaxic centre** in the **pons varolii**, which regulates expiration (see Figure 2.27). Both these control centres are located in the **respiratory centre** in the brainstem.

During exercise

The major regulatory mechanisms that affect rate and depth of breathing are illustrated in Figure 2.27. Increases in respiratory rates and depth of breathing are brought about as a direct result of increases in blood acidity levels (**pH**) and carbon dioxide content of the blood (**pCO$_2$**).

Central and **peripheral chemoreceptors** react to changes in pCO$_2$, pO$_2$ and pH in the cerebrospinal fluid and blood respectively. Increases in blood lactate

levels are the direct result of anaerobic energy production within working muscles. The highest level of exercise that can be performed without a significant change in blood pH is called the **anaerobic threshold**. Carbon dioxide is produced as a waste product of aerobic respiration and is the **main regulator** of breathing at rest and during bouts of physical activity.

Because changes in carbon dioxide levels can change pH, the respiratory system plays an important role in maintaining the **acid–base balance**. During exercise, increased amounts of carbon dioxide exert their influence by changing the hydrogen ion levels, as shown by the following reaction:

$$H_2CO_3 \quad \rightarrow \quad H^+ + HCO_3^-$$
$$\text{(carbonic acid)} \qquad \text{(bicarbonate ion)}$$

A small drop in blood pH is detected by **chemoreceptors** and so the respiratory centre stimulates an increase in rate and depth of breathing. The net result is the elimination of carbon dioxide and an increase in pH back to normal levels. As exercise levels get progressively harder, any further increases in minute ventilation are the direct result of increases in respiratory frequencies (refer to Investigation 2.16, p. 85).

Other minor regulatory mechanisms include the use of **proprioceptors** (sensors which feed information to the brain about joint angles, muscle stretch and body balance – see p. 35), **psychological factors** (such as anxiety and alertness) and **lung stretch receptors**. Lung stretch receptors, located within bronchi and bronchioles, are stimulated by overstretching, as experienced in hyperventilation. Impulses travel via the vagus nerve to the respiratory centre where inspiration is inhibited and expiration is stimulated. This mechanism is called the **Hering–Breuer reflex**.

During recovery

As soon as exercise stops there is a sudden decrease in minute ventilation, followed by a slower decrease towards rest (refer to your results from Investigation 2.16 on p. 85). This response is due to a decrease in stimulation from the respiratory centres, as pCO$_2$ and pH levels in the cerebrospinal fluid and blood return to pre-exercise levels (refer to p.80 for details of CO$_2$ transportation). Hence there is a reduction in the stimulation of the phrenic and intercostal nerves that innervate the diaphragm and intercostal muscles respectively.

The effect of exercise stress and recovery is that of a **continual** balance between **excitatory** (positive) and **inhibitory** (negative) factors, some of which are shown in Figure 2.27.

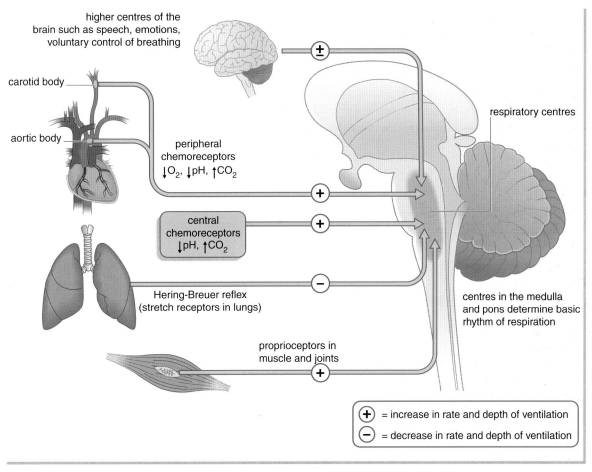

higher centres of the
brain such as speech, emotions,
voluntary control of breathing

carotid body

aortic body

peripheral
chemoreceptors
$\downarrow O_2$, $\downarrow pH$, $\uparrow CO_2$

central
chemoreceptors
$\downarrow pH$, $\uparrow CO_2$

Hering-Breuer reflex
(stretch receptors in lungs)

proprioceptors in
muscle and joints

respiratory centres

centres in the medulla
and pons determine basic
rhythm of respiration

$\oplus$ = increase in rate and depth of ventilation

$\ominus$ = decrease in rate and depth of ventilation

Fig. 2.27 The major regulatory mechanisms that affect rate and depth of ventilation. A plus sign (+) indicates an increase in ventilation and a minus sign (−) indicates a decrease in ventilation (after reference [2]).

Review questions

1. Complete Table 2.4, which investigates the muscles that are involved in breathing at rest and during exercise.

2. Describe the mechanism of inspiration during physical activity.

3. a. Identify the chemical stimuli that control the rate and depth of breathing. Which chemical stimulator is the main regulator?

   b. How do these stimuli control respiration during exercise?

   c. What other stimuli control ventilation during exercise?

Table 2.4 Muscles involved in breathing		
Respiratory phase	*Muscle acting*	*Action*
Inspiration		
at rest	diaphragm	flattens
during exercise		
Expiration		
at rest		
during exercise		

1. Identify and describe some of the long-term effects of an aerobic training programme on the respiratory system? *(8 marks)*

For help in answering question 1, refer to section 4.2 and references[4, 8].

2. During exercise, ventilation rates may increase 10-fold. How is this achieved? *(6 marks)*

3. An increase in the concentration of carbonic acid (HCO_3^-) causes a rise in blood pH. Briefly outline how the body resists pH change during exercise. *(4 marks)*

Other references that expand this section on lung structure, breathing mechanics and regulation are[1, 2, 4–6, 10].

2.5 Gas exchange in the lungs

Learning objectives

On completion of this section, you will be able to:

1. Understand the function of the breathing system in respect of gaseous exchange with the blood.

2. Describe how the breathing system adapts as a result of physical activity.

3. Summarise the concept of the partial pressures of gases and how the partial pressures of oxygen (pO_2) and carbon dioxide (pCO_2) affect the oxygen-carrying capacity of haemoglobin.

4. Appreciate how changes in pCO_2 affect the delivery of oxygen from haemoglobin to tissue sites.

5. Understand how the oxygen dissociation curve aids the release of oxygen from haemoglobin into muscle cell tissue.

6. Understand the concept of arteriovenous difference (a-$\bar{v}O_2$ diff).

Keywords

- arteriovenous oxygen difference (a-$\bar{v}O_2$ diff)
- Böhr effect
- carbamino-haemoglobin
- carbon dioxide
- carbonic acid
- exhaled air
- gaseous exchange
- haemoglobin
- haemoglobinic acid
- inhaled air
- myoglobin
- diffusion
- oxygen dissociation curve
- oxyhaemoglobin
- partial pressure (p)
- pulmonary blood pressure
- quiet breathing
- tissue respiration

One of the main functions of the breathing system is to operate in conjunction with the vascular system in the process of **gaseous exchange**.

This section will help you to understand how it is possible for two-way traffic to exist. **Oxygen** is transported in one direction from lung alveoli to tissue cell sites for intracellular use in the **mitochondria** (during **tissue respiration**) whilst **carbon dioxide** travels at the same time and in the same place in the opposite direction.

How gaseous exchange is achieved

During inspiration, alveolar pressure is lower than atmospheric pressure; therefore, air rushes in via the respiratory tract until the gas pressures are equalised. During expiration, the opposite occurs.

Also, despite a dense pulmonary capillary network, some alveoli have a poor or even non-existent blood supply. How do the lungs overcome this problem? At rest, inspired air goes to those alveoli with a good capillary network. The effect of regular exercise is to improve the capillary bed surrounding the alveoli and therefore increase the surface area available for gaseous exchange.

The movement of gases in and out of the circulatory system occurs by the process of **diffusion** (gas molecules moving from a region of high concentration to a region of low concentration) across the **epithelium** (membrane) that separates alveoli from lung circulatory capillaries. This is due to differences in **partial pressures** of carbon dioxide and oxygen in the pulmonary systems.

Partial pressures

The **partial pressure (p)** of a gas refers to its actual pressure as it exists within a mixture of gases. At

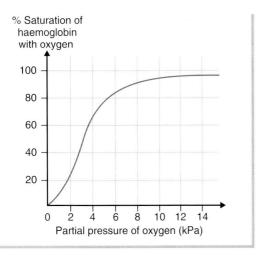

Fig. 2.28 Haemoglobin–oxygen dissociation curve. Standard conditions: 37°C, CO_2 = 5.26 kPa, pH = 7.4.

sea level, the partial pressure of oxygen (**pO₂**) in the atmosphere is about 20 kPa, which therefore means that oxygen contributes about 20% of the gas pressure in atmospheric air, the total pressure of which is 100 kPa. An oxygen partial pressure of 20 kPa represents a **concentration** of gas molecules equivalent to its normal atmosphere concentration. The partial pressure of oxygen in **alveolar air** is about 13 kPa and from Figure 2.28, you can see that this oxygen pressure will force about 98% of haemoglobin in blood passing through the alveolar capillary bed to become oxygenated. At altitude the ability to perform physical work is decreased by hypoxia (lowered pO₂). How the body copes with the difficulties experienced at **altitude** and the physiological changes that take place during acclimatisation are covered in section 4.3 on p. 161.

Oxygenation of haemoglobin (Figure 2.29A)
As blood is pumped through the pulmonary capillaries by pressure created by the heart, the red corpuscles are squeezed out of shape. This is the effect of the pressure of blood trying to force tiny corpuscles through tiny capillaries. This has the effect of forcing greater surface contact of the corpuscles with the capillary walls, which means that the oxygen diffusing across from the alveoli can more readily reach the haemoglobin in the red corpuscles.

Exercise increases the rate of expiration of air V̇E or the volume of expired air per minute) 10-fold, which means that up to 10 times the resting amount of oxygen is exchanged. This is achieved by the heart increasing **pulmonary blood pressure** (the driving pressure of blood in the lung–alveoli transport system) by a small amount. The effect is to cause a much greater distortion of the red corpuscles in the pulmonary capillaries and thus a much more rapid take-up of oxygen by the haemoglobin in the corpuscles.

Oxygen attaches to haemoglobin in red corpuscles in the following manner:

$$Hb \quad + \quad O_2 \quad \rightarrow \quad HbO_2$$

haemoglobin   oxygen   oxyhaemoglobin

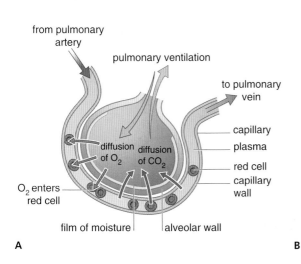

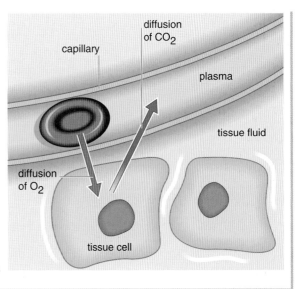

Fig. 2.29 A. Oxygenation of haemoglobin. **B.** Tissue respiration.

Blood then carries oxyhaemoglobin to the tissue sites where the oxygen is released and used in the process known as tissue respiration.

$$HbO_2 \rightarrow Hb + O_2$$

Tissue respiration

Oxygen

When **oxyhaemoglobin** reaches tissue cells, where the oxygen is required for energy release, the process of **diffusion** of **oxygen** across the tissue capillary walls **into** the tissue cells occurs (as illustrated in Figures 2.16H and 2.29B). This diffusion process is helped by a lower oxygen molecular concentration in the tissue cells (because energy creation uses up oxygen stored in the cells) and a relatively higher oxygen molecular concentration in the haemoglobin in the capillary.

Muscle cells contain a substance called **myoglobin** (a molecule similar to haemoglobin but which has a greater affinity for oxygen), which is depleted of oxygen by energy-creating processes in the cells. Oxygen therefore diffuses via the myoglobin across muscle cells to cell **mitochondria**, where it is used to produce the adenosine triphosphate (ATP) needed for muscle contraction (see Section 3.2 for a description of this aerobic process).

The absorption and utilisation of oxygen from the blood lead to a difference in the oxygen content of arterial and venous blood. **At rest**, as blood moves from arteries to veins, its oxygen content varies from 20 ml of oxygen per 100 ml of arterial blood to 15 ml of oxygen per 100 ml of venous blood. The difference between these two values (20 ml – 15 ml = 5 ml) is referred to as the **arteriovenous oxygen difference (a-$\bar{v}O_2$ diff)** (Note that the bar over the v in a-$\bar{v}O_2$ diff refers to an average based on calculations for mixed venous return.) This value represents the extent to which oxygen has been removed from the blood as it passes through the body, which means that, **at rest**, about 75% of the blood's original oxygen load remains bonded to the haemoglobin.

With increasing rates of exercise, the a-$\bar{v}O_2$ diff increases up to values of 15–16 ml per 100 ml of blood. This means that up to 80% of the available oxygen is extracted from arterial blood during intense exercise. In reality even more oxygen is released for tissue cell respiration in working muscles because the value of a-$\bar{v}O_2$ diff reflects an average based on calculations for mixed venous blood (i.e. blood returning from both active and inactive tissue). These two models are illustrated in Figure 2.30. Therefore an increase in a-$\bar{v}O_2$ diff reflects an increased extraction of oxygen from blood, as greater amounts of oxygen are required by active muscles.

Note that cardiac output indicates how much blood leaves the heart in one minute, whereas the a-$\bar{v}O_2$ diff indicates how much oxygen has been extracted from the blood by the tissues. The product of these two values gives the rate of cellular oxygen consumption.

$\dot{V}O_2$	= SV	× HR	× a-$\bar{v}O_2$ diff
oxygen consumed in cells	= stroke volume	× heart rate	× arteriovenous O_2 difference

The arteriovenous oxygen difference **in a trained sportsperson** increases with training, reflecting greater oxygen extraction at the tissue level and a more effective distribution of total blood volume (i.e. more blood going to active sites). This in turn can account for increases in $\dot{V}O_2$max.

Carbon dioxide

As energy is released in muscle cells, **carbon dioxide** is produced with the result that the concentration of carbon dioxide in the muscle cells is higher than that in the blood flowing through adjacent capillaries. Therefore, carbon dioxide **diffuses** across cell and

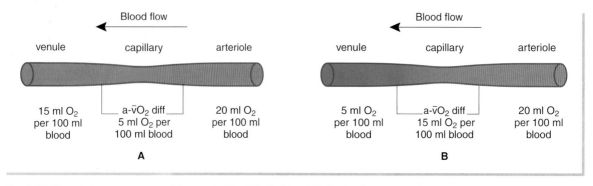

Fig. 2.30 The arteriovenous oxygen difference (a-$\bar{v}O_2$ diff). **A.** At rest. **B.** During intense exercise.

capillary walls into the blood (see Figures 2.16H and 2.29B). Blood carbon dioxide loading increases as blood reaches the venous end of the capillary bed.

There are **three** ways in which carbon dioxide can be carried by the blood: dissolved in plasma, as bicarbonate ion and as carbaminohaemoglobin.

Carbon dioxide dissolved in plasma

Approximately 7% is transported as carbon dioxide dissolved in blood plasma.

Bicarbonate ion

About 70% of carbon dioxide produced is transported in the plasma as **bicarbonate ions**. Carbon dioxide and water molecules combine to form carbonic acid (H_2CO_3) within the red blood cell (RBC), assisted by the enzyme carbonic anhydrase, which acts as a catalyst. This acid is very unstable and so quickly dissociates, freeing the hydrogen ion (H^+) and forming a bicarbonate ion (HCO_3^-) (see Step 1 below), thereby lowering the pH of venous return. The H^+ reacts with oxygenated haemoglobin to form haemoglobinic acid, which triggers the release of oxygen for tissue cell respiration (see Step 2 below).

Step 1:

$$H_2O + CO_2 \rightarrow H_2CO_3 \rightarrow H^+ + HCO_3^-$$

(carbonic anhydrase catalyst) (leaves RBC)

Step 2:

$$H^+ + HbO_2 \rightarrow HHb + O_2$$

(remains in RBC) (haemoglobinic acid) (for tissue respiration)

This is one of the mechanisms by which increased carbon dioxide in the blood causes the release of oxygen from haemoglobin. The binding of H^+ to haemoglobin triggers the **Böhr effect**, which shifts the oxygen–haemoglobin dissociation curve significantly downwards and to the right. A further drop in pH caused by lactic acid accumulation during intense exercise will additionally stimulate oxygen release by the same process.

Carbaminohaemoglobin

About 23% of carbon dioxide produced chemically combines with haemoglobin, once the haemoglobin has released its oxygen at the tissue site.

$$CO_2 + HbO_2 \rightarrow HbCO_2 + O_2$$

(carbaminohaemoglobin)

The carbon dioxide is not absorbed at the same molecular site as oxygen but still stimulates the release of oxygen for further tissue respiration.

These processes are in effect reversible when conditions of carbon dioxide and oxygen partial pressures are changed. For example, when venous blood carrying carbon dioxide reaches pulmonary capillaries in contact with oxygenated alveoli, pulmonary blood carbon dioxide partial pressure (pCO_2) is higher than that in the alveoli. Carbon dioxide dissolved in plasma comes out of solution, the H^+ and bicarbonate ions combine to form carbonic acid, which then splits into carbon dioxide and water, and carbon dioxide is released from haemoglobin. Carbon dioxide diffuses from the blood into the alveoli and is expired out of the lungs (Figure 2.29A).

Efficiency of gas process

Steep diffusion gradients of oxygen and carbon dioxide are maintained by:

- good lung ventilation
- the vast surface area of alveoli
- the very short distance between alveolar lining and blood (only 0.5 µm in thickness)
- constant blood flow
- the large amount of red corpuscles and muscle myoglobin
- moist lining.

At rest, approximately 250 ml of oxygen diffuses per minute. The effects of exercise can increase this volume to around 2–2.5 litres per minute. One of the effects of training is to increase alveolar ventilation by increasing the surface area of alveoli available for diffusion; another is to strengthen the musculature involved in breathing so that lung capacity becomes larger and the rates of breathing become higher.

Investigation 2.12   Differences between inhaled and exhaled air

Task 1

Consider the information in Table 2.5. What conclusions can you draw from the figures given in this table?

Task 2 – the oxygen dissociation curve (data in Table 2.6)

Exercise displaces the oxygen dissociation curve to the right as blood pH falls due to increased carbon dioxide pressure (concentration) and temperature increases.

1. Plot both sets of data in the same way as the oxygen dissociation curve. On the y-axis, plot % saturation of haemoglobin with oxygen and oxygen partial pressure on the x-axis.

2. Draw a vertical line at a spot on the x-axis where the oxygen partial pressure is at 5 kPa and follow the line up through the curves. What do you notice about the saturation of haemoglobin with oxygen for the two curves?

3. What effect does the increased pCO_2 in venous blood, as it passes through muscle tissue, have on the release of oxygen from haemoglobin into muscle cell tissue? (Note that pO_2 is about 5 kPa in venous haemoglobin.)

4. Relative to both rest and exercise, explain the significance of the shape of the oxyhaemoglobin curve with respect to gas exchange and transport.

5. On leaving the lungs, blood again has an oxygen partial pressure of 13 kPa. Trace the passage of the blood from this point through the circulatory system (see Table 2.7), highlighting:
   a. oxygen partial pressure
   b. carbon dioxide partial pressure
   c. haemoglobin oxygen saturation until the blood returns through the complete circuit.

Table 2.5 Proportion of O_2 and CO_2 breathed during exercise, compared to at rest

	Inhaled air	Exhaled air during quiet breathing	Exhaled air during exercise
%O_2	21	17	15
%CO_2	0.03	3	6

Table 2.6 Oxygen dissociation data

Partial pressure of O_2 (kPa)	% saturation of haemoglobin with oxygen for	
	$pCO_2 = 5.3$ kPa	$pCO_2 = 9.3$ kPa
1.3	7	4
2.6	27	15
3.9	53	35
5.3	70	58
6.6	79	71
7.9	85	82
9.3	90	88
10.5	95	94
11.8	98	98
13.0	100	100

Table 2.7 Partial pressures in the circulatory system

Location of blood	pO_2 (kPa)	pCO_2	%HbO_2
Leaving lungs	13	5.3	100
Entering muscle tissue	13	5.3	100
Leaving muscle tissue – venous	5	9.3	35
Venous blood arriving at lungs	5	9.3	35

Review questions

1. The lungs have no skeletal tissue, so how do they increase in size on breathing in?

2. Identify the major vascular substance that determines the amount of oxygen that can be delivered to body tissues and explain how it functions.

3. Describe how alveolar ventilation changes during exercise.

4. What **three** factors affect oxygen dissociation during exercise and how?

5. Describe the relationships between haemoglobin, pO_2, acidity, pCO_2 and temperature.

6. Explain how CO_2 is picked up by the tissue capillary blood and then released into the alveoli.

Exam-style questions

1. a. Distinguish between cardiac output and arteriovenous difference. *(2 marks)*

   b. Briefly identify and account for the changes that occur in cardiac output and arteriovenous difference from rest to maximal exercise. *(4 marks)*

   (Total 6 marks)

2. Figure 2.31 shows the relative partial pressure (amount) of oxygen (pO_2) and carbon dioxide (pCO_2) in the atmosphere, in the alveoli of the lungs and in the blood vessels of the pulmonary circulation. Use the information given in Figure 2.31 to answer the following questions.

   a. Explain, in terms of diffusion, how the changes in pO_2 and pCO_2 between the pulmonary artery and the pulmonary vein are brought about. *(4 marks)*

   b. What are the barriers to diffusion between the air in the alveoli and the haemoglobin in the blood, through which the oxygen must pass? *(5 marks)*

   c. How could you deduce from the data that gas exchange occurring in the alveoli is at an optimum? *(3 marks)*

   d. i. Explain briefly the purpose of a sports performer breathing pure oxygen immediately before competing. *(2 marks)*

      ii. Comment on the value of this procedure at sea level and at altitude. *(3 marks)*

   e. With reference to the information in the diagram, what changes in blood composition will occur during strenuous exercise? *(3 marks)*

   (Total 20 marks)

3. The long-term effects of aerobic exercise on arteriovenous oxygen difference (a-$\bar{v}O_2$ diff), for trained as opposed to untrained subjects, are illustrated in Figure 2.32.

   a. Work out the percentage increases in arteriovenous oxygen difference, from

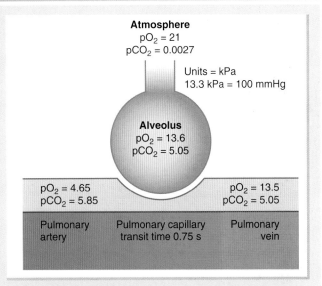

Fig. 2.31 Relative partial pressure of oxygen and carbon dioxide in the atmosphere, alveolus and pulmonary blood vessels.

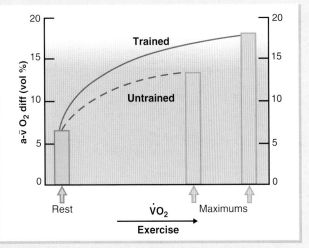

Fig. 2.32 Effects of exercise on arteriovenous oxygen difference (a-$\bar{v}O_2$ diff) for trained and untrained subjects. During exercise, the muscles extract a greater amount of O_2 from a given quantity of arterial blood. Training improves this capacity.

resting values to maximal values, for both untrained and trained subjects. (*4 marks*)

b. Using your knowledge of circulatory and respiratory dynamics, account for the differences in a-v̄O$_2$ diff maximal values between untrained and trained subjects. (*8 marks*)

(Total 12 marks)

4. Figure 2.28 on p. 77 shows the haemoglobin–oxygen dissociation curve. During exercise this curve shifts significantly downwards and to the right. Explain the causes of this change and the effect that this has on oxygen delivery to the muscles. (*4 marks*)

(Total 4 marks)

Good references that expand this section on gaseous exchange are[1, 2, 4–6, 8, 10, 11].

2.6 Lung volumes and physical activity

Learning objectives

On completion of this section, you will be able to:

1. Be familiar with the concepts of, and be able to measure, lung volumes and capacities.

2. Understand the concepts of minute ventilation, tidal volume and ventilation rates during quiet breathing and during exercise.

3. Account for the differences in lung volumes and capacities between untrained and trained sportspersons.

Keywords

- alveolar ventilation
- anatomical dead space
- expiratory reserve volume (ERV)
- expiratory capacity (EC)
- frequency of breaths (*f*)
- functional residual capacity (FRC)
- inspiratory reserve volume (IRV)
- inspiratory capacity (IC)
- minute ventilation: V̇E and V̇I
- quiet breathing
- residual volume (RV)
- spirometer
- tidal volume (TV)
- total lung capacity (TLC)
- vital capacity (VC)

During **quiet breathing**, we exchange about 0.5 litres (0.5 dm^3) of air per breath (the **tidal volume** or TV), of which 350 ml is **alveolar ventilation** and 150 ml is **anatomical dead space** air. Anatomical dead space

represents the volume of the trachea, bronchi and other structures that do not take part in gas exchange. **Tidal volume** is the volume of air inspired **or** expired per breath.

Minute ventilation, or minute volume, is the amount of air inspired **or** expired in one minute. Minute ventilation is expressed as:

$$\dot{V}E = \text{volume of air expired in a minute}$$

or

$$\dot{V}I = \text{volume of air inspired in a minute}$$

The **inspiratory reserve volume** (IRV) is the volume of air that can be forcibly inspired after a normal quiet breath. Similarly, the **expiratory reserve volume** (ERV) is that volume of air that can be forcibly expired over and above resting tidal volume. **Residual volume (RV)** is the volume of air remaining in the lungs after maximum expiration. These lung volumes are illustrated in Figure 2.33.

Vital capacity (VC) is the maximal volume of air that can forcefully be expired after maximal inspiration in one breath. **Total lung capacity** (TLC) is the volume of air in the lungs following maximal inspiration and can be between 4 and 8 litres in healthy adults. **Inspiratory capacity** (IC) is the tidal volume plus inspiratory reserve volume, **expiratory capacity** (EC) is the tidal volume plus expiratory reserve volume and the **functional residual capacity** (FRC) is a combination of the expiratory reserve volume and the residual volume.

Lung volumes and capacities can be measured by using a **spirometer** (Figure 2.34A), which produces a trace as illustrated in Figure 2.34B. Note in Figure 2.33 how tidal volume increases during exercise.

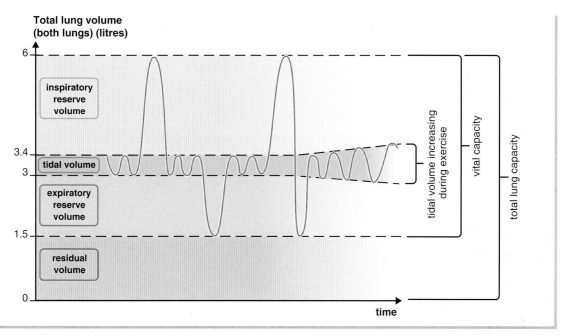

Fig. 2.33 Diagram of lung volumes and capacities.

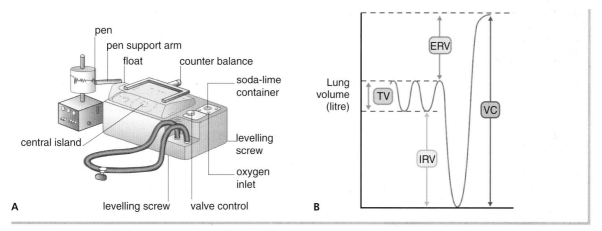

Fig. 2.34 A. Spirometer. **B.** Spirometer trace.

Investigation 2.13   To determine lung volumes using a spirometer

Materials: spirometer with graph paper attached, wide-bore flexible tube, mouthpiece and noseclip, scales and tape measure, disinfectant.

Task 1
1. Weigh yourself and measure your height.
2. Sitting down, clip on the noseclip and insert a freshly disinfected mouthpiece. Breathe normally and set the cylinder in motion so that you are inspiring and expiring into the spirometer.

3. Now take a maximal breath in and out. Repeat three normal breaths followed again by maximal inspiration and expiration. (The rotating cylinder records the different lung volumes described earlier; however, unless the rotating cylinder is suitably calibrated, the printout is only qualitative.)

4. Remove the graph paper and, using the descriptions on lung volumes, mark on the graph your TV, IRV, ERV and VC. Figure 2.34B should assist you with this exercise.

▶ **Task 2**
1. Assuming that your tidal volume in quiet breathing is 0.5 litres or 0.5 dm³, work out your IRV and ERV.
2. Calculate your VC using the following equation:

   VC = TV (at rest) + IRV + ERV

Task 3 – collation of results
1. Record your results in Table 2.8.
2. Collate the results of other students in your class.

Task 4 – analysis of results
1. Comment on the differing vital capacities. Discuss the relationship between vital capacity and height, weight and gender.
2. Describe two experimental errors that could have affected the results.
3. What volume of gas remains in the lungs at the end of maximal expiration?

Table 2.8 Results table

Name of subject	Height (metres)	Weight (kg)	TV (litres)	IRV (litres)	ERV (litres)	VC (litres)
Self						

Investigation 2.14   The measurement of lung volumes

Materials: a 5-litre calibrated plastic bottle, rubber tubing, disinfectant.

A simple method of determining **vital capacity** and **tidal volume** is to use a calibrated plastic bottle, illustrated in Figure 2.35.

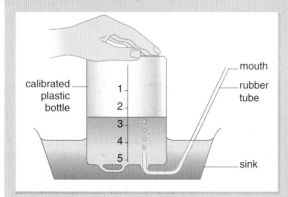

Fig. 2.35 Measurement of lung volumes.

Task 1
1. Calibrate a large plastic bottle up to 5 litres by filling it with water, 1 litre at a time, marking the levels.
2. Fill a sink with water and invert the bottle (full of water up to the 5-litre mark) into the sink.
3. Insert one end of the disinfected rubber tube into the neck of the bottle.
4. Take a deep breath and then exhale as hard as you can through the disinfected tubing so that the exhaled air displaces the water in the bottle.
5. The level of the water left in the bottle will give you your **vital capacity**.

Task 2
1. Push the rubber tubing halfway up inside the bottle, making sure that it is clear of the waterline.
2. Breathe in and out normally through the rubber tubing. The rise and fall in the water line with each breath accounts for the volume of air that is exchanged during quiet breathing. This volume is known as **tidal volume**.

Investigation 2.15   To consider minute ventilation (V̄E), tidal volume (TV) and frequency of breaths (f) during quiet breathing

This investigation is best done in groups with each member having a specific job.

Materials: Douglas bag, gasmeter, mouthpiece, tubing, noseclip and stopclock, disinfectant.

Task 1
1. Evacuate the Douglas bag, then connect a freshly disinfected mouthpiece to the Douglas bag via the rubber tubing.

2. Sit quietly and insert the mouthpiece in your mouth and fit the noseclip.

3. Start the stopclock and collect expired air in the Douglas bag for a 5-minute period, counting the number of breaths (f) taken for each minute.

4. Evacuate the Douglas bag into the gasmeter and determine the volume of air expired in 5 minutes.

5. Work out the minute volume:

$$\dot{V}E = \frac{\text{volume of air in 5 minutes}}{5}$$

6. Work out the tidal volume at rest:

$$TV = \frac{\dot{V}E}{f}$$

Task 2 – collation of results

Record your results, and those of other students in your class, in Table 2.9.

Table 2.9 Results table			
Name of subject	f	$\dot{V}E$ (litres)	TV (litres)
Self			

Task 3 – analysis of results

Compare the group's results. Explain any differences in $\dot{V}E$ and TV between members of your group.

Investigation 2.16   To determine minute ventilation, respiratory frequency and tidal volume during a progressively hard exercise test

This investigation is best achieved in a group, with each group member allocated a specific job.

Materials: as for Investigation 2.15, plus cycle ergometer, heart-rate monitor.

Task 1

1. The subject is seated on the bike and, while he/she is resting, expired air is collected for 1 minute in an evacuated Douglas bag. The number of breaths taken is also counted.

2. The volume of expired air passing through the gasmeter is measured and recorded.

3. The same subject begins to ride the cycle ergometer at a low work intensity. After 2 minutes, the subject's air is collected in an evacuated Douglas bag for a 1-minute period. During this time the number of expirations is counted and the volume of expired air passing through the gasmeter is measured and recorded.

4. In the meantime the subject continues to ride for a further 3 minutes at an increased medium work intensity. During the sixth minute of the investigation (i.e. the third of the 3 minutes at this workload) a further minute of air is collected, measured and the number of breaths counted.

5. This is repeated at a final maximal workload.

Note that work intensities need to be calculated prior to the investigation. This could be achieved by using appropriate heart-rate values, e.g. low intensity 130 bpm, medium intensity 160 bpm and high intensity in excess of 190 bpm. Hence the use of a heart-rate monitor is recommended.

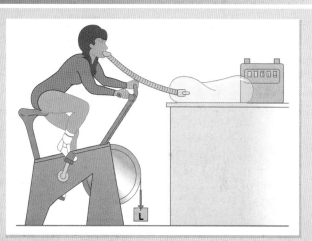

Fig. 2.36

Task 2

Record the results in Table 2.10. Work out the minute ventilation for each stage of the investigation:

$$\dot{V}E = TV \times f$$

Task 3 – analysis of results

1. On a piece of graph paper, draw curves of:
   a. minute ventilation ($\dot{V}E$)
   b. respiratory frequency (f)
   c. tidal volume (TV) on the y-axis, against work intensity on the x-axis. (Divide your graph paper into thirds and plot one graph under the next.)

2. Discuss the relationships between work intensity and minute ventilation ($\dot{V}E$), respiratory frequency (f) and tidal volume (TV).

3. Compare tidal volume (during maximum work intensity) and the subject's vital capacity. Account for these differences.

4. Identify the muscles acting during inspiration and expiration when you are exercising to your maximal workload.

5. As one moves from light to moderate to heavy exercise, explain how the respiratory system helps regulate the acid–base balance (refer to Section 2.4).

6. How reliable are the results of your investigation? Does your investigation test what you set out to

test? Does your investigation produce a consistent pattern of figures?

The answers to these questions will outline the reliability and validity of your scientific investigations.

Task 4

1. Sketch a graph comparing resting lung volumes of untrained and trained subjects. Show clearly the changes in the inspiratory reserve volume, expiratory reserve volume, vital capacity, residual volume and total lung capacity.

2. Explain why tidal volume remains unchanged at rest.

Table 2.10 Results

Work intensity	$\dot{V}E$ (litres)	f	TV (litres)
1. sitting on a bike			
2. light intensity			
3. medium intensity			
4. high intensity			

Review questions

1. Define tidal volume, breathing frequency, vital capacity, residual volume and total lung capacity. Using data from Investigations 2.15 and 2.16, how are tidal volume and breathing frequency changed during exercise?

2. What contribution do expiratory reserve volume and inspiratory reserve volume make to the changes in tidal volume that you have described in question 1?

3. Define alveolar ventilation and anatomical dead space. Explain their roles in providing adequate ventilation.

Exam-style questions

1. Figure 2.37 shows a diagram of lung volumes of an 18-year-old student at rest.

   a. Identify the four lung volumes **A, B, C, D** and indicate their approximate values and units. (*4 marks*)

   b. What happens to the volumes **C** and **D** during submaximal exercise? (*2 marks*)

   c. Which letters make up the inspiratory capacity? (*2 marks*)

   d. Which letters make up the functional residual capacity? (*2 marks*)

   e. Lung volumes vary with age, gender and body size. Discuss. (*10 marks*)

(*Total 20 marks*)

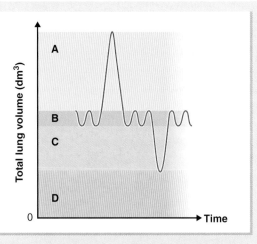

Fig. 2.37 Lung volumes of an 18-year-old student at rest.

2. Figure 2.38 shows the responses of ventilation and heart rate to exercise that might occur when running in a 3000 m track race.

   a. Using the information in Figure 2.38, explain why both heart rate and ventilation curves follow similar trends. (*6 marks*)

   b. Discuss how the **sympathetic** and **parasympathetic** nervous systems affect heart and ventilation rates. (*4 marks*)

   (*Total 10 marks*)

3. Describe and account for some of the long-term effects of regular exercise on the respiratory volumes. (*6 marks*)

4. A person's minute ventilation during exercise is 100 l min^{-1}, anatomical dead space is 0.4 l min^{-1} and tidal volume is 2.0 l breath^{-1}. Work out the breathing frequency and alveolar ventilation? (*4 marks*)

Good references that expand this section on lung volumes are [1, 2, 4–6, 10, 11].

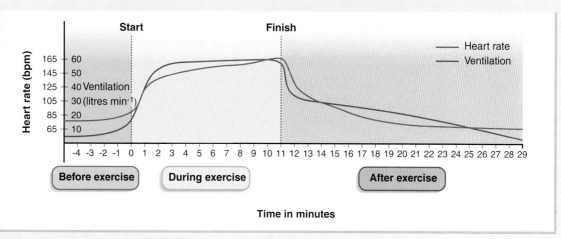

Fig. 2.38 Ventilation and heart rate responses when running a 3000 metre track race.

References

1. McKenna B R, Callendar R 1996 *Illustrated physiology*, 6th edn. Churchill Livingstone, Edinburgh
2. Seeley R R, Stephens T D, Tate P 2003 *Anatomy and physiology*, 6th edn. McGraw Hill, New York
3. Bastian G F 1993 *An illustrated review of anatomy and physiology: the cardiovascular system*. HarperCollins, New York
4. Foss M L, Keteyian S J 1998 *Fox's physiological basis for exercise and sport*, 6th edn. McGraw Hill, New York
5. McArdle W D, Katch F I, Katch V L 2004 *Essentials of exercise physiology*, 2nd edn. With Primer CD. Lippincott, Williams and Wilkins, New York
6. Tortora G 2003 *Principles of anatomy and physiology*, 10th edn. John Wiley, Toronto
7. Green J H 1986 *An introduction to human physiology*. Oxford University Press, Oxford
8. Wilmore J H 2004 *Physiology of sport and exercise*, 3rd edn. Human Kinetics, Champaign, Illinois
9. St John Ambulance 1998 *Young people's first aid*, 2nd edn. Mosby, London
10. Bastian G F 1993 *An illustrated review of anatomy and physiology: the respiratory system*. HarperCollins, London
11. Clegg C 1995 *Exercise physiology*. Feltham Press, New Milton

Further reading

James R, Thompson G, Wiggins-James N 2003 *Complete A–Z physical education handbook*, 2nd edn. Hodder and Stoughton, London

Roscoe D A, Roscoe J V, Honeybourne J, Davis R J, Galligan F 2003 *Physical education and sports studies AS/A2 level student revision guide*, 3rd edn. Jan Roscoe Publications, Widnes

MULTIMEDIA

Video

Functional Anatomy – The Sports Science Series, The University of Western Australia 1988. UK supplier Boulton and Hawker Films Ltd

CD-ROMs

Adams *Interactive Physiology – Cardiovascular System.* Benjamin/Cummings, California 2004

Adams *Interactive Physiology – Respiratory System* Benjamin/Cummings California 2004

Roscoe D A 2004 *Teacher's guide to physical education and the study of sport, CD-Rom 5th edn. Part I, the performer in action, anatomy and physiology.* Jan Roscoe Publications, Widnes

Roscoe D A, Roscoe J V 2002 *OCR/AQA/Edexcel Science and Sport Psychology Powerpoint Classroom Presentation CD-ROM.* Jan Roscoe Publications, Widnes

Roscoe D A, Roscoe J V, Honeybourne J, Davis R J, Galligan F 2003 *Physical Education and Sports Studies AS/A2 Level Student Revision Guide*, 3rd edn. Jan Roscoe Publications, Widnes

Energy for exercise

3.1 Energy and work

Learning objectives

On completion of this section, you will be able to:

1. Understand the concepts of work and energy and particularly the definition:

   work = force × distance
   = weight × height

2. Be aware of the joule as the unit of measurement of work and energy. 1 kilojoule (kJ) = 1000 joules.

3. Understand the concept of power as defined by:

   $$\text{power} = \frac{\text{energy used or work done}}{\text{time taken}}$$
   = force × velocity

   and that the **watt** is the unit of power.

4. Be familiar with the concept of chemical energy in respect of the energy store in muscles and its relationship to actual food consumption and oxygen consumption.

5. Be familiar with the concept of respiratory exchange ratio as an indication of the energy being oxidised during cellular respiration.

6. Be aware of the concept of efficiency defined by:

   $$\% \text{ efficiency} = \frac{\text{useful work done} \times 100}{\text{energy used doing that work}}$$

7. Appreciate that gains in skill development rather than strength development are more likely to improve efficiency of the human machine.

Keywords

➤ basal metabolic rate (BMR)
➤ chemical energy
➤ direct energy measurement
➤ efficiency
➤ energy
➤ energy expenditure
➤ gravitational field strength
➤ indirect energy measurement
➤ joule
➤ net oxygen cost
➤ power
➤ respiratory exchange ratio (RER)
➤ watt
➤ weight
➤ work

In scientific terms, energy and work mean the same thing and are interchangeable as concepts, energy being the capacity or ability of a system to do work.

The definition of **work** is:

work = force × distance moved (by the system acted upon by the force) in the direction of the force.

The unit of **work** and therefore of **energy** is the **joule** (J), which is defined as the work done (or energy used) when a force of **one newton** (N) acts through a distance of **one metre** (m).

This formula can be used to measure human energy output or work done – this will be illustrated by the following two investigations.

Investigation 3.1   Energy output of a person running upstairs

This investigation uses the **weight** of the athlete as the **force** used and the **vertical height** moved as the **distance** through which the force is applied. Here the energy output by the body equals the work done in climbing the stairs and is an approximate value, not taking into account the motion of the student's body.

Task 1 – the experiment

1. The student should find his/her **weight** in **newtons** using bathroom scales. To convert from kilograms, multiply by 10 to obtain the weight in newtons. (This is because the earth pulls down with a force of 10 N for every kilogram mass – the force of

▶

gravity is called the **weight**.) Refer to p. 209 for a further discussion about weight and mass.

2. Measure the **height** of the stairs to be climbed in **metres**, i.e. the height of each step × the number of steps.

3. The student should run up the stairs as fast as possible – the **time in seconds** is recorded for this activity.

Task 2 – analysis of results
Calculate the energy output of the student using:

$$\text{energy} = \text{force} \times \text{distance}$$
$$= \text{weight} \times \text{height}$$
$$= mg \times h$$

(The answer will be in **joules**).

Task 3 – calculation of power output
1. **Power** is defined as:

   Energy (or **work**) used per **second**

2. The values from Task 2 are therefore placed in the equation:

$$\text{power} = \frac{\text{energy (joules)}}{\text{time (seconds)}}$$

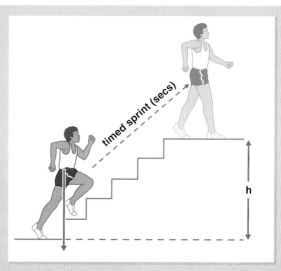

Fig. 3.1 Running upstairs.

The answer will be in **watts**, where **one watt** is defined as the power produced when **one joule** of energy is used per **second**.

Investigation 3.2 Energy output of a person operating a bicycle ergometer

Task 1 – the activity
1. The **force** setting on the bike (load on bike wheel – marked L in Figure 3.2) is noted and the distance (on the milometer) set to zero. If the force setting is in kilograms, this needs converting into **newtons** using the information that the weight of one kilogram mass is 10 N.

2. The student then pedals as fast as possible for 30 seconds and the **distance** travelled in metres (as recorded on the milometer) is noted. If the machine has no milometer, the distance travelled by the outer rim of the bike wheel as it turns past the friction belt is measured. This can be calculated by multiplying the circumference of the wheel by the number of revolutions done by the wheel in the time of the experiment. (Remember the answer to this should be in metres.)

Task 2 – analysis of results
Energy output is now calculated using the formula:

energy = force × distance

(The answer will be in **joules**).

Task 3 – calculation of power output
Using the definition of **power** in the investigation of energy output of a person running upstairs, this can be calculated using the formula:

$$\text{power} = \frac{\text{energy (joules)}}{\text{time taken (seconds)}}$$

(Answer in **watts**).

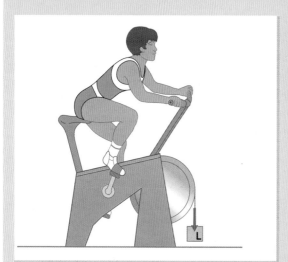

Fig. 3.2 A bicycle ergometer.

▶ **Extension of investigation**
With more sophisticated apparatus, the speed of the bike wheel can be monitored by a computer sensor and a full profile of power output with time obtained. Alternatively, power measurements can be made over 10 seconds, 20 seconds and 30 seconds by using the bicycle ergometer method above. It is then possible to observe maximal power output and how the power output changes as the athlete becomes more fatigued. This can be related to anaerobic power as discussed on p. 110–111.

Chemical energy

The question of where the energy produced by the human machine comes from now arises and it is fairly obvious that the original source of the energy is the food eaten by the person doing the exercise.

In fact, the energy is produced by a complex series of **chemical reactions** (to be discussed in detail below) and is then made available for contraction of muscles and other body functions.

This type of energy is called **chemical energy** since the energy is produced by chemical reactions and is converted into **work** by the contraction of muscle.

If we were able to calculate the full energy value of all food eaten by a person and compare this with measured energy output (as in the investigations above), we would find that only a small proportion of this energy is converted into useful work.

The power needs of sporting activity

From the definition of power in the investigations above, we have:

$$\text{power} = \frac{\text{energy}}{\text{time}} = \frac{\text{force} \times \text{distance}}{\text{time}}$$

But $\dfrac{\text{distance}}{\text{time}}$ is a definition of speed, therefore:

$$\text{power} = \frac{\text{force} \times \text{distance}}{\text{time}} = \text{force} \times \text{speed}$$

or, if the direction of the speed is fully taken into consideration:

$$\textbf{power = force} \times \textbf{velocity}$$

So it can be seen that power is a measure of force being applied at speed and therefore is the appropriate concept in the bulk of sports requiring fast dynamic movements, such as jumping, throwing, sprinting, weightlifting and most games.

It is suggested that another convenient activity (highly correlated with the two activities discussed in Investigations 3.1 and 3.2) that could be used to assess athletic power would be a timed 30 m sprint. Each of the three activities would assess a slightly different athletic **capability** but would be a measure of the individual's **power**.

Measurement of chemical energy stored in food as fuel

There are two ways of measuring the amounts of chemical energy stored in food (which would then be available for conversion into useful forms of energy – such as mechanical energy – by the person who eats the food). The chemical process that releases the stored energy amounts to the combination of food with oxygen – a process identical to the burning of food fuel in air.

The first method (called the **direct** method, since it directly measures energy produced by combination of the food with oxygen) involves the burning of the food in a controlled way and measuring the heat energy produced. This heat energy is measured by observing the rise in temperature of a quantity of water heated by the burning food. An alternative direct method that can measure energy usage during exercise is to measure the body's heat production in a calorimeter chamber. Such a unit is illustrated in Figure 3.3. The heat energy that is created by the subject radiates to the walls and warms the water. The temperatures of the incoming and outgoing water and air are recorded and used to calculate **basal metabolic rate** (**BMR** = rate of energy production of the body while at rest) and **total energy expenditure** (while exercising). This method is rarely used today since the apparatus is very costly, takes up considerable space and is slow in generating results.

The second method is called the **indirect** method, since it uses the fact that every atom of carbon in food combines with a molecule of oxygen (during the chemical reactions in body tissues), to produce one molecule of carbon dioxide and release a definite and constant amount of energy. Similarly, two hydrogen atoms in food combine with one atom of oxygen to produce one molecule of water and release a different but also constant amount of energy. The method involves the measurement of the **amount of oxygen**

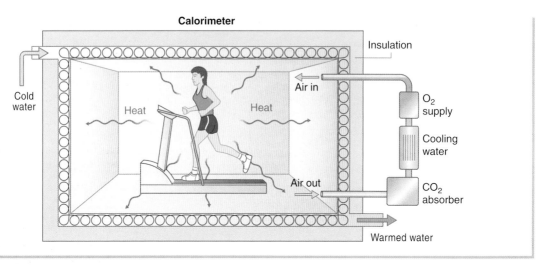

Fig. 3.3 Human calorimeter used to measure heat production.

consumed which can therefore be related to the amount of energy released by food.

For example, 134.4 litres of oxygen will oxidise 180 g of glycogen to release 2867 kJ of heat energy (1 kJ = 1 kilojoule = 1000 joules). Therefore, for all food fuels, one litre of oxygen produces 22 kJ of heat energy.

Figure 3.4 gives an idea of the equipment used to measure carbon dioxide production and oxygen consumption by calculating the respiratory exchange ratio (RER). (For further details of this method refer to specialist texts such as references[1,2] and for a detailed discussion on **oxygen consumption**, see Section 3.4.)

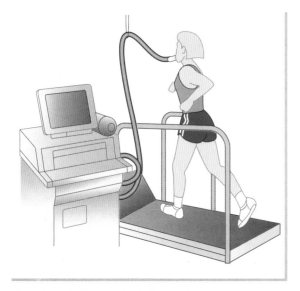

Fig. 3.4 The indirect method of measuring energy usage, using open circuit indirect calorimetry.

The respiratory exchange ratio

The energy released for a given volume of oxygen depends on whether carbohydrates, fats or proteins are being oxidised. This is because there are inherent chemical differences in the composition of carbohydrates, fats and proteins and therefore different amounts of oxygen are required to completely oxidise the carbon and hydrogen to carbon dioxide and water. In general, the amount of oxygen needed to completely oxidise a molecule of carbohydrate or fat is proportional to the amount of carbon in that fuel.

It is possible to estimate which particular type of food fuel – carbohydrate, fat or protein – is being oxidised by calculating the **respiratory exchange ratio** (RER) or the ratio of carbon dioxide (CO_2) produced to oxygen (O_2) consumed. This concept is also known as the **respiratory quotient** (RQ).

Thus, if carbohydrates are completely oxidised to CO_2 and water (H_2O) the relationship can be described as:

$$6O_2 + C_6H_{12}O_6 \rightarrow 6CO_2 + 6H_2O + 38ATP$$

(ATP = adenosine triphosphate) and it follows that:

$$RER = \frac{\text{volume of carbon dioxide given off}}{\text{volume of oxygen consumed}}$$

$$= \frac{6CO_2}{6O_2} = 1.00$$

If fat is used as a source of energy the ratio is different. For example, a typical fat, such as palmitic acid, being oxidised into carbon dioxide and water can be summarised by the following equation:

$$C_{16}H32O_2 + 23O_2 \rightarrow 16CO_2 + 16H_2O + 129ATP$$

$$RER = \frac{16}{23} = 0.70$$

The RER for protein metabolism is estimated as approximately 0.80. However, protein plays a very small part in energy metabolism and therefore is not important to the present discussion. A value between 0.70 and 1.00 indicates a mixture of fat and carbohydrate being burnt. A value over 1.00 indicates anaerobic respiration due to more CO_2 being produced than O_2 being consumed.

The efficiency of the human machine

The human body is a machine performing work but all machines use more fuel energy than they need for the task. The **mechanical efficiency** of any machine, including the human body, can be defined as:

$$\% \text{ efficiency} = \frac{\text{useful work done} \times 100}{\text{energy used doing that work}}$$

Energy expenditure refers to the total amount of energy required to perform an activity measured by oxygen consumption in the way outlined above.

However, there will be a difference between the total oxygen consumed during the exercise (and subsequent recovery) and the resting oxygen consumption which would have been consumed for the period of time involved without any exercise taking place. This difference gives the **net oxygen cost** of the exercise which will tell us the energy used to perform the exercise at 22 kJ per litre of oxygen consumed.

The resting oxygen consumption would enable us to calculate the basal metabolic rate, again at 22 kJ per litre of oxygen consumed: BMR = resting energy expenditure per kilogram of body mass divided by time taken for measurements – see p. 174.

With respect to the investigations above, in which amounts of **useful work done** are measured for students running up stairs or cycling on a bicycle ergometer, if the net oxygen cost is measured, it would be possible to compute the **efficiency** of the exercise process.

The percentage efficiency is usually within the range of 12–25% for the human body. This means that for every movement made, only 12–25% of the energy consumed is used doing the actual movement (above that which is needed for the basal metabolic rate) and the other 75–88% is converted into heat energy. Part of this heat energy is used to keep the body temperature above that of the surroundings (and stable at about 37°C) and the rest is lost to the surroundings. This means that whenever exercise is taken a lot of heat energy is produced, which can be used to raise body temperature (refer to your answers to p. 67, Task 6). This is why shivering occurs (muscles contract involuntarily as a response to low temperatures) and why people clap their hands and stamp their feet when cold.

In activities such as walking or running, the efficiency level is around 20–25%. In swimming it is around 2%.

A study of stair climbing has shown that the maximum efficiency (lowest energy costs) occurs at a speed of 50 steps per minute. As soon as this rate increases, efficiency is reduced. One can say that running even a fraction faster up the stairs means large increases in energy expenditure and rapid exhaustion. Conversely, tiny increases in efficiency, as a result of changes in technique or improved skill, will bring large reductions in energy expenditure. Therefore, improving skill levels is a much more profitable approach to improving performance than a simple increase in muscle strength.

Review questions

1. Describe the main features of a cycle ergometer and how it can be used to calculate power output as a fitness measurement.

2. A student has been asked to estimate the extra energy costs when playing a game of hockey, lasting one hour and 10 minutes. His body mass at the start of the game is 69 kg. The energy expenditure for the hockey game is 0.8 kJ kg^{-1} min^{-1} above his basal metabolic rate. Calculate his energy requirements above his basal metabolic rate during the hockey game.

3. What is the respiratory exchange ratio (RER)?

4. Explain how you would determine the oxidation of carbohydrate and fat.

3.2 Energy creation and release within muscle

Keywords

- adenosine diphosphate (ADP)
- adenosine triphosphate (ATP)
- aerobic system
- alactic anaerobic system (ATP–PC)
- coupled reaction
- duration
- electron transport chain
- endothermic reaction
- energy
- energy continuum
- energy systems
- exothermic reaction
- glycogen
- glycolysis
- intensity
- Kreb's cycle
- lactic acid anaerobic system
- metabolism
- mitochondria
- oxidation of hydrogen atoms
- phosphocreatine (PC)
- pyruvic acid
- sarcoplasm
- tissue respiration
- threshold

Adenosine triphosphate (ATP) is the means of energy generation in **all** cells but its supply is limited by the **intensity** and **duration** of physical activity.

The human body has developed **three** distinct mechanisms for the transfer of food to energy within muscle. These mechanisms are commonly known as **energy systems**.

1. In the first few seconds of physical activity, energy is freed **anaerobically (anaerobic** means **without oxygen)** from the energy bonds in phosphates stored in muscles.
2. Glucose is **anaerobically** split to release energy within the muscle.
3. Energy is released **aerobically (aerobic** means **with oxygen)** from the oxidation of glucose and fatty acids, achieved as a result of oxygen being transferred to the muscle via the cardiovascular-respiratory systems.

This chapter will help you to understand how these three mechanisms function to create and supply energy within muscle.

All chemical reactions either give out energy (**exothermic reaction**) or take in energy (**endothermic reaction**). This energy is what is referred to as **chemical energy** in the discussion above. The clever way that the biological system works is to **take in** energy (endothermic) with a series of chemical reactions from food and fuel and **give out** the same energy (exothermic) with a **different** series of chemical reactions in order to provide energy for muscular contractions and other bodily functions. In muscle tissue, **chemical energy** is converted into **mechanical** energy when the muscle contracts.

This section describes the exothermic half of the energy system. The endothermic reactions of acquiring energy and forming complex molecules within the system, such as glucose, are described in Section 3.5.

Tissue respiration

The chemical reactions taking place inside tissue cell sites, such as **sarcoplasm** and **mitochondria**, can be expressed by the following chemical equation:

$$C_6H_{12}O_6 \;+\; 6O_2 \;\rightarrow\; 6CO_2 \;+\; 6H_2O \;+\; \text{energy}$$

glucose   oxygen   carbon   water
                        dioxide

(This chemical reaction summarises **aerobic respiration**. Note the energy released is always constant for a given quantity of glucose.)

The process of energy release in muscle tissue cells

The chemical energy released in tissue respiration is stored in the chemical bonds of **ATP** until it is required for **metabolism** (the term metabolism is used to describe **all** the chemical reactions that take place inside the body). Only the energy released from the breakdown of ATP can be used for tissue cell respiration. ATP consists of adenosine and three phosphate groups. When the bond between the adenosine group and one of the phosphate groups is broken (by the enzyme ATPase), energy is released. This freed energy is used to drive metabolic functions including muscle contraction. This means that every time a muscle contracts, whether it be in involuntary or voluntary muscle tissue, it can only use energy that is derived from the breakdown of ATP. This exothermic reaction can be expressed as:

$$\text{ATP} \xrightarrow{\text{ATPase}} \text{ADP} + P_i + \text{energy}$$

ADP = adenosine diphosphate

P_i = free phosphate

The clever way that chemical energy is converted into mechanical energy is achieved by the delivery of free energy to the muscle proteins actin and myosin, to enable the cross-bridges (in Huxley's Sliding Filament Theory of Muscle Contraction) to connect and reconnect. The freed energy enables actin (thin) filaments to slide over myosin (thick) filaments during muscle contraction (refer to the discussion on muscle contraction in Chapter 1, p. 42).

But muscles have only a limited supply of ATP, which lasts about 2 seconds. After this time, ATP is **recreated** via one of the three different energy systems as mentioned above:

1. the **alactic anaerobic** or ATP/PC system
2. the **lactic acid** system
3. the **aerobic** system.

Energy from one of these systems is used to promote the reverse reaction:

$$\text{energy} + \text{ADP} + P_i \rightarrow \text{ATP}$$

i.e. to recreate ATP from the ADP and P_i which were produced when energy was released.

The alactic anaerobic system (ATP/PC system)
In activity lasting longer than about 2 seconds, the resynthesis of ATP relies on a substance called **phosphocreatine** (PC), which is also stored in our muscles. PC is similar to ATP in that when its phosphagen (a general term referring to phosphates, such as ADP, ATP and PC) group is removed, a large amount of energy is liberated. The amount of phosphagens stored is small and therefore this system has a limited capacity of under 10 seconds when exercise is taken at maximum capacity.

The process for this mechanism involves two immediate consecutive reactions occurring within muscle cell sarcoplasm.

Step 1. $\text{PC} \xrightarrow{\text{creatine kinase}} P_i + C + \text{energy}$

Step 2. $\qquad\qquad\qquad \text{energy} + \text{ADP} + P_i \rightarrow \text{ATP}$

The net effect of these reactions is:

$$\text{PC} + \text{ADP} \rightarrow \text{ATP} + C$$

(note that C is an abbreviation for creatine)

You can see that the chemical bond between the P_i and the C in PC holds energy. The enzyme that speeds up the breakdown of PC and the release of energy is **creatine kinase** (as illustrated in step 1 – an exothermic reaction). Step 2 shows the freed phosphate (P_i) combining with ADP to form ATP (an endothermic reaction). This energy is re-stored between the third P_i bond in the ATP. This combined process is known as a **coupled reaction** since the energy released from PC is coupled with the energy required when ADP is converted into ATP. The breakdown of PC is achieved **anaerobically** (without oxygen). Creatine (C) remains available for subsequent involvement in these reactions.

During flat-out exercise, such as sprinting, jumping and weightlifting, which lasts under 10 seconds, ATP is replenished by this system. Since no oxygen is used and there is no lactic acid formed, this system is called the **alactic anaerobic system**, usually abbreviated to the **ATP–PC** system. The main use of this system is that it provides an immediate source of energy.

When hard physical activity exceeds the time limit or **threshold** up to which the ATP–PC system operates (i.e. all the PC is used up), ATP is regenerated by a process which consumes carbohydrates. This process is known as the **lactic acid system** and the threshold between ATP–PC and lactic systems is called the **alactic–lactic threshold** (refer to Figure 4.21 on p. 137).

A major feature of training for speed endurance and power athletes would be anaerobic work whose purpose would be to delay the onset of the alactic–lactic threshold. This training would create biological adaptations which would enable muscle cell sarcoplasm to contain more ATP and larger creatine stores, to ensure that the ATP–PC system provides energy for longer periods of time at the highest possible rate. Also, a regular daily intake of small amounts of creatine is thought to increase total muscle creatine content and hence PC stores. This would then be available for alactic anaerobic exercise and would also delay the alactic–lactic threshold.

The lactic acid system

The **lactic acid system** depends on a chemical process known as **glycolysis** or the incomplete breakdown of sugar (Figure 3.5).

Carbohydrate is stored in the muscle as **glycogen**. Like the ATP–PC system, glycogen can be used to recreate ATP rapidly but again, only small amounts of glycogen and therefore energy-creating capacity is stored in muscle. Note that fast-twitch muscle fibres hold more glycogen than slow-twitch muscle fibres, which is one of the reasons that FT muscle can produce energy more rapidly than ST muscle.

It is the breakdown of glycogen that provides the energy to rebuild ADP into ATP. Glycolysis is far more complex than the ATP–PC system since it requires 10 enzyme controlled reactions for the breakdown of glucose to **lactic acid** ($C_3H_6O_3$). Three key enzymes are **glycogen phosphorylase** (GPP) and **phosphofructo-kinase** (PFK) (which are involved in the addition of phosphate groups in the breakdown of the glucose to form pyruvic acid) and **lactate dehydrogenase** (LDH). Since there is no oxygen present, **anaerobic metabolism** takes place. **Pyruvic acid**, formed during glycolysis, is converted by the enzyme lactate dehydrogenase (LDH) into **lactic acid**. The **net yield** from one molecule of glucose is **two** molecules of ATP.

As the lactic acid accumulates, muscle fatigue and pain occur. This is because the resultant low pH within the cell inhibits **enzyme** action in the cell **mitochondria**, which normally promotes the change of glycogen into energy. Hence the effect of lactic acid fatigue is to inhibit muscle action so that physical performance deteriorates. All anaerobic processes occur in the **sarcoplasm**, whereas aerobic processes take place within the confines of the cell **mitochondria** (see Figure 3.6).

Events such as a 400 metres race (lasting between 43 and 60 seconds of flat-out effort) rely heavily on the lactic acid system. After exercise has stopped extra oxygen is taken in to remove the lactic acid by changing it back into pyruvic acid. This is known as repaying the **oxygen debt** and is described in detail in Section 3.3.

The aerobic system

The **aerobic system** (Figure 3.6) relies on the presence of oxygen to break down carbohydrates and fats completely into carbon dioxide, water and energy. The energy yield is high – one molecule of glucose yields **36** molecules of ATP (note that in the lactic acid process the yield is **two** molecules of ATP!).

The first stage of the **aerobic** process is the same as that in the anaerobic lactic acid system: **glycolysis**, i.e. the conversion of glycogen into two molecules of pyruvic acid (see Figure 3.5), two ATP molecules and a number of **hydrogen atoms**. This process occurs via a series of 10 chemical reactions within the cell **sarcoplasm**.

From this point on, all chemical reactions involved in the aerobic system take place within the muscle cell **mitochondria** (see p. 40). The mitochondrion is often referred to as the **power house** of the cell, since it is the site of most energy production. Figure 3.7 shows the microscopic detail of a mitochondrion. The functions of these structures, labelled in Figure 3.7, are discussed below.

Krebs' cycle or the citric acid cycle

The two molecules of pyruvic acid are converted into a form of **acetyl coenzyme A (acetyl CoA)** (a 2-carbon compound), which enters the citric acid cycle by combining with **oxaloacetic acid** (to create a 6-carbon compound).

This process takes place in the inner fluid-filled matrix of the mitochondrion, which contains the enzymes of the citric acid cycle. Within this cycle there are a large number of reactions in which the two molecules go through a series of changes until they are degraded into pairs of hydrogen atoms and carbon dioxide and two ATP molecules. Fatty acids are taken up by the cycle at this point. (Hence the total release of energy from acetyl CoA, as a result of fat metabolism, is 34 ATPs.)

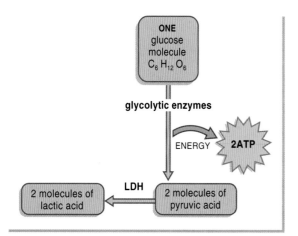

Fig. 3.5 The lactic acid system.

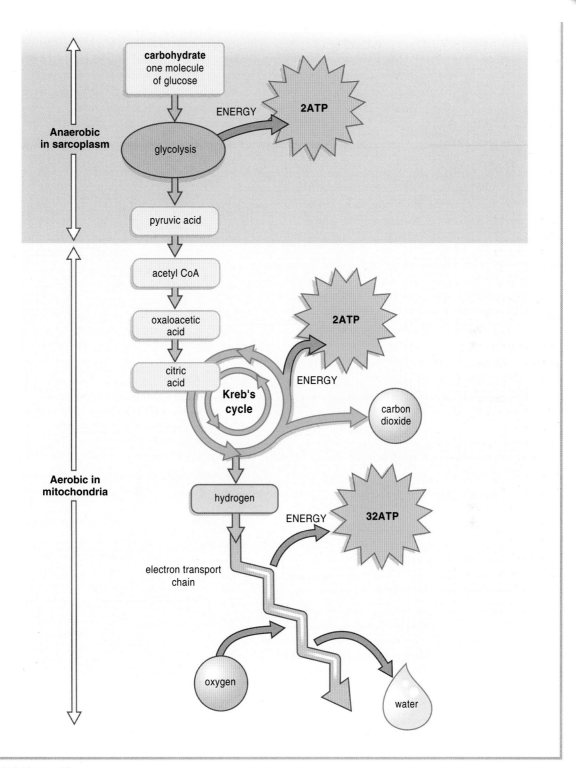

Fig. 3.6 The aerobic system.

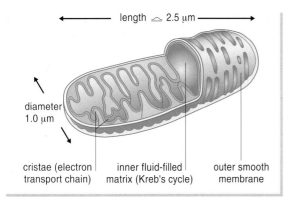

Fig. 3.7 The mitochondrion – the organelle of respiration.

The electron transport chain

Oxygen is given off from the muscle myoglobin or made available from blood haemoglobin and is taken in by the **mitochondria** to be used to oxidise hydrogen atoms:

H	$\rightarrow$	H$^+$	+	e$^-$
(hydrogen atom)		(hydrogen ion)		(electron)

The hydrogen ions and electrons are charged with potential energy. The electron transport chain consists of a chain of hydrogen ion–electron pairs, linked to the folds of the inner membrane (**cristae**) of the cell mitochondria. Energy is released in a controlled step-by-step manner as the hydrogen ion–electron pairs are passed downwards from a higher level of energy to a lower level of energy (each reaction is exothermic). For each pair of hydrogen atoms that enter this pathway, the net effect is the production of **three** molecules of ATP (an endothermic reaction) and one molecule of water. This is an **aerobic process**, because the hydrogen ion–electron pair is finally accepted by molecular oxygen, which combines with H$^+$ to produce water. Therefore the electron transport chain yields **32–34** molecules of ATP and several molecules of water.

The total possible yield produced by the aerobic metabolism is **36** or **38** molecules of **ATP** – the total energy yield is dependent on the biochemical pathway taken by the food fuel (i.e. whether the food fuel is carbohydrate, fat or protein). This is the maximum possible ATP yield from the complete oxidation of one molecule of glucose. The overall equation that expresses **aerobic respiration** is:

$$C_6H_{12}O_6 + 36ADP + 36P_i + 6O_2$$
$$\rightarrow 6CO_2 + 36ATP + 6H_2O$$

The aerobic route is 18 or 19 times more efficient than the anaerobic route, depending on the food fuel biochemical pathway.

Provided there is an adequate supply of oxygen to the working muscles, glucose and free fatty acids can be metabolised to produce the energy to recreate ATP. The major advantage of fat fuels is that there is a much larger supply available to sustain steady-state endurance activities, such as marathon running.

The effects of overload training significantly enhance the functional capacities of the three energy systems. A full account of these training adaptations is discussed in Section 4.2 on p. 136.

The energy continuum

So far, we have discussed the relevance of energy systems in terms of short-term, high-intensity work (the ATP–PC and lactic acid systems) or long-term, low-intensity work (the aerobic system). However, many physical activities require a mixture of both anaerobic and aerobic metabolism, for example a rugby or netball game. In these activities the anaerobic systems will create a limited supply of ATP for fast explosive work, with the aerobic system providing the majority of ATP during recovery phases and relatively less intense periods of activity.

The term **energy continuum** is used to describe the type of respiration demanded by physical activities. For example, Figure 3.8 shows that those activities

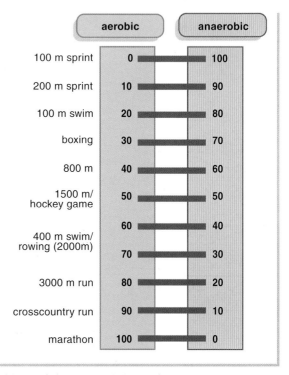

Fig. 3.8 The energy continuum and various activities.

which require 100% **anaerobic** respiration are at one end of the continuum (for example in sprinting), whereas those activities requiring 100% **aerobic** respiration are at the other end of this continuum (for example, in marathon running). In between these extremes are activities which require various proportions of anaerobic and aerobic respiration (most team sports would be located within the middle of the energy continuum). Within the context of training for a selected sport, it is important for the coach and sportsperson to devise training schedules that stress the energy system(s) relevant to his/her sport, otherwise physiological adaptations which improve performance will not take place.

For further details on ATP resynthesis, refer to references[1-6].

Investigation 3.3   To determine the energy sources for practical activities

(The material for this investigation was devised by Kevin Sykes, Principal Lecturer at Chester College of Higher Education, as part of an AEB 'A' level course.)

Materials: tape measure and stopwatch.

Task 1 – a standing long jump (Figure 3.9)
1. Crouch down low with flexed knees and prepare to take off from both feet. Spring forwards as far as possible and measure the distance achieved.
2. The distance is measured between the front of the toes at take-off and the rear of the heels on landing.
3. Record the maximum distance from three attempts in Table 3.1.

Task 2 – a flat-out shuttle sprint (Figure 3.10)
1. Identify the two baselines of a badminton court in your gym or sportshall. Start at one end and on the command 'GO' sprint as fast as you can to the far baseline and back three times altogether, making a total of six shuttle sprints. Use a partner to record your time.
2. Record your time in Table 3.1.

Task 3 – shuttle runs
1. Using the same baselines, perform a 30-length shuttle run at a steady pace. Use a partner to record your split times at 5, 10, 15, 20, 25 and 30 lengths.
2. During your run, make a subjective assessment of how your body is coping with the demands of this activity.
3. Record your split times in Table 3.1.

Task 4
1. Comment on the split times during the shuttle runs.

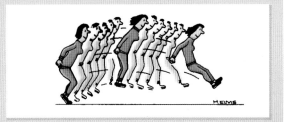

Fig. 3.9 A standing long jump.

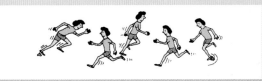

Fig. 3.10 A shuttle sprint.

2. How did you feel at various stages of the run and at the finish?
3. Roughly how long did it take you to recover?
4. Which of the energy systems is dominant in each of the three tasks?

Task 5 – collation of results
Collate your own results and those of five other students in your class in Table 3.1.

Task 6 – analysis of results
1. Discuss your group results in relation to gender, height, weight and sporting interests.
2. Discuss the meaningfulness of these results and the limitations of such measurements.
3. How would these results differ as you become fitter? Explain your answer.

Table 3.1 Results table								
Name	Standing broad jump (metres)	Shuttle sprint (seconds)	Shuttle runs (split times min/s)					
			5	10	15	20	25	30
Self								

Review questions

1. Write an equation which summarises:
   a. aerobic respiration
   b. anaerobic respiration.

2. a. What do the initials ATP stand for?
   b. What role does ATP play in energy release?

3. Describe the relationship between phosphocreatine (PC) and muscle ATP during a 100 metre sprint.

4. Describe the special role mitochondria play in energy release.

5. During any event of low or high intensity, all three energy systems are used. However, the physical demands of the event will determine the relative proportions of the energy system(s) being used. Complete the gaps in Table 3.2, identifying the major energy systems and examples in sporting activities in relation to performance time.

Table 3.2 Performance, energy systems and activity

Area	Performance time	Major energy system(s) related to performance time	Examples of type of activity
1	Less than 10 s	ATP–PC	100 m sprint, gymnastics vault
2	10–30 s		
3	30 s–1.5 minutes		
4	1.5–3 minutes		
5	Greater than 3 minutes		

Exam-style questions

1. Describe the **predominant** energy system being used in the following activities (remember this will be related to the time of the activity and the effort involved): shot put, marathon, 200 metres breaststroke, a game of hockey, 100 metres hurdles race, gymnastics vault, modern pentathlon, a brisk walk. *(7 marks)*

2. Figure 3.11 represents the energy systems used during the following athletic events: 100 metres, 400 metres, 1500 metres and marathon, but not necessarily in that order.
   a. Identify each event with an energy block and comment briefly on the reasons for your choice. *(4 marks)*
   b. Using the same key, complete a block to show the approximate proportions of aerobic and/or anaerobic work during a basketball game. *(2 marks)*

   (Total 6 marks)

3. The energy sources for a 1500 metre race are very specific. During the first 10 seconds the ATP–PC system is used, followed by a transition to the lactic acid system during the next minute. The pace settles into a short aerobic phase, followed by a return to the lactic acid system during the final sprint for the line. Using the same format, but in

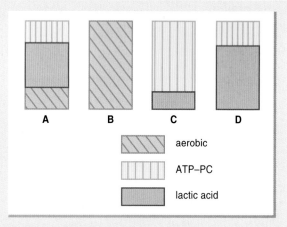

Fig. 3.11 Energy blocks.

more detail, analyse the energy sources used in a game of hockey. *(12 marks)*

4. a. Select a sport (other than hockey) with which you are familiar and briefly describe the energy systems used in your selected sport. *(4 marks)*
   b. How can a knowledge of the three energy systems assist you in devising a training programme for your selected sport? *(5 marks)*

   (Total 9 marks)

3.3 The recovery process after exercise

Learning objectives

On completion of this section, you will be able to:

1. Understand what is meant by the concept of oxygen deficit.

2. Understand what is meant by the concept of excess post-exercise oxygen consumption or EPOC or oxygen recovery or oxygen debt.

3. Understand what is meant by the concept of onset of blood lactate accumulation (OBLA).

4. Appreciate the importance of cool-down in the removal of lactic acid and in the reduction of muscle soreness.

5. Understand the role of oxygenated myoglobin during recovery from intensive exercise.

6. Understand the significance of the time factor and the effects of diet on the restoration of muscle phosphagen and muscle and liver glycogen levels.

7. Appreciate the causes of muscle soreness and muscle fatigue.

Keywords

➤ alactacid oxygen debt component
➤ delayed onset of muscle soreness (DOMS)
➤ excess post-exercise oxygen consumption (EPOC) or oxygen recovery or oxygen debt
➤ gluconeogenesis
➤ lactacid oxygen debt component
➤ lactate

➤ lactate shuttle
➤ muscle fatigue
➤ muscle glycogen stores
➤ muscle soreness
➤ onset of blood lactate accumulation (OBLA) or lactate threshold
➤ oxymyoglobin
➤ oxygen deficit
➤ phosphagen restoration

Normally, provided the effort or duration of exercise has not been too large, breathing and pulse rates rise as the need for oxygen rises to levels that enable ATP to be regenerated in muscles at the same rate as it is consumed. This is a continuous process, which varies according to the work or energy performed by muscles during a sportsperson's day.

Initially, as exercise begins, ATP is consumed directly, then replaced via the ATP–PC anaerobic energy system, **as well as** glycolysis and aerobic conversion of carbohydrates to provide energy for ATP manufacture. The important point to note is that **all three mechanisms** of ATP manufacture occur continuously but the **proportion** produced by the mechanisms changes as the exercise continues, as illustrated in Figures 3.11 and 4.21.

If exercise is intense enough, active cells rapidly run out of PC, so replacement of ATP by the ATP–PC mechanism stops as the alactic–lactic threshold is reached. Not enough ATP is produced aerobically, so **glycolysis** takes over as the predominant method of ATP supply, with its rapid depletion of muscle glycogen and production of lactic acid. (**Oxymyoglobin** stores supply a limited amount of oxygen to muscle cells to generate ATP aerobically.)

Eventually, ATP production via the anaerobic energy systems will be cease and exercise must stop or the sportsperson will collapse! During the exercise period an **oxygen deficit** is created (Figure 3.12). This is because the muscle requirement for oxygen is larger than the oxygen supply. The oxygen deficit for a specific exercise regime is calculated as the difference between oxygen required and oxygen actually consumed.

Again, the important issue to stress is that **all mechanisms for manufacture of ATP are continuous** (see Figure 4.21) and, of course, will continue when exercise stops, the aim of these mechanisms being then to replace ATP and glycogen as quickly as possible so that further exercise is possible.

Oxygen consumption during recovery

After every strenuous exercise, therefore, there are **five** tasks that need to be completed before the exhausted muscle can operate at full efficiency again:

1. replacement of ATP
2. reformation of phosphocreatine
3. removal of lactic acid
4. replenishment of myoglobin with oxygen
5. replacement of glycogen.

Items 1, 3 and 4 of these require oxygen in substantial quantities, hence the need for rapid breathing and high pulse rate to carry oxygen to the muscle cells. This need for oxygen to rapidly replace ATP and remove lactic

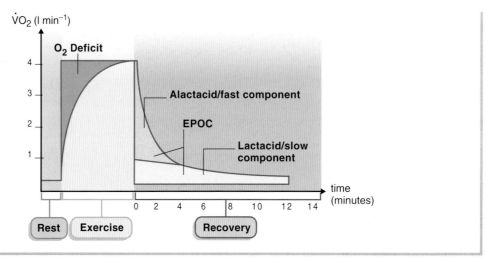

Fig. 3.12 The relationship between oxygen deficit, oxygen consumption and the time before, during and after maximal exercise.

acid is known as the **oxygen debt**. More contemporary terms for oxygen debt are **excess post-exercise oxygen consumption (EPOC)** or **oxygen recovery**, which represents the elevation of the metabolic rate above resting values which occurs after exercise during the recovery period.

Item (5) (replacement of glycogen) is a long-term process which can take 24–48 hours depending on the fitness level, diet of the sportsperson and the intensity and duration of the exercise.

In addition, there are many other processes (than the five listed above) involved in oxygen recovery: for example, restoration of cardiac and/or pulmonary functioning to resting values, reversal of the high phosphate breakdown and return of body temperature to normal. All these processes need additional oxygen (although substantially less than that used during the alactacid and lactacid components illustrated in Figure 3.12), and therefore additional time, to complete the paying back of the total oxygen deficit to pre-exercise oxygen consumption levels.

Figure 3.12 shows how the need for oxygen falls following cessation of exercise. Obviously, the more rapidly this process is completed, the quicker the sportsperson can resume exercise.

The **two** major traditional components of oxygen recovery are:

1. **alactacid oxygen debt** (or fast component)
2. **lactacid oxygen debt** (or slow component).

The contribution made by each to the overall process of oxygen recovery is marked on Figure 3.12 but note that both processes will occur initially, even though the alactic process is more rapid and is completed more quickly.

Alactacid oxygen debt component

The **alactacid oxygen debt** or **fast component** represents that portion of oxygen used to synthesise and restore muscle phosphagen stores (ATP and PC) which have been almost completely exhausted during high-intensity exercise. It is a rapid process achieved mainly by using the aerobic energy system and it is commonly known as the **restoration of muscle phosphagen stores**. **Three** mechanisms contribute to the regeneration of phosphocreatines.

1. Energy from aerobic conversion of carbohydrate into carbon dioxide and water is used to manufacture ATP from ADP and P_i (the products of ATP consumption).
2. Some of this ATP is immediately utilised to create PC using the coupled reaction:

$$ATP \rightarrow ADP + P_i + energy$$

$$energy + P_i + C \rightarrow PC$$

3. A very small percentage of ATP, derived from lactic acid production, is made available for phosphagen replenishment.

The size of the alactacid oxygen debt
The size of the alactacid oxygen debt is within a range of 1–4 litres, depending on the intensity of the exercise

and the fitness of the sportsperson. The volume of the **fast component** of oxygen recovery can be calculated from working out the area under the curve for O_2 uptake rates, $l\ min^{-1}$, plotted against time in minutes (Figure 3.12, labelled alactacid/fast component). One of the long-term adaptations resulting from anaerobic training is to increase ATP and PC stores within

muscle cell sarcoplasm (refer to p. 136). The long-term effects of aerobic training are to supply oxygen more rapidly to active tissue cells, by improved capillarisation and improved cardiovascular-respiratory systems. These adaptations increase the possible size of the EPOC in the fitter sportsperson and reduce the recovery time.

Investigation 3.4 Phosphagen restoration

This investigation asks the student to plot and interpret data relevant to the alactacid oxygen recovery.

Task 1
Consider the results (Table 3.3) of experiments on phosphagen recovery. Plot a graph of these data with recovery time on the *x*-axis and percentage phosphagen restored on the *y*-axis.

1. What would be the effect of restarting exercise after 30 seconds?

2. What resting interval would you recommend for full recovery?

Task 2 – implications for interval training
Assuming that it takes about 30 seconds to deplete ATP and PC stores by 50% in a particular muscle group doing flat-out exercise:

1. sketch a graph showing levels of muscle phosphagen (ATP and PC content) against time (x-axis) for this exercise period, followed by a full recovery.

Table 3.3 Phosphagen recovery

Recovery time (seconds)	Muscle phosphagen restored
10	10%
30	50%
60	75%
90	87%
120	93%
150	97%
180	99%
210	101%
240	102%

2. sketch a similar graph for three periods of exercise, each of 30 seconds followed by 60 seconds rest. What happens to the level of phosphagen store just at the end of the third exercise period (i.e. 210 seconds after the start of the session)?

The function of oxymyoglobin in purging oxygen debt

Part of the recovery mechanism following anaerobic exercise involves **myoglobin**, whose presence in muscle cells (particularly slow-twitch red muscle) is discussed in Section 1.6 on p. 40. During recovery from intense exercise, the absence of sufficient oxygen to continue the provision of energy in muscles means that myoglobin becomes an important, if small-scale carrier of oxygen from blood haemoglobin to the cell mitochondria, a process more rapid than natural diffusion of molecular oxygen.

Complete resaturation of muscle myoglobin with oxygen is thought to be completed within the time period needed to recover the alactacid oxygen debt component.

Lactacid oxygen debt component

The **lactacid oxygen debt** component, also known as the 'slow component' of recovery, represents the amount of oxygen consumed in order to remove accumulated lactic acid from muscle cells and blood, following intense exercise. The speed of lactate removal depends on the severity of the exercise and whether the subject rests during recovery (known as passive recovery) or performs light exercise (known as active recovery).

Again, it should be stressed that this process will begin as soon as lactic acid appears in muscle cell sites (i.e. as soon as exercise begins). The lactic acid produced quickly dissociates into hydrogen ions (H^+) and lactate. The lactate is a component of a salt formed when it combines with sodium (Na^+) or potassium

(K$^+$) ions. This process will continue utilising breathed oxygen until recovery is complete, as indicated in Figure 3.12.

Table 3.4 shows what happens to the lactate during lactacid oxygen recovery. A high proportion of lactate is oxidised to form carbon dioxide and water. The liver converts most of the remaining lactate back into glucose, in an ATP-requiring process called **gluco-neogenesis**. Muscle tissue also has this property but to a less extent than the liver. It is thought that some of the lactic acid dealt with in this way to produce glucose would immediately reenter glycolysis and create further lactic acid on production of the energy for creation of two ATP molecules. This continual recycling of lactate is called the **lactate shuttle**. However, most of the recycled glucose is used to top up blood glucose levels or is returned to muscle and liver tissue where it is converted and stored as glycogen. A small proportion of the recycled glucose is converted in the liver to form protein.

The normal amount of lactate circulating in the blood is about 1–2 millimoles of lactate per litre of blood (mmol l^{-1}). In aerobic exercise this amount remains the same. However, in medium-intensity workouts, such as a 30-minute run, this amount doubles to 4 mmol l^{-1}. This latter amount represents the anaerobic or **lactate threshold** (LT) or the point at which blood lactate begins to accumulate above resting values. Researchers often set an arbitrary value of between 2.0 and 4.0 mmol l^{-1} to represent the point at which blood lactate accumulation begins.[7] This standard point of reference is also known as the **onset of blood lactate accumulation (OBLA)**. By definition, the lactate threshold has been thought to reflect the change in dominance between the aerobic and anaerobic energy systems. In untrained people the lactate threshold occurs at around 50–60% of their V̇O$_2$max, whereas elite endurance athletes may not reach their lactate threshold until around 70–80% of their V̇O$_2$max. During high-intensity training, such as

a 300 metre flat-out run, lactate levels can reach up to 15–20 times resting values.

Most research into the speed of lactate removal suggests that 50% of the debt is repaid in the first 15 minutes after exercise[8] and at least one hour is required for full recovery depending on the intensity of the exercise and fitness of the performer. Secondly, active recovery between exercise repetitions and at the end of a session speeds up the removal of lactate.[9] Active recovery could take the form of jogging, walking or stretching between runs or light swimming between high-intensity swims.

Muscle soreness

Muscle soreness is often present during the latter stages of an exercise period, the following day after strenuous exercise or at both times. Possible explanations of this muscle soreness are the muscle spasm theory, the lactate theory and the damaged muscle and connective tissue theory.

Muscle spasms are the result of sudden involuntary muscle twitches, causing local muscle tearing, to generate the inflammatory response discussed below.

During intense exercise it has been found that the pH level of the blood is low due to the accumulation of H$^+$ or lactate. It is thought that this type of muscle soreness is due to the effect of pH (acidity) acting upon pain receptors. Active recovery or **cool-down** will reduce the effects of muscle soreness after strenuous exercise by keeping blood capillaries dilated and flushing oxygenated blood through muscle tissue to remove lactic acid.

Muscle soreness felt the day after strenuous exercise (for example, the delayed muscle soreness experienced by a novice weightlifter) is known as **delayed onset muscle soreness** or **DOMS**. Based on current evidence, it appears that DOMS is due to tissue injury caused by excessive mechanical forces that have been applied to muscle and connective tissue. DOMS is often the result of eccentric work and may occur because of structural damage within the muscle membranes.[10] The breakdown of muscle proteins causes an inflammatory response or tissue oedema, created as fluid shifts from blood plasma to damaged tissues. Local pain receptors are then stimulated by this excess fluid.

Muscle soreness can be minimised by building up training intensity gradually. Aerobic training also increases capillarisation within the muscle, which additionally allows oxygenated blood to reach the lactic acid in muscle cells. This means that the fitter sportsperson should suffer less from muscle soreness.

Table 3.4 Lactic acid utilisation during lactacid oxygen recovery

Destination	Approximate % lactic acid involved
Oxidation into carbon dioxide and water	65
Conversion into glycogen, then stored in muscles or liver	20
Conversion into protein	10
Conversion into glucose	5

Muscle fatigue

Many bodily systems contribute to fatigue levels; however, in this section we shall restrict our interest to muscle fatigue. **Muscle fatigue** can be defined as a reduction in muscular performance or a failure to maintain expected power output.

Within Sections 1.5 and 1.6 of this textbook, there is a full description of how nerve impulses are transmitted across the motor end-plate to activate the sarcoplasmic reticulum and release calcium, which binds with troponin to initiate muscle contraction. It is thought that the interruption of these neuromuscular events could contribute towards muscle fatigue. Fatigue could occur at the motor end-plate (refer to Figure 1.37, p. 33), since a delay in the release and synthesis of acetylcholine reduces the conduction of the action potential and in turn decreases the release of Ca^{++} available for muscle contraction. The voluntary part of the central nervous system might perceive fatigue prior to physiological fatigue and therefore act as a protective mechanism.

Other proposed theories of muscle fatigue are that it is due to depletion of high-energy phosphates (for example, PC) and glycogen stores and to the accumulation of metabolites, such as lactate and carbon dioxide. There is considerable evidence that supports the importance of accumulation of H^+ (released from lactic acid and carbonic acid) as a limiting factor in performance.

Experimental work has shown that fast-twitch fibres are capable of generating large forces but **local muscular fatigue** occurs more rapidly in FT fibres (as opposed to slow-twitch low-force fibres), and is confined to the contractile mechanism. This is probably due to their low aerobic capacity and energy creation via glycolysis, which leads to lactic acid accumulation.

Fatigue resulting from endurance-based exercise is probably due to depletion of muscle glycogen stores in both fast-twitch and slow-twitch fibres. **Total body fatigue** (that is often visible in marathon events) includes local muscular fatigue, plus additional factors such as low blood glucose levels, liver glycogen depletion and electrolyte loss in sweat (for example, sodium chloride and potassium are filtered out of blood plasma). Fluid loss decreases plasma volume and therefore blood pressure, which in turn reduces blood flow to the skin and muscles. To overcome a reduction in plasma volume the heart has to work harder and, because blood flow to the skin is reduced, the body retains more heat energy and the muscle temperature will rise. The optimal muscle temperature is somewhere between 37 and 40°C and fatigue occurs at a much greater rate either above or below these values.

Restoration of muscle glycogen stores

There are about 350 g of glycogen in the body, some stored as muscle glycogen, the remainder in the liver. During strenuous exercise, blood glucose levels increase as the liver and muscle tissues metabolise their glycogen stores (converting glycogen into glucose). Depletion of muscle glycogen stores appears to be a significant factor in muscular fatigue.

For short-distance, high-intensity exercise, such as an 800 metre race, muscle glycogen stores are replenished within about 2 hours.

In long-distance endurance activities, such as marathon racing, a **glycogen-loaded diet** prior to the competition enhances muscle and liver glycogen levels. However, during prolonged exercise, muscle and liver glycogen levels fall until a state of exhaustion is reached.[4]

Complete restoration of muscle and liver glycogen stores is accelerated by a high carbohydrate diet.[4] A detailed account of carbohydrate loading and its effect on performance is described on p. 115. It has been found that replenishment of muscle glycogen stores is most rapid during the first few hours after exercise and then can take several days to complete.

Another factor that may account for the speed of recovery of muscle glycogen stores after high-intensity exercise, as compared with low-intensity exercise, is that restoration of muscle glycogen is quicker in fast-twitch fibres than in slow-twitch fibres.

The discussion above is important to both sportspersons and coaches. They must understand the need to plan their training sessions and competitions or games so that recovery has occurred and ensure that high intake of carbohydrates enables complete resynthesis of glycogen stores.

Review questions

1. **a.** What is the physiological basis for muscle soreness?

   b. How could the information on lactic acid removal be of use to an athlete and coach in the design of training sessions? ▶

c. Explain the importance of cool-down in the assistance of lactacid oxygen recovery and in the avoidance of muscle soreness.

2. Using the information in the sections on energy systems and oxygen recovery, complete the spaces in Table 3.5 with the major characteristics of the three energy systems in relation to the speed of running.

Table 3.5 Phosphagen, lactic acid and oxygen systems

ATP-PC (phosphagen) system	Lactic acid system	Oxygen system
	Anaerobic	Aerobic
Very rapid		
Chemical fuel:	Food fuel	Food fuel
PC	Limited ATP production	
Muscular stores limited	By-product, lactic acid causes muscular pain	
Used with sprint or any high-power, short-duration work up to 10 s after reference[11]		Used with endurance or long-duration activities over 2–3 min duration

Exam-style questions

1. a. A student performs a flat-out 50 metre freestyle swim in 50 seconds.

   i. Describe how **most** of the ATP is regenerated during the swim. *(6 marks)*

   ii. Sketch a graph that shows the use of the appropriate energy systems against time during the swim. *(3 marks)*

   b. i. What is **muscle fatigue**? *(2 marks)*

   ii. Explain the process of **lactate conversion** that takes place during recovery from a swim. *(3 marks)*

   (Total 14 marks)

2. a. The data in Table 3.6 illustrate the relationship between the concentration of blood lactate and rate of working.

   i. Using the data in Table 3.6, plot a graph to illustrate the relationship between blood lactate concentration and rate of working (watts). *(3 marks)*

   ii. Using the data, explain how you would deduce that at around 200 watts most of the work is done aerobically and at around 900 watts most of the work is done anaerobically. Identify the approximate point at which the lactate threshold or OBLA occurs on your graph. *(3 marks)*

   iii. What processes are involved in excess post-exercise oxygen consumption? *(5 marks)*

   b. i. Discuss the fate of lactate removal during recovery. *(4 marks)*

   ii. What organs and tissues are involved in this process? *(2 marks)*

   c. How does light exercise influence lactate removal? *(3 marks)*

   (Total 20 marks)

3. Describe the possible causes of fatigue during:

   a. maximal exercise lasting between 2 and 10 seconds *(3 marks)*

   b. submaximal exercise lasting from between 2 and 4 hours. *(3 marks)*

   (Total 6 marks)

For further reading on the recovery process see references[1, 2, 4, 11–13].

Table 3.6 Blood lactate and rate of working

Blood lactate (mmol l^{-1})	Rate of working (watts)
1	100
1.2	200
1.5	400
2.2	600
4.5	800
6.5	900
8.5	1000

3.4 Maximal aerobic and anaerobic capacities

Keywords

- aerobic testing
- anaerobic capacity
- mean anaerobic power (MP)
- fatigue index (FI)
- minimum anaerobic power
- maximum oxygen uptake ($\dot{V}O_2$max) or aerobic power
- oxygen consumption or oxygen uptake
- peak anaerobic power (PP)
- power decline (PD)
- steady state
- Wingate anaerobic power test

Oxygen consumption, or **oxygen uptake**, is defined as the amount of oxygen a person consumes per unit of time (usually one minute). This concept is expressed as $\dot{V}O_2$, where V is volume, O_2 is oxygen and the dot over the V means **per unit of time**.

The oxidation of fuel foods requires a definite amount of oxygen per unit mass of fuel (per kg of fuel). This amount can be measured indirectly by collecting expired air and comparing it with the composition of inspired air (by measuring the amount of **oxygen** that has been removed from the atmosphere and the amount of **carbon dioxide** that has been produced by the body, as illustrated and described in Section 3.1).

At rest, oxygen uptake varies between 0.2 and 0.3 litres per minute. These figures mean that the

BMR converts to between 4.4 and 6.6 kJ per minute based on the fact that 1 litre of oxygen liberates 22 kJ of energy from glycogen. For a 60 kg person, the BMR would therefore be between 0.073 and 0.110 kJ per minute per kg of body mass. However, once an individual starts to exercise, the total body oxygen uptake increases proportionately to the intensity of the exercise, until a maximal work rate is reached. The highest $\dot{V}O_2$ achieved is expressed as $\dot{V}O_2$max. This concept of **maximum oxygen uptake** ($\dot{V}O_2$max) is also known as **aerobic power**.

$\dot{V}O_2$max can therefore be quantitatively represented as the maximum amount of oxygen that a person can consume per minute during a progressive exercise test to exhaustion. This highest value represents the individual's maximal physiological capacity to transport and use oxygen.

A mean value of $\dot{V}O_2$max for male students is about 3.5 litres per minute and for females it is about 2.7 litres per minute. Endurance athletes, such as those who participate regularly in middle- and long-distance running, rowing and cross-country skiing, may reach between 4 and 6 litres per minute. However, $\dot{V}O_2$max depends on body mass as well as physical fitness, so it is often expressed in millilitres per kilogram of body mass per minute (ml kg^{-1} min^{-1}) so that comparisons can be made between individuals of different body mass.

Factors affecting maximum aerobic power

The availability of oxygen in the tissues is the limiting factor in any exercise. The physical limitations that restrict the rate at which energy can be released aerobically are dependent upon the chemical ability of the muscular cellular tissue system to use oxygen in breaking down fuels and the combined ability of cardiovascular and pulmonary systems to transport oxygen to the muscular tissue system.

Simple aerobic tests

Aerobic tests that are used as indicators of aerobic fitness include the Physical Work Capacity Test (PWC 170), the Cooper Run Test described on p. 131, the NCF Multistage Shuttle Run,[14] the Fitech Step Test,[15] the Chester Step Test[16] and the Queen's College Step Test.

Investigation 3.5   To measure maximum aerobic power. The Queen's College Step Test

This investigation is a very simple method of determining maximum aerobic power. The data used to predict $\dot{V}O_2max$ (ml kg^{-1} min^{-1}) was based on the results of male and female college students at Queen's College in New York. The students had their $\dot{V}O_2max$ measured using a treadmill test procedure and measuring actual oxygen consumed. The same students then completed the step test procedure outlined below and their recovery heart rate scores (in beats per minute – bpm) were tabulated against $\dot{V}O_2max$ measurements from the treadmill procedure. So, a given student had his/her actual $\dot{V}O_2max$ correlated against his/her heart rate score as shown in Table 3.7. This test procedure has been validated using a large number of individuals, each individual being tested on several occasions.

Materials: stepping bench (41 cm high), stopwatch, metronome.

Task 1

1. Establish the step cadence: for females set the metronome at 88 beats per minute, for males at 96 beats per minute. Practise the step rhythm to adjust to the cadence of the metronome. The sequence is left up/right up/left down/right down – each element to a single metronome beat.

2. Take a rest and when you are ready, begin to step for 3 minutes at the set step cadence.

3. At the end of the exercise period remain standing for 5 seconds. Then take your pulse count at the carotid artery for a 15-second count. Multiply by four to give the heart rate score in beats per minute (bpm).

4. Using the information in Table 3.7, work out your predicted $\dot{V}O_2max$ and percentile ranking, based on your recovery heart rate value.

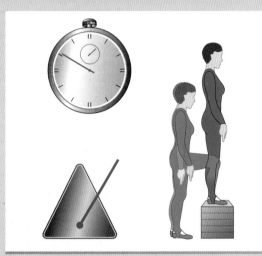

Fig. 3.13 The Queen's College Step Test.

Table 3.7 Queen's College Step Test

Percentile ranking	Recovery HR, female (bpm)	Predicted $\dot{V}O_2max$ (ml kg^{-1} min^{-1})	Recovery HR, male (bpm)	Predicted $\dot{V}O_2max$ (ml kg^{-1} min^{-1})
100	128	42.2	120	60.9
95	140	40.0	124	59.3
90	148	38.5	128	57.6
85	152	37.7	136	54.2
80	156	37.0	140	52.5
75	158	36.6	144	50.9
70	160	36.3	148	49.2
65	162	35.9	149	48.8
60	163	35.7	152	47.5
55	164	35.5	154	46.7
50	166	35.1	156	45.8
45	168	34.8	160	44.1
40	170	34.4	162	43.3
35	171	34.2	164	42.5
30	172	34.0	166	41.6
25	176	33.3	168	40.8
20	180	32.6	172	39.1
15	182	32.2	176	37.4
10	184	31.8	178	36.6
5	196	29.6	184	34.1

Table 3.8 Results table

Table	Percentile ranking	Recovery HR	Predicted $\dot{V}O_2max$ $(ml\ kg^{-1}\ min^{-1})$
Self			

Task 2 – collation of results

1. Record your results and those of male and female students in your class in Table 3.8.
2. Compare group results. Work out the percentage differences between male and female values. Are there any differences within your group? Account for these differences.
3. Work out your predicted $\dot{V}O_2max$ for your total body mass by multiplying $\dot{V}O_2max$ (ml kg⁻¹ min⁻¹) by your body weight (kg). How does this value relate to the values given earlier in this unit?

Task 3

1. Describe the two main factors that limit aerobic power.
2. Describe some of the ways in which aerobic capacity could be improved.
3. Which muscle fibre type is used predominantly in aerobic work?
4. Discuss the purpose of testing aerobic power with respect to endurance events.
5. Describe the energy systems used during the step test.
6. Identify **two** limitations of this test.

Task 4

Figure 3.14 shows how oxygen consumption changes as an athlete runs at a constant pace up a series of hills increasing in slope.

1. Describe and account for the pattern of oxygen consumption from the level ground until the end of the third hill.
2. Why does oxygen consumption begin to level off after the third hill?
3. The athlete is only just able to run up the final sixth hill where he/she achieves his/her $\dot{V}O_2max$. Explain what this concept means and why the athlete is unable to continue running at the set pace.
4. How would this pattern of oxygen consumption change if the athlete trained regularly over this terrain? Suggest possible reasons in your answer.

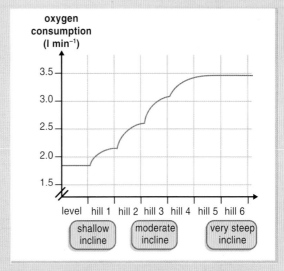

Fig. 3.14 Change in oxygen consumption as an athlete runs, at a constant pace, up a series of hills increasing in slope.

Task 5

1. Sketch a graph that illustrates the amount of oxygen consumed in litres per minute (on the y-axis) against time (on the x-axis) for a jogger, who at rest consumes 0.3 litres per minute. The jogger then starts to run at a steady pace for 20 minutes, having reached a 'steady state' of oxygen consumption at 1.75 litres per minute, 5 minutes into the run.
2. Label on your graph the part of the curve that is referred to as **'steady state'** and explain what this concept means.

Task 6

$\dot{V}O_2max$ decreases by about 10% per decade with ageing, starting in the late teens for women and in the mid-20s for men. Account for the effects of age on $\dot{V}O_2max$ values.

Oxygen consumption as an indirect way of measuring energy costs: a hypothetical example

Consider the following calculation as an example of how to go about estimating energy costs indirectly.

First, work out the **net oxygen cost** (the oxygen consumed during exercise above that which is needed at rest) from the resting and exercise rates of consumption. In our example these values are 0.4 litres per minute and 2.15 litres per minute, respectively, thereby giving a net oxygen cost total of 1.75 litres per minute.

Next, let us assume that the person undertaking the exercise works for a 10-minute period at this rate. The net oxygen cost for the 10 minutes will be $10 \times 1.75 = 17.5$ litres. As 1 litre of oxygen produces 22 kJ of heat energy by combination with food fuel in the body, the energy cost of the exercise will be:

$$22 \times 17.5 = 385 \text{ kJ}$$

In practice the net oxygen cost will always be greater than that calculated for the duration of exercise, as the net oxygen cost continues after exercise stops until oxygen consumption reaches its resting value.

You may wish to work out your own hypothetical example.

Anaerobic capacity

In addition to the assessment of aerobic fitness, the measurement of **anaerobic capacity** (the ability to do physical work, which is dependent upon the anaerobic mechanisms of energy supply) may also be of interest to those who are interested in short, explosive physical activities.

Investigation 3.6 Anaerobic capacity measurements

The **Wingate Anaerobic Cycling Test** (Figure 3.15) was devised at the Wingate Institute in Israel.[17] This test is a 30-second all-out cycling test, which is used to determine **peak anaerobic power** and **anaerobic capacity**. Anaerobic **power** is the ability to produce energy by the ATP–PC system. Anaerobic **capacity** is the combined ability of both anaerobic systems to produce energy and so is shown as the average power output during this 30 s test.

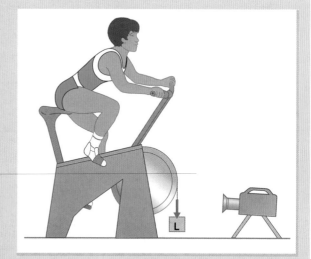

Fig. 3.15 The cycle ergometer.

Task 1
1. The subject warms up for a 2–3 minute cycling period to raise heart rate to 150 bpm.

2. The **workload** or bike resistance mass is worked out using the following information:
   a. **aged under 15 years**: 35 g kg^{-1} (grams of bike resistance mass per kilogram) of body weight
   b. **adult**: 45 g kg^{-1} of body weight for the Fleisch ergometer; 75 g kg^{-1} of body weight for the Monark ergometer. Set the cycle ergometer at the prescribed workload expressed in kg.

3. On the command 'GO' the subject pedals flat out for a period of **30 seconds**. During the first 2 seconds the resistance is adjusted and the timed flat-out cycling commences. For each 5 seconds of the investigation, a member of the group counts the number of pedal revolutions. Usually, the flywheel turns too quickly to count revolutions by eye, in which case a video recording or photo cell may assist the flywheel counting operation.

4. The subject pedals at a light load during a cool-down period.

5. The results for each 5-second period are recorded in watts according to the following equation:

   Power (watts) = loadmass (kg)
   × revolutions of flywheel in 5 seconds
   × radius of flywheel (metres)
   × 12.33.
   (12.33 = $\dfrac{2 \times 9.81 \times \pi}{5}$)

6. Record your results in Table 3.9.

Task 2 – analysis of results
1. Plot a graph of power (watts) (y-axis) against time in seconds (x-axis).

2. Identify the **peak anaerobic power (PP)** or the maximal power per kilogram of body mass achieved in a 5-second period (watt kg^{-1}). PP represents the maximum power created by the ATP–PC system.

3. Work out the **minimum anaerobic power** during the test, i.e. the minimum power recorded and the time at which this happens.

4. At what times in the investigation were peak and minimum anaerobic power attained?

Table 3.9 Results table

Time (s)	No. of revolutions of flywheel	Power (watts)	Power per kg of body mass
0–2			
2–7			
7–12			
12–17			
17–22			
22–27			
27–32			

5. **Power decline** is a measure of fatigue that can be calculated as a percentage of the peak power using this formula:

$$\frac{\text{Power}}{\text{decline}} = \frac{(\text{peak power} - \text{minimum power})}{\text{peak power}} \times 100$$

For example:

Peak power $= 1000$ W kg^{-1}
Minimum power $= 500$ W kg^{-1}

Time interval between peak and minimum power = 20 s

Power decline would be:

$$\frac{100 \times (1000 - 500)}{1000} = 50\%$$

6. A further interesting concept is the **fatigue index**. It can be calculated by using the formula:

$$\text{fatigue index} = \frac{\text{power decline}}{\text{time interval between peak and min. power (s)}}$$

In the example above (Task 2, item 5), the time interval was 20 s and the power decline was 50%. This gives a fatigue index of $\frac{50}{20} = 2.5\%$ s^{-1}.

Work out the subject's **fatigue index**.

7. Identify the **mean anaerobic capacity (MP)** or the average power over the 30-second period in **watts** per kilogram of body mass. This will be the area under the graph of power against time (in seconds) for the 30 seconds of the test divided by the time of the test (30 seconds).

Task 3

1. What do you think will be the effects on **anaerobic power** of:
   a. sprint interval training
   b. weight training
   c. jogging?

2. Which muscle fibre type is predominantly used during anaerobic exercise?

3. Give examples of **three** sporting activities that depend on anaerobic energy sources. Other examples of anaerobic capacity tests include the stair climb described in Investigation 3.1 (Figure 3.1), short sprints such as a 30-metre sprint, and the number of repetitions achieved in exercises such as squat-thrusts, press-ups, squat-jumps, dips or pull-ups. Alternatively, you could use static tests such as holding a weight at a fixed angle, as illustrated in the Strongest Man in the World competitions.

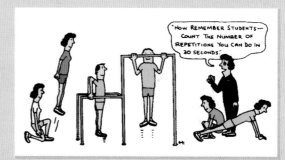

Fig. 3.16

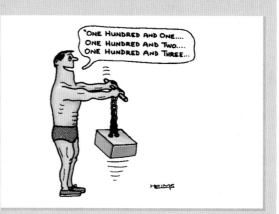

Fig. 3.17

Exam-style questions

1. Explain what is meant by $\dot{V}O_2$max and **anaerobic capacity.** *(2 marks)*
2. List **three** examples of physical activities that rely predominantly on aerobic metabolism for their energy supply. *(3 marks)*
3. Figure 3.18 shows variations in $\dot{V}O_2$max observed between different sports.
   a. Suggest reasons for variations in $\dot{V}O_2$max between these three sports. *(6 marks)*
   b. Explain the potential physiological advantages for endurance athletes having:
      i. a high $\dot{V}O_2$max *(2 marks)*
      ii. a low resting heart rate. *(2 marks)*
   c. What factors can account for the observation that $\dot{V}O_2$max is generally lower in females than in males? *(6 marks)*
   d. What is possibly the most important adaptation the body makes in response to endurance training that allows for an increase in $\dot{V}O_2$max and performance? *(2 marks)*
   e. Define **validity of testing** and comment on the validity of $\dot{V}O_2$max as a predictor of performance in sport. *(4 marks)*
   f. How would cardiovascular endurance conditioning be important in anaerobic sports? *(2 marks)*
   (Total 24 marks)

4. Briefly describe tests that can be used to evaluate one's capacity when performing:
   a. i. aerobic work *(3 marks)*
      ii. anaerobic work. *(3 marks)*
   b. Show how your selected tests can be evaluated. *(4 marks)*
   c. Comment on the advantages and disadvantages of the tests you have described. *(4 marks)*
   (Total 14 marks)

For further reading on maximal aerobic and anaerobic capacities see references[1, 4, 18–21].

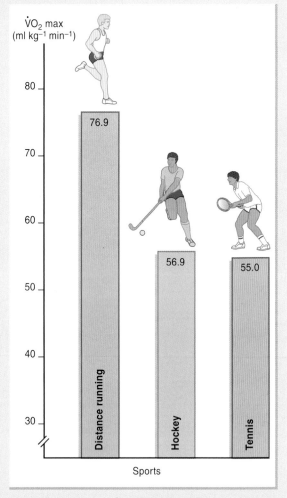

Fig. 3.18 Variations in $\dot{V}O_2$ between different sports.

3.5 Nutrition for exercise

Learning objectives

On completion of this section, you will be able to:

1. Understand the functions of carbohydrates, fats, proteins, minerals, vitamins, roughage and water in the context of a balanced diet.

2. Appreciate the role of carbohydrates and fats in relation to intensity and duration of the exercise period.

3. Understand the effects of carbo-loading on performance.

4. Appreciate the use of dietary supplements as an aid to performance enhancement.

Keywords

- balanced diet
- carbo-loading
- carbohydrates
- dietary supplements: sports drinks, creatine, glutamine
- energy metabolism
- fats
- fatty acids and glycerol
- glucose
- glycogen
- lipids
- minerals
- proteins
- roughage
- triglyceride
- vitamins
- water

The food and drink a sportsperson consumes daily provide the energy, mainly from carbohydrates and fats, to maintain bodily functions in addition to giving all the energy needed for training, competition and any other physical activity. Food also contain other nutrients, namely proteins, minerals, vitamins, water and roughage.

This section will help you to understand how these nutrients are vital to life processes and how carbohydrates and fats are the main energy providers for physical activity.

A **balanced diet** containing the correct proportions of carbohydrates, fats and proteins, together with minerals, vitamins, water and roughage, is important to an individual, whether active in sport or not, in order to maintain good health.

Proteins

Protein is present in most foods and occurs in large quantities in meat, eggs and milk. It is needed for growth and body building. For example, protein is used to increase the strength of muscle fibres, described in Chapter 1 (p. 42). Damaged tissues (resulting from fracture, dislocations, sprains, muscle strains and bruising – often incurred during physical activity) need proteins to repair injury sites. Proteins are also essential in the manufacture of enzymes required for metabolic functioning **but** they are used as an **energy source** only when the body is **depleted** of almost **all** carbohydrates and fat sources.

Minerals

Minerals are essential because they contain elements or small groups of elements needed to form part of the molecular structure of substances required by the body for life processes. For example, haemoglobin and muscle myoglobin contain an **iron** atom without which synthesis of haemoglobin would be impossible (lack of haemoglobin causes anaemia).

Vitamins

Vitamins perform a similar role as minerals except that they consist of **complex organic radicals** which are needed for the synthesis of molecules that participate in life processes. Such radicals cannot be manufactured by the body and therefore have to be ingested as part of the nutrition process (a radical is a stable group of atoms which forms part of a complex molecule). For example, ascorbic acid, otherwise known as vitamin C, contains the radical **ascorbate**, which is needed as part of the physiological **process** that prevents scurvy.

(See a specialist text on nutrition, e.g. references[22, 23], for a full list of vitamins and their effects on human health.)

Water

Water accounts for two-thirds of body weight. It is an essential ingredient in a daily diet because it dissolves more substances than anything else. As a result, nearly all chemical reactions essential to life take place in a watery medium. It also allows materials to move from one part of the body to another. For example, blood plasma consists of 90% water and transports a variety of substances, such as glucose, all around the body.

Water is very important as a heat regulator (heat is released as a result of tissue respiration). For example, blood plasma is able to take up heat and transport it to the body surface where it can be radiated away from the body. Another method of losing heat energy from the body surface involves water being excreted through the skin (sweating). As the water evaporates, the energy necessary to do this is extracted from the skin itself, thereby causing the skin to cool. Water is also lost as water vapour during expiration.

It therefore would be very important for a sportsperson to ensure that sufficient water is taken in during and immediately after exercise, particularly to replace fluid lost through sweating. In hot climates and for long-duration activities (triathlon, marathon, cycle touring, mountain activities), it will be essential to consume many litres of water to maintain hydration levels. Note that even in a 10 000 m race lasting 30 minutes or less, drinking stations are now provided during the race.

Roughage

Roughage or dietary fibre, found for example in cereals, provides bulk needed for the functioning of the large intestine.

Carbohydrates and fats: the energy givers

The bulk of chemical energy released by the chemical reactions involved in tissue respiration comes from carbohydrates and fats. Carbohydrates are the body's principal fuel, yielding 75% of our energy requirements; fats provide the remainder.

Carbohydrates

Carbohydrates include sugar, starch and cellulose. The sugars can be either **simple sugars** (**monosaccharides**; for example, glucose and fructose, both having the chemical formula $C_6H_{12}O_6$) or **complex sugars** (**disaccharides**; e.g. sucrose, maltose and lactose, all having the chemical formula $C_{12}H_{22}O_{11}$). Starch (found in food sources such as rice and potatoes) and cellulose are **polysaccharides**, since their molecular structures are chain-like multiples of glucose, and have the formula $(C_6H_{10}O_5)_n$ where n represents the number of glucose units in the molecule. This number varies between 100 and 1000 depending on the biological origin of the starch. Most of the carbohydrates we ingest are in the form of starch and cellulose.

Cellulose does not provide energy but is the main constituent of dietary fibre important for peristalsis in the large intestine. Peristalsis is a chain of muscular contractions that drives food along, thus preventing constipation.

Within the digestive tract, polysaccharides are hydrolysed to glucose and are stored as glycogen in both liver and muscle cells (the liver also has the function of converting glycogen into glucose when it is needed for tissue respiration).

One gram of carbohydrate provides 17 kJ of energy.

Fats

Fats have both animal and vegetable sources and should provide about 25% of energy requirements. Foods such as butter and bacon contain animal fats, with nuts and soya beans containing vegetable fats.

Within the digestive system, fats or **lipids** are converted by the enzyme **lipase** into **fatty acids** and **glycerol**.

Fats provide twice the energy yield of carbohydrates at 39 kJ g^{-1}.

In the bloodstream, glucose (derived from fats and carbohydrates) can be sent directly to muscles for energy release by direct involvement in the ADP to ATP conversion reaction or the PC-coupled reaction for the creation of ATP. Otherwise surplus glucose, not needed by these reactions, is converted (by the actions of the hormone **insulin**) into glycogen. This is stored in the liver (as **liver glycogen**) or in the muscle cell sarcoplasm (as **muscle glycogen**). If the body does not need the glucose, it enters the **fat metabolic system**, where it is converted into fatty acids and glycerol. These are then stored in the body as **triglycerides** (body fat) in adipose tissue (under the skin) and skeletal muscle (which would then contain strands of fat and be coated in a layer of fat). When energy is required from fat fuels, the contents of each individual adipose cell or muscle triglyceride are broken down into glycerol and free fatty acids. These are then transported by the circulatory system to the liver, where conversion into glucose takes place.

Other hormones that take part in the conversion of fat into carbohydrate are **glucagon** and **adrenaline** (insulin and glucagon are secreted by the islets of Langerhans in the pancreas and adrenaline is secreted from the adrenal glands situated on the top of each kidney).

The layer of fat formed under the skin (adipose tissue) acts as a heat insulator and, in a sporting context such as long-distance swimming, can be created and made thicker as an adaptation to cold conditions (and also by the eating of suitably large amounts of carbohydrates).

Energy metabolism

The total intake of food must be sufficient to supply enough energy to keep cells alive, their systems

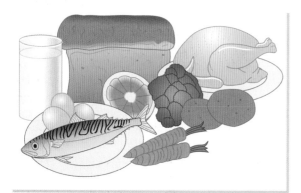

Fig. 3.19 A balanced diet.

working and to meet the demands of any activity that the body undertakes. The **basal metabolic rate** is the body's basic rate of energy required when resting and the **total metabolic rate** is the sum of the basal metabolic rate plus all the energy needed to carry out all daily activities. The energy requirements of an individual vary according to age, size, metabolic rate, gender, environment and lifestyle and they are discussed in Chapter 5.

Fuel foods for action

Both carbohydrates and fats are used to supply **glycogen** necessary for all forms of physical activity. However, the utilisation of carbohydrates and fats as nutrient fuels for muscle contraction during physical activity depends on the types of muscular activity. This means that differing amounts and types of fuel are used depending on whether the work is intermittent, prolonged, light or heavy – in other words, the **exercise duration** and **exercise intensity**. Table 3.10 describes these relationships.

Training and fuel use

The influence of endurance training on metabolic mixture and rate of energy utilisation is illustrated in Figure 3.20. This chart shows that untrained sportspersons who exercise at a low intensity will obtain the majority of their energy requirements from carbohydrates (column A). But if they continue to exercise long term at the same intensity, their metabolic systems will adapt by using more fat from the diet (and therefore less carbohydrate proportionately, column B). Hence, once the person has been training for some while, more carbohydrate is available for the energy needed for increased effort during aerobic exercise (column C). Therefore, the total energy available to the adapted metabolism from both fats and carbohydrates increases and the sportsperson becomes fitter and capable of more exercise.

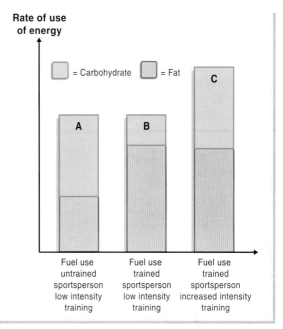

Fig. 3.20 Endurance training and fuel use.

Carbo-loading and performance

The concept of a **glycogen-loaded diet** was first devised in the 1960s and aimed to supercharge glycogen stores in muscle fibres ready for a long-duration activity such as a marathon (or triathlon or cycle touring race). This can be achieved by using an intensive training run that **depletes** muscle glycogen levels 7 days prior to a major event. At this point and for the next 3 days, the athlete eats mainly fats and proteins to deprive the muscle of carbohydrates. This has the effect of **increasing** the activity of glycogen synthase (the enzyme responsible for **glycogen synthesis**). During this period, the training intensity is reduced to prevent total glycogen depletion and possible injury. In the final 3–4-day period prior to the major event (during which low-intensity training is undertaken) the athlete switches to a carbohydrate-rich diet, restricts intake of fats and proteins but increases fluid intake. Because glycogen synthase activity has been boosted during the previous period, carbohydrate dietary intake now results in increased muscle glycogen storage. The overall effect is for performance times to improve significantly. However, there are **disadvantages** in using this dietary regime, since some athletes observe an increase in body weight (since more water is needed to store the increased glycogen stores) and during the depletion phase many athletes feel weak, depressed and irritable.

More recently, athletes have found alternative methods when preparing for major long-duration

Table 3.10 Fuel and exercise		
Exercise intensity	*Exercise duration*	*Fuel used*
Maximal sprint	Short	Carbohydrate
Low to moderate	Moderate Up to 2 hours, e.g. jogging	Carbohydrate and fat equally
Severe	Prolonged, e.g. cycling	Less carbohydrate, more fat

events. For example, following depletion of glycogen stores, athletes have reduced the period of low carbohydrate dietary intake to a single day or skipped it completely. They then have followed this by a 3–4-day period during which a carbohydrate-rich diet is taken. Recent studies have shown that a gradual tapering off in training alongside increased carbohydrate intake offers similar ergogenic benefits to those observed in early studies (which utilised the full programme as outlined above).

The best time to eat on the competition day is 2–3 hours prior to the event and meals should be of low volume and contain carbohydrates and plenty of fluids. This is because liver glycogen stores need topping up, even in a well-nourished, glycogen-laden athlete.

It is possible to measure the rate of respiration using simple respirometers and calculate respiratory quotients for proteins, fats and carbohydrates, as described on pp. 90–91.

Dietary supplements

By definition, food supplementation is an aid to performance and not a substitute for a balanced diet.

Fluid supplementation

Sports drinks are commercially very profitable and popular amongst young active sportspeople. There are two main categories of **sports drinks**: **fluid replacement drinks** and **carbohydrate (energy) drinks**, but there is often confusion about when to use each type of drink.

Fluid replacement drinks, such as Isostar and Gatorade, consist of dilute solutions of electrolytes (such as sodium) and sugars (between 4% and 8%). Their aim is to replace fluid very quickly. The addition of sugars, such as glucose, fructose and maltodextrins, helps maintain blood glucose levels. Most commercial fluid replacement drinks are **isotonic** (an isotonic drink has the same concentration of dissolved substances as our body fluids) and therefore are easily absorbed into the bloodstream. Research studies[24] have shown conclusively that regular ingestion of isotonic fluids **during** prolonged exercise prevents dehydration, whilst supplementing energy reserves.

Carbohydrate or **hypertonic** drinks are intended for consumption **well before** exercise commences and immediately **after** exercise. This is because the carbohydrate/electrolyte supplements contain increased sugar concentrations that take longer to digest, resulting in a slower release of additional sugars. This

will top up blood glucose levels but then may cause a fall in blood glucose due to a rise in insulin (which is produced as a response to high blood glucose). Excess blood glucose will replenish depleted glycogen stores, and the water in the drinks will maintain hydration. The purpose of **isotonic** drinks is to maintain blood glucose levels during exercise only.

Creatine supplementation

As mentioned above in respect of the maintenance of PC stores in muscle tissue (p. 95), **creatine** can be taken to delay the alactic–lactic threshold. Creatine is used by power athletes, for example, sprinters and all sportspeople who sprint during their games, weightlifters, gymnasts and combat sportspeople, as a training aid for training efforts of longer than 2 seconds.

Glutamine supplementation

Glutamine is an amino acid which is required by the immune system to build the T-lymphocyte cells which have a major role in the body's resistance to infection. Glutamine is also a constituent of skeletal muscle and is required when muscle is put under stress by hard training. Studies have found that sportspeople are most vulnerable to infections (colds, flu, etc.) immediately after hard physical effort and that a small amount of glutamine taken at this time may reduce the risk of infection.

Review questions

1. What are the purposes of each of the three basic groups of food?

2. How can high-carbohydrate diets influence metabolism?

3. How do you think different types of exercise could alter food intake?

4. Select **two** physical activities, one of short duration and high intensity and one of long duration and low intensity.

   a. Describe, with the aid of a bar chart, the relative contributions of carbohydrates and fats as fuel foods for your two chosen activities.

   b. Account for the differences between fuel usage for your two chosen activities.

   c. Sketch a graph to illustrate the relationship between short, high-intensity exercise and prolonged low-intensity exercise and food fuel usage (see Bowers,[11] Figure 4.1).

Exam-style questions

1. The digestion of fats results in the release of glycerol and fatty acids into the bloodstream.

   a. With reference to both short-term and long-term provision of energy for muscle contraction, describe what can happen to these compounds once they are released into the bloodstream. *(5 marks)*

   b. Very little fat is stored in muscle fibres yet fat is a main source during aerobic exercise. Explain how the fat stores of the body become available to working muscles. *(4 marks)*

   c. What are the disadvantages of fat as an energy source during exercise? *(2 marks)*

   d. After prolonged, continuous exercise there can be a severe drop in available energy, even though the body still has considerable fat reserves. Explain why this is so. *(5 marks)*

   e. Although fat reserves have value as a source of energy for exercise, in other ways they can be detrimental to sport performance. Explain why this is so. *(4 marks)*

   (Total 20 marks)

2. a. Explain how marathon runners can overcome the following problems:

      i. depletion of carbohydrate reserves *(3 marks)*

      ii. temperature regulation *(3 marks)*

      iii. reduce the risk of infection after a race. *(3 marks)*

   b. Describe and justify a preferred precompetition meal prior to a marathon. *(5 marks)*

   (Total 14 marks)

3. Give a brief outline and comment critically upon the effects of glycogen loading on the enhancement of sport performance. *(12 marks)*

For further reading on nutrition for exercise see references[1, 25, 26].

References

1. McArdle W D, Katch F I, Katch V L 2004 *Essentials of exercise physiology,* 2nd edn with Primal CD-ROM. Lippincott, Williams and Wilkins, New York
2. Wilmore J H 2004 *Physiology of sport and exercise*, 3rd edn. Human Kinetics, Champaign, Illinois
3. Bastian G F 1993 *An illustrated review of anatomy and physiology: the respiratory system*. HarperCollins, New York
4. Foss M L, Keteyian S J 1998 *Fox's physiological basis for exercise and sport*, 6th edn. McGraw Hill, New York
5. Seeley R R, Stephens T D, Tate P 2003 *Anatomy and physiology*, 6th edn. McGraw Hill, New York
6. Tortora G 2003 *Principles of anatomy and physiology*, 10th edn. John Wiley, New York
7. Karlsson J 1971 *Lactate and phosphagen concentrations in working muscles of man*. Acta Physiologica Scandinavica 358: 1–72
8. Karlsson J, Saltin B 1971 *Oxygen deficit and muscle metabolites in intermittent exercise*. Acta Physiologica Scandinavica 82:115–122
9. Bonen A, Belcastro A N 1976 *Comparison of self-selected recovery methods in lactic acid removal rates*. Medicine and Science in Sport and Exercise 8(3):176–178
10. Armstrong R 1984 *Mechanisms of exercise-induced delayed onset of muscle soreness. A brief review*. Medicine and Science in Sport and Exercise 16:529–538
11. Bowers R W, Fox E L 1992 *Sports physiology*. McGraw Hill, New York
12. Clegg C 1999 *Images and performance data for exercise physiology*. Feltham Press, New Milton
13. Newsholme E, Leech T, Duester G 1994 *Keep on running*. John Wiley, Chichester
14. NCF 1988 *Multistage fitness test*. NCF, Leeds
15. Sykes K 1987 *The FITECH fitness test*. Fitech, Chester
16. Sykes K 1998 *The Chester step test*. Assist Resources, Chester
17. Inbar O, Bar-Or O, Skinner J S 1996 *The Wingate anaerobic test*. Human Kinetics, Champaign, Illinois
18. Adam G M 1998 *Exercise physiology laboratory manual*. McGraw Hill, New York
19. Clegg C 1998 *Measurement and testing of physical performance*. Feltham Press, New Milton
20. Clegg C 1999 *Teaching support graphs for exercise physiology*. Feltham Press, New Milton
21. Sharkey B J 1991 *New dimensions in aerobic fitness*. Human Kinetics, Champaign, Illinois
22. Bean A 2003 *Sports Nutrition*. A & C Black, Huntingdon
23. Katch F I, McArdle W D 1993 *Introduction to nutrition, exercise and health*, 4th edn. Lea and Febiger, Philadelphia
24. Murray R G, Eddy D E, Murray T W 1987 *The effect of fluid and CHO feedings during intermittent cycling exercise*. Medicine and Science in Sport and Exercise 19: 597–604
25. Paish W 1990 *Nutrition for sport*. Crowood Press, Marlborough
26. Williams M H 1995 *Nutrition for fitness and sport*, 4th edn. Brown and Benchmark, London

Further reading

Bean A 2002 *Food for fitness,* 2nd edn. A&C Black, London
James R, Thompson G, Wiggins-James N 2003 *Complete A–Z physical education handbook*, 2nd edn. Hodder and Stoughton, London
Powers S K, Howley E J 2004 *Exercise Physiology theory and application to fitness and performance,* 5th edn. McGraw Hill, New York
Roscoe D A, Roscoe J V, Honeybourne J, Davis R J, Galligan F 2003 *Physical education and sports studies AS/A2 level student revision guide,* 3rd edn. Jan Roscoe Publications, Widnes

Wilmore J H, Costill D L 2004 *Physiology of sport and exercise,* 3rd edn. Human Kinetics, Champaign, Illinois.

MULTIMEDIA

CD-ROM

Mentor body systems – interactive physical education and teacher's manual. Department of Human Movement, The University of Western Australia 1987. UK supplier Boulton and Hawker Films Ltd

Roscoe D A 2002 *A Level Physical Education/Sports Studies OHPs for OCR/AQA/Edexcel syllabuses.* Jan Roscoe Publications, Widnes

Roscoe D A 2004 *Teacher's guide to physical education and the study of sport, CD-Rom, 5th edn. Part I, the performer in action, exercise physiology.* Jan Roscoe Publications, Widnes

Roscoe D A, Roscoe J V, Honeybourne J, Davis R J, Galligan F 2003 *Physical Education and Sports Studies AS/A2 Level Student Revision Guide,* 3rd edn. Jan Roscoe Publications, Widnes

Videos

Exercise Physiology. The Sports Science Series, Queensland Department of Education, Australia 1988. UK supplier Boulton and Hawker Films Ltd

Testing for Aerobic Fitness. Video Education, Australia 1997. UK supplier Boulton and Hawker Films Ltd

Food for Sport. Australian Sports Medicine 1999. UK supplier Boulton and Hawker Films Ltd

Sport and Nutrition. Video Education Australasia 2000. UK supplier Boulton and Hawker Films Ltd

Training for physical performance

4.1 Physical fitness and fitness testing

Keywords

- agility
- balance
- body composition
- cardiovascular endurance
- construct validation
- Cooper's 12-minute test
- coordination
- dynamic balance
- endurance
- fitness
- flexibility
- local muscle endurance
- motor fitness
- physical fitness
- power
- PWC-170 test
- reaction time
- speed
- static balance
- strength

Physical fitness is one of the basic requirements of life. Broadly speaking, it means the ability to carry out our daily tasks without undue fatigue. In the sporting context it is difficult to define since it can refer to psychological, physiological or anatomical states of the body. Most physical education teachers see it as a concept obtained by measuring and evaluating a person's state of fitness by using a battery of tests.

This section will help you to understand those aspects of **fitness** that are important to physical performance and good health.

Types of fitness test

1. **Motor fitness tests** aim to look at neuromuscular components of fitness and therefore consider skill-related exercises and the capacity of the individual to repeat a particular exercise.
2. **Physical fitness tests** aim to look at anatomical and physiological components that determine a person's physical performance capacity. These tests make direct measurements of physiological parameters such as heart rate, oxygen uptake and flexibility.

The ability of a person to perform successfully at a particular game may not be an indicator of physical fitness but an assessment of the motor fitness of the individual to perform the specific skills relevant to the game. Motor fitness refers to the **efficiency** of movements and, although including the **power** component, is mostly about **balance**, **agility** and **coordination**.

Physical fitness

The concept of **physical fitness**, in general athletic terms, means the capability of the individual to meet the varied physical and physiological demands made by a sporting activity, without reducing the person to an excessively fatigued state. Such a state would be one in which he/she can no longer perform the skills of the activity accurately and successfully.

The components of physical fitness are defined in Figure 4.1.

Strength
Strength is usually defined as the maximum force exerted by muscle groups during a sports movement. There are five types of strength.

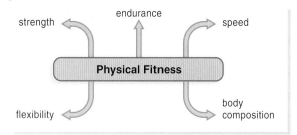

Fig. 4.1 Components of physical fitness.

Maximal strength is defined as the maximum force exerted by muscle groups during a **single maximal** muscle contraction. This is the sort of strength power (weight) lifters use in competition.

Static strength is maximal strength exerted without change of muscle length (see Chapter 1, p. 27); for example, holding a weight at arm's length or pushing hard in a stationary rugby scrum.

Dynamic strength is maximal strength exerted during a movement or exercise in which muscle length changes. Most sports use this type of maximal strength.

Explosive/elastic strength is defined as the ability to apply maximal force at a high speed of muscular contraction. This sort of strength is the most usual in sports situations: jumping, throwing, sprinting and most games or activities requiring flat-out movements.

Strength endurance is defined as the ability of muscles to undertake intense effort in order to repeat movements in spite of apparent fatigue. Examples of this sort of strength include doing a maximum number of chin-ups or performing shuttle runs flat out to failure.

Endurance

Endurance is the capacity to sustain movement or effort over a period of time. **Local muscle endurance** is the ability of the muscles to repeat movements without undue fatigue (this definition overlaps that of strength endurance to some extent), whilst **cardiovascular endurance** is the ability of the cardiovascular system to transport oxygen to muscles during sustained exercise.

Speed

Speed is the maximum rate at which a person is able to move his/her body. In physical terms, speed is the distance moved per second (see p. 194). In physical performance terms it refers to the speed of coordinated joint actions and whole-body movements.

Flexibility

Flexibility is the range of movement possible at a joint. It is affected by the type of joint and muscle attachment (refer to pp. 155–158 on types of flexibility).

Body composition

Body composition is a concept describing the relative percentage of muscle, fat and bone. This can be categorised by three extreme body types called somatotypes (after Sheldon[1]). Everybody can be characterised as a mixture of these three extremes. A somatotype is a numerical representation on a 1–7 scale of the degree to which a person possesses the three extremes.

Extreme **ectomorph**: a lean linear build with the appearance of long limbs with a low proportion of body fat and muscle. For example, a high jumper.

Extreme **endomorph**: a rounded appearance, often pear shaped with a high proportion of body fat. For example, a sumo wrestler.

Extreme **mesomorph**: broad shoulders, narrow hips and a higher percentage of lean muscle mass. For example, a male gymnast.

Although all three extreme morphs can be found in the sporting population, the majority of individuals are made up of a proportion of all three extreme body types.

Body composition analysis is a suitable tool for the assessment of a person's state of fitness.

Motor fitness

Motor fitness refers to the ability of a person to perform successfully at a particular game or activity. Although there is an overlap in the components essential to both physical fitness and motor fitness, there are specific components, identified in Figure 4.2, that enable a person to perform a skill successfully and that are more directly relevant to motor fitness.

Agility

Agility is the physical ability that enables a person rapidly to change body position and direction in a precise manner.

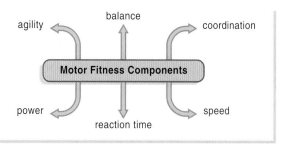

Fig. 4.2 Components of motor fitness.

Balance

Balance is the ability to retain the centre of mass of the body above the base of support. It is the awareness of the body's position in space and depends upon coordination between the inner ear, brain, skeleton and muscles. **Static balance** is the ability to hold a balance in a stationary position; **dynamic balance** is the ability to maintain balance under changing conditions of body movement, shape and orientation.

Coordination

Coordination is the ability to perform smooth and accurate motor tasks, often involving the use of the senses and a series of correlated muscular contractions that affect a range of joints and therefore relative limb and body positions.

Power

Power is a combination of **strength** and **speed**, previously described as a component of physical fitness (see p. 196 for a physical explanation of power and p. 130 for an investigation to evaluate a person's power). This definition overlaps that of elastic/explosive strength.

Reaction time

Reaction time is the interval of time between the presentation of a stimulus and the initiation of the muscular response to that stimulus.

Investigation 4.1   The measurement of fitness components

You are going to measure a number of indicators of your physical and motor fitness. The fitness ratings for each task are based on national norms for 16–19 year olds. Results and scores for each test should be recorded in Table 4.11.

Prior to testing, it is recommended that you assess your current state of health and fitness using a Physical Activity Readiness Questionnaire (**PARQ**). When you click onto this section located on the CD-ROM, there is a hyperlink to a suitable PARQ.

Before commencing this practical work, make sure that you warm up thoroughly.

Task 1 – self-evaluation of body strength

1. **Grip strength**: to test grip strength.

   Materials: hand grip dynamometer.

   Use a hand grip dynamometer (Figure 4.3) to measure grip strength. Record the maximum reading from three attempts from your dominant hand and the grip rating (Table 4.1).

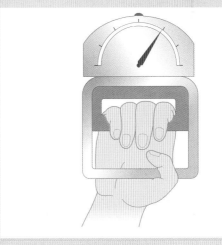

Fig. 4.3 Hand grip dynamometer.

Table 4.1 Grip rating

Dynamometer (kg)		Rating
males	*females*	
>56	>36	excellent
51–56	31–36	good
45–50	25–30	average
39–44	19–24	fair
<39	<19	poor

2. **Vertical jump**: to test the leg power vertically upwards (explosive strength).

    Materials: vertical jump board (Figure 4.4).

    Adjust the vertical jump board so that its lower edge touches your fingertips as both arms are held overhead at full body stretch with feet flat on the floor. Prepare to take off from both feet, flex your knees and then jump as high as you can, touching the calibrated scale with the fingertips of one hand. Record the maximum height from three attempts and jump rating (Table 4.2).

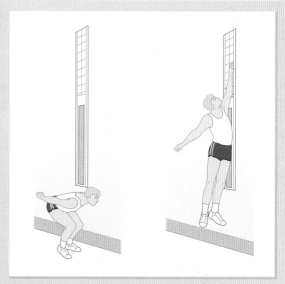

Fig. 4.4 Vertical jump.

Table 4.2 Vertical jump rating

Vertical (cm)		Rating
males	*females*	
>65	>58	excellent
50–65	47–58	good
40–49	36–46	average
30–39	26–35	fair
<30	<26	poor

Task 2 – self-evaluation of local muscular endurance

1. **Chins**: to test strength and muscular endurance of the arm and shoulder muscles.

    Materials: chinning bar (Figure 4.5).

    Hang from a bar with your palms facing away from your body. Pull up until your chin is level with the bar. Repeat as many chins as possible, ensuring that your arms reach a straight position between each effort. Record the number of chins achieved and the chin rating (Table 4.3).

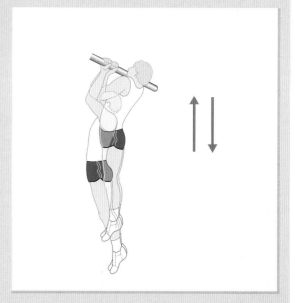

Fig. 4.5 Chinning bar.

Table 4.3 Chin rating

Number of chins		Rating
males	*females*	
>13	>6	excellent
9–13	5–6	good
6–8	3–4	average
3–5	1–2	fair
<3	0	poor

2. **Sit-ups**: to test the strength and muscular endurance of the abdominal muscles (Figure 4.6).

   Lie down on a mat with your knees flexed at right angles. Ask a partner to hold your feet and, on a signal, perform as many sit-ups (between your shoulders touching the ground and elbows touching your knees) as you can in 30 seconds. Have your partner count the number of sit-ups achieved at 30 seconds. Record the number achieved and sit-up rating (Table 4.4).

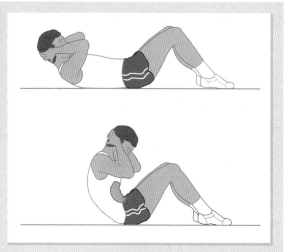

Fig. 4.6 Sit-ups.

Table 4.4 Sit-up rating

Number of sit-ups in 30s		Rating
males	females	
>30	>25	excellent
26–30	21–25	good
20–25	15–20	average
17–19	9–14	fair
<16	<8	poor

Task 3 – self-evaluation of cardiovascular endurance
The Queen's College Step Test: to test cardiovascular endurance (Figure 4.7).

Materials: stepping bench (41 cm high), stopwatch, metronome.

This test for cardiovascular fitness is described in detail in Investigation 3.5, p.108. The results have been extrapolated from the percentile rankings for recovery heart rate and predicted maximal oxygen consumption (Table 4.5).

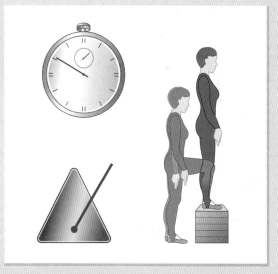

Fig. 4.7 The Queen's College Step Test.

Table 4.5 Step test rating

Heart rate in bpm		Rating
males	females	
<120	<128	excellent
148–121	158–129	good
156–149	166–159	average
162–157	170–167	fair
>162	>170	poor

▶ **Task 4 – self-evaluation of speed**
30 metres sprint: to test the speed of a performer over 30 metres (Figure 4.8).

Materials: 50 metre tape measure, stopwatch.

Mark out 30 m on your selected running surface. Using a flying start, sprint as hard as you can between the marked areas. Make sure that your sprint is timed by a partner from the start to the finish line. Record your time and speed rating (Table 4.6).

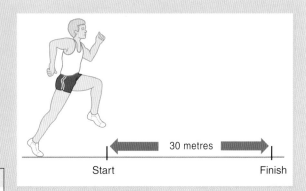

Fig. 4.8 Speed test.

Table 4.6 Speed rating

Time for 30 m sprint in seconds		Rating
males	females	
<4.0	<4.5	excellent
4.2–4.0	4.6–4.5	good
4.4–4.3	4.8–4.7	average
4.6–4.5	5.0–4.9	fair
>4.6	>5.0	poor

Task 5 – self-evaluation of flexibility
Sit and reach test: to test the flexibility of the hips.

Materials: gymnastics bench, metre ruler.

Turn a gymnastics bench on its side and sit on the floor with your legs straight and feet flat against the side of the secured bench. Place a ruler on the upturned bench so that it extends 15 cm over the end of the bench, with the zero end extending towards you. Reach slowly forwards as far as you can go and hold (Figure 4.9). Ask a partner to read off the distance, in centimetres, past your heels to the stretched distance that your fingertips have reached on the ruler. Record this distance and your flexibility rating (Table 4.7).

Note: The range of motion of a joint can be measured in degrees using a double arm goniometer.

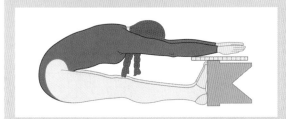

Fig. 4.9 Sit and reach test.

Table 4.7 Sit and reach rating

Flexibility (cm)		Rating
males	females	
>14	>15	excellent
11–13	12–14	good
7–10	7–11	average
4–6	4–6	fair
<3	<3	poor

► **Task 6 – self-evaluation of body fat composition: the Jackson & Pollock method**[2]

Skinfold measurements: to test skinfold measurements taken at three sites on the body.

Materials: skinfold calipers, Jackson–Pollock nomogram. The three sites for males are (A) thigh, (B) chest and (C) abdomen, whereas those for females are (A) thigh, (D) suprailium and (E) triceps as illustrated in Figure 4.10.

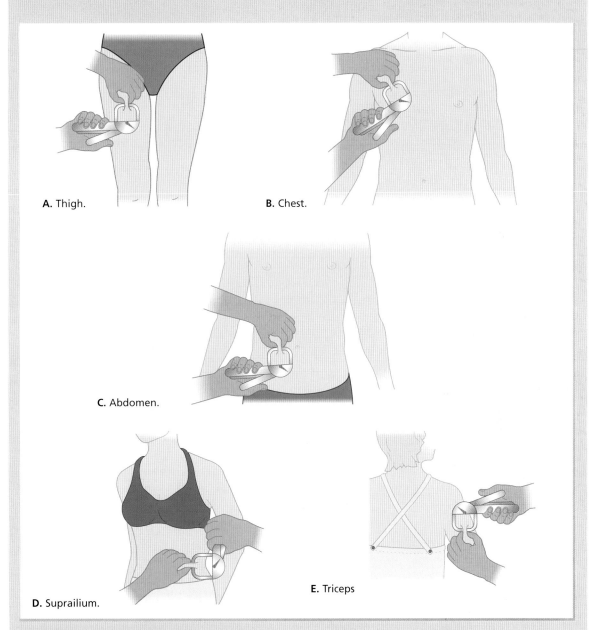

A. Thigh.

B. Chest.

C. Abdomen.

D. Suprailium.

E. Triceps

Fig. 4.10 Skinfold measurements.

Technique

Take skinfold measurements in a private area. Always use the right side of the body.

At the identified site, get a partner to grasp the skin to make a fold between thumb and forefinger.

Lift the fold of skin and engage the jaws of the caliper to measure the fold. Read off the dial to the nearest 0.5 millimetre, before removing the calipers. Repeat the measurement three times and record the mean score for the sum of the three skinfold measurements (mm). Find out your predicted percentage of body fat, by using the **Jackson–Pollock Equation** (Figure 4.11[3]) for predicting % body fat. The percentage body fat is found by placing a ruler at a point on the left vertical line that is closest to your age. The other end of the straight edge is pivoted to the approximate value on the far right vertical line, which contains the sum of your three skinfold measurements.

For example, a skinfold total of 35 mm for an 18-year-old male gives an 11% body fat composition.

Record the approximate percentage of body fat in Table 4.11 and evaluate your body fat rating in relation to the rating chart (Table 4.8).

Table 4.8 Body fat % rating		
Body fat % using the J–P nomogram		Rating
males	females	
<13	<18	excellent
18–13	23–18	good
22–19	29–24	average
26–23	34–30	fair
>26	>34	poor

An alternative method of measuring body fat percentage uses the BIA technique. **Bioelectrical Impedance Analysis** (BIA) sends a low, safe electrical current through the body. The current passes freely through the fluids contained in muscle tissue but encounters resistance (impedance) when it passes through fat tissue. This resistance is called bioelectrical impedance and is measured using a variety of apparatus similar to a bathroom scales. Percentage body fat can be read directly from the instrument. If such scales are used, body fat rating can be evaluated from Table 4.8 and recorded in Table 4.11.

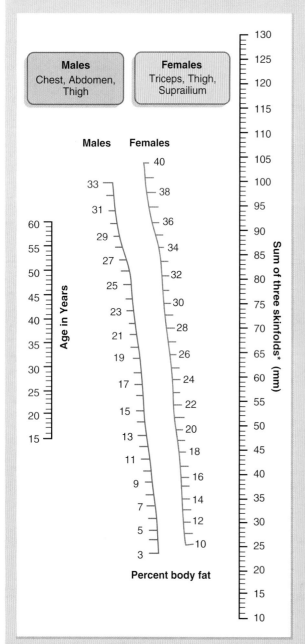

Fig. 4.11 The J–P nomogram for the estimate of percentage body fat.

▶ **Task 7 – self-evaluation of agility**
The Illinois Agility Run: to test speed and agility.

Materials: cones, tape measure, stopwatch.

Mark out a space 10 m in length and place four obstacles 3.3 m apart, as shown in Figure 4.12.

Lie prone, head to start line, hands beside your shoulders. On the command 'go' run the course as fast as possible. Have a member of your group issue the start command and time the run. Record your time and fitness rating (Table 4.9).

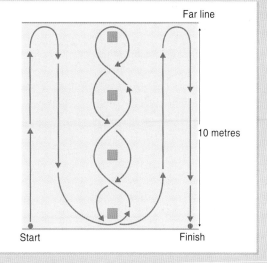

Fig. 4.12 Agility run.

Table 4.9 Agility run rating		
Time in seconds		*Rating*
males	*females*	
<15.2	<17.0	excellent
16.1–15.21	7.9–17.0	good
18.1–16.22	1.7–18.0	average
18.3–18.2	23.0–21.8	fair
>18.3	>23.0	poor

Task 8 – self-evaluation of static balance
Balancing on a beam: to test a timed static balance.

Materials: gymnastics bench (Figure 4.13), stopwatch.

Time how long balance can be maintained on one foot, with eyes closed, on a balance beam or inverted bench. Within your class use everyone's results to devise a rating scale.

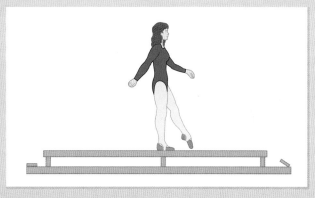

Fig. 4.13 Balancing on a beam.

▶ **Task 9 – self-evaluation of coordination**
Juggling: to test how long it takes you to learn how to juggle.

Materials: tennis balls, stopwatch.

Time how long it takes you to learn to juggle three balls as illustrated in Figure 4.14. Within your class use everyone's results to devise a rating scale. It is suggested that class members who have not learnt to juggle within 10 minutes stop after this time.

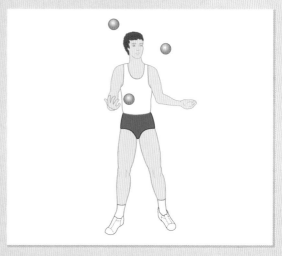

Fig. 4.14 Juggling.

Task 10 – self-evaluation of reaction time
The stick drop test: to test the time it takes you to catch a ruler.

Materials: metre ruler.

Place a metre ruler against the wall. Your partner holds the ruler against the wall at the zero end of the metre ruler. You place your preferred hand level with the 50 cm mark on the ruler but not touching it, as illustrated in Figure 4.15. Without warning, your partner lets go of the stick and you must catch it with thumb and index finger. Your score is the number just above your index finger. Record your best result from three attempts. Assess your rating with the results shown in Table 4.10.

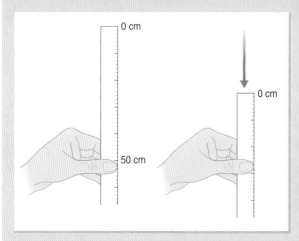

Fig. 4.15 Stick drop test.

Table 4.10 Stick drop test rating

Reaction time	Rating
>42.5	excellent
34.1–42.5	good
29.6–37.0	average
22.0–29.5	fair
<22	poor

▶ **Task 11**

1. Record all your results in Table 4.11 and, using these results, put together an assessment of your own personal physical and motor fitness profile.

2. How do your rating values compare with the given norms?

3. Describe the physiological value to the body of each of the tests you have done.

4. How could you use your results to best effect?

5. Apart from using a nomogram for predicting percentage body fat, identify other methods that are commonly used today.

6. Identify **one** advantage and **one** disadvantage for each test undertaken and results listed in Table 4.11.

7. Why is it important to evaluate test scores against normative data?

8. Why is it important to consider body composition in relation to sporting performance?

Table 4.11 Results table – physical fitness and motor fitness tests

Exercise	Score	Rating
grip strength		
vertical jump		
chins		
sit-ups		
step test		
30-metre sprint		
flexibility		
body fat percentage		
agility run		
static balance		
coordination		
reaction time		

Principles of maximal and submaximal fitness tests

Maximal fitness tests

Maximal means that the subject undertaking a test will make an all-out effort or take a test to exhaustion. In anaerobic work, 1 RM represents one maximal effort (refer to p. 138).

Examples of maximal anaerobic tests include a 30-metre sprint (refer to p. 124) and the Wingate 30-second cycle ergometer test (see p. 110). Examples of maximal aerobic tests include the NCF multi-stage shuttle run (which is performed to exhaustion) and the Cooper's 12-minute run test described on p. 131.

Submaximal fitness tests

Submaximal means that the subject will exercise below maximal effort. The data collected from submaximal tests can be extrapolated to **estimate** maximal capacities. Examples would be Investigation 4.2, the PWC-170 test (refer to p. 130), and the Queen's College Step Test outlined on p. 108.

Submaximal tests are often favoured over maximal tests because there is less stress on the performer and greater reliability of results.

Differences in fitness measures between males and females

Students will find considerable differences between **average** fitness measures for males and females in most of the tests above. The two major measures for which large differences are found to occur in both trained and untrained people are **strength** and **body composition** measures. This can be accounted for by the differences in gender-related hormones produced by the respective sexes. **Oestrogen** is responsible for extra insulating body fat in females and **testosterone** is responsible for the greater size and muscle mass of males. An effect of this is that the basal metabolic rate **(BMR)** is higher in males than in females, since males tend to lose heat through the skin more easily than females (see p. 174). However, training can reduce fat stores and increase strength in females and we should note that there are considerable individual differences within the female population such that some females can be bigger, stronger and less fat than some males. It should also be noted that females have the ability to perform at least as well if not better than males at some ultra-endurance activities. This could be because energy reserves (per unit mass of body weight) of females can be higher than energy reserves in males.

Validity and reliability of fitness testing

Validity in any kind of testing is always a key issue for discussion. The major problem is whether the actual test measures precisely what it aims to measure. Nearly all tests measure other aspects of physical and motor fitness that are not defined in the test criteria. For example, a sit-up test measures dynamic strength and could also be used to measure endurance and flexibility. A person may achieve a high score on the motor fitness components of the test and as a result inflate his/her overall test score, in spite of his/her possibly weak physical fitness abilities.

To overcome this problem, pioneers of battery testing devised the theory of **construct validation**. This theory accounts for any measure of an aspect of physical or motor fitness that is not defined in the objectivity of the test.[4]

Reliability in any kind of testing questions the accuracy of test results. A test is reliable when you undertake a retest under the same conditions as the original test and a similar result is obtained.

Simple tests, such as the 30-metre sprint, are also affected by the testing environment, motivation (particularly during a maximal fitness test) and previous experience. It is therefore important to recognise the **limitations** of such tests if they are to be used as assessment tools of physical and motor fitness.

Investigation 4.2   PWC-170 test

As the title suggests, the primary purpose of the **PWC-170** test is to predict the power output at a projected heart rate of 170 bpm. The subject performs two consecutive 6-minute bicycle ergometer rides in which the workloads are selected to produce heart rates between 120 and 140 bpm for the first power level and between 150 and 170 bpm for the second power level. An example of a graphic calculation of P-170 using heart rates of a conditioned subject at 600 kg min^{-1} (equivalent to 100 watts ergometer power output) and 900 kg min^{-1} (equivalent to 150 watts) is given in Figure 4.16. For this example, two points are plotted on the graph in Figure 4.16 for 130 bpm at 100 W and 153 bpm at 150 W.

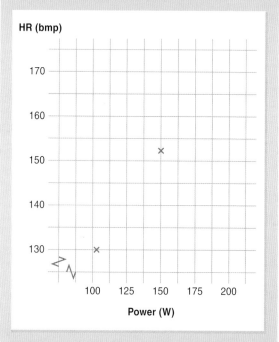

Fig. 4.16 Graphic estimation of PWC-170 test. ▶

▶ **Task 1**

1. Copy the graph in Figure 4.16 and then draw a line through the two points so that it is extended to a heart rate of 170 bpm. Now draw a perpendicular line from the point plotted at a heart rate of 170 bpm to the horizontal axis. Read off the projected power output in watts at this point.

2. Describe the relationship between heart rate and power output.

3. Draw a second line on your graph that would represent an estimated P-170 for an unconditioned subject.

4. Account for the differences between the conditioned and unconditioned subject.

5. What are the advantages of using submaximal as compared to maximal workloads in the assessment of fitness levels?

Review questions

1. Give concise definitions for each of the following:
   a. strength
   b. power
   c. stamina and/or endurance
   d. flexibility
   e. coordination.

2. Before commencing a testing session, there are a number of factors that need to be considered. Describe some very important pretest procedures.

3. Identify the specific physical fitness components in the following activities: gymnastics, sprint running, tennis, long-distance running.

4. In terms of fitness requirements, what is the difference between a squash player and a long-distance runner?

5. How could a knowledge of physical and motor tests assist you in assessing the general training needs of the individual sportsperson?

Exam-style questions

1. The aim of Cooper's 12-minute run/walk test is to run as far as possible in 12 minutes.
   a. i. Using an outdoor 400 m athletics track, describe a method that would give you an accurate result of the distance covered in 12 minutes. (*3 marks*)
      ii. What advantages and disadvantages would there be if this test were to be performed indoors? (*4 marks*)
      iii. What aspect of physical fitness does the 12-minute run/walk measure? Identify **two** other valid and reliable tests that measure the same aspect of fitness. (*3 marks*)
   b. Table 4.12 compares the results of the 12-minute run/walk test for males and females of differing levels of fitness and age.
      i. Using the data from Table 4.12, draw a graph which shows distances covered for the three fitness categories on the *y*-axis, against age on the *x*-axis for both males and females. (*4 marks*)
      ii. Discuss these results in relation to gender and levels of fitness. (*6 marks*)
      iii. Account for the decline in distance covered with age. (*4 marks*) (refer to Section 5.3, p. 185).

   (*Total 24 marks*)

2. a. **Validation** of **Cooper's 12-minute test** is done by correlating the distance covered in 12 minutes with maximal oxygen consumption ($\dot{V}O_2$max).

Table 4.12 12-minute run/walk test for males and females of differing fitness levels and age (distance measured in kilometres)

Fitness category	Age (years)		
	17	45	60+
	(distance covered in kilometres)		
Very poor			
(men)	2.09	1.83	1.40
(women)	1.61	1.42	1.25
Good			
(men)	2.64	2.35	2.03
(women)	2.19	1.90	1.67
Excellent			
(men)	2.88	2.56	2.32
(women)	2.36	2.08	1.83

Results from studies[5] show a direct or linear relationship between these two variables. Sketch a graph to show the relationship between these two variables. Put maximum oxygen consumption (ml kg^{-1} min^{-1}) on the *x*-axis and distance covered in kilometres on the *y*-axis. (*3 marks*)

   b. i. A reliable test generates a high correlation when values from repeated trials of the test are compared. However, reliability of a test may be affected by experimental errors. Identify **two** experimental errors that could have occurred during field trials. (*2 marks*)

▶   ii. Assuming that the 12-minute run/walk test was performed outdoors on a school field, identify some of the variables that could influence the validity and reliability of this test. *(4 marks)*

   (Total 9 marks)

3. A cycle ergometer can be used in simple fitness testing. Explain why its use in determining predicted $\dot{V}O_2$max is generally considered to be more accurate than a step test. *(8 marks)*

4. Discuss the fact that optimal body fat percentage differs between males and females at top performance level. *(8 marks)*

The following texts are recommended for further reading on physical and motor fitness testing: Adams 1998, Clegg 1996, Corbin 2002, Franks 1998, Prentice 2003 and Prentice 1998 as cited on p. 171.

4.2 Training

Learning objectives

On completion of this section, you will be able to:

1. Understand the aims and objectives of training with respect to enhancement of performance at sport or improvement of health.

2. Be familiar with the concepts of the principles of training.
   - duration
   - overload
   - regression
   - specificity
   - repetition
   - moderation
   - variance
   - individual response
   - warm-up
   - cool-down

3. Be aware of the physiological adaptations produced by aerobic and anaerobic training regimes.

4. Be aware of the neuromuscular adaptations produced by training.

5. Understand that when training stops the body regresses to fitness levels required by ongoing activities.

6. Appreciate the organisation of a training programme into a single and double periodised year.

Keywords

- ➤ aerobic adaptations
- ➤ agonist/antagonist response
- ➤ anaerobic adaptations
- ➤ bradycardia
- ➤ cool-down
- ➤ cyclical loading
- ➤ duration
- ➤ energy continuum
- ➤ frequency
- ➤ hypertrophy
- ➤ individual response
- ➤ inhibition
- ➤ intensity
- ➤ macrocycle
- ➤ mesocycle
- ➤ microcycle
- ➤ moderation
- ➤ 1 repetition maximum (1RM)
- ➤ overload
- ➤ periodisation
- ➤ progression
- ➤ regression or reversibility
- ➤ repetitions
- ➤ rest relief
- ➤ sets
- ➤ specificity
- ➤ threshold
- ➤ transfer
- ➤ variance
- ➤ warm-up

This is where the theoretical ideas involved in the discussion on the systems that provide the energy necessary for human exercise become directly related to day-to-day sporting activities. The idea is that we should use our knowledge of the scientific basis of exercise to help us improve performance at our sport and do this in a systematic and predictable way.

Unfortunately, nothing a human being does is ever thoroughly predictable and psychological, cultural and emotive factors tend to upset the true progress of science. However, it must be possible to enhance the aims of physical training by using what we know of physiology.

The aims and objectives of training are to improve performance, skill, game ability and motor and physical fitness. Some individuals will use training purely as a recreational activity in itself, in which case the outcome should be to enhance fitness and personal health without relation to any other skill or game. This latter case will not make the activity any less worthwhile but in the section below we aim to relate the needs of a sporting activity to the **extra** activities needed to enhance the quality of the sportsperson's performance.

The principles of training

Time – duration

The priority of training is that its aims must be long term. Biological, physiological, psychomotor, neuro-muscular and cardiovascular-respiratory changes all take time to develop and become consolidated within human structures.

This idea is **not** about how often or how intense the training is, since we know that light exercise or training done infrequently but regularly over a period of time has a beneficial effect on health and fitness. This is because the efficiency of the cardiovascular-respiratory systems and capability of the musculature to cope with day-to-day activities outside the sporting context are improved.

We have already discussed, and will discuss again below, how the human system responds to exercise – such **adaptive** responses do not take place instantly.

Training intensity – overload

Overload is the term used to describe training activities that are harder, more intense and/or lengthier than the normal physical activity undertaken by an individual and so this training principle applies to muscular endurance as well as to strength work.

Overload places the human system under **stress** and the human biological system responds by becoming more capable of coping with this stress. How does this happen? The following investigation gives a simple insight into one aspect of this effect.

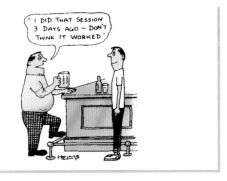

Fig. 4.17

Investigation 4.3   Response to overload in weight training

As mentioned above, it will not be possible to obtain any measurable effect of any training or exercise regime that takes place within the teaching context, i.e. within only a short period of time. It is therefore suggested that the activity described below takes place over at least 2 weeks and preferably longer.

At least two students should undertake this investigation together, so that safety procedures and monitoring of the activity of one by the other can be ensured.

Task 1 – initial assessment
1. The aim of this session is to assess the maximal strength of the student on four different exercises. These are shown in Figure 4.18.

2. The exercises have been chosen to be suitable for a multigym exercise machine. If one is not available, suitable free weight exercises should be used. If this is the case, take care over the safety of the lifter.

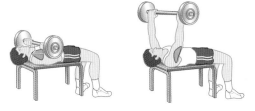

A

Fig. 4.18A Strength exercises.

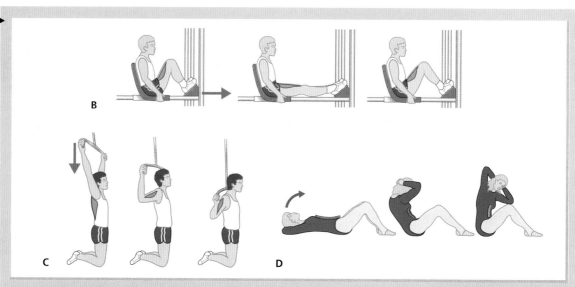

Fig. 4.18 B–D

3. Students should perform a warm-up consisting in 5 minutes jogging, 5 minutes general muscle stretching, five press-ups, five free squats and five sit-ups.

4. The exercises should be done in turn, starting at an easily achievable low level of weight or incline (sit-up) and then progressing by the smallest increases for each exercise until the student fails a lift. The highest successful lift is then recorded in Table 4.13. This lift is termed the **1 RM** or **one repetition maximum** for that exercise.

   For example, suppose the student starts at 20 kg for the bench press – he/she does this once, then progresses to 25 kg, does this once and progresses to 30 kg, does this once and so on, until

no further weight can be lifted. If the final weight actually lifted was 57.5 kg, then this would be this person's 1 RM for the bench press.

   In the case of the sit-ups, the student could begin on the flat and gradually increase the angle of the inclined sit-up board until he/she fails, the highest rung or angle achieved being recorded. Alternatively, a disc weight may be used in the same way as the other exercises and the biggest disc lifted recorded.

Task 2 – programme of exercise

1. The student then calculates 60% of the maximum and notes this in Table 4.13. This will be the load to be lifted for the first week of the programme.

Table 4.13 Results table

Session	Bench press	Leg press	Pull-down	Sit-up
assessment				
60%				
session 1				
session 2				
session 3				
final session				
final assessment				
% improvement				

▶ 2. The student performs five **sets** of six **repetitions** of each exercise at the 60% (or nearest possible below) level, with a 60-second interval between sets.

3. The schedule involves two sessions per week separated by at least 2 days; this must be continued for the period of the investigation.

Task 3 – progression
1. It will make things more interesting if the student increases the load as the weeks go by – this is called **progressive overload**.

2. This can be achieved by increasing the load by one weight on the multigym per week (or, say, 5 kg for a free weight exercise).

3. Weights lifted should be recorded in Table 4.13.

Task 4 – final assessment
1. The student should have at least 3 days' rest between the last session of the main programme and the final assessment.

2. The procedure of Task 1 above is now repeated and the resulting values of 1 RM for each exercise recorded in the final assessment row of Table 4.13.

Task 5 – analysis of results
1. Now compute the percentage improvement for each exercise and put results in the bottom row of Table 4.13.

2. Is the observed increase in measured strength a **real** increase in strength or could there be other factors enhancing the results?

3. What other noticeable effects can you observe on your body?

Task 6 – recovery after exercise
1. Comment on how your body has adapted to recovery between sets (of an exercise).

2. Make notes on breathing rates, pulse rates and whether or not you had recovered fully before the next set.

3. Did you have muscle soreness the next day?

4. What are the causes of muscle soreness (see p. 104)?

5. How could you reduce this type of muscle soreness (see p. 105)?

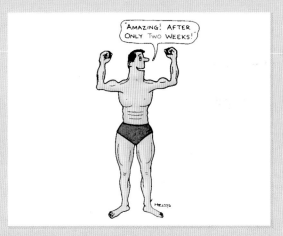

Fig. 4.19

Results of laboratory tests on strength training

Figure 4.20 shows the results of a strength training programme based on a single maximal contraction of a muscle group. Note that the measured strength gain is most rapid at the beginning of the programme, but lessens towards the sixth week; this is called 'plateauing out' and is an inevitable outcome of regular training of the same muscle groups with the same exercise.

The question is, how much of this observed strength gain is **real** and due to physiological adaptation (discussed below) and how much is a **learned response** due to use of the muscles and neuromuscular adaptation (of the brain and other parts of the nervous system)? Furthermore, would strength gain continue to increase if more stimulating and motivating exercises were substituted?

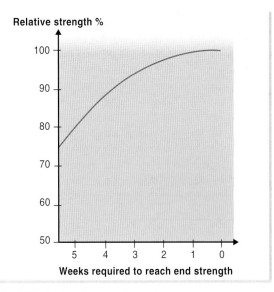

Fig. 4.20 Results of a strength training programme (after de Vries 1994[6]).

From this you will see that physiology is not the only consideration in producing training overload. Psychological and other motivational factors can contribute to making overload effective, in that the sportsperson needs to apply effort, without which overload is only apparent.

Effects of overload – adaptation

The simple investigation above aims to show the effects of stressing the body a certain way. There are many ways of stressing the body, each with different results. The effects of long-term training on the body are that physiological adaptations occur in almost every tissue or system and these changes allow the body to perform more effectively. **Overload training** significantly improves a variety of anaerobic and aerobic functional capacities, of which the most notable are discussed below.

Metabolic effects on energy systems within cells

Enhancement of the ATP-PC energy system

If exercises requiring large amounts of instant energy lasting less than 10 seconds are repeated, with full recovery between repetitions, then an adaptation occurs in which the stores of **ATP** and **PC** (and amounts of anaerobic muscle enzymes such as creatine kinase) within the muscle cell sarcoplasm are increased. This causes more energy to be available more rapidly and increases the maximum possible **peak power output** (see p. 111) of a muscle (refer to p. 95 for an explanation of the ATP-PC energy system). If the other energy systems are not stressed, then it is found that these **diminish** in comparison with the ATP-PC system.

Enhancement of the lactic anaerobic energy system

Again, if overloads are experienced for periods of up to 60 seconds (with only partial recovery between efforts), it is found that **glycogen stores** in muscle are enhanced (refer to p. 105 for an explanation of this energy system). This could be by virtue of an increase in **size** and **number** of **fast-twitch** muscle fibres and/or cells that preferentially and more rapidly store glycogen. The glycogen stores are also **more effectively utilised** through increases in the amount of glycogen-converting **enzymes** such as phosphofructokinase and glycogen phosphorylase and through increases in the enzyme lactate dehydrogenase which assists in the conversion of pyruvic acid into lactic acid as part of the glycolysis process. These enzymes are found in fast-twitch muscle fibres that control the anaerobic phase of glucose breakdown (the cells themselves being increased in size and number). This is in addition to larger amounts of ATP being stored. The **buffering capacity** of the muscle is increased because the muscle can work longer before the hydrogen ion concentration becomes sufficiently high to inhibit enzyme action and therefore inhibit muscle contraction. Such **improvements** in **anaerobic capacity** will cause performance gains.

Enhancement of the aerobic energy system

There are several major adaptations that occur in muscle as a result of aerobic training (refer to pp. 96–97 for an explanation of the aerobic energy system). Prolonged aerobic training improves the aerobic system by increasing the **number** and **size** of **mitochondria** and also the levels of mitochondrial **enzymes** in skeletal muscle, particularly within **slow-twitch** muscle fibres. This adaptation increases the ability of skeletal muscle to use oxygen at higher rates over longer periods of time.

Prolonged aerobic exercise increases **muscle glycogen stores** and the trained muscles' capacity to **mobilise** and **oxidise fats**. This is beneficial to endurance-based athletes because it conserves the carbohydrate stores (otherwise known as **glycogen sparing**) which are very important to successfully completing prolonged exercise.

The oxidative capacity of both slow-twitch and fast-twitch fibres is improved (particularly the slow-twitch fibres) as a result of an increase in muscle **myoglobin** which facilitates oxygen diffusion to the mitochondria. This is in addition to an increase in the numbers and size of mitochondria and mitochondrial oxidative enzymes mentioned above. If aerobic exercise **only** is done (i.e. a training regime with **no** fast dynamic exercises), it is found that ATP-PC stores within muscle are depleted and that toleration to lactic acid is reduced, thereby reducing the muscular capacity for strong rapid movements. This means, for example, that highly trained marathon runners rarely make good sprinters!

Threshold

This is the term used to describe the point at which the use of an energy system is exhausted (refer to Figure 4.21). The moment exercise begins for a particular muscle or group of muscles, **all mechanisms** for the remanufacture of ATP begin. Note that the residual ATP within muscle provides the immediate energy for

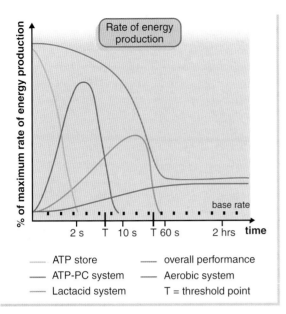

Fig. 4.21 Interrelationships of the energy systems and their threshold points.

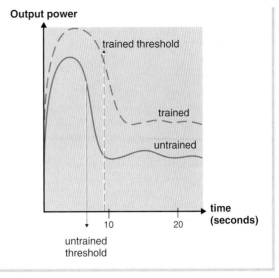

Fig. 4.22 Difference in ATP-PC to lactic thresholds between trained and untrained people.

performance but the ATP-PC system is quickly able to remanufacture this store after about 1.5 seconds. However, high-intensity exercise would deplete ATP so rapidly that the ATP-PC mechanism would be exhausted after a short period (usually less than 10 seconds). At this point, the lactic anaerobic mechanism would provide the bulk of the ATP regeneration with a consequent reduction in power output, as it takes longer for energy to become directly available to the muscle cell sarcoplasm via this system.

Under full effort, eventually (after about 45 seconds in the trained athlete) the lactic system can no longer provide enough energy for the demands made. The musculature either ceases functioning (collapse or tetanise) or requires adjustment of effort to levels compatible with aerobic functioning, so that the oxygen debt can be purged.

Figure 4.21 graphically expresses the way in which the **three** energy systems contribute to manufacture of ATP and hence overall performance level as time proceeds during full-out effort exercise. On this graph, **T** marks the points at which thresholds occur between systems, the first as the ATP-PC capability is exhausted, the second as the lactacid system becomes exhausted. Again, it should be stressed that all three systems begin operation at the beginning of the exercise but the timing and contribution (and hence the **thresholds**) of each vary between individuals and depend on the **effort** put into the exercise or on the rate at which energy is used.

It is found that thresholds are **delayed** by training, so the trained individual has greater capacity for ATP-PC and ATP regeneration, which means that high-power exercise can continue longer. This is a direct consequence of the adaptation that provides more ATP and PC in muscle sarcoplasm.

Figure 4.22 shows changes in ATP-PC to lactic thresholds between trained and untrained people. The unbroken line shows how power output at maximum effort changes with time for the untrained person. The point at which power rapidly falls is the point at which ATP-PC stores are used up and is therefore the **ATP-PC to lactic threshold** (at 7 seconds in this example).

On the other hand, the trained athlete (dashed line) has a higher maximum power output (**peak power**) and a delay in threshold (to about 10 seconds) due to larger ATP-PC stores.

Specific anaerobic adaptations to overload training

Muscle response

It is found that the most noticeable effect of **anaerobic** training in muscle fibres (particularly **fast-twitch**, which respond when large forces are applied to a given muscle) is **muscle hypertrophy**. This is due to an increase in muscle width because more actin and myosin are assimilated. This increases the strength of each fibre because more contractile protein allows for more cross-bridges to be formed (see p. 42), so the net effect is an **increase** in the **strength** of contraction. In addition, there is evidence that **more fibres** are generated, possibly by longitudinal splitting **(hyperplasia)** of existing fast-twitch fibres. The effect, therefore, is to make muscle bigger and stronger.

In highly trained anaerobic athletes, fast-twitch muscle fibres occupy a greater cross-sectional area when compared with the slow-twitch fibre content of a given muscle, whereas in highly trained aerobic athletes the reverse situation is found.

Neural response

In trained sportspersons there is a noticeable increase in the recruitment of fast-twitch motor units and improved coordination of the firing of fast-twitch motor units to allow increases in strength (see p. 34 and Investigation 4.3 above). This is in addition to the toughening of proprioceptors so that more force is required to stimulate inhibitory signals.

Specific aerobic adaptations to overload training

Vascular response

It has been found that **blood volume** and **haemoglobin** levels increase as a result of aerobic training, so the oxygen-carrying capacity of blood is enhanced. In addition, the blood supply to muscles (undertaking aerobic exercise) is enhanced by new capillaries being generated within the muscle bulk. An increase in capillary density results in a **shorter diffusion distance** between blood and muscle cells. This is in addition to increased **myoglobin** and **mitochondrial** density within slow-twitch muscle fibres. The net effect is an **increase** in the **arteriovenous oxygen difference (a-$\bar{\text{v}}$O$_2$ diff)**, as venous blood on returning from the working muscles to the heart is almost completely depleted of oxygen in the highly trained aerobic athlete (see Figure 2.30, p. 78).

A further adaptation of the vascular system is that the **smooth muscle** within artery and arteriole linings becomes stronger and more elastic (see pp. 61–63), thereby allowing greater and more efficient blood flow to working muscle. This is because the drag effect **(viscosity)** on a fluid flowing through a tube depends on the radius of the tube. Hence, the capability of a tube (artery or arteriole) to expand as the fluid (blood) flows through will reduce the drag effect, reduce peripheral resistance to blood flow and enable blood to flow more easily when under high pressure. Hence more oxygenated blood will be forced through the capillary network for tissue cell respiration.

Heart muscle is also subject to similar adaptations to the extent that capillaries within the myocardium are increased in number. Because the heart muscle **(myocardium)** is larger and stronger in the aerobically trained sportsperson (the condition known as **bradycardia**), blood flow via the coronary blood vessels to the myocardium will be substantially increased during intense exercise. This is because when the heart pumps rapidly, the myocardial tissue requires large amounts of oxygen. On the other hand, when the sportsperson is at rest, his/her heart muscle requires less oxygen than the untrained heart (since it beats much more slowly than the untrained heart) and hence blood flow to the trained heart at rest is reduced.

Bradycardia – the cardiac response

As mentioned above, one of the most obvious adaptations that occurs with endurance-based training is a **decrease** in resting **heart rate**. Endurance athletes often have resting heart rates in the low 40s (bpm). **Bradycardia** is a term that describes a reduction in heart rate to below 60 bpm. This is caused by the **enlargement** of the **heart muscle** in response to its increased rate of activity, in the same way that skeletal muscle **hypertrophy** occurs. An increase in the thickness and strength of the left ventricular wall causes an increase in the stroke volume and a lowering of resting pulse for a given cardiac output (see Figure 2.10, p. 57). This is the means by which greater blood volumes, and hence increased oxygen-carrying capacity, are available to the remaining skeletal musculature. Maximal cardiac output is increased to about the same extent as maximum stroke volume (see Figure 2.10, p. 57).

Respiratory response

In response to the demand for oxygen, more **lung alveoli** are utilised and hence the lungs have a greater surface for gaseous exchange. In addition, the **capillary network** surrounding the alveoli increases and therefore the alveolar capacity for oxygen transfer is enhanced.

Repeated aerobic exercise also has the effect of causing a slight increase in total lung capacity because the thoracic cavity becomes more capable of expanding and contracting by virtue of the increase in **strength** of the **respiratory musculature**. Furthermore, **tidal volume** (TV) is enhanced by enlarging the vital capacity at the expense of the residual volume. This enables air in larger volumes per intake (TV) to be breathed and exhaled more rapidly and has the effect of developing a more efficient breathing system and potentially **increasing** $\dot{\text{V}}$O$_2$**max.**

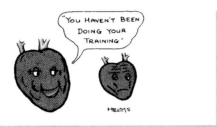

Fig. 4.23

Recovery enhancement

This is not a separate effect but more the combination of heart and lung adaptations that enable more oxygen to become available more rapidly during and immediately after exercise. Also, an enhanced capillary system supplies nutrients and glucose more efficiently to the muscle sites where they are needed. Improved oxygen recovery improves lactic acid removal, hence a reduction in muscle soreness and the more serious problem of reducing the effects of delayed onset of muscle soreness (DOMS – see p. 104).

The net effect of all these cardiovascular and respiratory aerobic training adaptations is the development of a more efficient oxygen transport system during prolonged exercise and immediately after exercise.

Muscle response

Many of the changes to slow-twitch fibres (that result from aerobic training) have been discussed above. Briefly, these adaptive responses are the result of increased myoglobin content, mitochondrial density, improved oxidation of carbohydrate (glycogen) and fat and changes within type I and type II muscle fibres (refer to Table 1.6 and Investigation 1.19).

Neural response

Better recruitment of slow-twitch motor units results in more efficient and controlled movement patterns.

General effects on tendons and other connective tissue

Aerobic and anaerobic training causes adaptations in tendons, ligaments and cartilage. **Tendon** thickness and **ligament** strength and thickness are **enhanced** by stress. This appears to be a process of gradual protein assimilation. **Articular cartilage** also becomes **thicker** and **more compressible** when large forces are repeatedly applied. This has the effect of providing more cushioning to the ends of long bones under impact.

General metabolic responses

The lactate threshold

Endurance training increases the ability of muscles to work harder and utilise more oxygen without bringing in the lactic acid energy system above the resting rate. In response to an increase in work rate above this point, the lactic acid would increase its output and muscle and blood lactate levels would rise. Endurance training therefore delays the onset of blood lactate accumulation (OBLA). Also, this type of training increases toleration of blood lactate (toleration of low blood pH – see p. 104) which means that even higher work rates can be achieved without fatigue.

Respiratory exchange ratio (RER)

The RER decreases at submaximal work rates, indicating greater use of free fatty acids. This concept is illustrated in Figure 3.20 on p. 115 and is known as **glycogen sparing**.

Sweating

Homeostasis is the maintenance of a constant internal bodily environment despite possible changes in external conditions. During exercise, the amount of heat energy produced is proportional to the intensity and duration of the exercise. The **thermoregulation centre**, which is situated in the **hypothalamus**, is sensitive to the temperature of the blood and sends out impulses to the skin, where appropriate action (for example, **sweating**) is taken. Another action is diversion of blood to the skin so that heat energy can be carried via blood from the musculature to the skin, where it is radiated away.

Sweating is therefore an evolutionary development that enables the human body to maintain approximately constant temperature. This is necessary because of the inefficient transformation of chemical energy to useful work energy in the musculature which creates so much unwanted heat.

Sweating provides moisture which evaporates from the skin surface. The energy required for this process is extracted from the skin, which therefore loses heat energy and cools down. This response is again

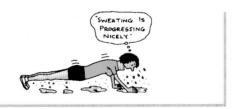

Fig. 4.24

subject to adaptation when the body generates more heat as more exercise is done. Therefore, the capability of sweat production is enhanced by training.

Gender differences in adaptations to training overload

Females tend to have lower levels of lactic acid in their blood following very heavy exercise than do males, which suggests that the capacity of female muscle for glycolysis is lower. This is one reason why females perform less well in high-power activities. However, most other differences seem to be related to body size and the fact that females on average are 15–25% smaller than males. For example, $\dot{V}O_2$max for total body mass in females is lower by this amount and this is due to females having less haemoglobin, less blood volume, smaller hearts and smaller lungs than males. However, $\dot{V}O_2$max measured per kilogram of body mass, and hence aerobic capacity for trained people, is comparable between males and females.

Investigation 4.4 Summary of adaptations to anaerobic and aerobic training

Task 1 Summarise the effects of physical exercise training-induced adaptations in Table 4.14

Table 4.14 Summary of expected anaerobic and aerobic physiological adaptations due to overload training

	Skeletal muscle	Soft tissues	Neural	Vascular	Cardiac	Respiratory
Anaerobic						
Aerobic						
General						

	Metabolic responses		Others
	Energy systems	General	
Anaerobic			
Aerobic			
General			

Task 2
Optional activity: place any other responses to training not covered in this book in the column headed 'Others'.

Regression or reversibility

It has been found that all the effects of training mentioned above revert or **regress** to their normal untrained state if training ceases. Interestingly, it is found that effects established by longer periods of training remain for longer after training stops. Figure 4.25 shows an example of this.

In Figure 4.25, time is measured from the point at which training stops, which is when peak performance is observed. What is found is that exercise regimes that begin a long time before this point (A on the graph) enable the body to retain the increased fitness for a long time after training stops. On the other hand, when training begins only a short while beforehand (B on the graph), even though high levels of performance may be achieved, fitness levels fall quickly after training stops.

This is because biological adaptation is a long-term process and most of the adaptations mentioned above take months or years to establish (A). Once established, these adaptations promote greater general and specific fitness which will remain with the sportsperson even if exercise stops. Eventually, most adaptations would return to the untrained state but again this would be a long-term process. Conversely, although intense daily

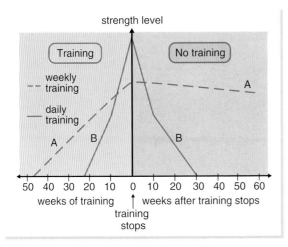

strength level

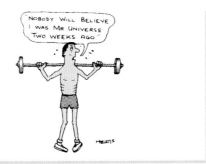

Fig. 4.25 Regression after training is stopped (after Hettinger 1961[7]).

Fig. 4.26

Table 4.15 Approximate percentage of contribution of aerobic and anaerobic energy sources in selected physical activities (adapted from reference[8])			
	% Emphasis according to energy system		
Sport/activity	ATP-PC and LA	LA–O$_2$	O$_2$
Basketball	60	20	20
Fencing	90	10	–
Field events	90	10	–
Golf swing	95	5	–
Gymnastics	80	15	5
Hockey	50	20	30
Long-distance running	10	20	70
Rowing	20	30	50
Skiing	33	33	33
Soccer	50	20	30
Sprints	90	10	–
Swimming 1500 m	10	20	70
Tennis	70	20	10
Volleyball	80	5	15

training can increase performance dramatically over a short period (B), there are no longer term biological adaptations which would maintain fitness once exercise stopped.

Specificity

This principle refers to the **relevance** of the **choice** of exercise to the activity to be improved. Choices to be made involve energy, strength, power, endurance and skill. This notion is thought to be very important for high performance in a chosen sport.

Energy systems

Which energy system is to be emphasised and therefore developed (see Table 4.15)? The main problem here concerns the accuracy of the percentage contributions. The values in Table 4.15 are approximate in value because it is very difficult to collect appropriate data accurately. The important point to stress when using Table 4.15 is that specific training programmes can be constructed. However, in activities that last

for longer than 3 minutes and in all game situations, quick bursts of highly intense activity are often interspersed with much longer periods of low activity. Therefore there is a need to develop aerobic conditioning with the ability to use the anaerobic mechanisms of energy supply when necessary.

Strength, power or endurance

Which type of muscle fibre is to be stressed and therefore made more efficient: fast-twitch for stronger, faster, more dynamic movements or slow-twitch for steady, low-force aerobic work?

Skill to be practised

Skills relevant to the sporting activity will need to be learnt. Perhaps some of the strength and/or endurance training can be done while skills are being practised.

The inference here is that the actual parts of the body to be used in the sport are to be stressed preferentially, leading to a direct improvement in the sport. This implies not only that their biology will be changed but that **skill learning** will occur. Such learning is a product of the development of a **link** between the use of muscles and a **stimulus** and also the development of more efficient use of the muscles in a sequence required by the stimulus. These changes occur in the brain and other parts of the nervous system.

Investigation 4.5   Training to learn a skill

Materials: tape measure, cones, stopwatch and relevant games equipment.

Choose one of the following activities:

1. **Soccer** (or field hockey): dribbling with the non-preferred foot (or reverse sticks for hockey).

2. **Tennis** (or other racket game): striking a ball with the non-preferred hand.

Note: non-preferred means the limb not normally used for the game. We assume ambidextrous people don't exist.

Soccer or hockey: complete a course dribbling the ball **entirely** with the non-preferred foot (or reverse sticks). The course could be set up using cones and lines as in Figure 4.27. The course would be completed twice and timed. (You may wish to adapt the distance between the cones depending on the availability of space.)

Tennis: hit a ball (completely free supply of balls) into a 1 metre square marked on the gymnasium wall positioned 1 metre from the floor, as in Figure 4.28. This should be done if possible by hit and return. If the hit ball goes astray, the player should be fed another ball to continue the exercise.

This should be done for **30 seconds** at each of 3 m, 6 m and 9 m from the wall, the total number of accurate hits being recorded.

Task 1 – initial assessment

1. The chosen activity should be completed and the score recorded in Table 4.16.

2. This should be done in pairs, with the non-active student recording time and/or score and, in the

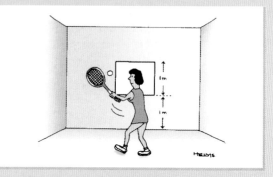

Fig. 4.28

case of tennis, feeding balls when necessary. He/she should also check that the non-preferred limb is used.

Task 2 – skill practice
The activity is repeated at least five times in 2 weeks (a total of six times in all) and the times and/or scores recorded in Table 4.16.

Task 3 – discussion of results

1. Have the scores improved over the period of the test?

2. If so, what factors have led to the improvement?

3. What other drills could you invent to enhance the skill chosen?

Table 4.16 Results table	
Session	*Time/score*
1	
2	
3	
4	
5	
6	

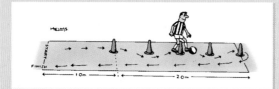

Fig. 4.27

Other changes that occur when muscles are used

Transfer

This is the idea that learning one skill will enhance the learning capability for another skill. For example, the practice of the skill of catching and throwing a ball rapidly and accurately may improve the sportsperson's ability to hit a ball with a racket firmly and accurately. This is discussed in more detail in Part 2, p. 340.

The agonist/antagonist response

There is evidence that when a muscle is used, its **inhibition** to use is lessened. This enables more fibres to be activated and more force to be exerted. The antagonist is able to stretch without inhibition as the stretch reflex is repressed. This means that movements will become more fluent and less jerky as they are practised. The normal awkwardness of the first attempt at a skill is in part due to contraction of antagonists when they should be relaxing.

Body awareness

With repeated use of the musculature, even without a skill-related learning element (as in weight training), it becomes possible to learn complex skills more easily. The sportsperson becomes aware of how to operate certain muscle groups efficiently and can relate this to certain skill demands.

Repetition

This principle underlies both overload and specificity. It seems essential to **repeat** an activity, both to apply stress in suitable amounts and to learn skills to a suitable degree of expertise. Generally speaking, it seems that the more often a system is stressed, the more rapidly it adapts to the stress. The **frequency** with which the exercise is repeated is therefore an important element of training.

Moderation – injury

Unfortunately, the biggest cause of injury in the fit sportsperson is overtraining. Initially, most people find that training produces very noticeable effects on health and fitness, so it is tempting to increase overloads rapidly. If this process continues indefinitely, eventually the musculature and more probably other soft tissue (tendons, ligaments or cartilage, which take longer to adapt to increased stress) break down and injury occurs.

There is obviously a limit to what the body can cope with. The aim of training is to increase this limit without exceeding it. Therefore it makes sense to apply the overload principle gradually and with moderation.

Variance

The idea of variance is that training loads and skill demands should be varied with time. It is thought that this principle provides a very important element for the training of the elite performer. There are two sets of reasons for this, physiological and psychological.

Physiological reasons

The effects of repeated and prolonged stress on biological systems are:

- fatigue
- depletion of energy reserves
- raising of response threshold to stimulus (muscles do not respond as they ought)
- muscle soreness
- injury.

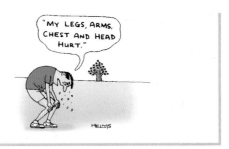

Fig. 4.29

It would therefore seem sensible to vary loads so that none of these factors causes regression.

Psychological reasons

Varying training patterns and loads tends to:

- remove the emotive stress of coping with large amounts of exhausting and painful work
- enable learning and activity targets to be reassessed
- improve motivation.

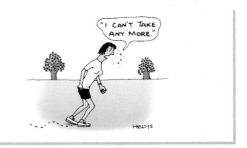

Fig. 4.30

Periodisation

Periodisation is a concept which is centred around a **cyclical load** design principle and enables the coach to vary intensity, duration and frequency of activity in a structured plan. Most training programmes will have medium- and long-term aims lasting, for example, 1 year and 4 years in the case of a sportsperson wanting to compete in the Olympic Games. Periodisation is based on the idea of developing sports performance capacity in **stages** and hence the development of general and specific fitness in stages. Each stage of development is referred to as a **cycle**.

When the programme extends over the whole training year with competitive aims in a single season, it is referred to as a **single periodised year** which in this case is divided into three periods:

1. **preparatory** period
2. **competition** period
3. **transition** period

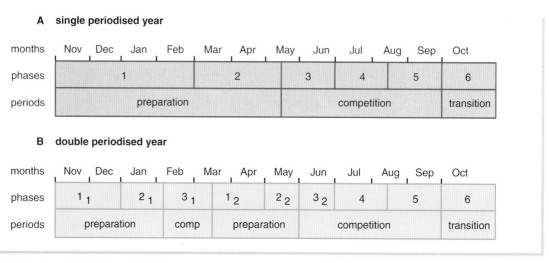

Fig. 4.31 A. Single and B. double periodised year.

In Figure 4.31A we show an example for a sports-person with a summer competitive season. The **single** periodised year is broken down into these three periods, each of which is subdivided into further cycles or stages. **Macrocycles** last from 4 to 6 weeks, **mesocycles** about 2 weeks and **microcycles** typically 1 week (daily cycles consisting of 1–3 sessions might be required). Each cycle would have specific aims in respect of skill learning and fitness and would aim to improve overall performance and prepare for a specific competitive peak.

Figure 4.31B shows how a training programme could be organised for a **double** periodised year, in which **two** competitive seasons are planned and therefore two peaks of skill and fitness required.

Figure 4.32 shows how a **microcyle** could be organised in terms of **variation** of training loads.

Investigation 4.10 (pp. 160–161) will lead you into the process of designing a training programme based on these principles.

Individual response

This training principle reflects the fact that no two individuals have the same training needs. The factors that need to be taken into account when designing a training programme are described below.

Fitness needs

Individuals will have differing fitness levels which mean that a different emphasis needs to be placed on the different fitness factors (endurance, strength or power) in training programmes aimed at the same sport. Fitness levels can be determined by a fitness testing assessment (see Section 4.1), which should also include measuring body composition.

Psychological needs

These include motivation, self-image, self-esteem and so on. The personal importance of these needs varies greatly between individuals.

Training should be organised so that clear goals are set and realistic targets for attainment agreed and understood.

Maturation

The individual's stage of development should be taken into account. It can be dangerous to subject physically immature people to high training loads. On the other hand, certain activities seem best learnt when young

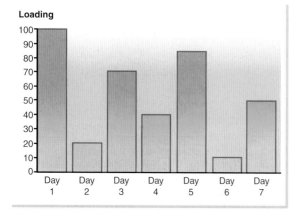

Fig. 4.32 Variation in loading over a microcycle.

and there is evidence that physical skill learning is a much slower process for older individuals.

Male/female

Size and strength are usually less in the female and therefore loads need to be adjusted accordingly. Menstruation can affect training loads, since there are body weight fluctuations as a result of monthly hormonal variations. There is also evidence that hormonal changes can affect joint stability. Generally, however, these effects are less important than size differences.

Cultural differences

Different attitudes to exercise and its place in one's lifestyle can play an important part in the effectiveness of training.

This applies particularly to female participation. Partner role, career prospects and self-image about size and muscularity still seem to be different between male and female sportspersons. The difference varies widely between societies and cultures. Roll on equal opportunities!

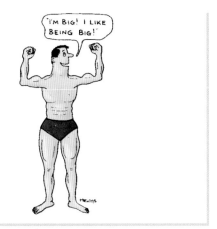

Fig. 4.33

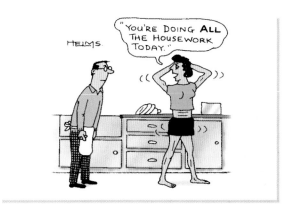

Fig. 4.34

Warm-up and cool-down

The final principles of training discussed here are preparation of the body for exercise and what to do immediately after exercise to minimise the risk of injury and muscle soreness.

Warm-up

Although anaerobic work can be done without using the oxygen-carrying and delivery capacity of the cardiovascular system, replenishment of ATP and muscle glycogen depends on an efficient blood capillary system. Therefore, recovery from the oxygen debt is improved if light aerobic exercise is undertaken before training. This dilates capillaries and raises the pulse rate, pumping blood around the body more quickly.

A further effect of warm-up is to raise the body temperature. It has been shown that ATP conversion, glycolytic enzyme action and muscle reaction response times are quicker at a slightly higher temperature.

Also, blood viscosity is slightly reduced at higher temperatures, so that the flow of blood (and its ability to pass through the capillary system) is improved. It is also found that light muscle stretching prepares the musculature for operation over its full range.

It is also found that an effective warm-up reduces the risk of injury.

Cool-down

It seems important to do a small amount of aerobic work immediately after completion of a training session. This has the purpose of flushing the capillary system with oxygenated blood, thereby enabling oxygen debt in muscles to be fully purged and lactic products of lactic anaerobic work to be converted and removed. This limits muscle soreness and enhances recovery.

1. a. What is meant by the **overload principle** as applied to anaerobic training programmes? (*8 marks*)

   b. Briefly explain how an organised fitness programme results in training effects. (*4 marks*)

   (*Total 12 marks*)

2. a. What is meant by **reversibility** of training effects? (*2 marks*)

   b. When an appropriate training programme stops, describe what happens to the cardiovascular system which helps to explain the reversibility of endurance training effects. (*7 marks*)

   c. Fast ball games require players to make quick decisions to cues and respond immediately with powerful movements. When training stops, what happens to the muscles and the nervous system which helps to explain the reversibility of these aspects of fitness? (*5 marks*)

   d. Compared with the effects of a continuous training programme, explain why it is possible to improve sports performance when training is resumed after a rest due to injury, despite the reversibility of training effects which will have occurred during the rest period. (*4 marks*)

   (*Total 18 marks*)

3. From a physiological standpoint, explain why warm-up and cool-down are important within an exercise programme. (*6 marks*)

4. 'Not all footballers are necessarily fit.' Discuss this statement in relation to **specificity** of training. (*10 marks*)

5. a. Define the concept of **periodisation** and identify **two** main objectives of such planning. (*4 marks*)

   b. Using the information in Figure 4.31A, prepare a single periodised year for a named winter sport. (*6 marks*)

   c. Individual periods are divided into macrocycles, mesocycles and microcycles. What advantage is there in choosing shorter mesocycles? (*3 marks*)

   (*Total 13 marks*)

For further reading on training, refer to texts cited on p. 171.

4.3 Types of training

On completion of this section, you will be able to:

1. Understand that continuous training methods mainly utilise and enhance aerobic energy systems.

2. Apply the concept of interval training to the development of all types of energy systems, its organisation in terms of repetitions, sets and intervals and how intervals are measured.

3. Understand the concepts of weight training as an intervalised progressive resistance form of training, some of the exercises used, how they can be used to enhance the different energy systems and the safety problems associated with this type of training.

4. Recall the organisation and principles of circuit, stage, mobility and skill-related training.

5. Construct a training programme for your personal fitness needs or those of a chosen sport.

6. Understand the effects on the body of a reduction in the partial pressure of oxygen in atmospheric air.

7. Understand the changes brought about by acclimatisation to altitude and the beneficial effects to the athlete competing at altitude.

8. Understand the benefits of altitude training on sea-level performance.

9. Discuss the issue of ergogenic aids in relation to performance.

Keywords

- ➤ acclimatisation
- ➤ active mobility
- ➤ altitude training
- ➤ barometric pressure
- ➤ blood doping
- ➤ circuit training
- ➤ continuous training
- ➤ duration
- ➤ ergogenic aids
- ➤ erythropoietin (EPO)
- ➤ frequency
- ➤ intensity
- ➤ interval
- ➤ interval training
- ➤ kinetic/ballistic mobility
- ➤ mobility training
- ➤ passive mobility
- ➤ proprioceptive neuromuscular facilitation (PNF)
- ➤ repetition
- ➤ rest relief
- ➤ safety
- ➤ set
- ➤ stage training

The following two investigations attempt to bring out the essential differences between types of training.

Investigation 4.6   Continuous training – jogging or swimming

Task 1 – initial assessment

1. Students should work in groups of at least two people, so that conversation can be held during the exercise. For the purposes of this investigation, the jogging should be done as quickly as is allowed by the holding of a conversation – hard breathing without breathlessness should be aimed at. A similar breathing regime should be adopted for swimming. This will stress your body's aerobic energy systems and we expect some adaptations to occur that will enhance aerobic capacity.

2. Pulse rate (beats per minute (bpm)) and respiration rate (breaths per minute (f)) are recorded before starting. Pulse rate is then recorded for the first 15 seconds after finishing and then for 15seconds after a rest of 60 seconds. Results are recorded in Table 4.17.

3. The initial jog is one mile (1600 m) in 10 minutes (the distance is a guide; the time is what is required), or a swim (any stroke) of 10 minutes.

This forms an initial assessment of pulse rates and recovery rate.

Task 2 – the exercise

1. The same measures are taken for three further sessions (at the times or approximate distances shown in Table 4.17) spread over a minimum of 2 weeks. Results should be recorded in Table 4.17.

2. Now work out the recovery rate for each session. Recovery rate can be expressed as:

Recovery rate = (pulse rate (bpm) at end of run/swim) – (pulse rate (bpm) after 60 s rest)

Recovery rate results should be recorded in Table 4.17.

Task 3 – conclusions

1. What effects are observed after the last session?

2. Make a direct comparison between the first and last sessions. Are any improvements found in either recovery or ability of the cardiovascular and respiratory systems to cope with the exercise?

Table 4.17 Results table

Pulse rate before activity (bpm)	Respiration rate before activity (f)	Approx. length of swim	Time to be taken	Approx. length of run	Pulse rate at finish (bpm)	Pulse rate 60 s after finish (bpm)	Recovery rate
		metres	min	metres			
		250	10	1600			
		375	15	2400			
		500	20	3200			
		250	10	1600			

Continuous exercise

Exercise regimes lasting longer than 60 seconds, involving low forces and where breathing is comfortable are essentially aerobic. The following types of exercise fall into this category:

- jogging, variation by changing distance and speed (as illustrated in Investigation 4.6)

- swimming, variation by changing stroke, distance and speed (Investigation 4.6)
- aerobics (a means of total body exercise, aerobically)
- rowing
- game or skill simulations without full effort
- fartlek – speed play without full effort.

Investigation 4.7 Interval training

Task 1 – sprint and/or swim interval training

1. The following session is attempted four times in 2 weeks. At least two students are needed to monitor each other's timing. The session is:

Running sprints

a. Five repetitions of a 40 m sprint with a 30-second interval between repetitions. (This is written as 5 × 40 m sprint at 30 seconds and is called a set.)

b. Followed by 5 minutes at rest.

c. Followed by a further set of 5 × 60 m sprints with 60-second intervals or rest relief.

Swimming

a. Five repetitions of 50 m (flat-out, choice of stroke), with a 30-second interval between repetitions.

b. Followed by 5 minutes at rest.

c. Followed by a further set of five repetitions at 75 m, with 60-second intervals.

These sessions will stress the lactic acid anaerobic energy system for the muscle groups involved and we will look for adaptations to thresholds and oxygen debt recovery.

2. Pulse rates are taken (for 15 seconds and then multiplied by four to obtain pulse count/bpm) before the session and immediately after completion of the exercise. A further count is taken after 60 seconds at rest and counts are entered in Table 4.18.

3. Now work out the recovery rate for each session (refer to p.150) and record results in Table 4.18.

Task 2 – results analysis

1. Have recovery rates been enhanced by this training regime? Use evidence from Table 4.18 to support your answer.

2. Identify the changes that occur in muscle which might reduce fatigue levels during this high-intensity exercise.

3. Discuss the long-term physiological effects of anaerobic sprint training on the human body.

4. Are there any advantages of this training system over the continuous exercise method?

Table 4.18 Results table

Session	Pulse rate before exercise (bpm)	Pulse rate at finish (bpm)	Pulse rate 60 s after finish (bpm)	Recovery rate
1				
2				
3				
4				

Interval training

As can be seen from Investigation 4.7, **interval training** is characterised by **repetitions** with an **interval** of time between; these are organised in **sets**, with a longer period of time between the sets (the rest period between sets is called **rest relief**). Figure 4.35 (p. 149) shows typical variations of a number of physiological indicators during interval training.

Figure 4.35 shows that this method can be more effective in establishing levels of fitness, and therefore biological changes, than the continuous exercise method. This is because of the repeated high-level stressing of anaerobic systems for energy production and the forcing of repetitions before full recovery is achieved (i.e. applying stress upon stress).

The idea can be used for acquiring fitness, utilising both anaerobic and aerobic energy mechanisms.

Types of training incorporating the interval concept include:

- weight training
- circuit training
- stage training
- sprint training
- endurance training
- training for a game utilising game skills but composed of sets and repetitions.

Examples of endurance training for 5000 metre runners could be:

- 4 × 1500 m at 80% 5000 m pace with 5 min intervals
- 20 × 400m in 65 s with 20 s intervals
- 3 × (8 × 200 m) with 30 s rest relief and 5 min between sets.

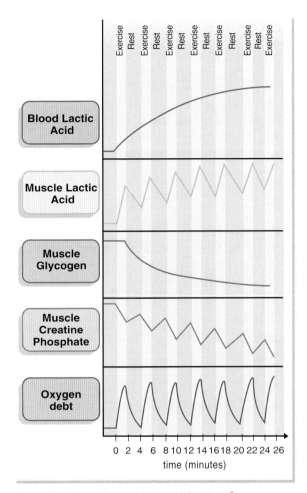

Fig. 4.35 Effects of interval training (after Lamb[9]).

Measurement of intervals

We have already mentioned the idea of using time for measuring the interval between repetitions and sets. Another way is to assess the pulse rate of the sportsperson immediately after a repetition. The next repetition is then begun when the pulse rate falls to a predetermined percentage of its value at the end of the effort or to a value set beforehand (say, 120 bpm).

For example, if the sportsperson has a pulse rate of 180 bpm at the end of an effort, then the next repetition would begin when his/her pulse rate falls to 70% of this value, i.e. 126 bpm.

This means that pulse rate needs to be continually monitored by the sportsperson after each exercise effort. This has the advantage that the interval is individualised and related to the person's recovery rate. As training progresses and the sportsperson becomes fitter, recovery rates become faster and the intervals smaller. This obviously enhances fitness even further, since now the individual is doing the same amount of work in a shorter time.

Training heart rate – the Karvonen method[9]

A training heart rate can be established by using the concept of maximal heart rate reserve, otherwise know as the **Karvonen method**. Maximal heart rate (HR_{max}) is calculated by this method using:

$$HR_{max} = 220 - age \text{ (of the performer)}$$

Maximal heart rate reserve ($HR_{max}R$) is then calculated using:

$$HR_{max}R = HR_{max} - HR_{rest}$$

where HR_{rest} is the resting heart rate of the performer.

Thus a training heart rate (THR – the heart rate at which optimal aerobic training effects can take place during continuous training) can be calculated by taking a percentage of the maximal heart rate reserve and adding it to the resting heart rate. For example, a training heart rate at 75% of maximal heart rate reserve would be calculated as follows:

$$THR_{75\%} = HR_{rest} + 0.75(HR_{max} - HR_{rest})$$

This gives a THR% which is approximately the same as the heart rate corresponding to 75% of the $\dot{V}O_{2max}$ at this exercise level.

Karvonen[9] suggests that an aerobic training zone of between 60% and 75% of maximal heart rate reserve should be used when designing aerobic training programmes for most athletes. The benefit of using a training heart rate range is that it confirms that work is being done at the correct intensity to ensure a training response and that a progression through the range of training heart rate percentages can be planned as the athlete improves his/her aerobic fitness.

Training activities – weight training

There are a range of activities under this heading, the basic features of which are:

- **exercises** with intervals arranged in repetitions and sets

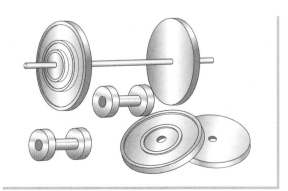

Fig. 4.36 Barbell, dumbbell and discs.

- **progressive resistance** exercises, in which the load can be increased by increasing either the forces applied or the number of repetitions.

Equipment that can be used includes:

- **free weights** with barbell, dumbbells and discs (Figure 4.36)

- **exercise machines** of the multigym or Nautilus type in which slotted weights are moved by levers (Figures 4.37 and 4.38)
- **hydraulic exercise machines** in which a system of levers operates a hydraulic dash pot, which can be set for different forces
- exercises using **body weight** as the load (see Figure 4.40).

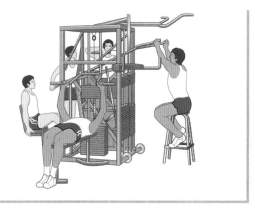

Fig. 4.37 Exercise machine.

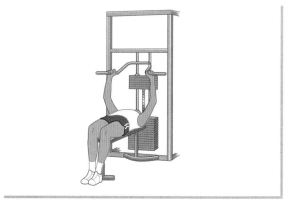

Fig. 4.38 Exercise machine.

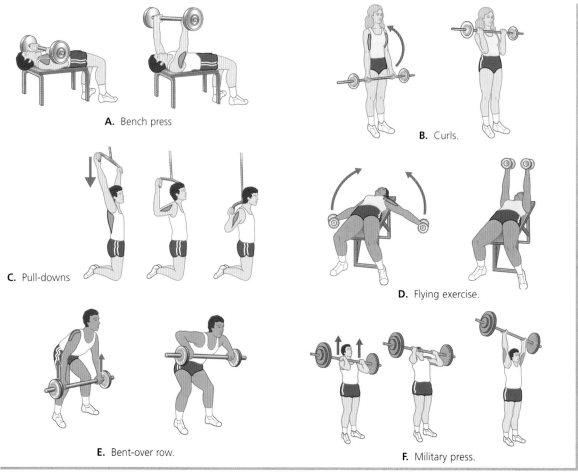

A. Bench press

B. Curls.

C. Pull-downs

D. Flying exercise.

E. Bent-over row.

F. Military press.

Fig. 4.39A–D Shoulders and arms.

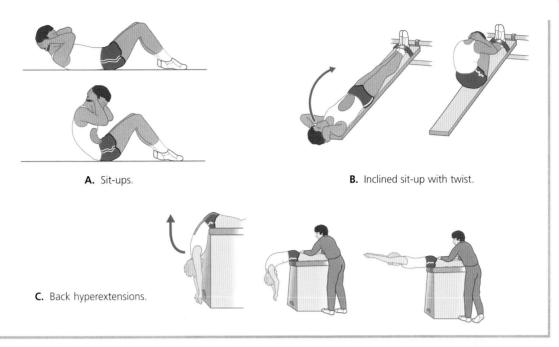

A. Sit-ups.

B. Inclined sit-up with twist.

C. Back hyperextensions.

Fig. 4.40 Trunk and back.

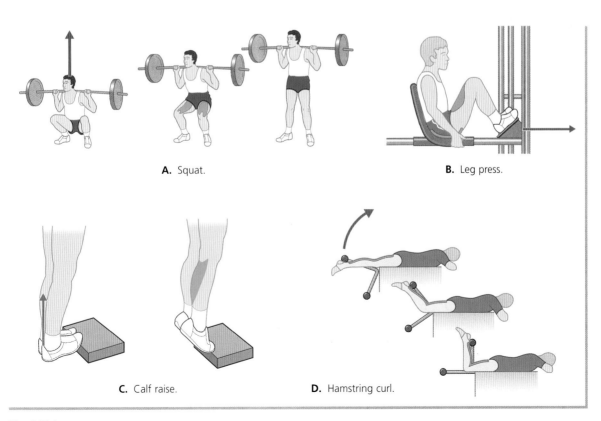

A. Squat.

B. Leg press.

C. Calf raise.

D. Hamstring curl.

Fig. 4.41 Legs.

The exercises

Exercises are usually classified into four groups, from which a few examples are given in Figures 4.39–4.42. If you need to know about more exercises than are shown here, refer to a specialist text on weight training (for example, references[11,12]).

'All-body' exercises

a. **Power clean** (Figure 4.42).

b. **Snatch**: the snatch is a variation of the same technique as the clean, except that the bar is lifted overhead to arm's length in a single movement.

c. **Dead lift**: the bar is again picked up in the same manner as the clean but the bar is lifted to thigh level only, with arms held straight at all times.

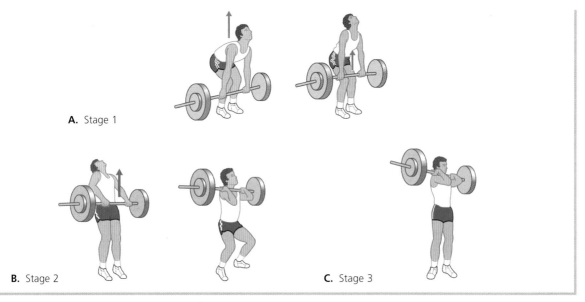

A. Stage 1

B. Stage 2

C. Stage 3

Fig. 4.42 Power clean.

Safety

First, it should be said that certain exercises can be dangerous if not performed correctly, particularly those in which the back is used (power clean, snatch, squat and dead lift). It is important for students to be aware that loadings at these exercises should be low until the skills of the activities are learnt.

Further injury can result from dropping the bars and discs on to the weight trainer. It is therefore essential for weight trainers to train in groups and to evolve a safety 'catching' protocol, wherever this danger is a possibility (exercises for which this is particularly important are the bench press, snatch, squat and military press).

Some exercises can involve very large loadings and can be dangerous if too large a weight is attempted (squat and bench press, for example).

Frequency and intensity

The beauty of weight training is that almost any combination of exercises can be chosen (specifically related to the sporting activity for which the training is being done), with any combination of load and repetitions.

If 100% represents the maximal force that can be exerted (see Investigation 4.3) for any given exercise, then the loadings and repetitions relevant to different requirements are suggested in the following. These suggestions are examples of how an exercise regime can be organised to develop a particular energy system; there are many other possibilities.

Alactic (ATP-PC) anaerobic energy system: fast-twitch muscle fibres

a. ● Three to five sets of up to six repetitions per set – between 80% and 100% load

- with full (60 s) recovery intervals between sets
- two to three times per week.
b. • Three sets of very fast dynamic work at 10–15 repetitions per set
- 60% load
- full recovery intervals
- three to four times per week.

Lactic anaerobic energy system: fast-twitch muscle fibres

a. • Five sets of 4–6 repetitions per set
- 80% load
- 60 s recovery
- three times per week.
b. • Five sets of 6–10 repetitions per set
- 60–80% load
- restricted intervals (60 s)
- two to three times per week.
c. • Three sets of 20 repetitions per set
- 50% load

- full recovery intervals
- three to five times per week.

Aerobic energy system: slow-twitch muscle fibres

Any exercise done slowly at less than 50% load; most training programmes would have between 10 and 20 repetitions per set.

- Three sets of 20 repetitions per set
- 40% load
- short recovery – 20–30 seconds
- three to five times per week.

Choice of exercise

It is usual to choose exercises that:

- relate to the muscle groups used in the sport
- exercise the antagonists to these muscle groups
- give all-round body fitness.

Investigation 4.8   The effects of circuit training

This investigation attempts to introduce the concepts of **circuit training** and its offshoot **stage training** (see Figure 4.43), within a mini fitness programme.

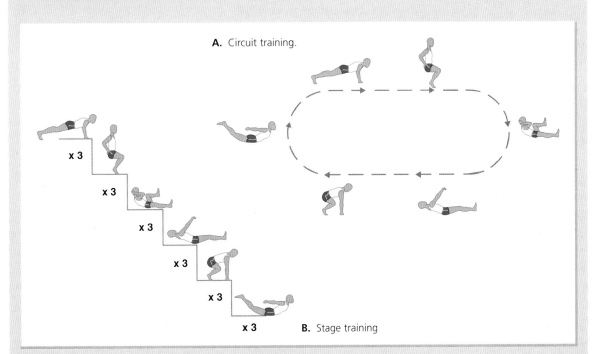

A. Circuit training.

x 3
x 3
x 3
x 3
x 3
x 3

B. Stage training

Fig. 4.43 Training regimens.

Task 1 – the exercises

1. As its name implies, circuit training involves a **circuit** of exercises (which could be the same ones mentioned in the section on weight training). The circuit is organised so that the different exercises are done one after the other, instead of in multiple sets of the same exercise (see Figure 4.43A).

2. So, for our example, we choose the body-weight exercises in Figure 4.44 for our circuit.

3. Sessions consist of a warm-up followed by one set each of press-ups, sit-ups, free squats, squat thrusts, pulls to bar and back hyperextensions – this would be one **circuit** of exercises.

4. Three circuits are then completed without rest between circuits.

Task 2 – determination of repetitions

1. Students should work in pairs, one scoring and timing the exercises while the other does the training.

2. The first session is used to assess the number of repetitions possible in 30 seconds for each exercise.

So, the exercises are done in turn for 30 seconds, with 3 minutes' rest between each exercise. The count is recorded in Table 4.19.

Task 3 – the training

1. Two further sessions are now done, with three circuits per session (as explained above). Each session is done continuously at **half** the 30-second loading per exercise.

2. For example, if the student achieves 30 press-ups in his 30-second assessment, he will perform 15 press-ups on each circuit (and so on for the other exercises).

3. Times for the second and third sessions are recorded. The aim is to improve on times.

Task 4 – final assessment

1. Repeat Task 2, record reassessed 30-second counts for each exercise in the 'session 4' row of Table 4.19.

2. This should be done at least 3 days after the previous session.

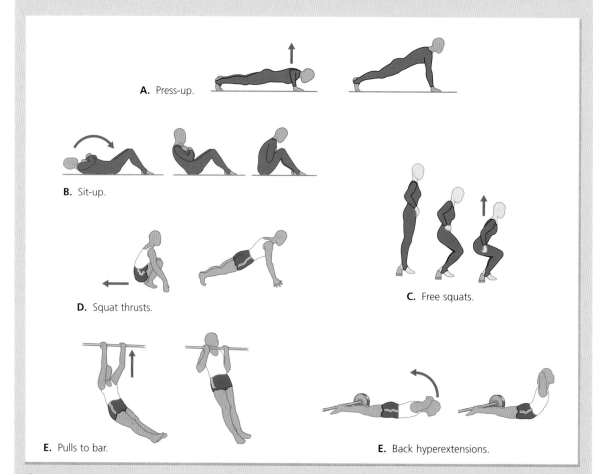

A. Press-up.

B. Sit-up.

D. Squat thrusts.

C. Free squats.

E. Pulls to bar.

E. Back hyperextensions.

Fig. 4.44 Circuit training.

▶ **Task 5 – conclusion**

1. What improvement has been made over the short period of this investigation?

2. What other measures could be taken to assess improved fitness?

3. Which energy system does this type of training develop?

4. What has been the effect of this type of training on your body?

Stage training (see Figure 4.43B)

This investigation could be modified by organising the exercises in sets with the same exercise (at one-third of the number of repetitions found in the initial 30-second test) done three times at 15-second intervals before moving to the next exercise. Stage training tends to stress the lactic acid energy system more than straight circuit training. It should be possible to detect differences between two groups of students, one performing circuits, the other performing stage training.

Table 4.19 Results table

Session	Press-up	Sit-up	Free squat	Squat thrust	Pulls to bar	Back hyper.
1						
2						
3						
4						

Time for session 2 =   min sec   Time for session 3 =   min   sec

Other circuit training exercises

Circuits can be organised using any combination of exercises that give all-body fitness; other exercises not already mentioned include:

- star jumps, bar jumping, straddle jumps to bench, full star jumps, bunny hops, shuttle runs, step-ups, box jumps, sergeant jumps
- bench dips, burpees, alternate dumbbell press, chins, rope climbs, V sit-ups, hip thrusts, chinnies, alternate-leg squat thrusts.

Categories of muscle use

The bulk of the discussion above has involved **muscle contractions**, in which the exercise is achieved by contracting the agonist (muscle that produces the desired body movement) more or less rapidly, depending on how vigorously the exercise is done and what the loading is.

It is possible, however, to exercise a muscle in several different ways, with different effects on strength gain (these aspects were discussed in detail in Chapter 1, p. 20, and Investigation 4.3, p. 133):

- **static contractions – isometric exercise**
- **concentric contractions – isotonic and isokinetic exercise**
- **eccentric contractions – plyometric exercises.**

During **static** contractions, the type of effort predominantly affects the ATP-PC anaerobic system. The main advantage of this **isometric** work is that it causes muscles to enlarge (**hypertrophy**). For further muscle development the training programme should include working the joint throughout a range of angles. However, despite the physiological benefits of increases in size and strength of muscles, the isometric training method does not enhance aerobic power and endurance, nor elevate heart rate values, to the same degree as does dynamic exercise. Whereas for **concentric** and **eccentric contractions**, the physiological benefits include increased capillarisation of skeletal and cardiac muscle tissues, improved **pulmonary** functioning and many other cardiovascular **adaptations** mentioned herein.

Track intervals

As discussed above, any exercise organised in **repetitions** and **sets** with time intervals between them (such time intervals are called **rest relief**) comes under the general heading of **interval training**. The proportions of interval training that develop the different energy systems are set out in Table 4.20 and linked to the athletic event for which they are most suitable.

Table 4.20 Percentage aerobic/anaerobic work within different interval training regime

Activity	% Aerobic	% Anaerobic
Continuous running	90	10
Fartlek running	75	25
Long slow running	60	40
Short fast intervals	40	60
Repetition intervals	25	75
Sprint running	10	90

Mobility training

The purpose of mobility training is not to enhance energy production muscles but to improve (or maintain) the **range of movement** over which muscles can act and joints can operate.

This works on the **stress–overload principle** in the same way as other types of training, only now the biological response is to make a muscle capable of operating more efficiently over a larger range of joint movement. This happens by **inhibiting** the **stretch reflex** (refer to p. 35) and by forcing the contraction processes to operate in conditions of full stretch, thereby bringing into play more contractile fibres.

It has been found that mobility training is best undertaken at the end of an anaerobic session, during cool down. This is because the muscular system is usually more relaxed at this time, with muscle temperatures slightly higher than during the warm-up phase of training. It has also been found that power training is less effective if performed after extensive mobility training.

Investigation 4.9 Mobility training

Task 1 – initial assessment
1. The four mobility tests shown in Figure 4.45 are completed.

2. Results are recorded in Table 4.21.

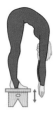

A. Hamstring stretch: distance of fingertips below soles of feet is measured.

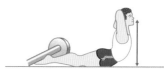

B. Spinal hyperextension: feet are held and height of nose above floor is measured

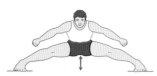

C. Hip mobility: height of pubic bone above floor is measured

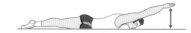

D. Shoulder mobility: nose in contact with ground; height of fingers above ground is measured.

Fig. 4.45 Mobility tests.

Table 4.21 Results table

	Hamstring stretch (cms)	Spinal mobility (cms)	Hip mobility (cms)	Shoulder mobility (cms)
Initial assessment				
Final assessment				

Task 2 – the exercises

1. About 15 minutes of exercises are completed per day for 2 weeks.

2. The mobility exercises can be put into three categories:

   • *Active mobility* (Figure 4.46): exercises in which joints are moved in as full a range as possible by the action of agonists and relaxation of antagonists. The exercise is done slowly **without** jerking or using body weight **or** a partner to extend the range of movement. Each exercise is performed five times by pulling, using muscle action only (hands must not grip another part of the body in the end position). The end position is held each time for a 5-second static stretch.

   • *Passive mobility* (Figure 4.47): again slow careful movements, but now by relaxation of all muscles, with increase of joint movement by a partner assisting **or** the sportsperson pulling him/herself into extended positions. Again, the end position is held for a 5-second static stretch for each of five repetitions per exercise. This method of improving joint mobility can be modified by stretching a muscle or muscle group, followed by an active contraction of the same muscle or muscle group, against a partner's resistance. This contraction is held for a few seconds and then is followed by a further passive stretch. The contract–reflex (C–R method) stretching of a muscle or muscle group is called **proprioceptive neuromuscular facilitation** or the **PNF method**. The aim of PNF is to toughen up or inhibit proprioceptors such as muscle spindles and Golgi tendons, in the relaxation of muscle tissue. As a result the stretch is greater and less painful.

   • *Kinetic or ballistic mobility* (Figure 4.48): this style of exercise uses body movement to extend joint range. Each movement is done five times per exercise.

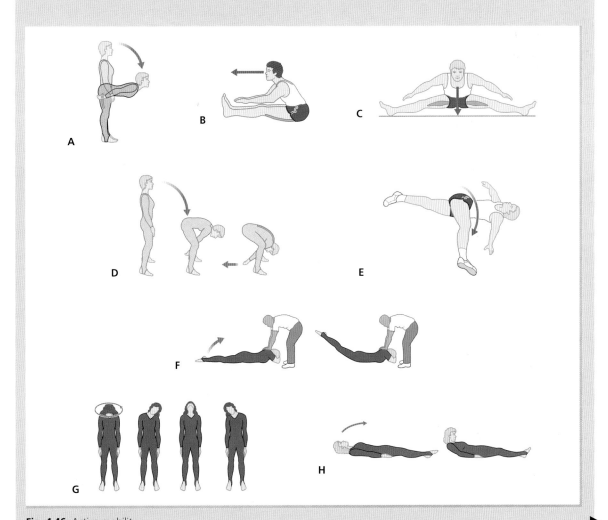

Fig. 4.46 Active mobility.

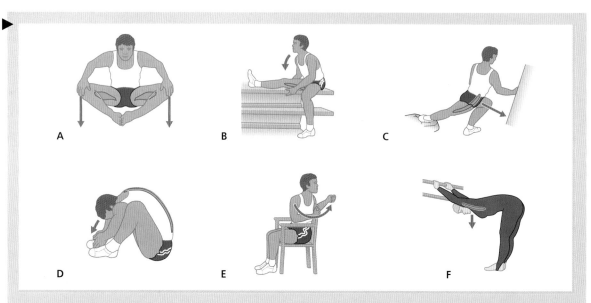

Fig. 4.47 Passive mobility.

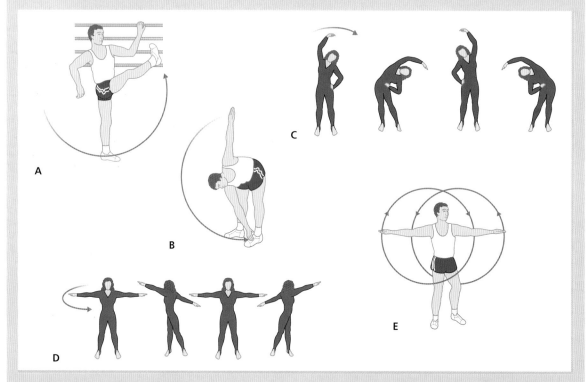

Fig. 4.48 Kinetic or ballistic mobility.

3. The exercises are done in sets of five without rest – a total of about 15 minutes per day.

Task 3 – final assessment

The mobility assessment test set out in Task 1 above is repeated and results are recorded in Table 4.21.

Task 4 – conclusions

1. Has there been an improvement in joint mobility? Use data from Table 4.21 to support your answer. Explain how the improvements in joint mobility have occurred.

2. Which type of mobility exercise would you think is most effective?

Review questions

1. With regard to strength training, what is meant by:
   a. 1 RM?
   b. the overload principle?
   c. progressive resistance exercises?

2. a. What are the principles of circuit training?

   b. Describe the stages you would go through in designing a circuit to develop the general strength of a sport performer such as a games player.

3. Discuss the advantages and disadvantages of active, passive and kinetic mobility.

Exam-style questions

1. Early increases in strength are more associated with neural adaptations but later long-term gains are almost solely the result of hypertrophy. Discuss. *(15 marks)*

2. a. What is meant by the term 1 repetition maximum (1 RM) and how would you assess an athlete's strength? *(3 marks)*

   b. You have been asked to devise a strength-training programme for a fit 18-year-old sprinter.

      i. Identify and explain the use of **four** important training principles that need to be considered when planning this athlete's training programme. *(4 marks)*

      ii. Describe the activities within one strength-training session for this athlete. *(4 marks)*

      iii. How is ATP regenerated during maximal strength work? *(3 marks)*

   c. i. What is the cause of muscle soreness after intense training? *(2 marks)*

      ii. How can muscle soreness be prevented? *(3 marks)*

   d. Explain the physiological advantages of a strength-training programme for a practising athlete. *(6 marks)*

   (Total 25 marks)

3. When male and female sports persons are compared for muscular strength by matching body size and training status, strength differences still persist between genders. Account for **three** possible factors which support this finding. *(6 marks)*

4. Study Table 4.22 which illustrates some outline interval training regimes for the training of different fitness components in a track athlete, before answering the questions which follow.

   a. Briefly explain the meaning and purpose of the term 'set' in interval training. *(4 marks)*

   b. What important information is missing from the outline interval training regimes in Table 4.22? *(3 marks)*

   c. Select **two** of the training regimes in Table 4.22 and briefly explain how their particular fitness components respond to such training. *(8 marks)*

   d. Identify the fuel foods used during each of these training regimes. *(3 marks)*

   e. Discuss the relative importance of these **three** fitness components for performance in a 'game' type activity such as football or hockey. *(5 marks)*

   (Total 23 marks)

Table 4.22 Outline interval training regimes

Component	Training regime
Alactic anaerobic	3 × (5 × 50m)
Lactic anaerobic	2 × (2 × 400m)
Aerobic	1 × (3 × 1000m)

Skill training and game simulation

This is the repeated practising of the skills involved in a sport or game. The aim is to improve **specific motor fitness**, that is, to improve effectiveness or capability at the sport by isolating skills and rehearsing game situations.

Although some skills can be practised in situations that do not need a substantial degree of fitness, it is more usual to incorporate the skills involved in a game into the anaerobic and aerobic training elements of a programme.

Investigation 4.10 Training programmes

This investigation puts into a practical situation the preparation of a training programme relevant to the student's own sporting interest and could form part of the student's **personal performance programme (PPP)** which is an assessed part of current syllabuses (refer to attached CD-ROM for more details).

Task 1 – selection of activities

1. Select *two* activities and/or games from:
   - athletics (choose an event)
   - basketball
   - tennis
   - gymnastics
   - swimming (select a stroke).

   You will set out a training programme for your chosen activities.

2. Time allocation is 5 hours in total per week. The age of the sportsperson is 16 or 17.

3. Analyse the energy system demands appropriate to the chosen sport by using Table 4.15. Enter the percentage contribution for each system in the first row of Table 4.23.

4. Decide the **general** training elements and activities for each energy system. Make a list of these in the second row of Table 4.23.

5. Decide the **specific** training elements and activities relevant to the sport and the energy system demands. Make a list of these in the third row of Table 4.23.

6. Allocate time for a warm-up and cool-down for each daily session.

7. Allocate time to each chosen activity over the weekly **microcycle**, according to the proportions required by the energy system demands of the sport (see first row of Table 4.23, as calculated at 3 above). List activities and times in the fourth row of Table 4.23.

Task 2 – choose details of activities

1. Decide on a battery of tests to determine what the loadings will be for each chosen activity.

2. Carry out the tests on yourself so that the actual loadings produced for the training programme are relevant to you.

3. Decide details of exercises, loadings, repetitions, distances run, rest, recovery times and so on.

4. Write down a programme of weekly activities to satisfy this; include a warm-up and cool-down in each daily session.

5. Table 4.23 is a suitable *pro forma* in which the details of this investigation can be recorded.

Task 3 – variations

1. Suggest *mesocycle* variations of loads for the schedule (a **mesocycle** is a training period of 3–8 weeks whose aim is to increase specific aspects of fitness and for which overload increases continuously).

2. Suggest variations in activities based on the mesocycle.

3. How would you modify the programme for progression to 17–18 and eventually 18–19 year olds?

Task 4 – self-evaluation of programme

1. Having carried out the pre-programme tests on yourself, now carry out the programme itself for a period of at least 2 weeks.

2. Carry out a post-programme test on yourself. Evaluate its effectiveness in terms of:
   - fitness benefit
   - skill learning
   - mobility and/or agility.

3. Explain your feeling of well-being and fatigue as the programme progresses in terms of:
   - energy system demands
   - matching with food intake.

Table 4.23 Results table

	ATP-PC energy system		Lactic acid energy system		Aerobic energy system	
% demand of sport						
Appropriate general activities						
Appropriate specific activities						
Time allocation to activities	activity	time	activity	time	activity	time
Weekly schedule of activities	activity	time/reps/load	activity	time/reps/load	activity	time/reps/load
Sun						
Mon						
Tue						
Wed						
Thur						
Fri						
Sat						

Altitude training

Since the beginning of the 20th century the effects of altitude on physical performance have been catalogued by mountaineers. The decision to hold the 1968 Olympic Games in Mexico City at an altitude of 2242 m (7450 feet) stimulated intense physiological research into human acclimatisation to living at altitude. More recently, data collected from many elite endurance athletes representing a variety of sports have shown that training at altitudes between 1800 and 3000 metres promotes improvement in endurance-based performances made at sea level.

Human difficulties experienced at altitude

Sportspeople training or competing at high altitude suffer from acute drops in performance in sports that rely on aerobic capacity. This is due to lack of oxygen. Figure 4.49 illustrates the oxygen transport system at sea level and at altitude before and after acclimatisation.

The degree to which **haemoglobin** is saturated with oxygen depends on the **partial pressure** of **oxygen** in the alveolar air (see Chapter 2, p. 77, to review the concept of the oxygen–haemoglobin dissociation curve). At sea level, the partial pressure of oxygen in inspired air is sufficient to ensure that the haemoglobin is fully saturated. At altitude, the partial pressure of oxygen in the atmosphere and pulmonary air is reduced. The result is that the haemoglobin is not fully saturated, therefore less oxygen is carried to muscle tissues and the aerobic working capacity of these tissues is reduced.

Physiological changes during acclimatisation to altitude

Three major physiological changes occur in the body as a result of acclimatisation, as outlined below.

Increase in blood haemoglobin concentrations

During acclimatisation to altitude there is an increase in **red blood cell count** (per ml of blood) and therefore an increase in haemoglobin concentration, but the haemoglobin remains unsaturated with

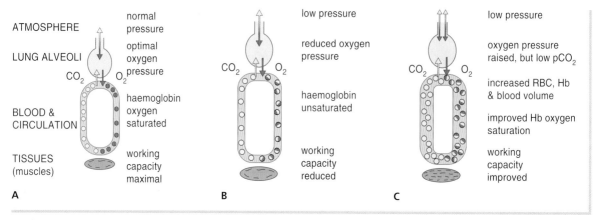

Fig. 4.49 The oxygen transport system at sea level and at altitude, both before and after acclimatisation. RBC = red blood cells; Hb = haemoglobin; pCO_2 = partial pressure of carbon dioxide. **A.** Sea level, normal. **B.** Altitude, unacclimatised. **C.** Altitude, acclimatised (after Brotherhood[13]).

oxygen. The increase in red blood cell count (called **polycythaemia**) is brought about by an increase in the **manufacture** of red blood cells (erythropoietin production), which is a rapid response made by the body to altitude. Also, there is a reduction in the plasma volume, which is a slow long-term response to training at altitude. Early studies[14] have shown that red cell count increases by 6% in men and 7.5% in women taking iron supplements, after 3 weeks' acclimatisation. More recent studies have shown that haemoglobin concentrations increase by 1% per week.[15] It has been found that the haemoglobin concentrations of healthy **residents** at altitude (which vary between 12% and 50% more than the healthy sea-level dweller) are inversely proportional to the prevailing barometric pressures.[16]

Increased rate of breathing

To compensate for a decrease in the partial pressure of oxygen in the alveoli, breathing rate increases. This response develops over several days.[17] Increased ventilation reduces the partial pressure of carbon dioxide, which makes the blood too alkaline. This problem is corrected by the kidneys, which excrete urine more alkaline than normal.

Cellular changes

There is an increase in the **myoglobin** content within muscle cells, as much as 16% above sea level values after acclimatisation at altitude. There is also an increase in numbers of **mitochondria** and **oxidative enzymes** within the mitochondria.[16,18]

Practical advice for optimal sea-level performance

The majority of the world's best endurance sportspeople prepare for major championships at altitude. Advice includes: dietary supplementation with iron and vitamin C (to increase gastrointestinal iron uptake), an adequate daily intake of protein (for erthyropoietin production) and polyunsaturated fats. Light training during the first few days will minimise any exercise-induced decrease in erythropoietin production. Such a programme will promote optimal short-term adaptations.

It is advisable to plan for two bouts of altitude training. The first visit to altitude should be close to the start of the competitive season for a 3-week period. Ideally, the second visit should be for 2 weeks and 7 weeks later than the first visit. This second visit should be planned to occur just before a major competition. It is generally agreed that the most improved competitive performances are within 3–4 days after descending from altitude. However, only experience can determine the optimum timing of descent from altitude for a superior competition performance at sea level.

Net effect

The net effect of human acclimatisation to altitude is to improve the **aerobic working capacity** of muscles to compensate for the reduced partial pressure of atmospheric oxygen and to improve the capacity of the **oxygen transport system** to purge the oxygen debt (refer to Investigation 4.11).

Blood doping and rhesus erythropoietin (rEPO)

Blood doping and rEPO are two illegal ways of simulating the effects of altitude training on the sportsperson. Both these methods produce higher than normal red blood cell counts which would increase the $\dot{V}O_2$max and hence oxygen uptake and energy delivery. This enables the sportsperson to work at a higher rate for longer and therefore considerably enhance aerobic performance.

Blood doping refers to the practice of augmenting a sportsperson's blood with extra amounts of his/her blood. It is reported that this practice involves withdrawing an amount of the athlete's own blood some weeks beforehand, storing it until just before a major competitive effort, then reinfusing the blood at this point. During the period after withdrawal of the blood, the sportsperson manufactures replacement blood cells so that normal haemoglobin levels are restored. Hence, immediately after the reinfusion, his/her blood count can be substantially higher than normal. This process carries a risk of a transfusion reaction in which a mismatching of blood could occur.

Erythropoietin (EPO) is a naturally occurring hormone (produced by the kidneys) which stimulates red blood cell production. Human erythropoietin can be cloned through genetic engineering and is commonly known as rEPO (rhesus erythropoietin). Subcutaneous injection of rEPO some 6 weeks before a planned major competition has been shown to produce a 10% increase in red cell count.

The risks of illegally using blood doping and rEPO are production of a dangerously low resting heart rate and a greater chance of blood clotting (thrombosis) since blood viscosity is increased, causing blood to flow more slowly than normal.

Ergogenic aids to performance

The Greek *ergon* means to work and *genon* to produce, hence an **ergogenic aid** is defined as any means of improving the efficiency and enhancing the quality of sporting performance. Such aids include:

- **physiological aids** which aim to augment physiological processes that naturally occur within the human body (examples include rational training methods like interval training or periodisation and illegal practices such as blood doping)
- **nutritional aids** which provide a natural way of enhancing performance (examples include the use of legal substance like creatine or protein and carbohydrate supplements)
- **mechanical aids** which are designed to improve energy efficiency and skill development (examples are modern sports equipment such as the design and construction of a racing bike and racing helmets and specialist footwear and throwing implements)
- **pharmacological/hormonal aids** which represent a very broad range of designer hormones and transmitter substances (for example, illegal drugs such as anabolic steroids and beta blockers)
- **psychological aids** which aim to improve the mental strength required to cope with the stress of competing, winning and losing (for example, the use of imagery, visualisation, hypnosis or focusing and goal setting).

Table 4.24 A summary of legal ergogenic aids, their effects and risks (as at January 2004)		
Ergogenic aid and brief description	*Benefits to performance*	*Associated risks*
Physiological aids		
Altitude training – training undertaken at altitude in order to benefit from the effects of altitude acclimatisation	Increased submaximal heart rate and rate of breathing, polycythaemia, increased capillarisation, muscle myoglobin and mitochondria increase in $\dot{V}O_2$max at sea level	Hypoxia, nausea, altitude sickness
Physiotherapy – use of physical methods which assist the recovery of damaged tissue	Injury treatment assists removal of metabolites such as lactic acid, reduces muscle soreness	Cost is a disadvantage
Acupuncture – Chinese therapy that uses needles inserted through skin at predetermined points	Increases healing process at injury site	Cost is a disadvantage
Herbal medicines (for example, arnica) – herb which stimulates anti-inflammatory response	Aids recovery to damaged tissue	

Table 4.24 *(cont'd)*

Ergogenic aid and brief description	Benefits to performance	Associated risks
Nutritional aids		
Creatine (refer to p. 116) – a substance found in skeletal muscle, stored as phosphocreatine	Supplements increase in PC levels to enhance ATP-PC energy system. Delay of alactic/lactic threshold	Muscle cramps, increase in body mass
Glutamine (refer to p. 116) – a constituent of skeletal muscle, also required by T lymphocytes, the immune system cells in blood	Reduces risk of infection if taken after training, when muscle building requires available glutamine	
Carboloading (refer to p. 115) – a procedure used to raise the glycogen content of muscle, based on depletion and repletion of CHO	Aids endurance-based activities. Shown to be very effective in boosting energy reserves after 90 minutes of running or other similar activity	Problem of fatigue, after depletion phase using classic 10-day method. Increased body weight since more water is needed to store increased glycogen
HMB (beta-hydroxy-beta-methylbutyrate) – natural component of mother's milk	Enhances strength and lean body mass	
Colostrum – the very rich protein liquid initially produced by a mammal at birth of an infant	Aids recovery between sessions, athlete can train longer	
Vitamins C and E – found in fresh fruit and vegetables	Antioxidants which collect free radicals produced during high-intensity exercise, furthering the recovery process	
Isotonic sports drink (refer to p. 116) – dilute solution of electrolytes (sodium) and sugars (4–8%)	Prevents dehydration, supplements energy reserve during exercise period	
Hypertonic sports drink – a carbohydrate and electrolyte supplement, with approximately 20% sugar concentration	Replenishes blood glucose and glycogen stores. Intended for consumption immediately after exercise has finished and well before exercise commences	
Caffeine – CNS stimulant	Increases mental alertness, free fatty acid mobilisation and use of muscle triglycerides to spare glycogen stores	A diuretic, can lead to dehydration and heat injury. Insomnia risk.
Mechanical aids		
Nasal strips – use of sticky plaster placed on bridge of nose to enlarge nasal cavity	Enables easier breathing by allowing more air to enter breathing mechanism	
Specialised equipment (examples): Carbon fibre bike frames	Lighter machine – shape of bike and position of rider more aerodynamically efficient	Cost is a possible disadvantage
Aerodynamic helmets	Aerodynamic efficiency	
Javelins/discuses	Greater stability in flight	
Poles (pole vault)	Elastic properties of pole enable greater height	
Training machines – weights machines, rugby scrum machines/tackle bags, tennis servers	Enable more effective and **specific** training practices	
Specialised clothing (examples): Lycra running and swim wear	Reduces drag (fluid friction) on person	
Footwear – spikes/studs	Increases friction with playing surface	
Psychological aids (refer to p. 413 onwards)		
Mental imagery/hypnosis – the practice of mentally rehearsing skills and strategies and mentally projecting effort and control of the sport to increase self-confidence	Neural pathways are stimulated as if muscle is actually active, hence reinforcement of skill and a confident approach to the competitive situation	

Table 4.25 A summary of illegal ergogenic aids, their effects and risks (as at January 2004)

Ergogenic aid and brief description	Benefits to performance	Associated risks
Physiological aids		
rEPO (rhesus erythropoietin) (refer to pp. 163) – injected EPO stimulates red blood cell production	Increases $\dot{V}O_2$max and oxygen uptake, therefore increases energy delivery to enhance aerobic performance	Reduces heart rate, heart failure possible. Increases blood viscosity which lowers rate of blood flow and increases risk of blood clotting. Reduces natural production of EPO
Blood doping (refer to p. 163) – another means by which a person's red blood cell count is increased by reinfusion of blood	Increases $\dot{V}O_2$max and oxygen uptake, therefore increases energy delivery to enhance aerobic performance	Reduces heart rate, heart failure possible. Increases blood viscosity which lowers rate of blood flow and increases risk of blood clotting. Possible mismatching of blood – a transfusion reaction
Pharmaceutical/hormonal aids **Amphetamine** – a CNS stimulant	Increased concentration, motivation and mental alertness, delays fatigue	Increased work = increased stress on heart, possible death, addictive
Beta blocker – blocks transmission of neural impulses from sensory nervous system	Reduction in heart rate and blood pressure. Useful in target sports	Dangerously low heart rate, could lead to heart failure
Human growth hormone (HGH) – naturally produced by the anterior pituitary gland. Synthetically produced by genetic engineering	Stimulation of protein and nucleic acid synthesis in muscle, hence increase in muscle mass. Stimulation of bone growth and length. More effective utilisation of body fat for energy. Aids healing process	Increases size of internal organs, weakens joints and muscles. Possibility of abnormal growth – acromegaly
Anabolic androgenic steroid – naturally produced in males and females as testosterone. Synthetically produced for medical conditions such as wasting diseases. Most common drug of abuse among bodybuilders and power sports performers. Examples: clostebol, nandrolone. The presence of testosterone (T) to epitestosterone (E) ratio greater than six to one in the urine sample of a performer constitutes an offence unless there is evidence that this ratio is due to a physiological or pathological condition, for example, low epitestosterone excretion.	Increased bone maturation and muscle mass = increased strength (androgenic). Aids recovery between heavy training sessions	Early closure of growth plates (stunts growth) **Females**: masculine effects – clitoris enlarges, breasts reduce, facial hair grows, voice deepens **Males**: testicular atrophy, enlarged prostate gland, reduction in sperm count **M & F**: reduced secretion of gonadotrophins. Increased high density lipoproteins (HDL) cholesterol levels = risk of heart attack, liver damage, personality changes (rage).
Masking agents – masking agents (some of which are diuretics) can mask the presence of another drug, such as a steroid group.	Hide banned substances that would normally be found in a urine sample produced for a dope test.	May give the athlete a false sense of security when faced with a dope test, when in fact the health hazards of taking the masked drugs could be extremely dangerous.
Diuretic – banned drug that increases urine flow which aids reduction in tissue fluids. Example, bumetanide.	Used in weight control by gymnasts and combat sportspeople. Also used as a masking agent to dilute the concentration of banned drugs in urine.	Loss of water leads to dehydration and heat loss impairment, loss of valuable water-soluble vitamins and minerals leads to impaired performance.

Investigation 4.11 To consider the results of running events in the Mexico Olympic Games, 1968, and the benefits of altitude training camps for sea-level performances, and various doping issues

Task 1
Consider the information in Figure 4.50. Suggest reasons why world records were broken at 100, 200 and 400 metres.

Task 2
In the endurance events above 1500 metres, there was a uniform reduction in performance of about 6%. Suggest reasons for this observation.

Task 3
The data in Table 4.26 refer to Olympic Games held at the sites stated. Carefully explain why acclimatised athletes were relatively successful during the 10 000 metres race at the Mexico Olympic Games.

Task 4
Haemoglobin reversal occurs between 3 and 8 days after return to sea level. Any respiratory changes are reversed immediately and cellular changes reverse within 1–2 weeks.
  Since the Mexico Olympic Games it has been common for endurance athletes to spend a period of several weeks at high-altitude training camps and then return to sea level to compete within about 3 days. How useful is the rationale of altitude camps to sea-level performances?

Task 5 – aids to performance
Acclimatisation is one way in which performance in sporting activities may be enhanced. What other methods are used by current sportsmen and women to aid performance?

Task 6 – the ethics of aids to performance
Doping is defined as the administration or use of substances in any form alien to the body or of physiological substances in abnormal amounts and with abnormal methods by healthy persons with the exclusive aim of attaining an artificial and unfair increase in performance in competition. Furthermore, various psychological measures to increase performance in sports must be regarded as doping.
(Statement by the International Olympic Committee)

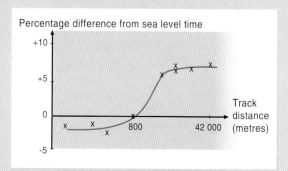

Fig. 4.50 Results of running events in the 1968 Olympic Games.

  Using this definition of doping and your answers to Task 5, decide whether you think there are any ethical objections to the use of such aids to enhance performance.

Table 4.26 Results of the 10 000 m race

Tokyo 1964 (200 m above sea level)	Mexico 1968 (2300 m above sea level)
1. M. Mills, USA	1. N. Temu, Kenya**
2. M. Gammoudi, Tunisia**	2. M. Wolde, Ethiopia**
3. R. Clarke, Australia	3. M. Gammoudi, Tunisia**
4. M. Wolde, Ethiopia**	4. J. Martinez, Mexico**
5. L. Evanov, Russia	5. N. Sviridov, Russia*
6. K. Tsudurova, Japan	6. R. Clarke, Australia*
7. M. Halberg, New Zealand	7. R. Hill, UK*
8. A. Cook, Australia	8. W. Masresha, Ethiopia*

**had lived at high altitude for most of their life
*trained at high altitude for an extended period prior to the Games

Exam-style questions

1. The data in Table 4.27 show the relationship between altitude and maximum oxygen uptake in suitably trained sports performers.

   a. Plot a graph to show the relationship between altitude and maximum oxygen uptake. *(4 marks)*

   b. The 1968 Olympic Games were held in Mexico City at an altitude of 2300 m.

      i. Using the graph, estimate the percentage decrease in maximum oxygen uptake in Mexico City. *(2 marks)*

      ii. With reference to Table 4.27, briefly state what implications arise from the data for race times of 5000 metres and longer. *(2 marks)*

      iii. At a height of 5450 m the amount of oxygen in 1 dm³ of air is 50% that at sea level. Using the graph, estimate the maximum oxygen uptake at 5450 m as a percentage of the maximum at sea level. With reference to physiological adaptations, account for the differences between the percentages. *(8 marks)*

      iv. What advantage is there for an altitude-trained athlete returning to sea level? *(2 marks)*

      v. What effect would altitude training have on the anaerobic processes of metabolism? *(2 marks)*

   (Total 20 marks)

2. a. What is the meaning of the term ergogenic aid? *(2 marks)*

   b. Under what circumstances might **beta blockers** be ergogenic aids? *(3 marks)*

   c. World class performances in many sports are due more to improvements in mechanical aids as opposed to improvements in physical fitness levels. Discuss. *(15 marks)*

   (Total 20 marks)

Table 4.27 Altitude and oxygen uptake	
Altitude in metres above sea level	*Oxygen uptake as % of maximum at sea level*
0	100
1000	98
2000	95
3000	90
4000	85
5000	75
6000	60
7000	40

3. Give a brief outline of, and comment critically upon, the following techniques which may be employed in the belief that they will enhance sport performance:

   a. the use of anabolic steroids *(5 marks)*

   b. ingestion of drinks containing caffeine *(5 marks)*

   c. blood doping *(5 marks)*

   d. physiotherapy. *(5 marks)*

   (Total 20 marks)

4. a. Certain sportspeople have been banned from sport for using illegal substances.

      i. What advantages does the use of steroids give to the performer? *(2 marks)*

      ii. What is a 'masking' agent and why is it significant? *(3 marks)*

   b. Discuss why sportspeople might wish to use banned substances. In your answer identify the hazards of taking such substances. *(15 marks)*

   (Total 20 marks)

An excellent resource for these questions is Wilmore J H 2004 Physiology of sport and exercise, 3rd edn. Human Kinetics.

For further reading on the topics of training and types of training refer to texts cited on p. 171.

4.4 Children and physical activity

Learning objectives

On completion of this section, you will be able to:

1. Understand that physical growth is a process associated with a steady increase in height, weight and muscle mass.

2. Understand how the physical limitations of a child's body affect physiological functioning.

3. Appreciate how anaerobic training can improve a child's anaerobic performance.

4. Appreciate how aerobic training can improve a child's aerobic performance.

5. Understand that the ability to perform anaerobically and aerobically increases as children approach physical maturity.

Keywords

➤ balance
➤ cardio/vascular/ respiratory functioning
➤ children
➤ coordination
➤ development
➤ flexibility
➤ growth
➤ motor skill
➤ myelination
➤ perceptual ability
➤ preadolescence
➤ puberty
➤ strength

Physical growth is a process that is associated with steady increases in height, weight and muscle mass. **Development** refers to the functional changes that occur with growth. With increasing popularity of sports, such as soccer, swimming, gymnastics and athletics, there is an increasing interest in paediatric (paediatric means dealing with children) exercise physiology. This section examines age-related changes that are associated with the young performer (Figure 4.51).

The annual growth during early childhood (ages 3–8 years) is about 5 cm per year and the corresponding weight gain around 2.5 kg per year. During these years boys and girls follow similar growth patterns, have similar amounts of muscle, bone mass and body proportions and progressively lose fat as they grow. During puberty, **growth** is under the influence of sex hormones. Increases in linear growth and skeletal muscle hypertrophy are responsible for increases in muscle strength and aerobic power. In addition, appropriate food intake is the most critical environmental factor that influences biological development. Physical activity is known to benefit growing bodies by reducing levels of body fat, increasing muscle mass and strengthening bone tissue. **Myelination**

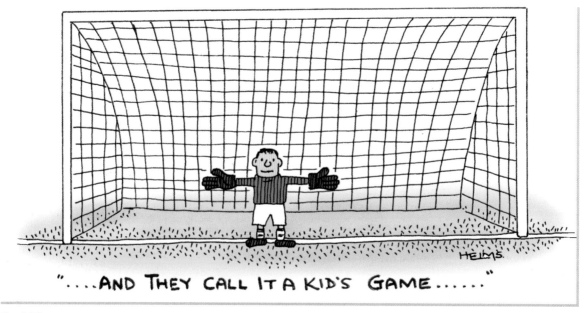

"....AND THEY CALL IT A KID'S GAME......"

Fig. 4.51

(the process of increasing the fatty substance within the sheath that surrounds neurones) is largely completed towards the end of early childhood; hence neural impulses are accelerated, thereby enabling the development of fast reactions and skilled movement. During late childhood (ages 8–12 years) the young performer progresses by improving **perceptual abilities**. Skills requiring visual acuity and tracking abilities (for example, the ability to strike a cricket ball) develop along with the motor organisation needed to accomplish the task.

Anaerobic aspects

The ability of young performers to work anaerobically is distinctly less than that of adolescents and adults, resulting in **reduced** peak and mean power outputs. This is because children do not have the capability of acquiring a large oxygen debt due to less capability of anaerobic glycolysis in working muscle. This means that young children can only work flat out for very short periods – they are not capable of exceeding quite low levels of oxygen debt – and so experience fatigue much more easily than older performers. Working **preadolescents** too hard in training sessions could lead to total exhaustion and injury as body systems become overstressed. Young people will therefore have fully depleted glycogen stores after quite short bouts of intense exercise and would be unable to continue exercising in the same way as an adult performer.

On the other hand, it is possible to improve anaerobic parameters by appropriate interval training. **Strength** is measurable in many ways, such as by isokinetic dynamometry and the vertical jump. In young children strength training can be achieved by using the child's own body weight as the resistance. A strength-training programme could be recommended at the frequency level of twice a week.

A typical strength-training routine for a young athlete would be:

- start with a good warm-up
- moderate flexibility exercises that work through the whole body
- 10 maximal-effort flat and hurdles relays over 20 m
- an introduction to long-jump technique
- finally a cool-down which could incorporate more extensive flexibility exercises.

The emphasis of the session would be on **strength** and **skill** development.

It is thought that any observable increases in strength that result from such a training regime are more likely to be the result of improved **motor skill coordination**, growth and increased **activation of motor units** rather than an increase in actual muscle mass.

Muscular strength improves with age and is a reflection of neural adaptation (as mentioned above) and increases in muscle size. During puberty, androgenic steroids, such as testosterone, cause a dramatic acceleration in muscle mass and associated strength in males and to a lesser extent in physically active females. The net result is that peak and mean anaerobic power rise and recovery times get less. The capability to acquire oxygen debt increases with age, as muscle tissue adapts by increasing glycogen stores and the capacity for glycolysis (refer to p. 134). These anaerobic adaptations are due in part to increased resting levels of ATP, PC and glycogen, increased phosphofructokinase activity and increased toleration to blood lactate.

During puberty, a strength session could involve:

- the use of circuit training using body mass
- light weight training
- stressing the lactic acid system
- therefore building up tolerance to muscle and blood lactate.

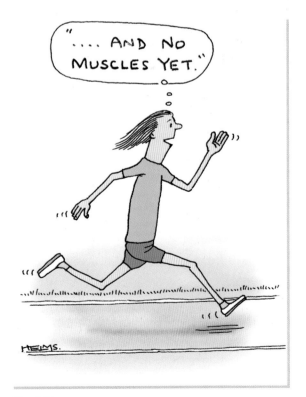

Fig. 4.52

Flexibility usually decreases with age, especially during the growth spurt when increases in bone length stretch the attached muscles. **Slow static stretching**, in which stretched positions are held for several seconds, is most suitable for the young performer. Children do have a better sense of **balance** and **coordination**, mainly due to their smaller body size and lower centre of gravity, and hence they have an enormous capacity to learn complicated skills such as those required for gymnastics.

Aerobic aspects

Cardiovascular-respiratory functioning is much the same in both sexes prior to puberty.

Blood pressure is directly related to size and so is lower in the child but progressively reaches adult values during adolescence. This is because of the child's **smaller heart** and **reduced stroke volume** and because there is **less peripheral resistance** offered by blood vessels. During submaximal exercise, a child's heart compensates by working harder than that of the adult performer and there is a bigger a-$\bar{v}O_2$ diff. This is because there is a greater tendency among children to transfer oxygen from blood to the tissue site where it is needed and this factor compensates for the reduced stroke volume. **Reduced haemoglobin** levels is another limiting factor which contributes towards a lower aerobic capacity.

Research evidence indicates that during puberty there are improvements in $\dot{V}O_2$max for both males and females, with lower values for females. This would suggest that the adolescent growth spurt is a critical period for the development of aerobic fitness as an effect of endurance-based training.

Lung volumes, such as vital capacity, are correlated to body mass and therefore increase alongside general growth. **Breathing rates** are therefore higher when compared with adolescents and adults at equivalent exercise workloads.

Children have a **higher metabolic rate** and therefore use up energy at a higher rate than adults, because they have a larger skin surface area to volume ratio than adults. This means that children lose more heat through their skin to the environment (per kilogram of body mass) than adults. Therefore children have greater difficulty in maintaining normal body temperature, particularly in cold conditions.

Aerobic training for young children produces small increases in aerobic capacity but must be limited by stroke volume, since any further increases in aerobic capacity depend on heart growth.

Examples of an **aerobic training programme** for young children (8–11 years old):

- a variety of games and individual activities, for example, soccer or hockey training including skill development and ball control, with a competitive element in a game situation
- including swimming in the context of lessons in which the skills are learnt
- three to four times per week
- up to an hour in duration
- emphasis on skill development and overall body awareness as well as fitness development
- encouragement of the use of bikes and walking as a means of transport and for fun.

For this age range, both anaerobic and aerobic activities should be encouraged.

When coaches are developing specific training programmes for young male and female performers, they must take into account their growth and development. Training programmes have been shown to improve anaerobic and aerobic capacities but they should be specifically designed for the appropriate age group.

For an excellent resource that enlarges this brief section, refer to Rowland.[19] This text provides a complete review of current knowledge about children's physiological responses to exercise. For further reading on children and physical activity refer to texts on p. 172.

Review questions

1. Identify some of the physiological changes that occur in children when training with submaximal and maximal workloads.
2. What advice would you give coaches wanting to improve the strength of young athletes within their coaching group?
3. How does regular training affect growth and maturation?
4. How do children differ from adults with respect to thermoregulation?

Exam-style questions

1. What factors are responsible for the dramatic improvements in endurance performance from childhood through to puberty? *(8 marks)*

2. Muscle strength progressively improves from childhood through to adolescence. Discuss. *(12 marks)*

References

1. Sheldon W H 1940 *The varieties of human physique*. Harper and Brothers, New York
2. Jackson A S, Pollock M I 1985 *Practical assessment of body composition*. Physician and Sports Medicine 13: 76–90
3. Baum W B 1981 *A nomogram for the estimate of percent body fat from generalized equations*. Research Quarterly for Exercise and Sport 52: 380–384
4. Fleishman E A 1964 *The structure and measurement of physical fitness*. Prentice Hall, New York
5. Cooper K H 1968 *Testing and developing cardiovascular fitness within United States Air Force*. Journal of Occupational Medicine 10: 636–639
6. de Vries H A 1994 *Physiology of exercise*. Brown and Benchmark, Maddison
7. Fox E L, Bower R W, Foss M L 1993 *The physiological basis for exercise and sport*, 5th edn. William C Brown, Dubuque
8. Hettinger L 1961 *Physiology of strength*. Charles C Thomas, Berlin
9. Lamb D R 1984 *Physiology of responses and adaptations*, 3rd edn. Macmillan, New York
10. Karvonen M J, Kentala E, Mustalo O 1957 *The effects of training heart rate. A longitudinal study*. Annales Medicine Experimentalis et Biologiae Femiae 35: 307–315
11. Jones M 1990 *Strength training*. BAAB, Birmingham
12. Cook B B, Stewart G W 1996 *Strength basics*. Human Kinetics, Champaign, Illinois
13. Brotherhood J R 1974 *Human acclimatisation to altitude*. British Journal of Sports Medicine 8:1
14. Hannon J P 1969 *Effects of altitude acclimatization on blood composition of women*. Journal of Applied Physiology 26: 540
15. Hartman U, Burrichter H, Glaser D, Mader A, Oette K 1990 *Changes in ergometer power outputs and peripheral blood during several high altitude camps of top class sportsmen and sportswomen*. Abstract from the 24th FIMS World Congress of Sports Medicine, Amsterdam
16. Pugh L G 1964 *Man at high altitude*. The scientific basis of medicine. Annual review, British Postgraduate Medical Federation, Athlone Press, London
17. Pugh L G 1967 *Athletes at altitude*. Journal of Physiology 192: 619–646
18. Tappen D V, Reynafarje B 1957 *Tissue pigment manifestations of adaptation to high altitudes*. American Journal of Physiology 190: 99–103
19. Rowland T W 1996 *Developmental exercise physiology*. Human Kinetics, Champaign, Illinois

Further reading

Physical and motor fitness testing

Adam G M 1998 *Exercise physiology laboratory manual*. McGraw-Hill, New York

Clegg C 1996 *Teaching support graphs for exercise physiology*. Feltham Press, New Milton

Corbin B C, Lindsey R 2002 *Fitness for life*, 4th edn. McGraw-Hill, New York

Franks D B 1998 *Fitness leader's handbook*, 2nd edn. Human Kinetics, Champaign, Illinois

Prentice W E 1998 *Fitness and wellness for life*, 6th edn. McGraw-Hill, New York

Prentice W E 2003 *Get fit, stay fit*, 3rd edn. McGraw-Hill, New York

Training

Bompa T 1999 *Periodization: theory and methodology of training*, 4th edn. Human Kinetics, Champaign, Illinois

Boyle M 2004 *Functional training for sports*. Human Kinetics, Champaign, Illinois

Dick F W 1991 *Training theory*. BAAB/AAA, Birmingham

McArdle W D, Katch F I, Katch V L 2004 *Essentials of exercise physiology, with primal CD*, 2nd edn. Lippincott, Williams and Wilkins, New York

Sharkey B J 2002 *Fitness and health*, 5th edn. Human Kinetics, Champaign, Illinois

Wilmore J H, Costill D L 2004 *Physiology of sport and exercise*, 3rd edn. Human Kinetics, Champaign, Illinois

Types of training

Alter M J 1998 *Sport stretch*, 2nd edn. Human Kinetics, Champaign, Illinois

Bompa T, Pasquale MD, Cornacchia LJ 2003 *Serious strength training*, 2nd edn. Human Kinetics, Champaign, Illinois

Brown L, Ferrigno V, Santana J 2000 *Training for speed, agility and quickness*. Human Kinetics, Champaign, Illinois

Corbin B C, Lindsey R 2002 *Fitness for life*, 4th edn. McGraw-Hill, New York

Dick F W 1991 *Training theory*. BAAB/AAA, Birmingham

Dintiman G B, Ward R D 1998 *Sport speed*, 2nd edn. Human Kinetics, Champaign, Illinois

Foss M L, Keteyian S J 1998 *Fox's physiological basis for exercise and sport*, 6th edn. McGraw Hill, New York

Nitti JT, Nitti K 2002 *Interval training for fitness*. A & C Black, London

Norris C M 1999 *The complete book of stretching*. A & C Black, London

Pearson P 1998 *Safe and effective exercise*. Crowood Press, Marlborough

Roscoe D A, Roscoe J V, Honeybourne J, Davis R J, Galligan F 2003 *Physical education and sports studies AS/A2 level student revision guide*, 3rd edn. Jan Roscoe Publications, Widnes

Williams M H 1998 *The ergogenic edge*. Human Kinetics, Champaign, Illinois

Wilmore J H, Costill D L 2004 *Physiology of sport and exercise*, 3rd edn. Human Kinetics, Champaign, Illinois

Wirhed R 1997 *Athletic ability and the anatomy of motion*, 2nd edn. Mosby, London

Yesalis C E 1998 *The steroid game*. Human Kinetics, Champaign, Illinois

Children and physical activity

Armstrong N 1996 *New directions in physical education*. Cassell, London

Maffulli N 1995 *Colour atlas and textbook of sports medicine in childhood and adolescence*. Mosby Wolfe, London

Wilmore J H, Costill D L 2004 *Physiology of sport and exercise*, 3rd edn. Human Kinetics, Champaign, Illinois

Multimedia

Videos

Exercise physiology. The Sports Science Series, Queensland Department of Education, Australia 1988. UK supplier Boulton and Hawker Films Ltd

Principles for training for fitness. Queensland Department of Education, Australia 1999. UK supplier Boulton and Hawker Films Ltd

Anabolic steroids – a quest for superman. Human Relations Media, USA 1990. UK supplier Boulton and Hawker Films Ltd

Ergogenic aids. Fitness Video Education, Australia 1999. UK supplier Boulton and Hawker Films Ltd

What is physical fitness? Video Education, Australia 1996. UK supplier Boulton and Hawker Films Ltd

Designing fitness programmes. Video Education, Australia 1996. UK supplier Boulton and Hawker Films Ltd

Pushing the limits in athletic performance. Video Education. Australia 2002. UK supplier Boulton and Hawker Films Ltd

The use of drugs in sport. Video Education. Australia 1998. UK supplier Boulton and Hawker Films Ltd

Body composition and flexibility. Human Relations Media 1999. UK supplier Boulton and Hawker Films Ltd

Cardiovascular fitness. Human Relations Media 1999. UK supplier Boulton and Hawker Films Ltd

Muscle strength and endurance. Human Relations Media 1999. UK supplier Boulton and Hawker Films Ltd

CD-ROMs

Roscoe D A, Roscoe J V 2002 *OCR/AQUA/Edexcel Science and Sport Psychology Powerpoint Classroom Presentation CD-ROM*. Jan Roscoe Publications, Widnes

Roscoe D A, Roscoe J V, Honeybourne J, Davis R J, Galligan F 2003 *Physical Education and Sports Studies AS/A2 Level Student Revision Guide*, 3rd edn. Jan Roscoe Publications, Widnes

Roscoe D A 2004 *teacher's guide to physical education and the study of sport, Part I, the performer in action, exercise physiology*, CD-Rom 5th edn. Jan Roscoe Publications, Widnes

Fitness for life 5

People who exercise regularly, whether walking, jogging, swimming, cycling or playing team sports, are more likely to be able to carry on exhausting work for longer periods of time than sedentary people. This is due to the **adaptive** responses made by the body as a result of regular exercise (see Chapter 4, p. 138 onwards, for details of the long-term effects of exercise on the body).

Today's mass participation in jogging and distance running is a strong indicator that people generally value good health and work hard to keep their bodies in 'good working order'. On the other hand, modern-day living, with its sedentary lifestyles and increased leisure time, has brought modern-day illnesses such as **obesity**, **heart disease** and **cancers**.

This chapter will help you to understand the causes and consequences of obesity and heart disease and the role that regular exercise can take in the pursuit of **fitness for life**.

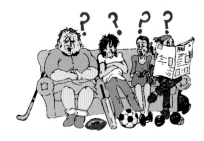

Fig. 5.1

5.1 Obesity

Learning objectives

On completion of this section, you will be able to:

1. Understand the causes, cures and effects of obesity on health.

2. Appreciate the long-term effects of exercise on weight control.

3. Understand the concepts of neutral, positive and negative energy balance.

4. Compare energy intake with energy output using investigational procedures.

5. Relate this information to the concepts of the role of exercise and nutrition in body weight control.

6. Understand what is meant by a 'balanced diet'.

7. Understand that body composition consists of two basic components – body fat and lean body mass.

Keywords

- balanced diet
- basal metabolic rate (BMR)
- energy input
- energy output
- glandular malfunction
- metabolic rate (MR)
- negative energy balance
- neutral energy balance
- nutritional balance
- obesity
- overeating
- positive energy balance
- specific dynamic action (SDA)
- total metabolic rate (TMR)
- underwater weighing

Obesity is a severe overweight condition of the body, defined as accumulation of body fat that is more than 20% above the norm for the person's height and build. It is a serious form of **malnutrition** of the body (*mal*, of course, meaning bad).

Physical effects of obesity on the body

Because of the increase in body size, the cardiovascular-respiratory systems have to work much harder since more energy is used in just moving the body mass.

In addition, an increase in **adipose tissue** (fat under the skin) and a decrease in sweat gland density make it much harder for the vascular system to remove waste heat energy. This waste heat is produced as part of the process of conversion of food fuel into useful work or energy in the body's muscles and organs and has to leave the body from the skin surface. Therefore, a thick insulating layer under the skin will tend to restrict flow of heat outwards. This means that the heart has to work harder to pump blood faster round the circulatory system, so that heat energy, carried by the blood, can be released more rapidly near the skin surface.

Also, a relatively poor circulatory system within adipose tissue means that the blood (and therefore heat energy) cannot reach the skin surface in large enough quantities to release its heat as effectively as it would in a thin person.

All these factors result in **heart overload** and **increased respiratory functioning**, to keep pace with the **increases** in total **metabolic functioning**.

Obesity and disease

Obesity has been strongly associated with a number of modern-day **cardiovascular diseases**, such as **atherosclerosis**, **hypertension** and **coronary** and **cerebral thrombosis**.

An obese person has an increased risk of suffering from **mature diabetes**, **hernia**, and **gall bladder diseases**, **cirrhosis of the liver** and mechanical injuries to the body, such as **backache** and **damage** to **joint structures** (leading to joint pain and arthritis). In addition, an obese person would be more at risk during surgery and an obese woman would be more likely to experience complications during pregnancy.

Causes of obesity

Positive energy balance

Carbohydrates and fats are the fuels needed for energy production (see Chapter 3, p. 114). The major cause of obesity is that **energy intake** (eating carbohydrate and fat) is **far greater** than **energy output**. In other words, there is a lack of energy expenditure, so the obese person will continue to gain weight. This concept

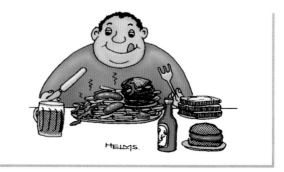

Fig. 5.2

is known as a **positive energy balance** and can be expressed as:

$$\text{ENERGY INPUT} > \text{ENERGY OUTPUT}$$

Excess carbohydrate is stored as glycogen. When all the glycogen stores are filled, **carbohydrate** (together with the excess fat content in the diet) is converted to **fatty acids** and **glycerol**. Excess fatty acids and glycerol are stored as **triglycerides** (fat) in adipose tissue around major organs such as the heart and stomach, underneath the skin and in skeletal muscle.

Glandular malfunction

A small percentage of obese people suffer from a **glandular malfunction**, which results in a hormonal imbalance in the body. This tends to create adipose tissue abnormally.

Overeating and overweight

There is a strong relationship between a positive energy balance and being **overweight**. The latter is often associated with poor eating habits and unbalanced diets containing a high proportion of fat. This results in an individual becoming exhausted through work (exercise) more quickly than someone with a higher proportion of carbohydrate in his/her diet.

Overindulgence in food is also associated with **psychological**, **social** and **cultural** factors. For example, the overeater may eat in an attempt to relieve anxieties. It has been shown that childhood obesity is strongly linked to adult obesity, i.e. the fat child grows into a fat adult!

The development of fat cells begins during the first 2 years of life. Numbers of fat cells in young overfed children may proliferate to **five times** the normal number of cells. So, as the child grows, she/he has thousands of extra fat cells just waiting to fill with fat. In the adult the number of fat cells remains constant but the cells increase in size as weight is gained. Once

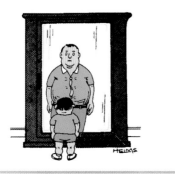

Fig. 5.3

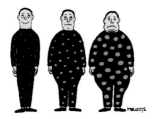

Fig. 5.4

this weight is gained it will be maintained unless a negative energy balance (described in detail below) is achieved.

Obesity and lack of exercise

There is strong evidence to suggest that overweight children and adults are far **less active** than their thinner counterparts. Obesity has the long-term effect of limiting the mobility of joints, thus restricting the person's ability to coordinate movements. It also places an additional strain on the cardiovascular and respiratory systems, as described earlier. Bodily strength, endurance and speed are impaired as a result of weight gain. So a combination of physical and psychological factors (such as poor self-esteem, learned helplessness caused by repeated failure at sporting activities (see p. 383) and unwillingness to expose the body to the scrutiny of others) often inhibit the person from participating in sport and leisure activities.

How to lose weight

The only method of controlling obesity is to shift the energy relationship so that energy output exceeds energy intake. This concept is known as a **negative energy balance** and can be expressed as:

ENERGY OUTPUT > ENERGY INPUT

The result is that the body will mobilise the potential **energy reserves** stored in the **fat deposits**.

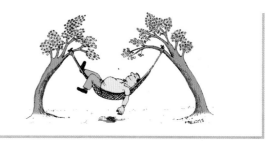

Fig. 5.5

A combination of **balanced diet** and **regular aerobic exercise** is known to be the most effective means of weight control.

A balanced diet

Whilst dieting may be one effective way of losing weight, **drastic dieting** often leads to **lethargy** and **illness** as energy levels drop and resistance to infection decreases, as a result of vitamin and mineral deficiencies. The key to dieting is that a diet must be **well balanced**, i.e. containing all the nutrients for good health. Weight reduction will be achieved only when the normal proportions of fats, carbohydrates and proteins (see pp. 113–114) are maintained but amounts are reduced.

Regular aerobic exercise

The long-term effects of aerobic exercise in alleviating obesity are well established. Long-term systematic exercise increases energy output, as **fat mobilisation** takes place in the liver. Exercise causes lipids (fat-like molecules, insoluble in water, which form large parts of fat cells) to decrease and metabolic rate to increase. For example, an increase of energy output of approximately 5000 kJ per day through exercise will burn off 1 kg of body fat in 1 week. The result of such an excess of **energy output** through exercise, against input via food, is a steady progressive **long-term weight loss**.

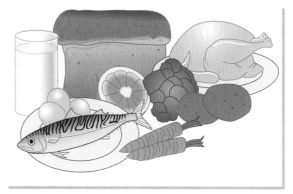

Fig. 5.6 A balanced diet.

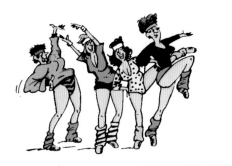

Fig. 5.7

As weight decreases, physiological functioning and physical fitness improve and so the obese person is able to increase the intensity, duration and frequency of exercise. In addition, there is a small reduction in the risk of **heart disease**.

Energy balance

When energy input is equal to energy output a **neutral energy balance** is achieved, as a result of which a person's weight remains constant. This concept can be expressed as:

$$\text{ENERGY INPUT} = \text{ENERGY OUTPUT}$$

Body fat and its measurement

Body composition has two basic components:

1. **body fat** or accumulated adipose tissue
2. **lean body mass** or the fat-free mass, including the mass of other tissues such as muscle, bone and skin.

Measurement of the proportion of body fat is one of the measures of physical fitness discussed in Chapter 4 (p. 125). It is also possible to estimate the proportions of body fat and lean body mass by underwater weighing. The subject is weighed in air and reweighed under water while breathing out (see McArdle[1] *Essentials of exercise physiology*, p. 507 onwards for details of this method).

Preparing a weight control programme

The principles of preparing a weight control programme involve a knowledge of the relationships between:

- the quantities and types of **nutrients** required by the individual for perfect health
- energy expenditure needed for **basal** and **total metabolic rates**
- the concept of energy balance and body weight.

Investigation 5.1   The preparation of a weight control programme

Task 1 – calculation of energy intake over 24 hours
Record all details of food and drink taken in 24 hours in Table 5.1. Quantities of each item will need to be estimated so that energy values can be calculated using food energy tables from a standard table or chart such as those found in references[2,3,4].

Task 2 – calculating energy expenditure over 24 hours
1. Using Table 5.2 and the information that the basal metabolic rate (BMR) for a male is 100 kJ kg^{-1} per day and for a female is 90 kJ kg^{-1} per day, calculate your total metabolic requirements and insert the value in Table 5.3.

Table 5.1 Kilojoule intake			
Meal	*Food*	*Quantity*	*Kilojoules*
Breakfast			
Snack			
Lunch			
Snack			
Evening meal			
		Energy total	**kJ**

Table 5.2 Energy expenditure for various activities

Subject's weight (kg) _____

Activity	kJ kg^{-1} min^{-1} over BMR requirements
Sitting at rest	0.14
Walking	0.2
Jogging and swimming (moderate)	0.6
Cycling (moderate)	0.46
Vigorous exercise	0.8

2. **Specific dynamic action (SDA)** accounts for the extra energy needed for digestion, absorption and transport of the nutrients to body cells. To calculate the SDA, refer to the food intake Table 5.1 and work out 10% of the kJ in food consumed.

Now add this value to Table 5.3. You will observe that the **total energy output** is the result of the BMR + *all* energy requirements **above** BMR and SDA added together. Hence:

Total metabolic rate = all energy requirements for activity + BMR + SDA.

3. Discuss the relationship between your energy intake and energy expenditure. What type of energy balance is there?

4. Using the information from Tables 5.1 and 5.3, describe the different ways in which positive and negative energy balances could be achieved.

Task 3
Write an equation reflecting energy relationships for:

a. maintaining body weight

b. losing weight

c. gaining weight.

Table 5.3 Energy expenditure table

Activity	Duration of activity	kJ kg^{-1} above BMR needs	Total kJ for body mass
			+SDA =
			+BMR =
			TOTAL MR _____

Review questions

1. What are the effects of **obesity** on **health** and what are its causes and its cure, based on energy considerations?

2. Describe the most effective way of **reducing** body weight.

3. What do you understand by '**healthy eating**'? How can this concept be applied to **dieting**?

4. How could an evaluation of body composition assist in:

   a. the control of body weight?

   b. aiding sportsmen and women preparing for competitions?

5. How can **exercise** be used as a means of weight control?

For further reading on aspects of obesity, refer to references on p. 187.

5.2 Cardiovascular diseases

Learning objectives

On completion of this section, you will be able to:

1. Appreciate the effects of changes in modern lifestyles on the general state of health of populations.

2. Understand what is meant by coronary heart disease, appreciate its risks and causes and be aware of the long-term effects of different types of exercise in protection from coronary heart disease.

Keywords

- ➤ angina
- ➤ atherosclerosis
- ➤ cardiac arrest
- ➤ cardiovascular disease
- ➤ coronary heart disease (CHD)
- ➤ coronary thrombosis
- ➤ hypertension

Cardiovascular diseases include diseases of the **heart** and **blood vessels**. The majority of patients suffering from cardiovascular diseases have hypertension or high blood pressure (hypertension is diagnosed when the diastolic pressure consistently reads over 95 mmHg or 11.9 kPa). Hypertension is a major contributing factor in atherosclerosis, coronary heart disease and strokes.

Atherosclerosis, commonly described as **furring up of the arteries**, is caused by lipid (fat) deposits accumulating in the inner lining of arteries, resulting in a narrowing of the arterial lumen, thereby impeding blood flow. When the deposits silt up one of the coronary arteries, a coronary heart attack results – illustrated in Figure 5.8B and C.

Coronary heart disease (CHD) is one of Britain's greatest killers and encompasses diseases such as **angina** and **heart attacks** or **coronary thrombosis**. The first symptoms of coronary heart disease are often manifested as a result of an increased heart rate caused by physical exertion or excitement. Heavy, cramp-like pains are experienced across the chest. This kind of pain is known as **angina** and is normally treated and controlled with drugs and relaxation. A person suffering from angina has a higher risk of suffering from a **coronary thrombosis**.

A **coronary thrombosis** or heart attack is a sudden severe blockage in one of the coronary arteries, cutting off the blood supply to the cardiac tissue. This blockage is often caused by a blood clot formed within slowly moving blood in an already damaged, furred-up coronary artery, as illustrated in Figure 5.8C. Heart attacks can be severe or mild, depending on the positioning of the blockage.

In Figure 5.9 a severe blockage has occurred in a descending coronary artery. The amount of heart tissue involved is great, causing a major heart attack. The figure also shows a mild blockage towards the end of the coronary artery in which the amount of heart tissue involved is minimal. In this instance the patient would have a better chance of full recovery.

In a severe blockage the heart may stop beating. This is called a **cardiac arrest**. About half of all cardiac arrest cases die.

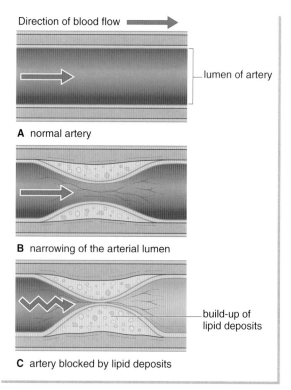

A normal artery

B narrowing of the arterial lumen

C artery blocked by lipid deposits

Fig. 5.8 A. Normal artery. **B.** Narrowing of the arterial lumen. **C.** Artery blocked by lipid deposits.

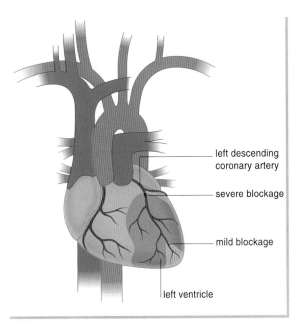

Fig. 5.9 Blockage in the descending coronary artery.

left descending coronary artery

severe blockage

mild blockage

left ventricle

Investigation 5.2 To examine death rates from coronary heart disease

Task 1
Coronary heart disease accounts for 30% of all UK deaths in people aged under 75 years. Suggest possible reasons and causes for this.

Task 2
Figure 5.10 shows different death rates from heart disease for those aged 35–74 years in different countries of the world.
1. Using examples from this chart, suggest reasons why the death rate from coronary heart disease varies so much from one country to another.
2. Suggest reasons why men are more likely than women to suffer from coronary heart disease.

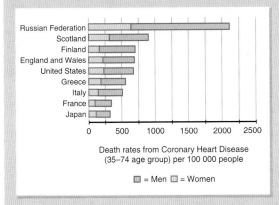

Death rates from Coronary Heart Disease (35–74 age group) per 100 000 people

☐ = Men ☐ = Women

Fig. 5.10 Death rates from coronary heart disease.

Protection against coronary heart disease

The advice usually given is to watch your **weight**, do not **smoke**, do not drink too much **alcohol**, reduce your **salt intake** and **relax**, but take **regular exercise**. This is because, although some individuals who smoke, eat too much and drink too much live to old age without heart trouble, a higher proportion contract heart disease than the average for the population as a whole. There is therefore a higher statistical risk of heart disease among people who drink, smoke, eat too much and take salt in their food.

Exercise and coronary heart disease

There is good evidence that **regular exercise** can have a protective effect on the heart. Stamina-building activities such as jogging, cycling and swimming will improve the efficiency of cardiac tissue and circulation within the heart muscle.

Regular exercise **reduces resting heart rate** and **increases stroke volume** because of a stronger, more efficient heart. Resting **blood pressure** is **lowered** and the **balance** of **cholesterol** (a constituent of animal fat in the diet) and triglycerides (fat) is **improved**. Amounts of cholesterol and triglycerides that reach the fuel transport system of the body are statistically associated with a high incidence of atherosclerosis and therefore there is an increased probability of heart disease and coronary thrombosis. Diets should therefore include less animal fat (saturated fats) to reduce this risk.

In addition to the positive physiological effects of exercise on the body, a person will feel and look better.

The type of exercise undertaken to protect your body from coronary heart disease will depend on your present physical condition. The major questions to be asked in devising an exercise programme are: how

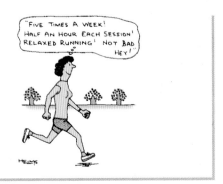

Fig. 5.11

often (**frequency**); how much (**intensity**); and how long (**duration**).

1. **Frequency**: at least two to three times a week.
2. **Intensity**: hard enough to make you breathless. This should mean that your heart rate should be at least 60% of your maximal heart rate and increase in proportion to your maximal heart rate as your fitness improves.

3. **Duration**: the length of each session will depend on the intensity of the exercise but should last between 20 and 60 minutes for it to be beneficial to the body.
4. Finally, **what activity**? Something that you enjoy doing! It is important that the selected mode of exercise is aerobic and uses large muscle groups so that stamina is improved.

Investigation 5.3   To devise an activity programme

Task 1
Consider the information in the stamina rating chart (Table 5.4) and devise two exercise programmes – one for a male and one for a female aged 42 years. Give reasons for your selection of activities, frequency, intensity and duration of the schedule.

Task 2
Why would a medical examination be advised for anyone who decides to start regular exercise at this age?

Task 3
Why should an exercise session be preceded with a warm-up and finished with a cool-down?

Table 5.4 Stamina rating chart

	Stamina rating		Stamina rating
Badminton	••	Mowing the lawn by hand	••
Canoeing	••••	Swimming	•••••
Golf	••	Tennis	••
Jogging	•••	Walking (briskly)	••
House work (moderate)	••	Yoga	•

KEY
not much effort	••	very good effort	•••
beneficial effort	•••	excellent effort	••••

Investigation 5.4   The application of energy concepts

Task 1
Select a team game and individual sport and briefly describe the ways in which energy is supplied to working muscles. How can an understanding of the ways in which energy is produced help you in devising a training programme for your selected activities (refer to pp. 94–100)?

Task 2
How can an understanding of energy production enable us to find out about the causes of fatigue and how it can be delayed or even avoided during competitive performance (p. 105 onwards)?

Task 3
How does information regarding nutrition and its potential energy supply assist performance (pp. 114–116)?

Task 4
What principles of body weight need to be applied to energy requirements of the body?

Task 5
Why is it important for the athlete to keep a stable body temperature (p. 139)?

Review questions

1. Describe the ways in which exercise can reduce the risk of getting coronary heart disease.

2. How might changes in lifestyle go some way to preventing coronary heart disease?

1. Regular exercise can positively influence several health risks.

   a. Identify **four** such risks and explain why exercise might reduce these risks. (*12 marks*)

   b. Briefly describe an outline for a week's exercise programme that would be suitable for an overweight and ageing adult. In your answer identify the major fitness components to be stressed. (*8 marks*)

   c. What principles of training would you incorporate in your plan to ensure that the person retained some fitness in 2 years' time? (*5 marks*)

   (*Total 25 marks*)

For further reading on cardiovascular diseases refer to references on p. 187.

5.3 Ageing and physical fitness

Learning objectives

On completion of this section, you will be able to:

1. Understand the physiological changes that occur during ageing.
2. Explain how physical activity produces adaptive responses that lessen the effects of ageing.
3. Devise an activity programme based on the criteria of duration, intensity and frequency, which would improve the health profile of a subject of your choice.

Keywords

➤ atrophy
➤ biological ageing
➤ blood cholesterol
➤ body composition
➤ flexibility
➤ HRmax
➤ osteoarthritis
➤ osteoporosis
➤ target zone
➤ $\dot{V}O_2$max

Ageing includes all the changes that occur in the body with the passage of time. A major problem for researchers in this field is to distinguish between **biological ageing** and physical inactivity. This section examines the effects of ageing on body systems and the effects of physical activity in slowing down the ageing process (Figures 5.12 and 5.13).

Ageing is often associated with quite dramatic physical changes. For example, both sexes lose height as a result of compression of the fibrocartilage between the vertebrae and loss in bone density. Often these changes are due to dietary deficiencies and lack of physical activity. In women this process occurs much faster following menopause when oestrogen levels fall, accelerating the onset of **osteoporosis**.

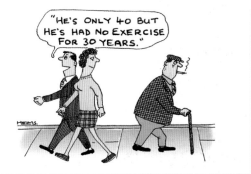

Fig. 5.12

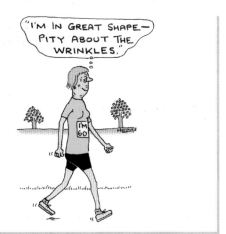

Fig. 5.13

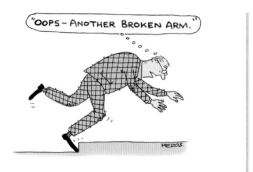

Fig. 5.14

Joint flexibility becomes severely restricted if mobility work is not done on a regular basis and diseases such a **osteoarthritis** cause abnormal thicknesses and fluid-filled pockets in joints, resulting in impaired joint functioning.

Body composition continues to change throughout life. Young males and females have roughly 15–25% body fat and around 35–45% of muscle, respectively. Over the following decades the ratio of body fat to muscle steadily changes until mean values for fat in men and women in their 70s are 25% and 40%, respectively. Increases in fat levels and decreases in muscle mass cause substantial decreases in anaerobic and aerobic capacities.

Such changes are in addition to the more obvious changes to the skin, voice, posture and gait (changes to gait depend on joint stability and spinal changes).

The rate of ageing is the change in function of organs and systems per unit of time. This rate will fluctuate depending on the state of health of the older person (whether or not he/she has had to fight an infection). The rate of ageing would also depend on the health of muscles and joints, as well as the physical efficiency or ability of the cardiovascular and respiratory systems to function at rest and during exercise.

Anaerobic aspects

From 30 years of age onwards, reduced strength output and speed of movement are largely attributed to:

- loss of muscle mass (in particular fast-twitch fibres)
- an increase in adipose tissue
- loss of fast-twitch motor units
- hence a higher proportion of slow-twitch motor units
- changes in synapse/neuromuscular junctions

- a reduced myelinated sheath (which surrounds the neurones).

Loss of central and peripheral neurones decreases the capacity for sending nerve impulses to and from the brain and hence the capacity for information processing, particularly affecting short-term memory (from loss of central neurones) and muscle coordination (from loss of peripheral neurones). An effect of nervous deterioration is that nerve conduction velocity decreases and therefore there is an associated increase in reaction time. The fact that the nervous control of muscle contractions is poorer in the older person means that muscle is not used as effectively or extensively as in the younger person, hence **muscle atrophy** occurs (muscle mass reduces with age) and muscular performance would decline. People who have undertaken physical training or exercise on a regular basis from the age of 40 onwards tend to show less decline in both muscle mass and function (Figure 5.15). The comparison between trained and untrained people from Figure 5.15 shows that the 40-year-old who continues training until he/she is 80 years old has far less decline in strength/ fitness between the ages of 40 and 60 compared with the untrained, very unfit person. This is followed by a similar decline between the ages of 60 and 80 but the decline begins from a higher strength/fitness level in the trained person. Obviously this situation would depend on general health factors but it is clear that exercise into old age provides a significant advantage to the musculature

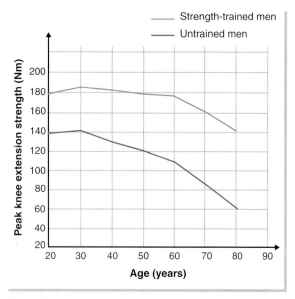

Fig. 5.15 A comparison of strength between trained and untrained men with age.

of such a person in comparison to the sedentary older person.

Aerobic aspects

Cardiovascular changes

The most observable physiological change that accompanies the ageing process is a decline in maximum heart rate, which can be estimated by using the following equation:

$$HRmax = 220 - age$$

(Depending on state of fitness, individual values can deviate by more than 20 beats per minute.)

Other changes are:

- an increase in resting pulse rate due to a decrease in stroke volume, which causes an increase in heart rate during rest and moderate exercise
- a reduction in cardiac muscle fibre size, which causes an increase in resting heart rate and a reduction in maximum heart rate (HRmax)
- this causes a reduction in maximal cardiac output and hence $\dot{V}O_2$max, leading to a reduced capacity to deliver oxygen to muscle sites at maximal effort
- during exercise the heart rate of older people remains higher and recovers more slowly following maximum exercise, because an oxygen debt takes longer to remove than in the younger person
- this is because of the lower rate of blood flow and hence lower oxygen-carrying capacity to working muscle
- an increase in resting systolic blood pressure (due primarily to a thickening and hardening and therefore loss of elasticity of the aorta and other main arteries), which would tend to increase the risk of stroke or cerebral haemorrhage
- an increase in peripheral resistance (often caused by diseases such as atherosclerosis), such that blood flow decreases by up to 15% in old age and hence produces an increased risk of thrombosis or clotting
- additionally maximum a-$\bar{v}O_2$diff (when exercising hard) is lower in older people because less oxygen is extracted by working muscles
- a reduction in blood flow to brain tissue which results in the death of brain cells, sometimes leading to severe reduction in cerebral functioning (senility)
- an increase in total blood cholesterol, particularly low-density lipoproteins (LDL), which increases the risk of CHD.

Respiratory changes

Changes to the respiratory system include:

- the airway and tissue of the respiratory tract including alveoli become less elastic and more rigid
- the chest wall becomes more rigid
- therefore there is a reduction in lung capacity, with vital capacity (VC) down by 35% by age 70
- total lung capacity (TLC) tends to remain the same but the residual volume (RV) increases, so that less air can be exchanged. RV is the part of the lung capacity which is not available for gaseous exchange (refer to p. 82)
- smoking tends to increase the RV and make shallow breathing even more likely
- a reduction in levels of oxygen in the blood, hence a reduction in alveolar macrophages and a reduction in the capacity of the cleaning mechanism of the lungs (refer to p. 70)
- therefore the older person is more susceptible to pneumonia, bronchitis and other pulmonary infections
- the capacity to undertake endurance training is reduced because of the reduced flexibility of the lungs and chest wall, so that older athletes have a reduction in pulmonary functioning.

Neuromuscular changes

Changes to the neuromuscular system include:

- a small reduction in oxidative enzyme activity in trained older athletes of between 10% and 15% compared with endurance-trained young athletes
- therefore ageing only has a small impact on mitochondrial performance for the trained performer
- loss of neurones has the effect of reducing muscular control and hence coordination
- reduction in nerve conduction velocity, which means that reaction times are increased, response

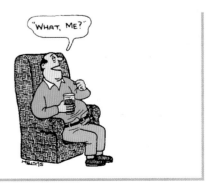

Fig. 5.16

to stimuli is slower and capacity to perform physical skills reduced

- a deterioration in glucose and lipid metabolism, which means that less energy is available for aerobic mechanisms.

All this is a wonderful list of things to look forward to if you opt for the sedentary lifestyle!

The effects of exercise on aerobic performance

$\dot{V}O_2$max declines at a rate of about 10% per decade (starting in late teens for inactive females and in the mid-20s for inactive males) mainly due to reductions in stroke volume and maximum heart rate. Within the physically active ageing group, maximal oxygen consumption can be maintained at much higher levels. Figure 5.17 illustrates the changes in $\dot{V}O_2$max which occur with age for three groups of individuals: trained males, male joggers and untrained males. It is clear that the trained individuals maintain a substantially higher $\dot{V}O_2$max than the other groups and although the rate of decline in aerobic capacity is similar for all three groups, the trained group has started at and maintained a higher level at least up to the age of 60.

When older people take regular aerobic (and anaerobic) exercise most of the changes associated with ageing are lessened. A summary of some of the benefits, insofar as adaptations to body systems produced by long-term exercise is concerned, can be found from p. 138 onwards.

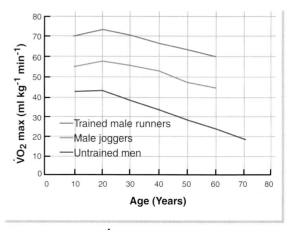

Fig. 5.17 Changes in $\dot{V}O_2$max in trained and untrained subjects.

Summary of the effects of training on older sportspeople

- Improved pulmonary functioning
- Improved cardiovascular functioning
- Hence improved $\dot{V}O_2$max
- Improved a-$\bar{v}O_2$diff
- Maintenance of strength and hypertrophy
- Reduced risk of cardiovascular diseases
- Additional health benefits, such as resistance to infection
- Reduced risk of injury
- Increased sense of well-being
- Increased ability to perform routine tasks in daily life.

Investigation 5.5   A training programme for health-related fitness

The aim of this investigation is to build an exercise/training programme based on improving fitness for health, as opposed to a particular sporting activity. The student should choose a single subject for the investigation from among parents, brothers/sisters or friends.

Task 1 – initial assessment
Decide on a battery of tests from Section 4.1 on fitness testing and energy balance that would determine the fitness levels of the chosen subject. Take into account:

- age and sex
- general build of individual
- physical fitness assessment (the duration of any step test must not be so long as to initiate heart failure!)
- body composition tests

- dietary intake
- energy demands of occupation.

Task 2 – the programme
1. Decide on a gradual, progressive exercise regime that would help the health needs of your subject without overstrain. You can calculate your subject's maximum heart rate (220 – age) and then select an appropriate working intensity within the target zone from Figure 5.18 (selection of the target zone will depend on your subject's current state of health and personal fitness goals). When your subject begins the exercise programme, start at the lower end of the target zone and, as his/her fitness levels improve, vary the exercise intensity within the selected target zone. Work within the target zone for 20–30 minutes.

▶

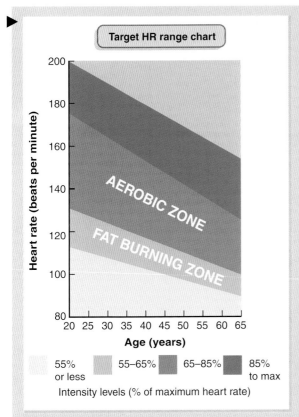

Fig. 5.18 Chart showing target heart rates.

2. Research one of the many available texts to help in sorting this out, such as Corbin & Lindsey,[5] Corbin,[6] Franks,[7] Prentice,[4,8] Wilmore & Costill.[9]

3. Set out in detail the day-to-day activity programme for the subject for a period of 4 weeks. Make this realistic for the subject to achieve. It is unlikely that he/she would cooperate with an exercise regime thought to be too difficult or time consuming.

DO NOT TRY TO IMPLEMENT THE PROGRAMME BEFORE CONSULTATION WITH YOUR TEACHER – WE DON'T WANT FATALITIES AS A RESULT OF YOUR EFFORTS!

4. Explain in your programme how warm-up and cool-down are incorporated.

5. Using the information in Figure 5.18, sketch a graph to show the expected changes in your subject's heart rate, from resting through to: warm-up; target (HR) zone exercise period; cool-down; and resting for the duration of one training session. Indicate on your graph the fat-burning zone, aerobic zone and maximum heart rate.

6. Draw a second curve on your graph to indicate expected changes in exercise heart rate values following 3 months of regular aerobic training.

Task 3 – evaluation
1. If it is possible to implement the suggested regime with your subject, then do so after consultation with her/his doctor if necessary!

2. How would you assess the effectiveness of your programme?

3. Devise a before-and-after questionnaire that would assess the impact of the programme on:
   - physiological factors: pulse rate, breathlessness, circulation, recovery
   - body composition
   - feeling of well-being
   - feeling of coping with the physical demands of life: work, hobbies, sex
   - feeling of coping with emotive stress-related demands: coping with workload, interpersonal relationships
   - states of exhaustion
   - sleep patterns
   - eating habits
   - personal cleanliness habits and so on.

Review questions

1. How does ageing affect resting and maximal stroke volume and cardiac output? What mechanisms can explain these changes?

2. What muscular changes occur with ageing? How do they affect physical activity?

3. When older people are physically active, most of the changes associated with ageing are lessened. What changes produced by aerobic exercise would be helpful to the ageing process?

Exam-style questions

1. A fitness trail is an exercise circuit consisting of exercise stations along a jogging path. A fitness trail is versatile, since it offers safe, healthy exercise regardless of age or condition. Progress is at the individual's own rate and as few or as many repetitions of the exercises and circuits can be done. ▶

a. Using the information in the map of the trail (Figure 5.19), explain the principles you would apply in devising a training session for a 49-year-old male or female who is obese and unfit. (*5 marks*)

b. Explain the methods you would employ and give an example of the amount of activity you would expect from this 49-year-old person. (*2 marks*)

c. Describe the physical and motor fitness components you would stress. (*3 marks*)

d. Describe the predominant energy system being used in this training session. (*6 marks*)

e. Identify the food fuels being used at different stages of the session. (*2 marks*)

(*Total 18 marks*)

2. a. How does physical training affect the biology of ageing? (*6 marks*)

b. What influence does ageing and training have on body composition? (*6 marks*)

(*Total 12 marks*)

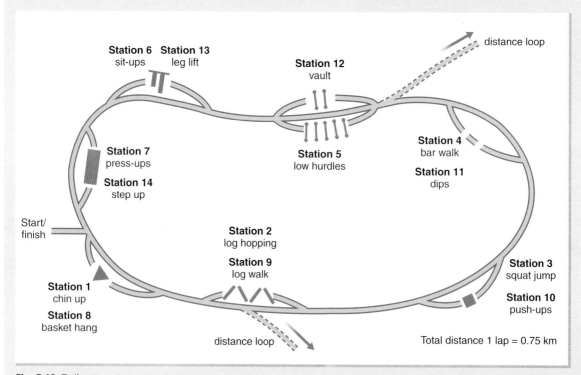

Fig. 5.19 Trail map.

References

1. McArdle W D, Katch F I, Katch V L 2004 *Essentials of exercise physiology, with primal CD*, 3rd edn. Lippincott, Williams and Wilkins, New York
2. McArdle W D 2001 *Exercise physiology, energy, nutrition and human performance*, 5th edn. Lippincott, Williams and Wilkins, Baltimore
3. Anspaugh D J, Hamrick M H, Rosato F D 1997 *Wellness concepts and applications*, 3rd edn. Mosby, St Louis
4. Prentice W E 2004 *Get fit, stay fit*, 3rd edn. McGraw Hill, New York
5. Corbin B C, Lindsey R 2002 *Fitness for life*, 4th edn. Human Kinetics, Champaign, Illinois
6. Corbin B C, Walk G, Lindsey R, Corbin W 2003 *Concepts of fitness and wellness: a comprehensive life-style approach with free Health Quest CD-ROM*, 5th edn. McGraw Hill, New York
7. Franks D B 1998 *Fitness leader's handbook*, 2nd edn. Human Kinetics, Champaign, Illinois
8. Prentice W E 1998 *Fitness and wellness for life*, 6th edn. McGraw Hill, New York
9. Wilmore J H, Costill D L 2004 *Physiology of sport and exercise*, 3rd edn. Human Kinetics, Champaign, Illinois

Further reading

Obesity and cardiovascular diseases

Allsen H V 1997 *Fitness for life*, 6th edn. Brown and Benchmark, Madison

Franks D B 1998 *Fitness leader's handbook*, 2nd edn. Human Kinetics, Champaign, Illinois

Jackson A W, Morrow J R, Hill D W, Dishman R 1999 *Physical activity for health and fitness – an individualised lifetime approach*. Human Kinetics, Champaign, Illinois

McArdle W D, Katch F I, Katch V L 2004 *Essentials of exercise physiology, with primal CD,* 2nd edn. Lippincott, Williams and Wilkins, New York

Prentice W E 1998 *Fitness for college and life*, 6th edn. McGraw Hill, New York

Prentice W E 2004 *Get fit, stay fit,* 3rd edn. McGraw Hill, New York

Roscoe D A, Roscoe J V, Honeybourne J, Davis R J, Galligan F 2003 *Physical education and sports studies AS/A2 level student revision guide,* 3rd edn. Jan Roscoe Publications, Widnes

Sharkey B J 2002 *Fitness and health*, 5th edn. Human Kinetics, Champaign, Illinois

Wilmore J H, Costill D L 2004 *Physiology of sport and exercise*, 3rd edn. Human Kinetics, Champaign, Illinois (pp. 634–688)

Ageing and physical performance

Allsen H V 1997 *Fitness for life*, 6th edn. Brown and Benchmark, Madison

Anspaugh D J, Hamrick M H, Rosato F D 1997 *Wellness concepts and applications*, 3rd edn. Mosby, St Louis

Corbin C B, Lindsey R 1997 *Concepts of fitness and wellness with laboratories*. Brown and Benchmark, Madison

Franks D B 1998 *Fitness leader's handbook*, 2nd edn. Human Kinetics, Champaign, Illinois

Jackson A W, Morrow J R, Hill D W, Dishman R 1999 *Physical activity for health and fitness – an individualised lifetime approach*. Human Kinetics, Champaign, Illinois

Prentice W E 1998 *Fitness for college and life*, 6th edn. McGraw Hill, New York

Prentice W E 2004 *Get fit, stay fit,* 3rd edn. McGraw Hill, New York

Robbins G, Powers D, Burgess S 1997 *A wellness of life*. Brown and Benchmark, Madison

Sharkey B J 2002 *Fitness and health*, 5th edn. Human Kinetics, Champaign, Illinois

Spirduso W W 1995 *Physical dimensions of aging*. Human Kinetics, Champaign, Illinois

Sykes K 1999 *The Chester step test version 3*. ASSIST Creative Resources, Chester

Wilmore J H, Costill D L 2004 *Physiology of sport and exercise*, 3rd edn. Human Kinetics, Champaign, Illinois (pp. 538–539)

Multimedia

CD-ROMs

Roscoe D A, Roscoe J V, Honeybourne J, Davis R J, Galligan F 2003 *Physical Education and Sports Studies AS/A2 Level Student Revision Guide, 3rd edn.* Jan Roscoe Publications, Widnes

Roscoe D A, Roscoe J V 2002 OCR/AQA/Edexcel Science and Sport Psychology Powerpoint Classroom Presentation CD-Rom. Jan Roscoe Publications, Widnes

Roscoe D A 2004 *Teacher's guide to physical education and the study of sport. Part I, the performer in action, exercise physiology,* CD-Rom, 5th edn. Jan Roscoe Publications, Widnes

Sykes K 1999 *The Chester step test version 3*. ASSIST Creative Resources, Chester

Videos

Human Relations Media USA 2001 *Ten Reasons to Get and Stay in Shape*. UK Supplier Boulton and Hawker Films Ltd.

Human Relations Media USA 1999 *Total Health Series: Becoming Physically Fit.- Set of 3 videos:Body Composition and Flexibility, Muscle Strength and Endurance, Cardiovascular Fitness*. UK Supplier Boulton and Hawker Films Ltd.

Biomechanics: linear motion

6

Chapters 6–8 deal with the study of **biomechanics**. This area of study applies the concepts of physics and mechanics to the way in which the human body moves and how it applies forces to itself and other objects with which it comes into contact.

Linear means **in a straight line**. Chapter 6 attempts to put into perspective concepts involving movement in a single direction such as speed, velocity, acceleration and force (through Newton's Second Law of Motion). Chapter 8 deals with **rotating systems**, which involves sportspeople spinning, twisting or turning. In practice most sports movements consist of a mixture of linear and rotational motion and this is termed **general motion**. For example, a sprinter running down a track is moving **linearly** as a whole, but has his arms and legs **rotating** about shoulder and hip joints. In this text we attempt to simplify a particular sports situation by referring to linear and rotational movements separately.

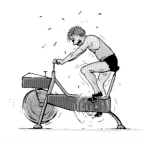

Fig. 6.1 All motion and no speed!

6.1 Linear motion

Learning objectives

On completion of this section, you will be able to:

1. Calculate speed, acceleration and deceleration from primary data taken from moving sports people or objects:

$$\text{speed} = \frac{\text{distance moved}}{\text{time taken}}$$

$$v = \frac{s}{t}$$

$$\text{acceleration} = \text{change of speed per second}$$

$$a = \frac{v-u}{t}$$

2. Plot distance–time and speed–time graphs and understand the meaning of the slope (gradient) of each.

3. Apply Newton's Second Law to accelerating sportspeople and objects, where a net force acts.

$$\text{force} = \text{mass} \times \text{acceleration}$$
$$F = m \times a$$

4. Apply Newton's First Law to stationary or constant velocity sports people or objects, where there is **zero** net force.

5. Understand Newton's Third Law and how this leads to the idea of reaction forces applied to sports situations.

6. Appreciate the place of air resistance and streamlining applied to moving sports people or objects.

7. Distinguish between the concepts of speed and velocity.

8. Be familiar with the concept of the conservation of energy as applied to thrown objects and be aware that:

$$\text{kinetic energy} = \tfrac{1}{2} \times \text{mass} \times (\text{velocity})^2$$
$$KE = \tfrac{1}{2} \times m \times v^2$$

9. Be familiar with the concept of power as the rate of energy conversion or expenditure as applied to sports situations.

$$\text{Power} = \frac{\text{energy used}}{\text{time taken}} = \text{force} \times \text{velocity}$$

Keywords

- acceleration
- air resistance
- deceleration
- displacement
- distance
- fluid friction
- force
- friction forces
- general motion
- linear motion
- kinetic energy
- position
- power
- reaction forces
- rotating systems
- speed
- streamlining
- velocity
- weight
- work

Distance, position and displacement

Speed and **velocity** (see p. 194 for an explanation of the difference between these two concepts) are ideas that involve a body or object changing its **position**. For example, if an athlete starts a race – the stopwatch or electronic timer starts also – and he runs 10 m in 2 seconds, his **position** has changed by 10 m from the start line, the **distance** moved is 10 m and the average speed over this distance is 5 metres per second.

The same idea could be used in a game situation but now the **position** of the centre-forward might be 20 m out from the opposing goal, on a line 10 m to the left of the left-hand post. At this point he might shoot for goal and the ball travels 25 m – the **distance** from the striker to the net at the back of the goal – in 0.5 seconds. In this case the speed of the ball would be 50 metres per second.

So, you can see that **distance** is usually measured from one point to another point and the **position** of the points tells us where they are in space (or on a pitch or court). This distinction becomes important in races or games where starts and finishes are fixed. The **displacement** of a sportsperson from the start of an event may also be important in some cases. For example, a triathlete may swim, cycle and run huge distances but he/she may only be displaced at most 2 km from the start position. So the displacement of the triathlete is the distance (as the crow flies!) between the start position and the position of the triathlete – usually the **direction** is also taken into account.

Investigation 6.1 attempts to apply the ideas of distance, time, speed, velocity, acceleration and force to a practical situation. The student will describe the motion of a running athlete, attempt to understand how force affects the athlete and explain how we conclude what causes the forces which act, and discuss the way force is represented (in a diagram of the activity).

Investigation 6.1   Motion of a sprinter during a 100 m run

This investigation comprises the bulk of the work in this chapter and requires the use of a video camera (with on-screen timing facility), a tape measure (50 m), 10 traffic cones or markers, bathroom scales and a video playback machine with slow and stop facilities.

Task 1 – production of video film
Work in groups of at least four.

1. Mark out a 100 m (or 50 m) stretch of straight track with cones (or other easily visible objects) at 10 m intervals down the track.
2. Set up your video camera, viewing at right angles to the screen, at about 50 m from the track.
3. Student A then performs the run from a standing start (flat out from the start, otherwise important features of the exercise will be lost; Figure 6.2); Student B calls the start commands; Student C operates the video camera (which will need to follow the runner as he/she runs down the track); Student D has the very important task of operating the timer start on the on-screen timer display of the camera.

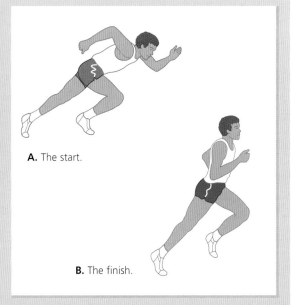

A. The start.

B. The finish.

Fig. 6.2 Performing the exercise.

▶ 4. The latter facility is essential for all practical uses of a video camera in measuring the motion of a sportsperson.

5. Trial runs of the investigation showed that only a couple of 'takes' were needed to obtain very usable film.

6. An alternative method of obtaining the data is to station students armed with a stopwatch at each cone, who then measure the time from the start to the moment the runner passes.

Task 2 – production of primary data from the film

1. Locate the beginning of a suitable run on the film.

2. Using the pause and frame advance facility on the video machine, move the film forwards until the runner is level with the first 10 m marker (i.e. at 10 m from the start line) and record the time in the second column of Table 6.1.

3. Continue this process, moving the film so that the runner is at successive 10 m points down the track and recording the times on the chart. Note that it will be important to allow for the fact that the camera is not alongside the runner. Therefore you will have to estimate when he/she passes each marker and then not line up the marker with her/him in the field of view.

4. Now complete the third column of Table 6.1, 'time interval for the previous 10 m' (by subtraction of times).

Task 3 – graph of distance against time

1. Plot a graph of distance (y-axis) against time (x-axis) from the second column of Table 6.1. *Note*: For the purpose of this text the y-axis is the vertical axis and the x-axis is the horizontal axis of a graph (Figure 6.3).

2. Mark on your graph any straight (or almost straight) portions; note that when drawing a line

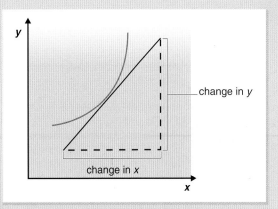

Fig. 6.3 Sketch graph of a gradient.

through your graph points, **do not** connect up the points but draw a smooth curve or line that best fits the motion that is represented.

3. Mark on your graph any obviously curved portions.

4. Write a brief description of what you understand may be happening during the straight and curved parts of the graph.

5. Using the equation below, work out the slope (gradient) of the graph at 1.0 and 5.0 seconds after the start. What do these values tell you about the motion of the runner?

$$\text{gradient} = \frac{\text{change in } y \text{ value of graph}}{\text{corresponding change in } x \text{ value}}$$

Task 4 – computation of the speed of the runner

1. Using a calculator and the information that:

$$\text{speed} = \frac{\text{distance moved}}{\text{time taken}}$$

[units – metres per second (ms^{-1})] calculate the speeds of the runner for successive 10 m intervals. Record these values in the second column of Table 6.2.

Table 6.1 Times at 10 m intervals during the run

Distance moved (m)	Time at this point (s)	Time interval for previous 10 m (s)
0	0.0	
10		
20		
30		
40		
50		
60		
70		
80		
90		
100		

Table 6.2 Speed against time for the runner

Section of race (m)	Speed for the section (m s⁻¹)	Time at the middle (s)
0–10		
10–20		
20–30		
30–40		
40–50		
50–60		
60–70		
70–80		
80–90		
90–100		

2. Now work out the average time at which each speed was reached. For example, for the 10–20 m section of Table 6.2, calculate the time halfway between the 10 m and the 20 m times. This should be done for all sections of the run and entered in column three of Table 6.2. This can also be done approximately by taking the times at 5 m, 15 m, 25 m, 35 m and so on from the **distance–time** graph produced in Task 3 above.

3. This may seem complicated but it is necessary so that the average speed over each 10 m distance is linked to the average time at which this speed was achieved.

Task 5 – speed–time graph

1. Now plot a graph of the speed of the runner (y-axis) against the time at the middle of the section (x-axis), using the data from columns two and three of Table 6.2.

2. Try to make the graph as large as possible within your paper; include the origin of the graph (0.0).

Note: remember that the distance moved is always 10 m and the time taken is the time recorded in the third column of Table 6.1. Also, you should draw a smooth curving line of best fit to your points on the graph; **don't** connect up the points (as this will result in a graph showing rapid and sharp changes in speed, which cannot be the case). A smooth curve of this construction averages out the errors made in taking measurements.

Task 6 – analysis of motion

Now put into writing what you understand, on the basis of your graph, actually happens to the athlete during the run. This should be between half and one side of A4 paper in length and include comments on the following:

1. What happens between 0 and 2 seconds after the start?

2. When does the athlete reach maximum speed?

3. What happens to the athlete in the last three-quarters of the run?

4. Does the athlete slow down at any time during the run in spite of maximum effort?

5. When is the biggest **net** force being applied to the runner (to enable him/her to accelerate)?

Task 7 – calculation of initial acceleration

1. From your speed–time graph, write down the speed at time = 0.0 seconds and time = 1.0 seconds.

2. These two values give you the change of speed in 1 second, which is the acceleration of the athlete at the start of the run. Write down the value of this acceleration:

acceleration = change of speed per second
unit of answer = metres per second per
second ($m\ s^{-2}$)

Task 8 – calculation of final deceleration

1. During the last part of the run the runner will be slowing down. Why do you think this is?

2. Deceleration is very similar in definition to acceleration, only slowing down instead of speeding up. Complete the following sequence to calculate the final deceleration of the runner. Use values from your speed–time graph.

3. Calculate the speed at 2.0 seconds from the end of the run and the speed at the end of the run. Calculate the deceleration using:

deceleration = change of speed per second

Task 9 – forward force at start of run

1. Use Newton's Second Law of Motion to compute the accelerating force on the athlete at the start of the run. Newton's Second Law of Motion says:

force (in newtons) = mass (kg) × acceleration ($m\ s^{-2}$)

(provided the mass that is accelerating remains constant, which in this case it does).

2. Find the mass of the runner in kilograms (using bathroom scales).

3. Compute the force at the start of the run using:

force = mass × acceleration
[unit of answer – newtons (N)]

4. What is the nature of this forward force acting on the athlete? *Note*: it must be a forward force since the athlete is accelerating forwards, but the athlete pushes **backwards** on the ground.

5. Does friction play a part in this force? *Note*: the runner probably would not be able to accelerate as quickly if he/she wore flat shoes instead of spiked ones. How could we test if friction is the cause of this forward force and in any case, how does this friction force manage to push the runner forwards when he/she obviously pushes backwards?

Task 10 – forces acting on the runner

1. Consider Figure 6.4 – our runner is 1 second into the run. Copy this diagram and sketch on him/her the forces that might be acting.

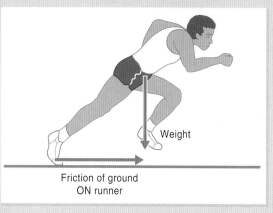

Weight

Friction of ground
ON runner

Fig. 6.4 Forces that might be acting on the runner.

2. To extend the list a little, remember that gravity acts downwards (towards the centre of the earth) on all objects on the surface of the earth and the **force** due to gravity is called **weight**.

3. Newton's First Law of Motion says that an object that is not accelerating has **no net force** acting on it. Our runner is not accelerating vertically, therefore there can be **no net** vertical force acting on him/her.

4. Using the bathroom scales again, stand still on them and read the force (or, better still, have a partner read the force) you are exerting on them.

5. Bend your knees very slowly until they are at about 90°, then jump violently upwards (making sure you don't land on the scales, thereby breaking them or your ankle!).

   a. What do the scales read during the act of jumping? (It will be important here to have a partner read the scales.) More or less than your weight?

   b. Why should the scales read more, since your weight obviously remains the same?

   c. Perhaps the fact that you push hard down on the scales means that the scales push hard up on you and enable you to accelerate upwards off the ground?

This is Newton's Third Law of Motion – that for every action there is an equal and opposite reaction.

6. This means that when the athlete pushes hard against the ground during the start, the ground pushes back on the runner with an exactly equal force but in the opposite direction.

Now extend your force drawing to include all the forces that might be acting on the runner (Figure 6.5).

Task 11 – does air resistance affect the runner?

1. Near the end of the race (when the runner is moving at considerable speed) another force may come into play. What could this force be and how does it depend on the speed of the runner?

2. Air resistance (or fluid friction) crops up in various forms in other sports and sporting situations. Write about one side of A4 paper to describe this, mentioning as many examples as you can. (*Hint* – water has a much bigger fluid friction than air and very fast-moving objects, such as golf balls or motor cars, generate much more fluid friction.)

3. What about the shape of the moving object? Streamlining occurs naturally in fish, birds and some animals and less naturally in cars and planes; boats also are streamlined to reduce water fluid friction.

4. Look at the drawing of our runner (Figure 6.6), which includes the forces acting on the runner near the end of the run. Will the friction force now be as large as it was at the start? *Note*: since the runner is running at almost constant speed, Newton's First Law of Motion can be used to answer this question.

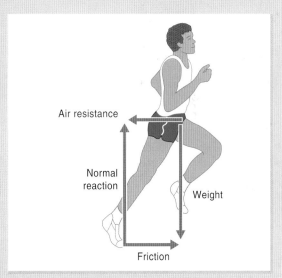

Fig. 6.6 Forces acting on the runner near the end of the run.

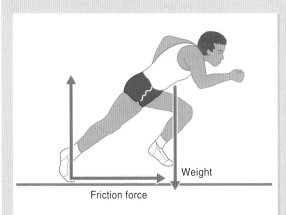

Fig. 6.5 Forces acting on the runner.

At the end of the run, the fact that the runner is going at almost constant speed means that although each force is large, they cancel out to produce almost zero net (or resultant) force.

Speed and velocity

At this point it is worthwhile explaining the difference between these two apparently similar concepts.

Although both are expressed as metres per second and are defined by the same formula (v = distance/time), **velocity** is a **vector** and has value and direction whereas **speed** is a **scalar** and has value only. There is a discussion on vectors in Chapter 7 (p. 200 onwards), when we look at the concept of force, which is also a vector.

In Investigation 6.1, it doesn't actually make any difference whether we use speed or velocity to describe the motion of our sprinter, because he/she always moves in the same direction. But once the direction changes, then it is important to use **velocity** to describe the motion. This is because the definition of acceleration is:

change of VELOCITY per second

So if the **direction** changes, so will the velocity and there will be an acceleration and a force (by Newton's Second Law).

Newton's Laws of Motion

Remember **Newton's First Law**, which says that an object on which **no net forces are acting** has no change in velocity, i.e. it will remain stationary (at rest) or will move at constant velocity (in a straight line). This law is therefore applicable when any sportsperson is stationary (without any upward or downward motion) or when a sportsperson moves at constant speed, however quickly, in a fixed direction, as a cyclist travelling flat out near the end of a sprint might be. The implication here is that if the cyclist is travelling at constant velocity, then all forces acting on him/her **must** cancel out.

Newton's Second Law, which gives a value for the force needed to provide an acceleration (using **F = m × a**, when a force does act), describes what happens when a **net force** causes change of **velocity** and an **acceleration** (which can include a **change of direction** and usually a **change of speed**). The situation is straightforward when speed changes without change of direction (as the sprinter accelerating or decelerating down the track in Investigation 6.1 above, when **F = m × a** enables you to directly calculate the acceleration from the measured values of the change of speed). However, when direction changes the application of Newton's Second Law is more complex.

For example, imagine a football, soccer, tennis or rugby player swerving (Figure 6.7). The friction force of the ground on his/her feet (which is sideways to the direction of travel) causes a change of direction but **no change of speed**. The fact that there has been a change of direction means that there has been an acceleration in the **direction of the force**, i.e. sideways to the direction of travel.

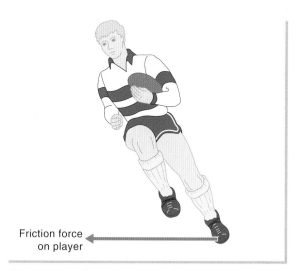

Friction force on player

Fig. 6.7 Friction force on a swerving player.

Another sporting example in which this idea is important is the hammer throw (Figure 6.8). As the hammer head moves in a circle, its direction is continually changing, so there is a force causing this change **along the hammer wire towards the thrower**. This means that the hammer head is continuously accelerating towards the thrower, as the hammer head continuously changes **direction** towards the thrower, although the

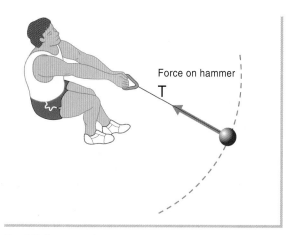

Force on hammer
T

Fig. 6.8 Force on a hammer.

direction of travel of the hammer head at any instant is along a tangent to its arc of motion. Generally, if a force is acting at right angles to a direction of motion (as for the hammer throw example above), then the effect is to change the direction of travel, without changing the speed.

Newton's Third Law describes what happens when one body exerts a force on another body, as for example an athlete pushing hard on the ground. This leads to reaction forces (which in this case would cause the athlete's body to jump upwards) and will be discussed in more detail on p. 209.

Review questions

1. Sketch a pin-man drawing of a sportsperson standing still, showing all the forces acting on him/her.
2. Sketch a second diagram showing all the forces acting on a runner accelerating.
3. Sketch a third diagram showing the vertical forces acting on a high jumper just before take-off. Clearly mark the relative sizes of any forces you show, representing the size of the force by the length of arrow.

4. Use this third diagram and your understanding of Newton's Laws of Motion to explain why the high jumper is able to take off.
5. If the vertical upward ground reaction force on the jumper is 1400 N and the weight of the jumper is 600 N, estimate the net upward force acting on him/her.
6. If the mass of the jumper is 60 kg, calculate his/her upward acceleration during this part of the jump.

Further optional reading on linear motion

Linear motion can be described by a set of equations called **equations of motion**, some of which we have come across already.

$$\text{speed/velocity} = \frac{\text{distance travelled}}{\text{time taken}} = v = \frac{s}{t}$$

$$\text{acceleration} = \frac{\text{change of velocity}}{\text{time taken}} = a = \frac{v-u}{t}$$

where s = distance travelled
          t = time taken
          u = starting velocity

v = finishing velocity
a = acceleration

Further equations can be derived from these:

$$v = u + at$$
$$s = ut + 0.5at^2$$
$$\text{average speed} = \frac{u + v}{2}$$
$$v^2 = u^2 + 2as$$

all of which apply to uniformly accelerating motion of acceleration **a** (without change of direction).

The student who wishes to use these formulae to describe the motion of people or objects should obtain advice from a physics text book since this is more a physics matter than a biomechanics matter.

Review questions

1. Define the terms force, mass, velocity and acceleration and give the unit of measurement for each.
2. State Newton's First Law of Motion.
3. An ice hockey puck is struck by a player and travels across the ice to rebound from the far wall of the rink.
   Assuming that both the friction between puck and ice and the air resistance are negligible and

that the puck travels from right to left as you look at it, sketch force diagrams to show what forces act in each of the following situations.

a. While the puck is stationary before being struck.
b. While the stick is in contact with the puck.
c. While the puck is travelling across the ice before it hits the wall.
d. While the puck is in contact with the wall.

Work, energy and motion

The discussion in Chapter 3 (p. 94) on human energy systems outlines the ways in which the human body as a machine can transform energy from food as fuel (from chemical energy) into movement of the skeleton. The implication is that energy can be neither created nor destroyed but only transformed from one form to another (this is the Law of Conservation of Energy). One of the forms into which energy can be transformed is **motion energy** or **kinetic energy**.

    Kinetic energy (KE) is mechanical energy possessed by any moving object or body **by virtue of its motion**. This motion can be **linear** (in a straight line) or **rotational** (spinning or turning). A formula for KE can be derived from the **work** definition:

$$\text{work} = \text{force} \times \text{distance moved in the direction of the force}$$

$$\text{KE} = \tfrac{1}{2} \times \text{mass} \times (\text{velocity})^2$$
$$= \tfrac{1}{2} \times m \times v^2$$

(Answer in joules)

Note that this concept includes dependence on the mass as well as the speed of the moving body.

    An application of this idea to a sporting context is in the throwing of an implement (such as a shot or javelin or ball). Mechanical work is done by the thrower, who applies a force over a distance in order to accelerate the thrown object:

$$\text{work} = \text{force} \times \text{distance}$$
$$= F \times s$$

At the point of release, this energy has been transferred into kinetic energy:

$$\text{KE} = \tfrac{1}{2} \times m \times v^2$$

So it can be seen that in order to make the release velocity (*v*) of the thrown object as large as possible, it is necessary to **increase** the **force** (*F*) or **distance** (*s*) over which the force is applied. This is the reason throwers do so much weight training (to increase strength and hence *F*) and mobility and skill training (to improve the distance over which force is applied).

    Looking at Figure 6.9, it can be seen that the skilful shot putter starts applying force on the shot from a position where the shot lies on a vertical line that passes outside the back of the circle to a point on a vertical line that passes outside the front of the circle and therefore applies force over the greatest distance possible.

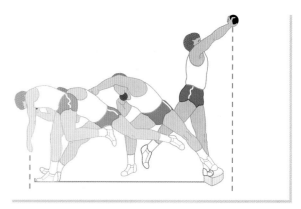

Fig. 6.9 Action of a skilful shot putter.

Power

Another concept useful in the above context is that of **power**. Power is defined scientifically as the rate at which energy is used or created from other forms or:

$$\text{Power} = \text{energy used/second} = \frac{\text{energy used}}{\text{time taken}}$$

(measured in watts or joules per second) and following from the equivalence of energy and work:

$$\text{Power} = \frac{\text{work done per second}}{} = \frac{\text{force} \times \text{distance}}{\text{time taken}} = \text{force} \times \text{velocity}$$

$$\text{since velocity} = \frac{\text{distance}}{\text{time taken}}$$

So this means that power is not only a measure of how much energy is created (in a movement or activity) in each second that passes but also a measure of the size of force applied and the velocity at which it is applied. In the example of the shot putter, large forces applied at high speed are required to put the shot a long way, i.e. the most powerful athlete is one who can apply the largest force at the highest possible speed – the objectives of training for throwers are to maximise both force and speed during training movements.

    Power is also the relevant concept when discussing anaerobic capacity. Therefore, when undertaking the Wingate anaerobic power cycling test, the output measure is that of the maximum power output of the sportsperson taking the test measured in watts, i.e. the maximum energy expenditure per second (see Chapter 3, p. 90).

Exam-style questions

1. Consider the data in Table 6.3, obtained during an athlete's 100 metres sprint race at an international championship meeting in 1987.

a. i. Work out the athlete's average speed over successive 10 m sections of the race and complete the blank column E of Table 6.3. (*3 marks*)

$$\text{speed (E)} = \frac{10}{\text{time (C)}}$$

ii. Plot a speed–time graph (with time along the x-axis) of this motion using the last two columns of Table 6.3 (*3 marks*)

iii. Explain what the shape of the graph means. (*3 marks*)

iv. By using the data at time = 0 seconds and at time = 0.93 seconds (or otherwise), calculate the athlete's initial acceleration. (*2 marks*)

b. The athlete has a mass of 75 kg.

i. Calculate the net force acting on him at the start of the race. (*2 marks*)

ii. Draw a pin diagram to show all the forces acting on him at the start of the race and explain the nature of these forces. (*4 marks*)

c. Before 1968 all major athletic championships were held on a cinder surface. How do you think this might have affected this athlete's performance and explain how the wearing of flat shoes instead of spikes might have affected his acceleration? (*3 marks*)

d. Later in the race, from 6 to 8 seconds, a different pattern of forces acted upon him.

i. Draw a pin diagram to show all the forces acting on him at this later stage and explain the nature of any extra forces now acting which were not evident at the start of the race. (*3 marks*)

ii. What can you say about the resultant (net) force acting in a forwards direction on him during this later part of the race? (*2 marks*)

(*Total 25 marks*)

Table 6.3 Data for 100 metres sprint

A Distance	B Time at this distance (s)	C Time for previous 10 m	D Average distance at which measurement is taken (m)	E Speed at this point (m s⁻¹)	F Time at this point (c)
0	0	–	0	0	0
10	1.86	1.86	5		0.93
20	2.87	1.01	15		2.37
30	3.80	0.93	25		3.34
40	4.66	0.86	35		4.23
50	5.55	0.89	45		5.11
60	6.38	0.83	55		5.97
70	7.21	0.83	65		6.80
80	8.11	0.90	75		7.66
90	8.98	0.87	85		8.55
100	9.83	0.85	95		9.41

Note: the time shown in column F is halfway along each 10 m section

2. Table 6.4 shows the speed of an 18-year-old female sprinter during a 200 m race.
   a. i. Plot a graph of speed against time during this race. (*5 marks*)
      ii. When does she reach maximum speed and what happens to her speed between 8 and 27 seconds? (*2 marks*)
      iii. Use the graph to establish her speed at 0.5 seconds and 1.5 seconds and calculate the average acceleration between these times. (*3 marks*)
      iv. If her mass was 50 kg, what was the net forwards force acting on her between 0.5 and 1.5 seconds? What is the nature of this force? (*3 marks*)
      v. Sketch pin diagrams of the athlete to show the forces acting on her at the start and end of the race. (*5 marks*)
   b. What physiological reason could you give for the fact that she begins to slow down from about 7 seconds after the start, assuming that she is going 'flat out' all the way? (*2 marks*)
   c. A hockey player at constant speed is able to swerve and change direction.
      i. Sketch a diagram to show the direction of the force acting on her which would have this effect. (Show on your diagram the direction of the force relative to the direction of travel.) What is the nature of this force? (*3 marks*)
      ii. What factors would enable her to swerve more effectively? (*2 marks*)

   (*Total 25 marks*)

3. a. i. Define the term 'velocity'.
      ii. For movements that take place along a single line of motion, what is the significance of positive and negative velocity values? (*2 marks*)
   b. The diagram (Figure 6.10) shows a linear velocity curve (of the centre of gravity – centre of mass) for a volleyball blocker during the take-off ground contact phase of a vertical jump. Examine the curve and explain what is happening to the jumper at points **P, Q, R** and **S**. (*8 marks*)
   c. Copy the diagram and sketch a continuation of the graph to show what would happen to the player's velocity during the period of flight. (*2 marks*)
   d. If it is assumed that air resistance is negligible, identify which forces will cause the changes in velocity when the jumper is:
      i. on the ground
      ii. in the air. (*4 marks*)
   e. At which points on the graph is the net force acting on the jumper zero? Explain your answer. (*4 marks*)

   (*Total 20 marks*)

Table 6.4 Data for 200 m sprint	
Speed (m s⁻¹)	Time (s)
0.0	0
5.0	1
7.1	2
7.8	3
8.0	4
8.1	5
8.1	7
8.0	8
7.9	10
7.8	13
7.7	18
7.6	22
7.5	27

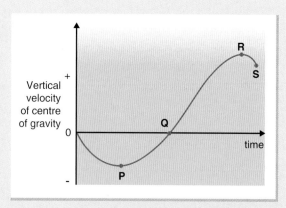

Fig. 6.10 Linear velocity curve for a volleyball player.

The nature and application of force

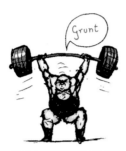

Grunt

Fig. 7.1 'Grunt'.

Very broadly speaking, force involves the idea of 'pushing' or 'pulling', the idea that one object exerts a force on another object and the idea that a force will cause motion (that is, accelerated motion).

7.1 The nature of force

Learning objectives

On completion of this section, you will be able to:

1. Understand the concept of force as applied to a sports person or object and be aware of the unit of measurement of force – the **newton**.

2. Understand the concept of force as a vector and the idea of a vector as a quantity with **direction** as well as size. Also, you should understand the way in which several forces acting on a sports person or object in different directions can combine to form a **net** force or **resultant** force.

3. Distinguish between **weight** and **mass** and use the formula:

   weight = **mass × gravitational field strength**
   = **mass × g**
   = **mass × 10 (newtons)**

4. Understand the nature of **reaction forces**:
   a. applied on the sportsperson by his/her surroundings
   b. applied by one part of the body to another.

5. Understand the nature of **friction** forces when applied to a sports person or object and the factors affecting them.

6. Be aware of **air resistance** and **fluid friction** acting on objects and the human body moving through fluid, and the factors affecting them.

7. Be aware of the **Bernoulli effect** (and the Magnus effect) as it affects spinning balls in flight.

8. Use the concepts of **momentum** and **impulse** in respect of the analysis of forces of impact between bat and ball and foot and ground.

   Momentum = **mass × velocity**
   = $m \times v$

   impulse = **force × time**
   = $F \times t$

   impulse = **change of momentum**
   $F \times t = mv - mu$

9. Be aware of the **Law of Conservation of Momentum** as applied to collisions between objects or sportspeople and that this law can lead to the **transfer of momentum** between bodies involved in collisions.

Keywords

- air resistance
- Bernoulli effect
- component
- drag
- fluid friction
- force
- friction forces
- gravitational field strength
- gravity field
- impulse
- laminar flow
- Magnus effect
- mass
- momentum
- net force
- reaction force
- resultant force
- scalar
- streamlining
- the newton
- vector
- weight

Force as a vector

Force is also a **vector** and therefore has a **direction** as well as a size or value. This point is very important to anyone thinking about what happens when forces are applied, because it enables a force in one direction to cancel out completely an equal force in the opposite direction so that, in spite of very large forces being involved in a given situation, forces can cancel out to give a zero (or very small) **net** or **resultant** force.

For example, consider the weightlifter in Figure 7.2. As he pulls upwards on the bar, he exerts a force of 1000 newtons (N) **upwards** on the bar and gravity exerts a force of 980 newtons **downwards** on the bar. (See section on measurement of force, p. 202, for a definition of the newton as the unit of force.)

The **resultant** or **net** force acting on the actual bar is therefore only about 20 N **upwards**, just enough to accelerate the bar off the floor.

The idea that **net** force causes **acceleration** is linked with Newton's First and Second Laws of Motion and is a fundamental property of force.

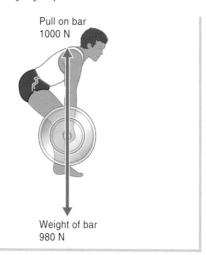

Pull on bar
1000 N

Weight of bar
980 N

Fig. 7.2 Forces acting on a weights bar.

Also, it is possible for many forces acting in all sorts of different directions to cancel one another out. When this happens, from Newton's First Law we know that the object (or sportsperson) on which the forces act will either be stationary or moving at constant velocity (in a straight line). This situation is called **equilibrium**: where the object is stationary this is **static equilibrium** and where it is moving at constant velocity this is **dynamic equilibrium**.

Further notes on vectors

There are specific mathematical rules that enable you to add together vectors that are **not in the same direction**. You may notice from Figures 7.3A and B that the **resultant** of two forces at an angle has been drawn by completing a parallelogram (in Figure 7.3A) or a rectangle (in Figure 7.3B, where the forces are at right angles). The **resultant** then lies along the **diagonal** of the parallelogram.

It is also possible to calculate the size and direction of resultant vectors using trigonometry. Looking at Figure 7.3D, in which R (the reaction force) and F (the total friction force) are at right angles, we note that angle α lies between F and the resultant X of the two vectors as drawn.

Using Pythagoras' theorem:

$$X^2 = R^2 + F^2$$

and

$$X = \sqrt{(R^2 + F^2)}$$

= **the magnitude or size** of the resultant ($\sqrt{} =$ 'square root of').

Also:

$$\tan \alpha = \frac{R}{F}$$

and

$$\alpha = \tan^{-1} \frac{R}{F}$$

= the **angle** between X and R, which gives the **direction** of the resultant.

Example

Looking at Figure 7.3E, the normal reaction force on the sprinter's foot has the value 700 N and the forward friction force 200 N, so that the resultant total reaction force on his/her foot, X, has the magnitude:

$$
\begin{aligned}
X &= \sqrt{(700^2 + 200^2)} \\
&= \sqrt{(530\,000)} \\
&= 728 \text{ N}
\end{aligned}
$$

The angle α between X and the 700 N force will be:

$$
\begin{aligned}
\alpha &= \tan^{-1} \frac{700}{200} \\
&= \tan^{-1} 3.500 \\
&= 74.06°
\end{aligned}
$$

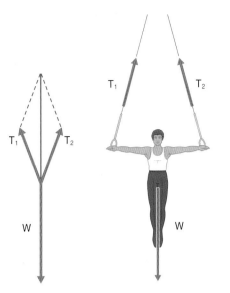

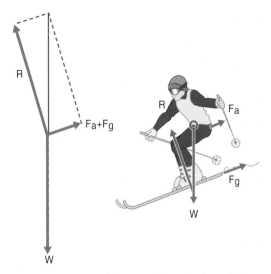

B. Again, the resultant of the normal reaction force (*R*) and the combined friction forces (air resistance and friction with the ground) exactly cancels out the weight of the skier – note the geometric vector diagram (dynamic equilibrium).

A. The resultant of the forces in the wires (*T₁* and *T₂*) supporting the gymnast upwards cancels out exactly his/her weight (*W*) downwards (static equilibrium).

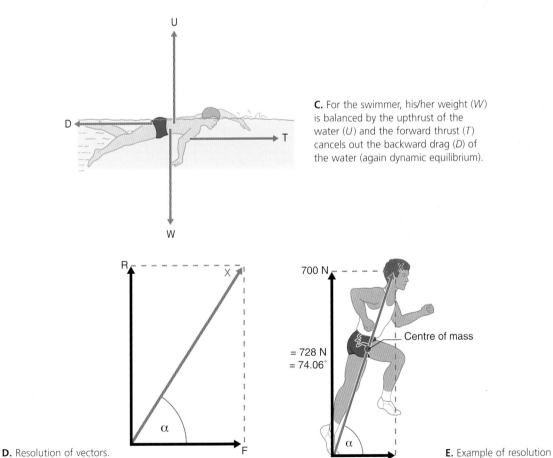

C. For the swimmer, his/her weight (*W*) is balanced by the upthrust of the water (*U*) and the forward thrust (*T*) cancels out the backward drag (*D*) of the water (again dynamic equilibrium).

D. Resolution of vectors.

= 728 N
= 74.06°

E. Example of resolution of vectors.

Fig. 7.3 Resultants of forces.

Hence the resultant force has a value of 728 N acting at an angle of 74.06° to the 200 N force (horizontal). (Note that this force *X* passes through the centre of mass of the runner and therefore would cause no toppling or rotation of his/her body during the running action; see p. 235 on the effect of the net force **at** take-off on the motion of a jumper **after** take-off for a further explanation of this.)

Components of a vector

It turns out that it is possible to do the opposite of this process and split a **single** force into two parts at right angles to one another – this is called **taking components**. This is particularly useful when looking at vertical and horizontal components of a force; it might enable you to see how a complicated set of forces could add up or cancel out in relation to the **weight** of an object, which is always vertical.

The components together with the original force form a right-angled triangle (see Figure 7.4). Then we see that:

$$\frac{F_v}{F} = \sin\alpha \text{ and } F_v = F \times \sin\alpha$$

and

$$\frac{F_h}{F} = \cos\alpha \text{ and } F_h = F \times \cos\alpha$$

where F_v = the vertical component of F, F_h = the horizontal component of F (the original force) and α = the angle the original force makes with the horizontal.

Note that **either** the original force **or** the components can be used, but not **both together**.

Example

Looking at Figure 7.4B of a discus in flight with a velocity of 25 m s^{-1} at an angle of 35° to the horizontal (approximately the situation at the moment of release of an international-standard thrower), the vertical and horizontal **components** of this velocity can be calculated as for forces (velocity is a vector and obeys the same rules as forces):

$$\begin{aligned} &\text{vertical} \\ &\text{component} \quad V_v = 25 \times \sin 35° = 14.34 \text{ m s}^{-1} \\ &\text{of velocity} \end{aligned}$$

$$\begin{aligned} &\text{horizontal} \\ &\text{component} \quad V_h = 25 \times \cos 35° = 20.48 \text{ m s}^{-1} \\ &\text{of velocity} \end{aligned}$$

It is worth noting in this example that the vertical component changes with time (since gravity acts vertically downwards and will accelerate the discus – change its velocity – continuously in a downward direction), whereas the horizontal component hardly changes throughout the flight since the horizontal forces (i.e. air resistance) that would produce a change in horizontal velocity are small compared with the weight; see p. 206 (Investigation 7.1, Task 5, point 3) and the *Teachers' guide* for further explanation of this.

It is beyond the scope of this book to progress these ideas further (physics text books will provide many examples of the use and practice of the formulae) and the *Teachers' guide* to this text (5th edition) gives examples related specifically to sporting situations.

Measurement of force

Force is measured in **newtons**, one newton (N) being defined as that force which produces an acceleration of 1 metre per second squared (1 m s^{-2}) in a mass of 1 kilogram (1 kg). (This is linked with Newton's Second Law of Motion, mentioned in Task 9 of Investigation 6.1.)

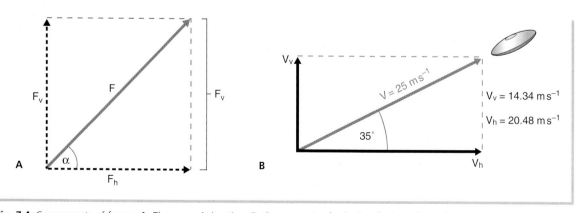

Fig. 7.4 Components of forces. **A.** The general situation. **B.** Components of velocity of release for a discus.

Review questions

1. What are the characteristics of a vector quantity?
2. A stationary snooker ball is struck by a cue and experiences a force of 60 N which is applied at an angle of 30° to the long side of the table. Sketch a diagram to show the direction of the ball relative to the long side of the table.

Calculate the components of the force which act parallel to the long and short sides of the table.
3. State Newton's Second Law of Motion.
4. If the mass of the ball is 0.1 kg, what was the acceleration of the ball during the time the cue was in contact with it?

A more convenient measure is that one newton is approximately one-tenth of the **weight** of a 1 kilogram mass, as shown in Figure 7.5.

The following paragraphs deal with the nature of force and how forces are applied.

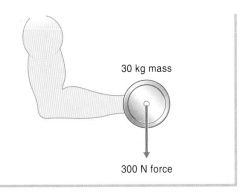

Fig. 7.5 The lifter lifts a **mass** of 30 kg and exerts a **force** of 300 N.

Weight

Gravity is an example of a **force field** (others occurring in nature are electromagnetic and nuclear fields which are not relevant to this text).

A force field is a means by which a force can be exerted **without touching**. So, for example, a ball in flight is accelerated towards the earth's centre continuously and therefore has a net force acting on it without being in contact with the earth.

When thinking about this, you may be confused by the fact that the air **surrounds** the ball (since the ball is in contact with the air, which in turn is in contact with the earth). However, experiments on falling objects have been done in a vacuum, which confirm the concept of the 'non-touching' force.

For our purposes, what is relevant is the gravity field at the earth's surface. This field exerts a force of 10 N for every kilogram of mass; this figure is known as the **gravitational field strength** (g) (the actual figure is $9.81 \ \text{N kg}^{-1}$ but it is usual to approximate this to $10 \ \text{N kg}^{-1}$ to simplify calculations). In other words,

every kilogram mass has a force of 10 N acting on it towards the earth's centre, regardless of whether the mass is in contact with the ground or other surface or whether it is moving through the air without contact (Figure 7.6). Newton first introduced the notion that

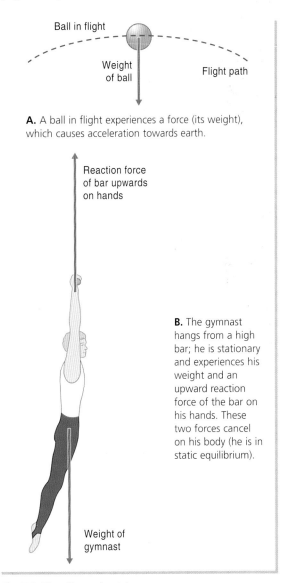

A. A ball in flight experiences a force (its weight), which causes acceleration towards earth.

B. The gymnast hangs from a high bar; he is stationary and experiences his weight and an upward reaction force of the bar on his hands. These two forces cancel on his body (he is in static equilibrium).

Fig. 7.6 The effects of weight.

the gravity force is proportional to the mass of an object, so the force on 1 kg would be 10 N, on 5 kg it would be 50 N and on 100 kg it would be 1000 N and so on.

The effects of altitude on weight

In fact, Newton's Universal Law of Gravitation says that the force of attraction between two objects is not only proportional to the masses of the objects but also inversely proportional to the square of the distance between the centres of the objects. This means that as we move away from the centre of the earth (as, for example, when athletes undertake altitude training or competition at altitude – the Mexico Olympic Games) there is a reduction in the weight of the sportsperson or thrown implement. The effect is small, however, and at an altitude of 3000 m above sea level the gravitational field strength decreases from 9.8100 N kg^{-1} at sea level to 9.8009 N kg^{-1}, a reduction of less than 0.1%, which is insignificant in the context of physical activity.

This effect must not be confused with the reduction in oxygen pressure due to altitude and the consequent potential reduction in performance due to reduced oxygen uptake. At 3000 m above sea level, O_2 pressure is reduced by more than 10% of the sea-level value, which definitely causes a reduction in **aerobic** capacity.

The difference between weight and mass

At this point it is worth mentioning that in scientific terms **weight** and **mass** are not the same.

The **mass** of a body is the same everywhere for that given object and does not change with, for example, the gravity field. So someone on the moon, where gravity is one-sixth that of earth, would have the same mass as on earth. Mass also depends on the quantity of matter present in the body and is related to the inertia.

Inertia is explained as resistance to acceleration. The more inertia an object has, the harder it is to accelerate when a given force is applied. This is why it is a good idea for any sportsperson who has to change speed or direction rapidly or accelerate from rest to have the least body mass possible consistent with the necessary strength (Figure 7.7).

The concept of inertia is derived from **Newton's First and Second Laws**; the quantity m in the formula $F = m \times a$ relates exactly to this, so inertia is therefore a property of mass and consequently a property of all objects. Inertia also applies to decelerating objects or people, so that, once moving, an object requires a

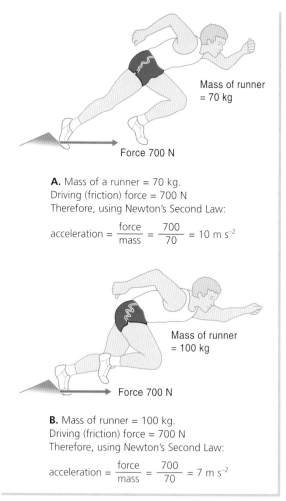

A. Mass of a runner = 70 kg.
Driving (friction) force = 700 N
Therefore, using Newton's Second Law:

$$\text{acceleration} = \frac{\text{force}}{\text{mass}} = \frac{700}{70} = 10 \text{ m s}^{-2}$$

B. Mass of runner = 100 kg.
Driving (friction) force = 700 N
Therefore, using Newton's Second Law:

$$\text{acceleration} = \frac{\text{force}}{\text{mass}} = \frac{700}{70} = 7 \text{ m s}^{-2}$$

Fig. 7.7 The effects of inertia. A bigger mass/inertia of the runner means a smaller acceleration for the same force.

force to slow it down or stop it. For example, at the end of an indoor 60 m sprint, runners have difficulty in stopping (Figure 7.8); this is because of the inertia of their mass.

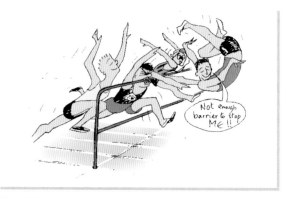

Fig. 7.8

Weight, in comparison, is the force due to the gravity field and changes with the gravity field (for example, on the moon). It is therefore always present as a vertical downward force acting on either a sportsperson or an object in flight. In most situations, it is very large relative to other forces such as air resistance, friction, the Bernoulli effect and so on. Weight can be calculated using the formula:

$$\text{weight} = \text{mass} \times \text{gravity field strength}$$
$$w = m \times g$$
$$\text{where } g = 10 \text{ N kg}^{-1}$$

As weight is proportional to mass, the acceleration produced by weight alone is always the same (i.e. the acceleration due to gravity is always 9.81 m s^{-2} or approximately 10 m s^{-2}). This means that sportspeople or objects in flight have weight as the predominant force.

The examples in Figure 7.9 assume air resistance to be small compared with the effect of weight. Note that in each case the flight is a parabolic arc – this is discussed in more detail in Investigation 7.1 (Figure 7.10 shows the precise shape of a parabolic arc).

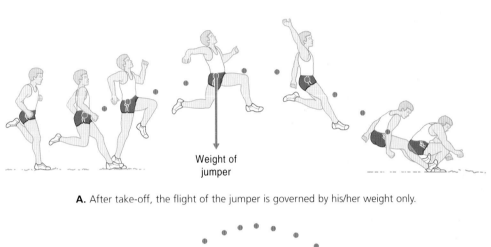

Weight of jumper

A. After take-off, the flight of the jumper is governed by his/her weight only.

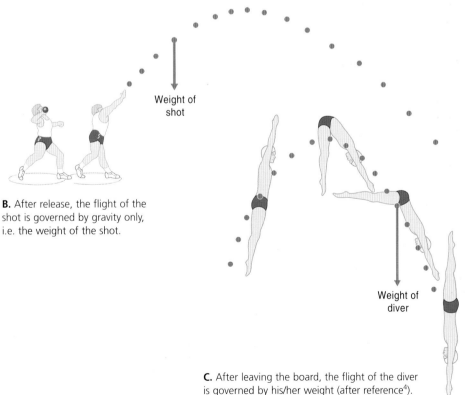

Weight of shot

B. After release, the flight of the shot is governed by gravity only, i.e. the weight of the shot.

Weight of diver

C. After leaving the board, the flight of the diver is governed by his/her weight (after reference[4]).

Fig. 7.9 Predominant force in flight.

Factors affecting the distance travelled by an object in flight

Once an object is in flight, gravity (and to a lesser extent the air) controls the situation but it might be useful to list the factors that affect the distance travelled by the object before it touches the ground again.

Velocity at start

Remembering that the concept of velocity includes both **speed** and **direction** (it is a vector), the important factors are **speed** value and the **angle** between the direction of flight and the horizontal; the optimum angle to ensure maximum distance would be 45° if the start of the flight was at the same height as the landing. This will be the crucial factor in optimising the distance travelled and will be determined by the timing of forces and the way in which they are applied to the object (shot, badminton shuttle, rugby ball, etc.) before release into the flight. The faster the object is launched into its flight, the further it will travel.

Height of release

This is the **height** of the starting position **above the landing position** and affects the optimum angle. For example, for a shot-put of 20 m and a release height of 2 m, the optimum angle (to ensure the maximum distance thrown) would be approximately 42°.

Air resistance

This is greater when the object travels faster (see section on air resistance and fluid friction, p. 214) and it applies throughout the flight. Most objects (shots, balls, people) travel slowly enough or are so shaped that this factor is small compared with gravity, but for others (badminton shuttle) this factor is larger than gravity, particularly when moving quickly at the start of flight (see the discussion in Investigation 7.1 and in the *Teachers' guide*).

Lift forces

These are caused by the aerodynamic shape of an object (discus, javelin, American football, etc.) and they also apply throughout the flight.

Spin

This causes swerving, dipping or soaring of a ball and is caused by the Bernoulli or Magnus effect – see p. 216 and the *Teacher's guide* on this topic.

Investigation 7.1   Flight of a ball or thrown or struck object

Aim: to consider the flight paths of different objects. The word 'object' is meant to include badminton shuttles, discuses and javelins, as well as light and heavy balls.

Task 1

Work in threes – one acting as thrower, one as catcher and the other as viewer and/or sketcher.

1. Throw or strike the following objects outdoors – remember that you are watching the flight path, not playing a game:

   a. shot
   b. discus
   c. football
   d. tennis ball
   e. golf ball
   f. cricket or hockey ball
   g. javelin
   h. frisbee.

   To obtain the most simple shapes, try to make the release height as near as possible to the landing or caught height.

2. In each case sketch the flight path as you see it **from a position some distance from the flight and observed at right angles to it**. The stress is laid on this because we want a view of the flight undistorted by the perspective of the thrower (or striker) or receiver of the ball or object.

3. It may be helpful to take a video film of these flights, so that the shape of the flight path can be assessed more carefully. This would then be viewed indoors later and corrected versions of the flight paths drawn up.

Task 2

1. The same sequence is repeated indoors, this time with a gently thrown or struck:

   a. badminton shuttle
   b. tennis ball
   c. indoor shot
   d. squash ball.

2. This lends itself more to observation by video film.

3. Drawings of flight paths should be sketched.

Task 3 – analysis of flight paths

1. Collect together drawings (from the whole group) into groups:

   a. flight paths almost exactly symmetrical or parabolic in shape
   b. flight paths nearly symmetrical but obviously not so
   c. flight paths definitely asymmetrical.

▶

2. i. What characterises groups **a**, **b** and **c**?

   ii. Make a list of factors that might affect the shape of flight for each group. Consider effects like: weight of the object, speed of the object, spin of the object and so on.

3. Create a chart of possible factors in the three categories above.

Figure 7.10 shows a typical shape of a symmetrical flight path. Note that the shape is parabolic and not circular and is that mentioned in the section on the effect of weight on objects.

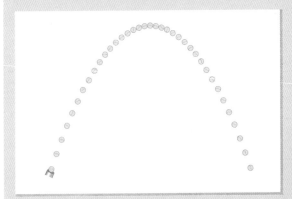

Fig. 7.10 A typical shape of a symmetrical flight path.

Task 4 – what forces affect the flight path?

1. Sketch a diagram of the flight path of:

   a. a shot
   b. a badminton shuttle
   c. a football (outdoors).

2. Indicate the forces acting on each object. Assume that the object is well clear of the ground and moving upwards (at an angle of about 45° to the vertical) with considerable speed.

3. Remember that once the object is in flight and moving with whatever velocity it started with (at whatever angle to the horizontal), the only things that can affect the flight are the earth's pull of gravity (force = its weight) and the effects of the atmosphere.

   a. In which direction will the gravity force (its weight) always act?

   b. In which direction will the air resistance force act (relative to the direction of motion at any given point in the flight path)?

Task 5 – how do the forces affect the flight path?

1. a. If gravity always acts in the same direction (downwards, towards the centre of the earth), what shape would this give the flight path if there were no air resistance? (Sketch your answer.)

   b. Would the shape of the flight path always be the same (regardless of the shape or mass of the object) if there were no air resistance?

2. a. What factors does the air resistance force depend on?

   b. Fluid friction (scientific term for air resistance) depends on the speed of the object (the faster it goes, the more the force) and on the shape of the object. How do these factors fit in with what happened to our real objects in flight?

3. What effect will air resistance have on the motion of our flying objects?

   This depends on the property of inertia (mass) of the object. The argument goes like this:

   a. For any two objects of the same size and shape moving at the same speed, the air resistance will be the same and in the same direction.

   b. If the two objects have different masses, then the effect of the same air resistance force on each would be different; the heavier (more massive) object would be decelerated less than the lighter (less massive) object. (This follows from Newton's Second Law of Motion, i.e. $F = m \times a$. For a given force, $m \times a$ remains the same, so if m is bigger, a must be smaller and vice versa.)

4. Write about one side of A4 to show how these ideas explain what you have observed in the first parts of this investigation.

Task 6 – the effects of spin during flight

You will now perform a series of experiments indoors with a table tennis ball.

1. Attempt to observe and draw diagrams of the flight paths for:

   a. side spin – left and right handed
   b. top spin
   c. underspin (backspin).

2. In each case mark on your diagram the direction (or sense) of spin – clockwise or anticlockwise to the direction of view; also show the direction of swerve or dip of the ball.

   The Bernoulli effect, which enables winged objects heavier than air to fly, is thought to be responsible for these effects. This is called the Magnus effect when applied to the air flow around a spinning ball and is discussed in more detail later in this section.

3. Go and practise (and then write an explanation of how you did it) the spinning and swerving of one or more of:

   a. a tennis ball
   b. a cricket ball
   c. a soccer ball
   d. a golf ball.

Shape of flight paths and forces acting on projectiles

The general rule is that the more symmetric (and therefore parabolic in shape) the flight path, the less effect that air resistance, lift or the Magnus effect has on the object in flight and the more dominant the weight of all forces acting. The opposite is true for highly asymmetric flight paths, where the air resistance (and possibly lift or Magnus effect forces) is dominant.

Figure 7.11 shows three examples of force diagrams and flight paths for (A) a shot, in which the dominant force is the **weight**, (B) a badminton shuttle, in which the dominant force is the **air resistance**, and (C) a spinning table tennis ball with backspin, in which air resistance and the **Magnus effect** are both important. In example (C) the Magnusk effect would be responsible for the soaring first part of the flight. In these diagrams, **A** represents the air resistance force, **W** the weight and **M** the Magnus effect force.

Note that flight paths for a slow-moving badminton shuttle could be nearly parabolic (symmetrical) because air resistance (which depends on its speed) would be low.

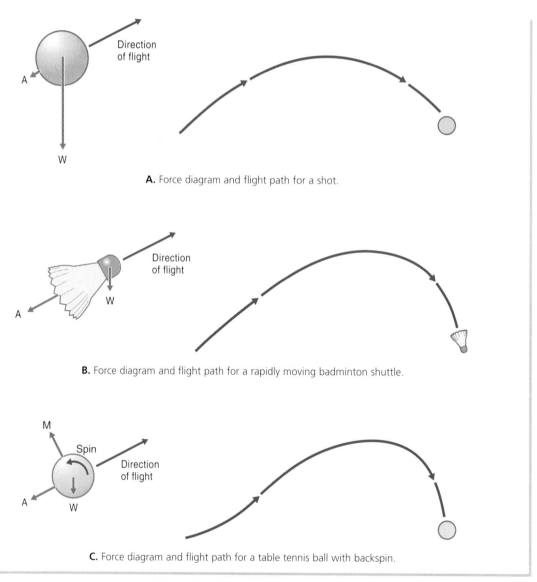

A. Force diagram and flight path for a shot.

B. Force diagram and flight path for a rapidly moving badminton shuttle.

C. Force diagram and flight path for a table tennis ball with backspin.

Fig. 7.11 Forces acting and flight paths for different objects in flight.

Review questions

1. Assuming air resistance to be negligible, what is the name of the path followed by a shot once in flight?

2. Sketch a diagram to show the flight path of the shot from the moment it leaves the putter's hand to the moment it lands.

3. Add arrows to your diagram to represent the horizontal and vertical components of the velocity of the shot at:

   a. the point it leaves the putter's hand
   b. the highest point of the flight path
   c. the point in the path level with the point of release
   d. the point just before landing.

4. State and briefly explain **three** factors (excluding air effects) which should be used by the putter to optimise the distance thrown.

Reaction forces

Reaction forces are those produced as a result of **Newton's Third Law of Motion** and were discussed in Investigation 6.1. This law states that when any object exerts a force on another, then it experiences an equal force exerted by the other but opposite in direction (Figure 7.12).

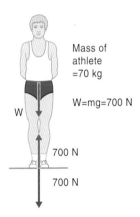

A. The athlete pushes **downwards** on the ground with a force of 700 N – the ground therefore pushes **upwards** on the athlete with a force of equal value.

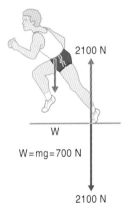

B. The athlete drives hard **into** the ground with a force of 2100 N – the ground therefore pushes **upwards** on the athlete with a force of 2100 N. Here the net upward force on the athlete is 1400 N, which causes an upwards acceleration of 20 m s^{-2} (using $F = m \times a$, with $F = 1400$ N and $m =$ mass of athlete = 70 kg).

Fig. 7.12 Reaction forces.

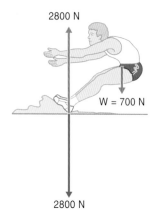

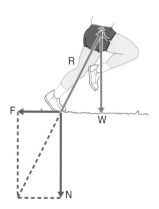

C. As the jumper lands, he pushes **into** the sand at 2800 N, which in turn pushes **upwards** on him at 2100 N. The net upwards force is now 2100 N, producing a deceleration of 30 m s^{-2} (again, using $F = m \times a$, with $m = 70$ kg).

D. The total reaction force is the resultant of the normal reaction (i.e. at right angles to the ground) and friction forces (parallel to the ground). In this example, the reaction resultant (R) on the athlete is a reaction to the athlete pushing both backwards (F) and downwards (N) on the ground.

Fig. 7.12 Reaction forces.

Reaction forces with the ground (or from the ground on the athlete) are caused as the athlete pushes hard downwards on the ground. These forces enable the ground to push upwards on the athlete and hence cause upward acceleration of the athlete. The skilful person can vary this force by swinging or moving any body segment, such as the trunk, arms or legs, as demonstrated in Figure 7.13.

A detailed discussion of reaction forces is to be found in reference[1].

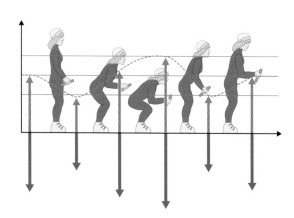

A. As the skier in this example moves her body down and then up, the **downward** force she exerts on the ground (black arrows) changes and hence the reaction force of the ground **upwards** on her (red arrows) varies.

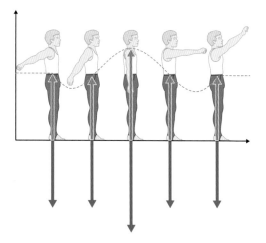

B. A similar example to that in **A** is of a person swinging his arms. As the arms accelerate downwards or decelerate upwards, the force exerted on the ground is less; as the arms swing violently at waist level the effect is to pull down on the shoulders and hence increase the force on the ground. The reaction force upwards on the body exactly mirrors this.

Fig. 7.13 Reaction forces on the body.

Reaction forces during the strike of a ball

Reaction forces can also be applied to the impact between sportsperson and ball, as in striking a ball with the foot, golf club, tennis racket, etc. The force forwards on the ball is equal and opposite in direction to the reaction force backwards on the foot and so on. In Figure 7.14, the force forwards on the ball is marked in red and the reaction in black.

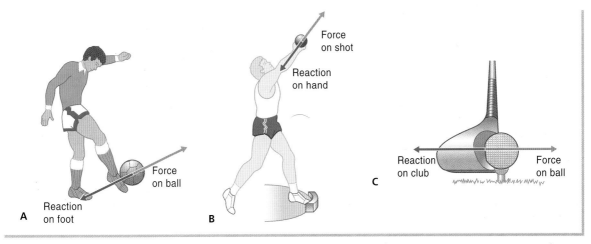

Fig. 7.14 Reaction forces during the strike of a ball. **A.** Kicking a ball (after reference[4]). **B.** Putting the shot (after reference[4]). **C.** Hitting a golf ball.

Reaction forces within the body

Action and reaction forces within the body are caused when any muscle contracts. The two ends of the muscle pull equally on one another. In Figure 7.15 the insertion of the muscle is pulled to the left and the origin to the right. The effect this has on the body shape or relative position of the different limbs and attachments depends on which of these are able to move.

Examples of muscle contraction causing changes in body shape, as origins and insertions are pulled towards one another, are shown in Figure 7.16.

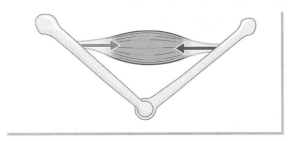

Fig. 7.15 Reaction forces within the body.

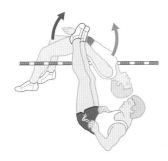

A. Bending over the bar during the high jump.

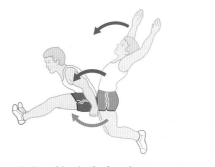

B. Stretching in the long jump.

Fig. 7.16 Muscle contractions causing changes in body shape.

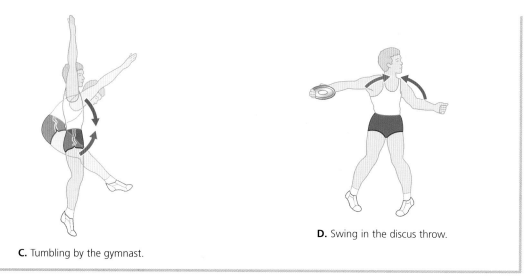

D. Swing in the discus throw.

C. Tumbling by the gymnast.

Fig. 7.16 Muscle contractions causing changes in body shape.

Friction forces

Friction forces act sideways to any two surfaces that are sliding or trying to slide or slip past each other.

Friction forces are extremely important to the athlete or sportsperson since even walking would be impossible without them (Figure 7.17). Forces that enable a person to accelerate, slow down or swerve and change direction are due to friction between the footwear and the ground (Figure 7.18). Therefore, anything that lowers the friction (mud, flat shoes, ice, etc.) drastically affects the ability of the person to do these things.

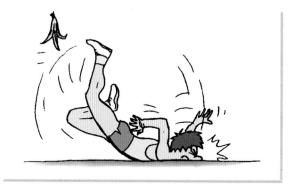

Fig. 7.17 'Ouch! No friction.'

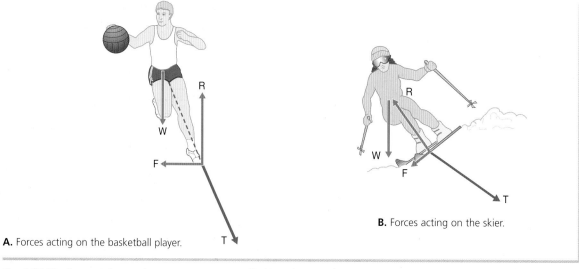

A. Forces acting on the basketball player.

B. Forces acting on the skier.

Fig. 7.18 The forces acting on the sportsperson are marked in red. Note that in each case the normal reaction force (at right angles to the ground) is marked R and the friction force F; T is the thrust of the athlete on the ground (marked in black), i.e. the force the athlete applies to the ground in order to achieve the swerve or acceleration required

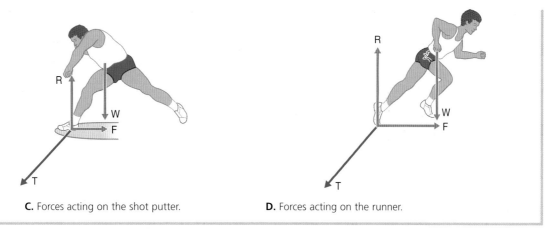

C. Forces acting on the shot putter.   **D.** Forces acting on the runner.

Fig. 7.18 The forces acting on the sportsperson are marked in red. Note that in each case the normal reaction force (at right angles to the ground) is marked R and the friction force F; T is the thrust of the athlete on the ground (marked in black), i.e. the force the athlete applies to the ground in order to achieve the swerve or acceleration required.

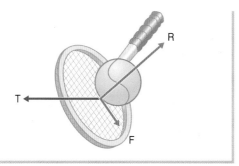

Fig. 7.19 Forces acting on the ball are marked in red and the thrust of the ball on the racket is marked in black. In this case the friction force F will cause the ball to spin.

In conclusion, the amount of friction that can be exerted depends on the nature of both the footwear and the surface and on the normal reaction forces between the footwear and the surface. This latter point is particularly significant in the case of the racing car with inverted wings, which force the car down onto the road, thereby increasing the reaction force on the car and therefore increasing cornering friction between tyres and road.

For an athlete, running spikes are an attempt to remove completely the differences between various footwear and surfaces and considerable research has been undertaken by shoe companies to find variations (bobbles, nylon barbs, spike plates, brush spikes, etc.) that would be more effective in this aim. Studs do the same job for games players and shoe companies lay great store by the efficiency of their shoe stud patterns for different conditions of playing surface.

Investigation 7.2   The effect of different footwear and surfaces on friction forces

Aim: to demonstrate how friction forces change as footwear and surface change.

Task 1
1. There is an almost unlimited number of combinations of the two factors; in fact, any combination from:

spikes	rubber track surface
flat trainers	shale track surface
studs	grass
ridged trainers	sand
walking boots	mud
climbing boots	ice
discus shoes	concrete
etc.	etc.

2. Some measure of comparability can be gained from a timed run over 20 m.
3. Each student can perform the 20 m run with a range of footwear and surfaces.

Task 2 – tabulation of results
Complete Table 7.1 by putting the fastest time at the top of the chart and the slowest at the bottom.

Task 3 – analysis of results
1. Obviously, it will be difficult to prove anything scientifically from this investigation, but it should be possible to place the footwear–surface combinations in some sort of grouped order, the most friction to the least.

▶

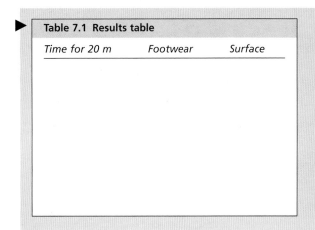

Table 7.1 Results table

Time for 20 m	Footwear	Surface

2. What factors increase friction?
   a. It would be simple to say clean, dry fixed surfaces (with no loose material), but is it always the case that ridged, spiked or studded shoes have the most friction?
   b. What about the effect of smooth-soled shoes on concrete?
   c. What effect does surface water have?
   d. Why are rock-climbing boots completely smooth soled?
   e. Does the area of contact between shoe and surface play a part?
   f. Do spikes completely eliminate the effect of surface?

Pressure

Another concept useful when looking at footwear and surfaces is that of **pressure**. Pressure connects together the force applied to a surface and the area of surface it is applied to.

For example, traditional snowshoes and skis have a **large surface area** which means that the person wearing them doesn't sink into the snow as readily as someone wearing ordinary shoes. This is because the pressure is less the larger the area of contact and the less the pressure, the less the tendency to sink into the snow. This can equally be applied to the sportsperson with big feet not sinking into the mud as easily as one with small feet (and having the same weight) and explains why spikes work so well on rubberised tracks.

The formula for pressure is:

pressure = force per unit area of surface
(applied at right angles to the surface)

$$= \frac{\text{force applied to surface}}{\text{surface area of contact}}$$

(unit = pascal = N m^{-2})

Take the example of a sportsperson of mass 60 kg (whose weight is therefore = 10 × 60 = 600 N) wearing size 9 training shoes. When running, the area of sole in contact with the ground is, say, 40 cm^2 (= 0.004 m^2). The pressure of his foot on the ground is given by:

$$\text{Pressure} = \frac{\text{his weight}}{\text{area of sole}} = \frac{600}{0.004}$$

$$= 150\,000 \text{ N m}^{-2} \text{ or } 150\,000 \text{ pascal (Pa)}$$

If, on the other hand, he were to wear spikes, the surface area of the point of the spike (this could be applied to studs or ripples also) is the area in immediate contact with the ground.

If we estimate this area as 6 mm^2, assuming six spikes each with a point of the area of 1 mm^2 (6 mm^2 = 0.000006 m^2, i.e. 6 millionths of a square metre), then the pressure now on the ground at the point of contact is given by:

$$\text{Pressure} = \frac{\text{his weight}}{\text{area of points of spikes}} = \frac{600}{0.000006}$$

$$= 100\,000\,000 \text{ Pa}$$

This new pressure is now large enough to penetrate the track surface so there is an enormously improved grip.

Air resistance and fluid friction

As discussed in Investigation 7.1, **fluid friction** is the scientific term used to describe resistance to motion of any object or body moving through a fluid – gas or liquid. This force (marked **A** in Figures 7.20–7.22) depends on the shape and speed of the moving object and acts in the opposite direction to that of its forwards motion. In each of the diagrams, the weight of the moving object or person is marked **W**.

Experiments have shown that a sphere moving through a fluid experiences a drag (fluid friction force) proportional to the speed of movement through the fluid and the radius of the sphere for slow-moving spheres. It also depends on the stickiness of the fluid (viscosity – the more viscous a fluid, the slower flowing it would be). This means that since air is far less viscous than water, the drag effects in air (runners, cyclists, cars, etc.) are far less than those in water (swimmers, waterskis, boats, etc.). Sportspeople are usually not spherical in shape but the fluid friction

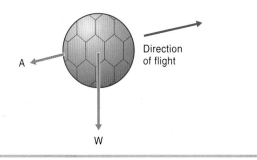

Fig. 7.20 Forces acting on a ball in flight. The most simple object has the shape of a sphere and in this case the fluid friction force is proportional to the radius of the sphere and to its forward velocity. So it can be guessed that the size of a swimmer, boat or freefall diver, as viewed from the front, affects the size of the fluid friction force.

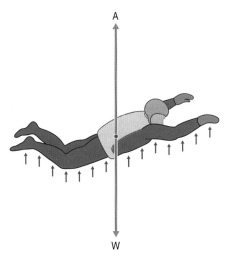

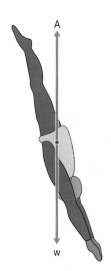

A. The freefaller moves at terminal (constant) velocity with the force of air resistance exactly balancing weight (after reference[4]).

B. In a diving position the freefaller would move faster because the air resistance force is too small to balance the weight at the slower speed. He would therefore accelerate and increase the fluid friction force until the two forces balanced again.

Fig. 7.21 Air resistance on the falling person.

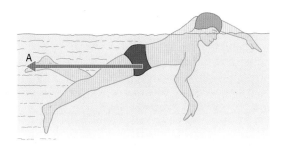

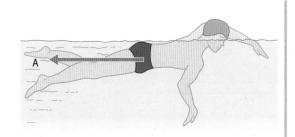

A. Swimmer hanging down in the water.

B. Swimmer lying more flat in the water.

Fig. 7.22 The swimmer in **A** has a bigger shape, when viewed from the front, than the swimmer in **B** and therefore has a larger fluid friction force A. As an object moves through the fluid, it has to push fluid out of its way, so obviously the more fluid that needs to be moved, the greater the fluid friction force.

effect still depends on the size – as observed from the forward direction – and the speed (some studies have shown that drag is proportional to the square of the speed). This means that the fluid friction gets very large very quickly as a sportsperson moves faster through a fluid, particularly water.

Streamlining

If we can make the fluid flow smoothly past the object, as opposed to being flung into vortices, then the fluid friction drag will be less. Smooth flow means that the fluid flows in layers (scientifically termed **laminar flow**). It is the design of the shape of wings, car bodies, racing cyclists' helmets, ski and speed-skating outfits and swimming gear that tries to reduce the tendency for fluid to be flung sideways into vortex patterns. The rough texture of certain types of cloth can also create vortices when moving through air. The two racing cyclists' helmets (seen from above) shown in Figure 7.23 are moving at the same speed and have the same profile if looked at from the front, but the helmet profiled in Figure 7.23B has less fluid friction because the air flows smoothly past in layers.

Helmet moves to the left

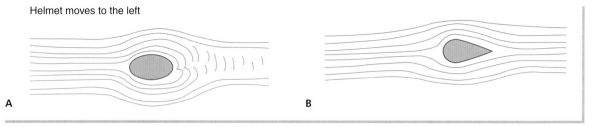

A   B

Fig. 7.23 Streamlining of racing helmets. **A.** Poorly streamlined, creating vortices. **B.** Streamlined to create laminar flow.

Review questions

1. What is the effect of air resistance on the flight path of an object?
2. Explain the effect of air resistance on the flight of two badminton shuttles, one of which has been struck hard and one gently.
3. Briefly explain why the flight of a shot in athletics is so different from the flight of a badminton shuttle.

Investigation 7.3   Drag on a swimmer in the pool

Aim: to look at how the shape and speed of a body (or boat) moving through water affect the fluid friction drag of the water. You will need a force meter that can measure up to 500 N.

Task 1 – towing the swimmer
1. Students should work in pairs, one towing and one in the water. The person doing the towing (A) will need to practise two speeds of moving (walking and trotting) and try to maintain these when actually towing.
2. Student A then tows the swimmer using a rope, either fastening it to the swimmer's wrist or to a body harness. The rope should be attached to a force meter.

3. Four different tows are suggested (see Figure 7.24).
4. Tow at the two speeds practised and tabulate the results.

Task 2 – discussions of observations
1. What effect does speed have on drag force?
2. What effect does shape or area of body, when viewed from the front, have on the drag force?
3. Look for water turbulence in the four situations – which has most and which least?
4. What conclusion would you draw about the best body shape and position when swimming?

▶

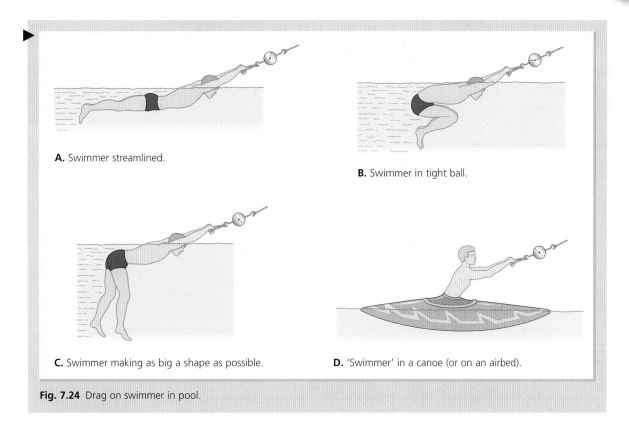

A. Swimmer streamlined.

B. Swimmer in tight ball.

C. Swimmer making as big a shape as possible.

D. 'Swimmer' in a canoe (or on an airbed).

Fig. 7.24 Drag on swimmer in pool.

Review questions

1. **a.** Identify three physical factors (not **skill** factors) which govern a swimmer's speed and explain how one of these occurs.
   b. Describe the factors which determine the amount of fluid friction acting on a swimmer.
   c. Explain how you would minimise **turbulent flow** (high-drag vortex creation) of the water past the swimmer's body.

2. **a.** Give three examples, each from a different sporting context, to show how fluid friction affects the sportsperson.
   b. Taking examples from a sport of your choice, explain three factors which would affect the size of the fluid friction force acting on the moving person or object (use diagrams in your answer).
   c. How would you attempt to reduce fluid friction?
   d. Sketch a vector diagram (with arrows representing the size and direction of the forces) to show all forces acting on a badminton shuttle in flight.
   e. Mark the **resultant** force on your diagram and briefly explain how the direction of the resultant force helps explain the path of the shuttle.

The Bernoulli effect

As mentioned briefly above, this is the effect that enables wings to fly and that can be applied to spinning and swerving balls in flight. Essentially, the pressure on a surface is reduced when a fluid flows past and the faster the flow, the greater the reduction in pressure. On a very simple level, this is because there is less chance of a fluid molecule striking the surface if the fluid is flowing rapidly; hence an effective reduction in pressure is created.

Application of this idea to a spinning ball is called the **Magnus effect** and concerns the way the air flows past the ball (Figure 7.25).

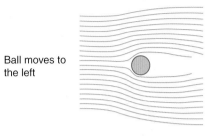

Ball moves to
the left

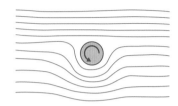

A. For a non-spinning ball, the air moves past symmetrically;
there is no sideways force.

B. For a spinning ball, air flows further past the lower edge
and therefore travels faster on this edge; hence pressure is
reduced on the bottom of the ball and the ball swerves
downwards.

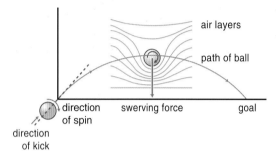

air layers

path of ball

direction
of spin

swerving force

goal

direction
of kick

C. This diagram shows how a
soccer corner kick can be made
to swerve into the goal.

Fig. 7.25 The Magnus effect.

Review questions

1. **a.** Using the ideas involved in the Magnus effect,
    draw a diagram which shows the direction of
    the force experienced on a ball with sidespin.
    b. Identify one sport, other than a ball game, in
    which the Bernoulli effect plays a part.
    c. When a spinning ball bounces, it exerts forces
    on the ground. Explain with a diagram what
    happens when a ball with **backspin** bounces.
2. **a.** The Bernoulli effect states that a faster flowing
    liquid or gas exerts less pressure than a slower

    moving liquid or gas. Using the diagram in
    Figure 7.25B, show how the Bernoulli/Magnus
    effect explains the swerve of a spinning ball.
    b. Show with diagrams how your explanation
    relates to the flight of a table tennis ball with
    side, back and topspin.
    c. Sketch a vector diagram of all the forces acting
    on a table tennis ball in flight with backspin
    and explain how the resultant force on the ball
    predicts its actual acceleration.

Impulse and impact

When a foot, bat or club strikes a ball, there are often
very large forces acting on the ball during the period
of contact. These cause correspondingly large
accelerations of the ball as it moves from rest to its
speed at the start of its flight. Since such forces act
over very short times, when dealing with such cases
it is convenient to use a different approach to that of
the straightforward definition of acceleration and
Newton's Second Law of Motion.

The same idea is applicable to tennis, squash,
cricket and baseball where the ball is already moving

rapidly on contact with the racket or bat. This new
approach is as follows.

Strictly, Newton's Second Law should read:

$$\frac{\text{Force applied}}{\text{to a body}} = \frac{\text{rate of change of}}{\text{momentum of the body}}$$

$$\text{Force} = \frac{\text{change of momentum}}{\text{per second}}$$

$$\text{Force} = \frac{\text{change of momentum}}{\text{time taken to change}}$$

or

$$\text{Force} \times \text{time} = \text{change of momentum}$$

This brings in two new constructs as below:

Momentum: defined by mass × velocity
or **momentum = $m \times v$**

Impulse: defined by force × time
or **impulse = $F \times t$**

Therefore Newton's Second Law becomes:

impulse = change of momentum
$F \times t$ = change of $(m \times v)$

Note: this formula is compatible with our original Newton's Second Law formula since:

change of $(m \times v)$ = $m \times$ (change of v)

therefore

$F \times t$ = $m \times$ (change of v)

or

$$F = m \times \frac{\text{(change of } v)}{t}$$

and

$F = m \times$ acceleration

Use of impulse in impacts

In Figure 7.26 we see the force of impact on the ball (F) and its reaction on the foot of the kicker (R). This force of impact lasts for a short time (*t* in the formula).

Figure 7.27 shows a graph of force of impact against time. It shows a force of 250 N lasting for 1/50 s. It can be seen that the product $F \times t$ has the value $250 \times 1/50 = 5$ Ns.

This can be equated to the area under the graph (shaded red). The area under a force–time graph is a convenient measure of impulse.

In practice, the force of impact is not constant but varies with time. It is possible to measure how F changes with time using a force sensor mounted on the ball or foot. Figure 7.28A shows how a graph of force (acting on the ball) against time would look.

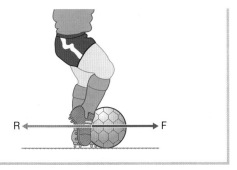

Fig. 7.26 Force (*F*) and reaction force (*R*) when a ball is kicked.

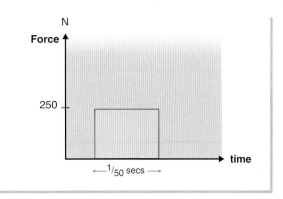

Fig. 7.27 Graphic measure of impulse.

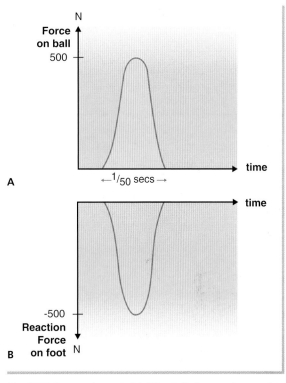

Fig. 7.28 Forces when a ball is kicked. **A.** Force acting on the ball against time. **B.** Reaction force acting on the foot against time.

Impulse is defined as the area under the graph (shaded red), which represents the total force × time added up over the time of contact. Note that the maximum force is large, 500 N, and the time of contact short, 1/50 s.

impulse = area under graph
= 1/2 × 1/50 × 500 approximately
= 5 Ns

(this assumes that the shape in Figure 7.28A is a triangle and its area = 1/2 × base × height).

If the mass of the ball, $m = 0.5$ kg, then the change of momentum

$$= m \times \text{change of velocity of the ball}$$
$$= 0.5 \times \text{final velocity}$$

Therefore

$$\text{impulse} = \text{change of momentum}$$
$$5 \text{ Ns} = 0.5 \times \text{final velocity}$$

and so

$$\text{final velocity} = 10 \text{ m s}^{-1}$$

Figure 7.28B shows the graph of the reaction force on the foot of the kicker with time. Note that the graph exactly mirrors that of the force on the ball – this fits in with Newton's Third Law, since at all times the reaction force must be exactly equal and opposite (and therefore negative) to the force on the ball.

Investigation 7.4   Impulse and impacts

Task 1
When a tennis ball is struck by a racket, as in Figure 7.29, the ball arrives with an incoming velocity of 15 m s^{-1} and leaves the racket with an outgoing velocity of 25 m s^{-1}. The mass of the ball is 200 g = 0.2 kg. Time of contact between ball and racket is 0.1 seconds.

1. Calculate the incoming momentum of the ball (remember: momentum = $m \times v$).

2. Calculate the outgoing momentum of the ball.

3. Calculate the change of momentum of the ball.

4. Using the formula:

   $F \times t$ = change of momentum

   calculate the average force of impact between ball and racket.

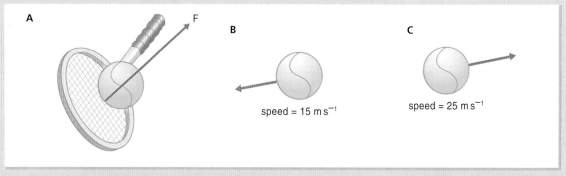

Fig. 7.29 Tennis ball struck by a racket. **A.** Force of the racket on the ball. **B.** Incoming velocity of the ball. **C.** Outgoing velocity of the ball.

Task 2
Look at the two graphs in Figure 7.30 of force of impact against time for a baseball bat striking a ball.

1. Explain why follow-through increases the outgoing velocity of the ball.

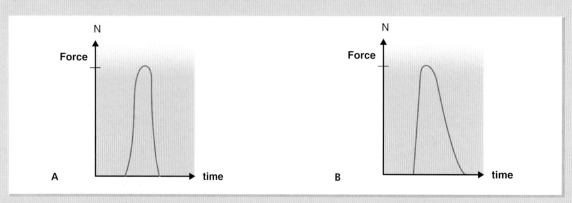

Fig. 7.30 Force of impact against time for a baseball bat striking a ball. **A.** The force acting on the ball without follow-through. **B.** The force acting on the ball with follow-through.

▶ **Task 3**
Explain why the catcher of a hard ball finds it more comfortable to let his hands ride with the ball on catching (Figure 7.31).

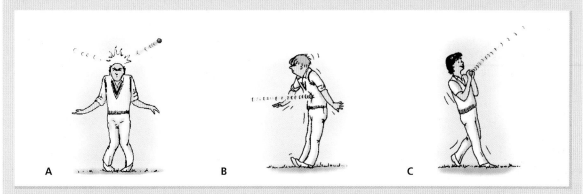

Fig. 7.31 Impact on catching a ball. **A.** Short time of impact – large force. **B.** Larger time of impact – moderate force. **C.** Long time of impact – …

Task 4
1. Look at the properties of ball and surface that may affect the outgoing velocity of the ball from an impact.

2. Where does the energy come from in ball–bat impacts?
3. What effect does spin of the incoming ball have on the outgoing spin, direction and velocity of the ball?

Applications of impulse

The reason that follow-through in striking a ball increases the outgoing velocity of the ball (not to mention better control of its direction) is because the **time of contact** is increased and therefore the **impulse** is increased.

When a ball is caught, the impulse is determined by the incoming mass and velocity of the ball (see Investigation 7.4, Figure 7.31) so an increase in the length of time over which force acts on the ball will reduce the force exerted during the catch. This is similar to the sprinter running into a barrier at the end of a 60 m indoor sprint – a padded barrier increases the time over which force is exerted and therefore reduces the force required to stop the sprinter (see Figure 7.32) and hence reduces the damage done to the sprinter on hitting the barrier.

Force platforms linked to a computer have been developed to analyse scientifically impacts between the foot and the ground during foot strike of a runner during a race or at the point of take-off for a high or long jumper or volleyball or basketball player when

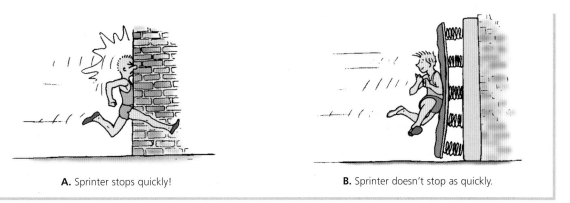

A. Sprinter stops quickly!   **B.** Sprinter doesn't stop as quickly.

Fig. 7.32 Impacts of a moving body against an object.

jumping. These produce graphs of force applied against the time of contact for both horizontal and vertical forces and allow comparison of the way in which force is applied for runners or jumpers of different standards and so point the way towards improvements in technique of the less competent performer.

Example of the application of impulse to foot impact in running

The interpretation of force–time graphs is crucial to understanding what happens in this case. For **horizontal forces**, graphs similar to those shown in Figure 7.33 would be produced. Examples are given for four different parts of a run: (A) when the runner is in contact with starting blocks or immediately at the start; (B) when he/she is accelerating during the first 2–3 seconds of a run; (C) when the runner is running at approximately constant speed during the middle of a run; and (D) during the slowing down at the end of a run.

In Figure 7.33A, the area under the force–time curve is above the horizontal axis (and hence positive), which means the force is acting **forwards** on the runner. The force lasts for a relatively long time,

therefore the impulse is high and positive and would cause large forward acceleration and change of forward velocity of the runner.

In Figure 7.33B, some of the area of the graph is below the horizontal axis and therefore negative but the overall impulse is positive, meaning that the runner is still accelerating forwards but not now as much as in case (A).

In Figure 7.33C, the positive area above the horizontal axis is exactly cancelled by the negative area under the axis. This means that the horizontal impulse is zero so the sprinter would not be accelerating or decelerating and would be running at constant speed.

In Figure 7.33D, the negative area below the axis of the graph is bigger than the positive part and hence the overall impulse is negative. This means that the runner will be experiencing an overall force (averaged over the stride) backwards and hence would be decelerating or losing speed.

In Figures 7.33B, C and D, the parts of the graphs which show a negative impulse (area below the horizontal axis of the graph) correspond to the situation where the foot placement is in front of the runner's centre of mass and so exerts a backwards force for a

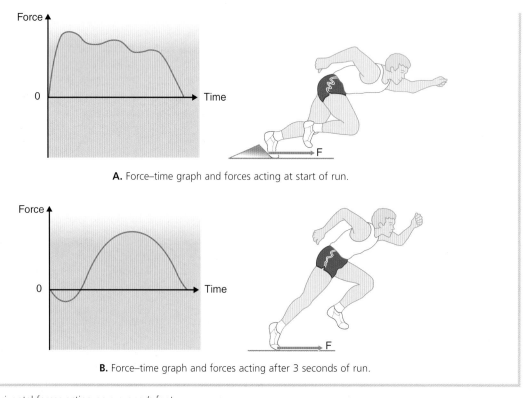

A. Force–time graph and forces acting at start of run.

B. Force–time graph and forces acting after 3 seconds of run.

Fig. 7.33 Horizontal forces acting on a runner's foot.

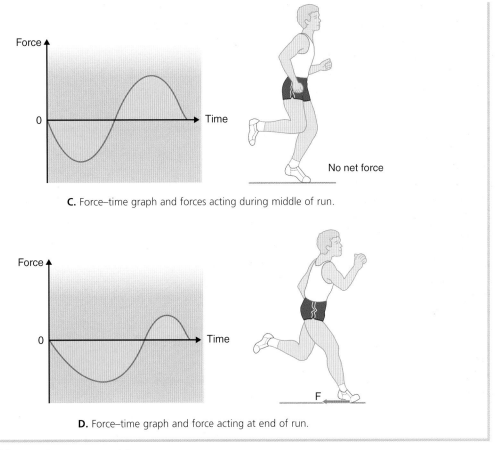

C. Force–time graph and forces acting during middle of run.

D. Force–time graph and force acting at end of run.

Fig. 7.33 Horizontal forces acting on a runner's foot.

short time. This is immediately followed by the centre of mass moving forward over the contact foot which then applies a forward force on the runner and hence a positive impulse for the latter part of the foot contact.

For vertical forces, a graph similar to that shown in Figure 7.34A would be produced. In this diagram, a positive impulse is shown (positive area above the horizontal axis of the graph) representing the upward vertical force exerted by the track on the athlete's foot (the reaction force). Figure 7.34B represents the **net upward force** acting on the runner, taking into account the **weight** of the runner acting downwards on his/her centre of mass. Now you can see that the total impulse is positive (upwards), since the area above the horizontal axis is bigger than the negative area. This happens because during the unsupported part of a stride (between foot placements), the centre of mass of a runner's body falls toward the ground requiring a net upward force from the foot to stop the fall and send his/her centre of mass back upwards during the unsupported phase of the next stride. On the force diagram of this situation in Figure 7.34B, the reaction force **R** is shown bigger than the weight of the runner **W**. See the *Teacher's guide* (5th edition) for a discussion of this and a calculation of the upward force exerted by a single foot placement during a sprint race.

Example of the application of impulse to a jumper taking off

Figure 7.35A shows a graph of the **vertical force** against time for the take-off foot of a volleyball player during the plant phase of his jump. The positive area above the horizontal axis of the graph represents the upwards impulse and hence force exerted by the floor on the jumper (reaction force). Figure 7.35B represents the **net force** acting on the jumper, again taking into account his/her **weight**. This is very similar to the runner's foot contact in Figure 7.34B above but note that now the impulse is positive, larger and lasts longer which tells us that there is a large average **net force** acting upwards on the jumper during take-off. This will cause the jumper to accelerate upwards and

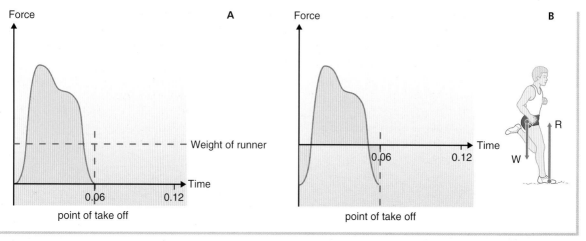

Fig. 7.34 Vertical forces acting on a runner's foot. **A.** Force–time graph for a single foot contact. **B.** Force–time graph of **net** force acting during single foot contact.

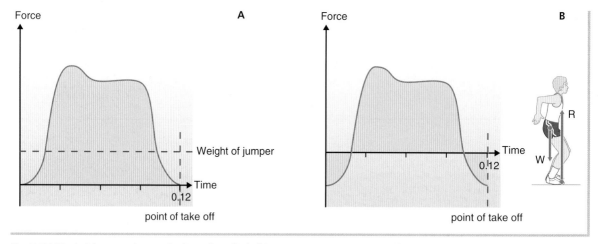

Fig. 7.35 Vertical forces acting on the feet of a volleyball jumper. **A.** Force–time graph for take-off phase. **B.** Force–time graph of **net** force acting on a jumper.

leave the ground; this upward acceleration needs to be larger and last for longer than the foot contact of the runner in order to send the jumper well off the ground. Now the reaction force **R** is much larger than **W** for most of the take-off process.

Conservation of momentum in collisions

In the above section the concept of **momentum** (**momentum = mass × velocity** of a moving object) was introduced as a way of looking at collisions and also as part of the fundamental description of Newton's Second Law of Motion.

Momentum is a **vector** (and has therefore both size and direction) and the same theory reproduced above can show that it is **conserved** in collisions in which no

external forces act. What this means is that if you were to calculate the momentum of two snooker balls (by adding together the values of mass × velocity, taking into account the direction) just before collision and then calculated it again just after the collision, you would find **exactly the same result**. The bit about no external forces means that the balls do not touch any other objects (cushion, cue, other balls, you) during the time of contact during the collision.

This law seems to apply everywhere in the universe and can be used to predict what happens during the collisions between planets and asteroids, spaceships and satellites and, on earth, rugby or football players and tacklers, moving racing cars and so on.

For example, a simple case is when a snooker cue ball strikes another head on **without spin**. This results in the object ball (the second ball) moving away from the collision at exactly the same velocity (speed and direction) that the cue ball had before the collision, with the cue ball stopping dead. Of course, all pool and snooker players use spin to position the cue ball after the collision, so what we have said here is a simplification. Another example is that of the running rugby (or football) player being able to brush off the tackle of a much bigger opponent. The momentum of the running player can be transferred to the tackler (and hence knock him/her over) with a skilful flick of the hips or a hand-off, particularly if the tackler is balanced, i.e. not leaning into the runner. This latter point is mentioned because the law of conservation of momentum in collisions does not apply if **external forces** are applied during the collision. If a tackler were to lean into the runner, then he/she would be exerting a force from the ground into the collision and hence preventing transfer of momentum from the runner.

Transfer of momentum

The case of the unspinning snooker ball striking another ball head on, causing the first ball to stop dead and the second ball to move with the same momentum as the original ball, is a direct case of transfer of momentum. The momentum of the cue ball is directly transferred to the object ball during the collision between the balls.

Most sporting situations in which collisions occur have some transfer of momentum. However, the amount of momentum transferred from a moving object (rugby player, for example) to the stationary object with which it collides (for example, the rugby tackler) depends on the relative mass of the two objects. The skill of the running player is to transfer as much momentum as possible to the tackler in order to evade tackling and the skill of the tackler is to apply as much force as possible from the surroundings to the runner in order to minimise transfer of momentum to himself and therefore successfully complete the tackle.

Another example of transfer of momentum would be when a racquet or bat strikes a ball. The momentum of the racquet would be much larger than that of a moving ball since its mass would be much larger. After the strike, some of the momentum of the racquet would be transferred to the ball, giving it substantial speed and direction in a way controlled by the player using the racquet.

Exam-style questions

1. a. The graph (Figure 7.36) shows the flight paths of three different types of projectiles found in sport:

    - **X** represents the flight path of a tennis ball with backspin
    - **Y** represents the flight path of a shot in athletics
    - **Z** represents the flight path of a badminton shuttle.

The force diagrams in Figure 7.37 represent the forces acting on the projectiles at the point in the path marked with a large dot in Figure 7.36.

   i.   Describe the nature of the forces labelled **A** and **B** in Figure 7.37. (*2 marks*)
   ii. Explain why each projectile has a different flight path. (*6 marks*)
   iii. What factors would affect the **distance** travelled by the shot? (*3 marks*)

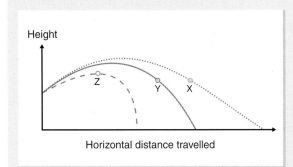

Fig. 7.36 Flight paths of tennis ball with backspin (X), shot in athletics (Y) and badminton shuttle (Z).

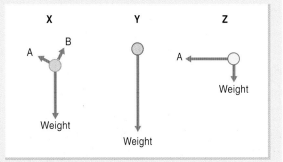

Fig. 7.37 Force diagrams for the tennis ball with backspin (X), shot in athletics (Y) and badminton shuttle (Z) at the points marked by a large dot in Figure 7.36.

b. Figure 7.38 illustrates the forces acting on a javelin. Force L is the **lift force** caused by aerodynamic forces acting on the javelin as a whole. Force W is the **weight** of the javelin.

i. How would the two forces affect the orientation of the javelin as it continues its flight? (*4 marks*)

ii. If the weight of the javelin cannot be changed, how could you alter the forces acting on the javelin other than throw it harder? (*4 marks*)

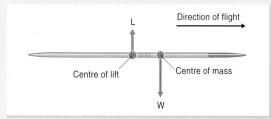

Fig. 7.38 Forces acting on a javelin in flight.

c. A hockey player strikes a ball.

i. Sketch a graph of the force applied to the ball (*y*-axis) against time (*x*-axis). (*2 marks*)

ii. Explain how using a follow-through would affect the motion of the struck ball. (*4 marks*)

(Total 25 marks)

2. a. Figure 7.39 shows a stationary golf ball about to be hit by a golf club. On impact, the club provides an impulse to the ball, as a result of which the ball gains momentum.

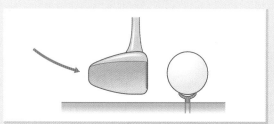

Fig. 7.39 Golf club about to hit a golf ball.

2. a. i. Explain the terms **impulse** and **momentum** with respect to the motion of the golf ball. (*2 marks*)

ii. The equation below defines the relationship between the variables involved in the motion of the golf ball from the tee as it is hit by the club:

$$Ft = m(v_1 - v_2)$$

Identify each variable in the equation. (*4 marks*)

iii. Assume the golf ball has a fixed mass of 0.046 kg and that the club head imparted a constant force of magnitude 6440 N to the ball for a period of 0.0005 seconds. Explaining your working, calculate how fast the ball will be travelling at the moment it leaves the face of the club. (*4 marks*)

b. Graphs **X**, **Y** and **Z** (Figure 7.40) show the **horizontal ground reaction force** versus **time** traces for three situations during a 100 metre sprint race. *Note:* Positive forces act on the runner in the direction of the run.

i. Explain how you can tell that graph **X** represents the horizontal force acting on the runner during a foot contact just after crossing the finish line. (*6 marks*)

ii. Each of the remaining two graphs represents the horizontal force acting on the runner during one of the following situations:

- the period of time during which the runner is leaving the starting blocks
- a foot contact in the middle of the race.

Match graphs **Y** and **Z** to each of these two situations. Describe and explain the reasons for your choices. (*4 marks*)

(Total 20 marks)

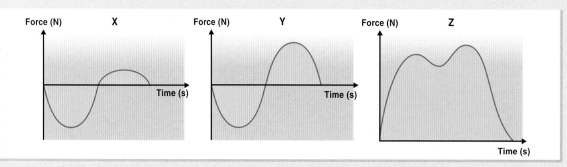

Fig. 7.40 Horizontal ground reaction forces versus time in a 100 metre sprint (after reference[3]).

3. a. When striking a ball:

   i. What factors govern the speed and direction of a tennis ball as it leaves the racquet? (*6 marks*)

   ii. Explain the importance of **follow-through** in striking a hockey or cricket ball. (*4 marks*)

b. An object in flight has a specific flight path due to the forces acting on it.

   i. Draw the flight path of a shot put. Make a sketch of the forces acting on it. (*2 marks*)

   ii. Draw the flight path of a badminton shuttle. Make a sketch of the forces acting upon it. (*2 marks*)

   iii. Explain the differences in the shape of the flight path of the two objects. (*4 marks*)

c. The **flight** of a ball is affected by spin.

   i. Illustrate the effects of topspin and backspin diagrammatically. (*2 marks*)

   ii. Explain the effect of sidespin, making sure that you indicate the direction of spin in relation to any swerving effect you may mention. (*2 marks*)

d. Explain the effect of spin on the bounce of a ball, illustrating your answer with a suitable example. (*3 marks*)

(*Total 25 marks*)

7.2 Internal forces

Learning objectives

On completion of this section, you will be able to:

1. Understand the concept of **moment** of a force applied to forces acting at a joint lever system in a sports person's body:

   moment of = force × perpendicular distance a force from fulcrum to line of action of force

2. Apply the **principle of moments** to lever systems and classify such lever systems:

   clockwise moment = anticlockwise moment

3. Describe some of the lever systems within joint complexes of a sports person's body.

4. Understand how **internal forces** are applied within a sports person's body and some of the effects produced by them.

5. Understand the concept of **centre of mass** and how its position in the body can be changed by changing the shape of the body.

6. Understand that the weight and mass both appear to act at the **centre of mass** and that the centre of mass of the body follows a parabolic path when in flight.

7. Understand that the **stability** of your body position depends on the position of your centre of mass relative to your base of support.

Keywords

- anticlockwise
- base of support
- centre of mass
- clockwise
- couple
- effort
- equilibrium
- fulcrum
- internal forces
- lever
- load
- moment of a force
- neutral equilibrium
- principle of moments
- stability
- stable equilibrium
- torque
- unstable equilibrium

Wirhed[1] uses the term **internal forces** to describe those forces exerted by one part of the body on another, via the musculature and internal system of ligaments and tendons of the body.

Simply, a muscle contracts when a suitable string of nerve impulses arrives and causes muscle fibres to shorten via a complex series of biochemical reactions, involving the consumption of glycogen and the release of energy. When this happens, both ends of the muscle, i.e. origin and insertion, are pulled towards each other in the manner described in the section on reaction forces and in Figure 7.41. The effect that this has on body shape, limb orientation and motion of the body or parts of it depends on the relationship

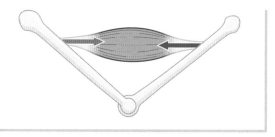

Fig. 7.41 Origin and insertion are pulled towards each other as the muscle contracts.

of the muscle insertion to the joint complex that enables movement in any particular case and whether or not the body is in contact with the surroundings. For example, consider the gymnast in Figure 7.42A who is performing a pike action while in flight. Here, both upper and lower body move **towards each other** as the abdominal muscles contract.

In Figure 7.42B the feet are fixed in position so that only the upper body moves when the stomach muscles contract.

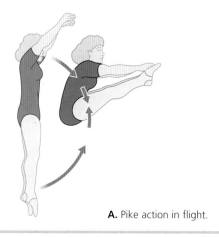

A. Pike action in flight.

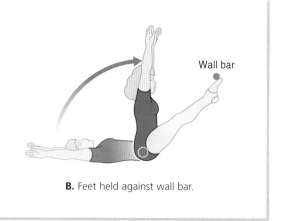

Wall bar

B. Feet held against wall bar.

Fig. 7.42 Effect of abdominal muscles contracting.

Investigation 7.5 Force developed in a muscle

This investigation uses the concepts involved in levers and the principle of moments applied to specific muscles in certain joint complexes. Since it is very difficult to isolate one muscle (or closely located group of muscles) in a body movement, two examples have been chosen. Others may be developed by the students but care must be taken when using these ideas that several muscle groups and joint complexes are not used. The simple technique here applies only to the simpler situations.

Materials: a range of force meters (or weight-training equipment) to measure forces up to 500 N and rulers or soft tape measures.

Task 1 – levers

1. Most of you will be familiar with the concept behind levers and what is meant by **pivot** or **fulcrum**. This is the balance point for the lever, the point about which the 'lever arm' turns or the **axis of rotation** of the lever system.

2. **Effort** is the force applied by the user of the lever to some point on the lever arm.

3. The **load** is the force applied by the lever system; this can be more than or less than the effort depending on the type of lever used.

4. Draw sketches of the following lever systems, identifying clearly the positions and directions of the **fulcrum, effort** and **load** in each case:
   a. a wheelbarrow
   b. nutcrackers
   c. a spade
   d. a screwdriver
   e. scissors or pliers
   f. a crowbar.

Task 2 – the principle of moments

1. The **moment of force** about a fulcrum is defined by:

   moment of force = force × distance to the fulcrum

   (Distance is measured at right angles to the force.)

   Moment of force is also known as **torque**.
   Couple is defined as the moment of a pair of equal ▶

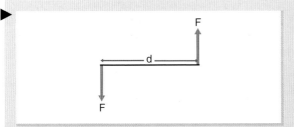

Fig. 7.43 A couple.

forces applied in opposite directions to a lever arm, as shown in Figure 7.43.

The couple = $F \times d$

2. Looking at Figure 7.44:

moment of force = force × distance to the fulcrum
(Distance is measured at right
angles to the force.)
= 200 (newtons) × 0.3 (metres)
= 60 Nm

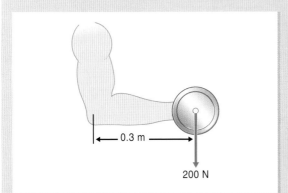

Fig. 7.44 Moment of force about a fulcrum.

3. The **moment** tends to turn the lever clockwise (the opposite direction of turn being anticlockwise). The **principle of moments** says that for a system of balanced forces about a fulcrum or pivot:

total
anticlockwise = total clockwise moment
moment   about the fulcrum

A system in balance in this way is said to be in **equilibrium**.

4. Consider the elbow joint complex in Figure 7.45. Calculate the moment of the weight held in the hand about the elbow joint as a fulcrum (this force, the weight, is the **load** on the lever) using:

moment of force = force × distance to the fulcrum
(fulcrum is at elbow)

This moment would be the **clockwise** moment, i.e. tending to turn the forearm in a clockwise direction.

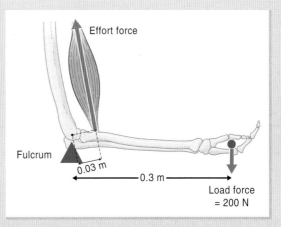

Fig. 7.45 The elbow joint complex as a lever.

5. The **anticlockwise** moment is provided by the force in the biceps muscle (this is the **effort** on the lever) as it pulls upwards to balance the force in the hand. Now calculate this force using the principle of moments:

anticlockwise = force × distance of biceps
moment   insertion from elbow joint

This must be equal to the final answer obtained in **4** above; therefore, we arrive at the equation:

anticlockwise moment = clockwise moment

Thus you can now calculate the force in the biceps muscle which is the only unknown quantity in the above equations.

Task 3 – calculation of the force in your own biceps muscle

1. You are now going to measure this force using the same method as above.

2. Make measurement with a ruler of the two distances marked in Figure 7.46, i.e. the distance of

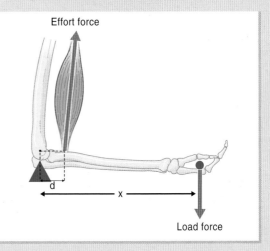

Fig. 7.46 Calculation of the force in the biceps muscle.

hand from the elbow (*x*) and distance of insertion of the biceps tendon to the elbow (*d*).

3. Measure the load force you can apply with your hand in the position shown in the diagram – the position is chosen so that the angles between the effort and the forearm and load and the forearm are both right angles. The force can be measured by using weights, a multigym or force meter.

   Remember: the weight of 1 kg is 10 N force.

4. Following exactly the procedure in Task 2 above, calculate the force developed in your biceps muscle.

Task 4 – force in Achilles' tendon and calf muscles
1. The aim now is to repeat this procedure for a further joint complex, i.e. the ankle.

2. From Figure 7.47, measure carefully **on yourself** the distances shown (it may be easier if a partner takes the measurements).

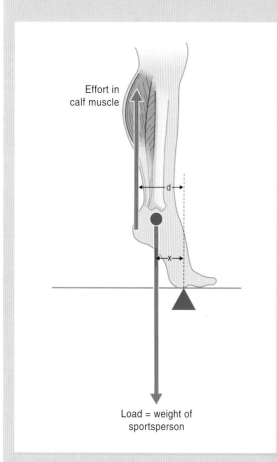

Fig. 7.47 Calculation of the force in the Achilles' tendon and calf muscle.

Note that the fulcrum is under the ball of your foot, i.e.:

Distance from tibia–ankle joint to fulcrum (*x*) and distance from Achilles' tendon to fulcrum (*d*).

Note: distances must be measured at right angles to the forces.

3. Calculate the force lifted by this system through your leg, adding together your weight (in newtons) to any weight or force exerted by your body (for example, a weight on your shoulders).

   Remember: 1 kg mass equals 10 N force

4. Now calculate the force in the Achilles' tendon using the same process as developed in Task 3.

Task 5 – another force in muscle calculation
Try to find another joint complex and range of muscles and an appropriate exercise that will enable you to calculate the force in the muscles in the same manner as in Tasks 3 and 4.

Task 6 – extension study
1. This further study examines the relationship between force developed in a muscle and the muscle girth or cross-section. It involves measurement of:

   a. muscle girth (using tape measure) **OR**

   b. cross-sectional area.

   Estimate maximum width of the muscle, *w*, assuming a circular cross-section and using the formula:

   $$A = \frac{\pi \times w^2}{4}$$

   find an approximate value for the area (**A**).

2. Create a table of force developed in a muscle used in Tasks 3, 4 and 5 and the girth or muscle cross-sectional area.

3. Next plot a graph of force developed in the muscle (*y*-axis) against muscle girth or cross-section (*x*-axis).

4. What can you conclude from the graph?

Task 7 – changing the angles
1. Taking the biceps group as an example, explore what happens when the angle between the effort and the lever arm (in this case the forearm) changes, as in Figure 7.48.

2. You will need to measure the angle between the 'pull' of the biceps and the forearm and note whether the force at the hand changes.

3. This task is left open for the student to explore the best method of displaying his/her results and deciding on a conclusion from these.

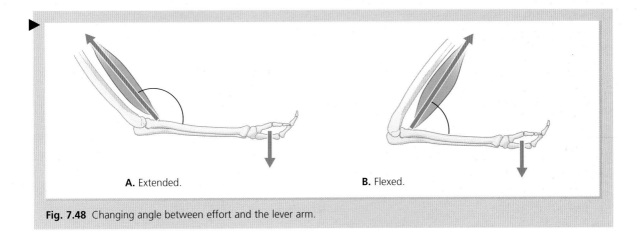

Fig. 7.48 Changing angle between effort and the lever arm.

A. Extended.

B. Flexed.

Classification of levers

Another way of looking at lever systems is to classify them in the following way.

Class 1 lever

The **fulcrum** lies **between** the **effort** and the **load**, as in Figure 7.49A. Note that if the system is in balance the principle of moments applies.

An example from a human joint complex is the action of the **triceps** muscle on the elbow joint; the **effort** lies in the muscle, the **fulcrum** at the elbow joint and the **load** at the hand exerting a force, as shown in Figure 7.49B. This particular arrangement has the load smaller than the effort (effort is closest to the fulcrum).

Class 2 lever

In this type of lever the **fulcrum** is at **one end** of the lever arm, the **effort** at the **other end** and the **load** is **between** fulcrum and the effort (Figure 7.50).

The example of this in the human body is the ankle joint, as discussed in Task 4 of Investigation 7.5. Here the load is larger than the effort (effort is further from the fulcrum).

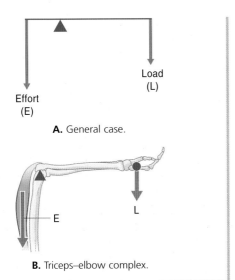

A. General case.

B. Triceps–elbow complex.

Fig. 7.49 Class 1 lever.

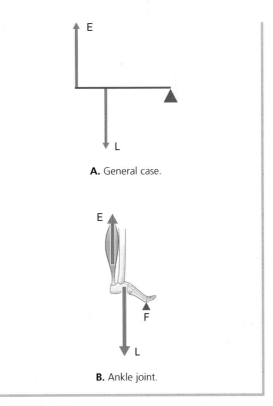

A. General case.

B. Ankle joint.

Fig. 7.50 Class 2 lever.

Class 3 lever

The **fulcrum** and **load** are at **opposite ends** of the lever arm, with the **effort** somewhere in the **middle**. In this case the effort is always larger than the load, since the effort is nearer the fulcrum (Figure 7.51A). This is the most common class of lever to be found in human joint complexes.

The simplest example from the human system is the biceps–elbow complex (Figure 7.51B), used frequently in the discussions above.

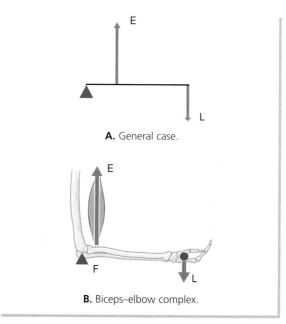

A. General case.

B. Biceps–elbow complex.

Fig. 7.51 Class 3 lever.

Review questions

1. Classify the lever systems mentioned in Task 1 of Investigation 7.5.
2. Research the human joint complexes and classify the lever class of as many groups as you can.

A more advanced lever representation

In the interests of simplicity, the discussion above has been restricted to those cases where the muscle (effort) action and the load direction are at right angles to the lever arm. This is because the definition of a moment includes the idea that all distances from the fulcrum are to be measured at right angles to the force involved.

In practice, of course, it rarely if ever happens that these angles are 90°, so it is necessary to be able to represent diagrammatically in a simple way real muscles and joints as they would naturally operate. From such diagrams it is possible to calculate the forces acting in muscles in the same way as in Investigation 7.5. Figures 7.52–7.55 show how this can be done.

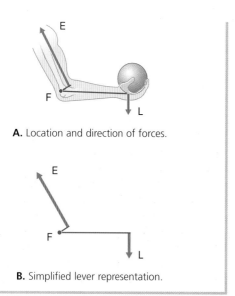

A. Location and direction of forces.

B. Simplified lever representation.

Fig. 7.52 The biceps–elbow system.

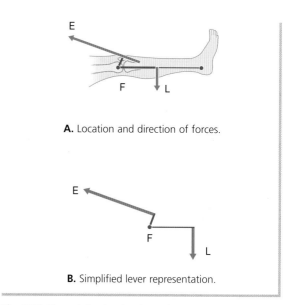

A. Location and direction of forces.

B. Simplified lever representation.

Fig. 7.53 The patellar tendon–lower leg system.

In each case:

'**A**' shows the location and directions of forces (**load** and **effort**) and **fulcrum**,

'**B**' shows the simplified lever representation. The load is, in each case, the weight of object, limb or head.

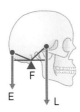

A. Location and direction of forces.

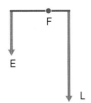

B. Simplified lever representation.

Fig. 7.54 The neck muscles–head system.

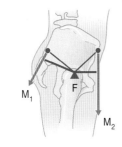

A. Location and direction of forces.

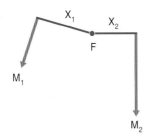

B. Simplified lever representation.

Fig. 7.55 The pelvic system.

In Figure 7.55, we have two antagonistic muscle groups working on opposite ends of the lever arm; the forces exerted by these muscles are marked M_1 and M_2, respectively and perpendicular distances from the fulcrum x_1 and x_2 (after reference[2]).

The effect of lever length on sporting applications

Individual differences between one sportsperson and another mean that it is difficult to make general comments on this issue. However, there are two fairly simple examples in which the effect of lever length could make a difference to sporting performance.

Shorter levers – the shortlimbed weightlifter

For a person with shorter arms but similar joint structure to, for example, the person discussed in Task 2 of Investigation 7.5, Figure 7.45 above, if the **same force** were exerted in the biceps muscle, then a **bigger force** would be exerted as the **load** at the hand. The same argument could be applied to triceps/elbow, quadriceps/knee and calf/ankle systems mentioned above. The reason for this is that the moment produced around the joint by the effort in the muscle is fixed by the joint anatomy and this moment is applied to the load via the lever arm. Since moment = force multiplied by distance from the fulcrum, the longer the lever arm, the smaller the load force produced and the **shorter the lever** arm, the **larger the load** force produced. This is why weightlifters tend to be shorter limbed than the average in the population.

Longer levers – the long-armed discus thrower

Spectators would note that the more effective discus thrower seems to have long arms (and is usually tall and long-limbed in general). The argument used to explain this is not really based on the force produced by the hand caused by the shoulder musculature but is to do with the speed of rotation of the limb system (arm rotating about the shoulder as an axis).

The argument goes like this. For a short-armed thrower, for example if the arm were to rotate through 30°, then his/her hand would move through a certain distance, whereas for a longer armed thrower, the hand would move further. This means the hand of the longer-armed thrower would be moving **faster** than that of the shorter arm for the **same rotational speed**.

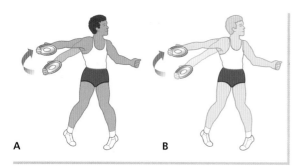

Fig. 7.56 A. The effect of lever arm on hand speed in a discus thrower. **B.** The discus moves further for the same angle rotated.

Figure 7.56 helps explain this idea. The point is that the longer-armed thrower could rotate (spin or turn) more slowly and therefore with more control and technical stability to produce the same release velocity of the discus or, by rotating at the same rate of spin, could produce a higher release velocity.

The effect of change of joint angle on load forces

This is discussed as part of Investigation 7.5, Task 7 above, with reference to Figure 7.48.

Most sportspeople will know that both elbow and knee joints appear to be substantially stronger when straight or almost straight. The comparison is most acute between the limb when straight and the limb whose joint is a right angle. This is because the lever arm between effort (in quadriceps for leg and triceps for arm) and fulcrum is more or less the same whatever the limb angle, because of the anatomy of each joint (see Figure 7.49B for the arm and 7.53A for the leg). Therefore the **moment** exerted by the muscles at maximum exertion will be more or less the **same** whatever the limb angle. This moment is then transmitted via the limb lever to the hand or foot and when the arm or leg is straight the lever arm is at a minimum and (since the moment = the load force multiplied by the length of lever arm) the load force would be at a maximum. Figure 7.57 helps to explain this – note that the lever arm is measured at right angles to the load force when computing the moment so although the hand is some considerable distance from the fulcrum, the line of action of the load force passes quite close to the joint fulcrum when the arm is straight.

Centre of gravity – centre of mass

This is the idea that the mass of a body behaves as if it is all at one point in the body instead of spread out across the arms, legs, torso, head, etc.

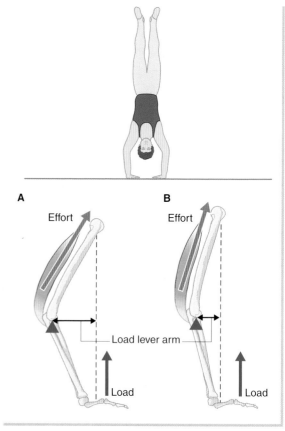

Fig. 7.57 The effect of joint angle on load force.
A. Larger load lever arm – small load force.
B. Small load lever arm – large load force.

Strictly speaking, the concept is **not** dependent on gravity and is relevant in weightless situations as well as on the surface of our planet. We therefore use the term **centre of mass** from now on.

Consider the simplified object in Figure 7.58 in balance (equilibrium) at the fulcrum marked. This is where the moment of the left-hand weight (anti-clockwise) balances the moment of the right-hand weight (clockwise). If we were now to apply a force to the system as a whole it would behave as if the mass were entirely at the balance point instead of in two parts.

Therefore, you can see that the definition of the position of the centre of mass is that at which the body would balance at any angle, if suspended at that position.

Also, if the body were suspended or hung from a point, the centre of mass would lie vertically below the point, since if it were not there would be a **moment** of the weight tending to turn it towards this position, as shown in Figure 7.59.

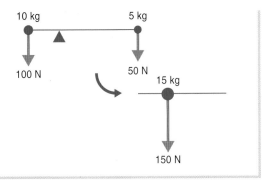

Fig. 7.58 Centre of mass is the balance point of all parts of the body.

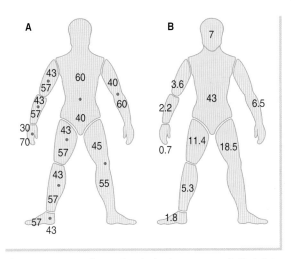

Fig. 7.60 Centre of mass for the body segments. **A.** Red dots mark centre of mass of the body segments, with percentage length shown on either side. **B.** Percentage of total body mass for each body segment.

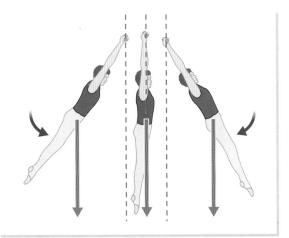

Fig. 7.59 In equilibrium, centre of mass lies vertically below point of suspension.

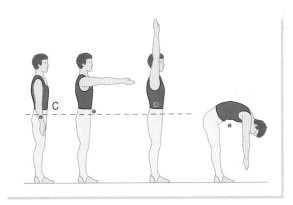

Fig. 7.61 Position of centre of mass (red dot) changes as body shape changes (after reference[4]).

The idea of **centre of mass** can be extended to any body (or object) spread out in space, such as the human body. This is obviously much more complicated than the simple example above but the same principle applies, only now with variable masses and distances from the fulcrum.

In Figure 7.60A the dots mark the approximate positions of the centre of mass of the body segment, with the numbers representing the percentage of the total length of the segment on each side of the centre of mass. Figure 7.60B shows the percentage of total body mass of each body segment (after reference[1]).

The application of the concept to the human body revolves around the fact that the position of the centre of mass will change as the shape of the body changes (Figure 7.61). The dots in Figure 7.61 mark the position of the centre of mass.

The detailed position of the centre of mass can be calculated (and computerised) using the methods of Wirhed[1] or Hochmuth[2].

It is also possible to use a mannequin (cardboard model, with jointed movable limbs weighted in proportion to actual body parts[3]) to simulate body shapes and discover the position of the centre of mass. This is done by hanging the mannequin from at least two points, determining a line vertically below the point of suspension and finding the intersection of the lines from each suspension.

It is now possible to simplify the mechanics of any given sporting situation to a single mass and a single **net** force (and a **couple**, which is a turning moment, as explained in Task 2 of Investigation 7.5).

Review questions

1. Explain the concept of **centre of mass** (centre of gravity). Illustrate your answer using sketches of the human body.
2. Research and describe an experiment you could use to determine the position of the centre of mass of a person who is adopting a sporting pose.
3. What effects do changes in body position have on the location of the centre of mass?
4. Explain with drawings how a high jumper changes the position of his/her centre of mass by changing body shape after take-off.

Motion of a jumper

We use the example of a jumper to illustrate how the **mechanics** of a sporting situation involving the human body can be simplified. Whether a high jumper, long jumper, basketball dunker, gymnast or trampoline tumbler, the mechanics can be split into two sections, **before take-off** and **flight after take-off**.

Before take-off

While in contact with the ground (or trampoline) the combination of **reaction force**, **friction force** and **weight** produces a **net** force on the jumper, as shown in Figure 7.62.

This **net** upward force produces an upward acceleration on the body, which can be increased by the skilful swinging or moving of trunk, arms and legs, as discussed in the section on reaction forces (p. 209), and in the section on impulse and the analysis of a force platform measurement for a jumper taking off (see Figure 7.35). We can therefore represent the vertical motion of the athlete on a velocity–time graph, as in Figure 7.63.

So at the instant of the foot leaving the ground the jumper has a velocity of just less than 4 m s^{-1} (in this example). In fact, the **centre of mass** of the jumper has an upward vertical velocity of 4 m s^{-1} and it will follow a flight path similar to (and following the same rules as) that of the objects in flight discussed in Investigation 7.2 above.

After take-off

In flight the force diagram (Figure 7.64) consists of just two forces: **weight** and **air resistance**. However, because the jumper is moving relatively slowly (so that air resistance is relatively small), the force is almost entirely the weight acting vertically downwards; hence the centre of mass of the jumper's body will accelerate vertically downwards at 10 m s^{-2} and will describe a parabolic path of the sort discussed in Investigation 7.2.

This is where the **flexibility** of the human body affects the pattern of the activity in the air. As you can see from Figure 7.64, the body changes shape considerably during flight, but the path of the centre of mass remains parabolic.

In the case of the high jumper, a skilful performer can actually have the centre of mass pass underneath the bar while clearing the bar with his/her body; in Figure 7.65 this is not quite achieved.

Similarly, the basketball dunker can gain extra height for his dunking hand by lowering the free arm and leg rapidly near the top of the jump (Figure 7.66).

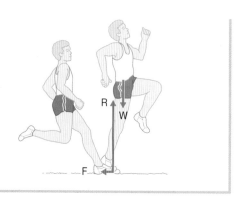

Fig. 7.62 The resultant of R, W and F will be upwards and slightly backwards.

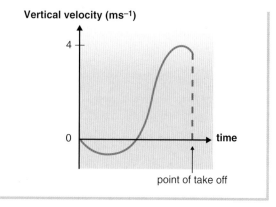

Fig. 7.63 Vertical motion of a jumping athlete on a velocity–time graph.

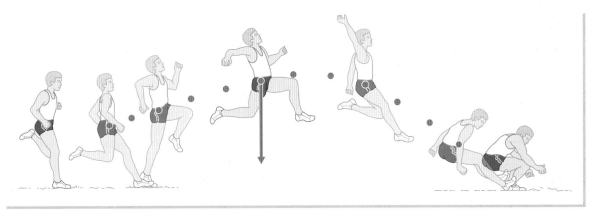

Fig. 7.64 Force diagram for a jumping athlete in flight.

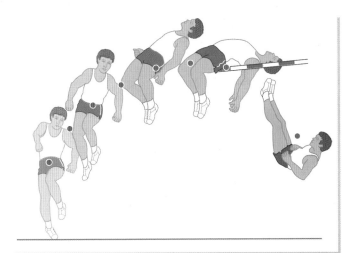

Fig. 7.65 Path of centre of mass (red dots) in a high jump.

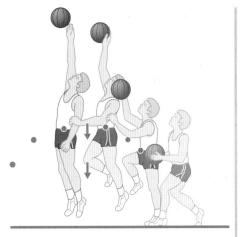

Fig. 7.66 Path of centre of mass (red dots) in a basketball dunk.

Note that the centre of mass still follows a parabolic path.

Effect of direction of net force on motion of jumper

In Figure 7.67, showing a jumper before take-off, the basketball player has the **resultant** (of reaction and friction) force of the ground on him/her acting in a direction **through** the centre of mass, whereas the high jumper has this force acting in a direction to the **left** of the centre of mass.

The effect of this is for the basketball player to keep the same body orientation throughout the jump, whereas the high jumper's body rotates in a clockwise direction.

In the case of the high jumper this is because the **net** force has a **moment** about the jumper's centre

of mass, which will cause rotation about this point as a fulcrum or axis of rotation.

More detail of this process is shown in Figure 7.67c, in which a tumbling gymnast applies force to the ground (which then applies force to him as shown – reaction force R and friction force F) which causes the take-off and subsequent tumbling motion. The resultant of these two forces (marked X on Figure 7.67c) lies to the left of the gymnast's centre of mass and causes upward acceleration (into the jump) and his somersault after take-off. The gymnast has to exert a large upward force on himself (and much larger than the weight so that the **net** force is still large and upward) to produce the upward acceleration necessary before take-off which will produce the height necessary to complete the somersault during flight. He also has to produce a large backward friction force, which will initiate the tumble process as violently as

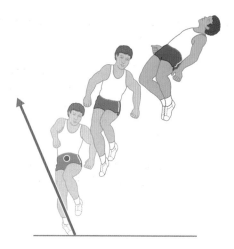

A. For the high jumper the resultant force acts in a direction away from the centre of mass.

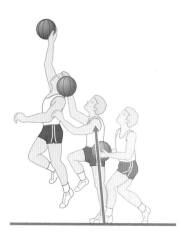

B. For the basketball player the resultant force acts in a direction through the centre of mass.

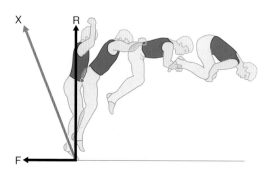

C. For the gymnast, backward friction force F and upward reaction force R combine to form a resultant X whose direction lies well behind the centre of mass.

Fig. 7.67 The jumper taking off.

possible and hence complete the somersault as quickly as possible. The more successful gymnast will initiate the timing of his drive into the ground **before take-off**, so that optimum somersault positions in flight and balance on landing will occur.

Once the athlete (jumper or gymnast) has taken off, then the path of the centre of mass and the **rotational momentum** of the body have been determined and **cannot be changed** (assuming the effect of air resistance can be ignored).

Review questions

1. Sport performers adopt strategies to improve height in situations such as basketball tip-off, rugby line-out, soccer header, etc. State the shape of the flight path of the centre of mass of the jumper once he/she has taken off and briefly explain why this cannot change once he/she is in the air (assume air resistance is so small as to be negligible).

2. How does the jumper change the position of his/her centre of mass relative to the centre of his/her torso during the jump?

3. The size and direction of forces applied before take-off can affect the subsequent flight. Sketch diagrams or briefly explain how this is done in the cases of a high jumper and of a basketball player executing a jump shot.

Stability

Another issue related to the concept of centre of mass is that of **stability**.

As mentioned above, a body suspended from a point will tend to hang so that the centre of mass is vertically below that point. This is called **stable equilibrium**, since whichever way the gymnast is pushed he/she will tend to return to the same position (Figure 7.68A).

On the other hand, a gymnast doing a handstand would fall over if pushed, although in balance (equilibrium) while he/she holds the handstand: this is called **unstable equilibrium** (Figure 7.68B).

Neutral equilibrium is where, on pushing the system, it immediately adopts a new equilibrium position – as for the gymnast lying on the floor (Figure 7.68C).

In practice, all sportspeople need to perform movements in balance, which is done by ensuring that the line of action of their weight lies between their **base of support**. In other words, the centre of mass lies **above** the base of support. If, on the other hand, the centre of mass lies above a point **outside** the base of support, then the sportsperson will lose balance and be unstable.

For example, in Figure 7.69 the martial arts performer adopts a stance with his feet wide apart, so that the opponent has to apply a large force to move his centre of mass to a position in which it lies over one of his feet; this is then unstable equilibrium and he can be thrown.

In order to increase stability the martial arts performer can bend his legs, thereby lowering his centre of mass and increasing the moment needed to tip him off balance.

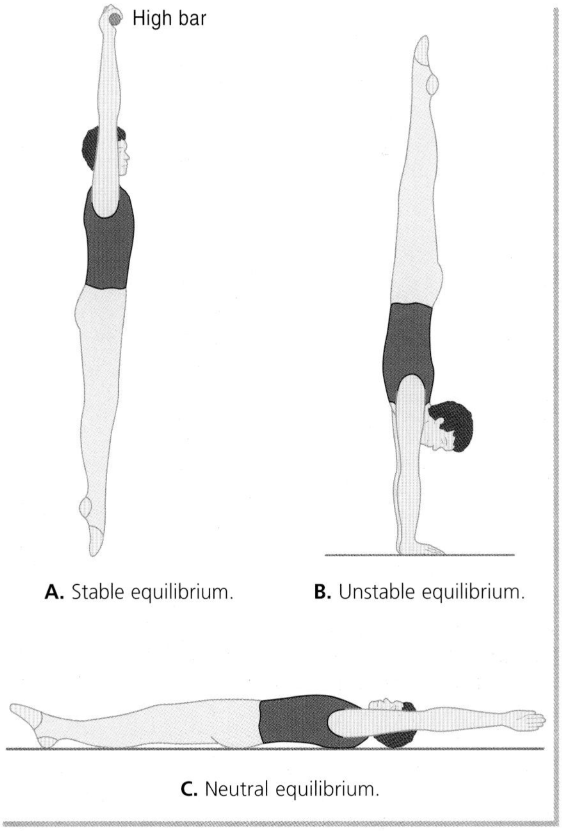

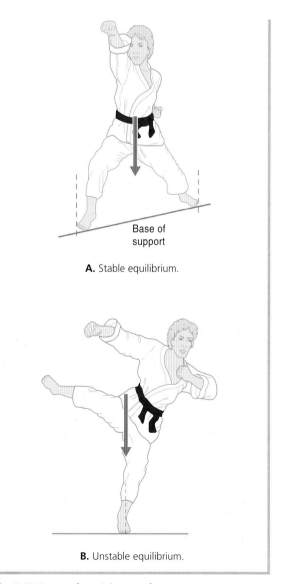

A. Stable equilibrium.

B. Unstable equilibrium.

Fig. 7.69 Stance of martial arts performer.

High bar

A. Stable equilibrium.   **B.** Unstable equilibrium.

C. Neutral equilibrium.

Fig. 7.68 Stability.

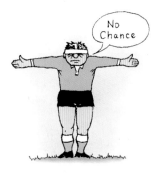

A. Easily made unstable.

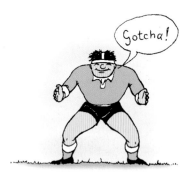

B. Difficult to make unstable.

Fig. 7.70 Stance of football or rugby player about to make a standing tackle.

Similarly, the rugby or football player about to make a standing tackle will adopt the stance in which the centre of mass must be moved further in order to be above a point outside the base of support (Figure 7.70).

A slightly more sophisticated example is that of the beam gymnast who needs careful control of the position of her centre of mass if she is not to fall off (Figure 7.71).

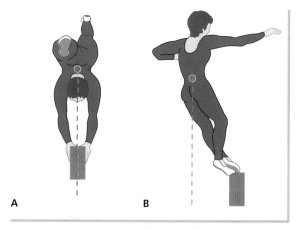

A   **B**

Fig. 7.71 Gymnast on beam. **A.** Centre of mass above beam but in unstable equilibrium. **B.** Centre of mass to side of beam and so off balance.

Exam-style questions

1. **a.** Figure 7.72 shows an elbow joint of a person performing an exercise. Work out the **clockwise moment** provided by the force of 160 N about the elbow as a pivot/fulcrum, then, assuming the arm is stationary, use the **principle of moments** to calculate the force F exerted by the biceps muscle. Show your working. (*6 marks*)

   b. The results from an experiment on various joints and muscles of the same person are given in Table 7.2.

     i. Plot a graph of force exerted by muscle against cross-sectional area of muscle using your answer *x* from **a** above. (*3 marks*)

     ii. What is the physiological reason for the shape of this graph? (*2 marks*)

   c. What feature of the ankle joint and its associated calf muscles makes it more efficient in exerting force to the body than almost any other joint? (*2 marks*)

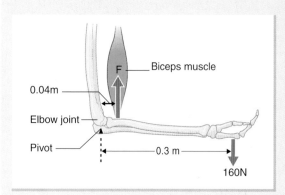

Fig. 7.72 Elbow joint of a person performing an exercise.

Table 7.2 Results table

Muscle	Force exerted by muscle/N	Cross-section of muscle/cm²
biceps	×	30
gastrocnemius	1400	40
triceps	1000	25
quadriceps	2000	70

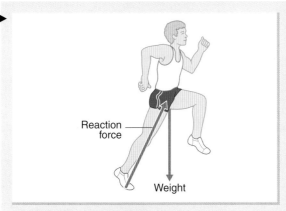

Fig. 7.73 Force diagram for a runner at the start of a race.

d. A sprinter uses his calf muscles to push hard on the blocks at the start of a run. Explain, using Newton's Laws, how this enables him to accelerate forwards out of the blocks. (*5 marks*)

e. Figure 7.73 shows the forces acting on the runner at the start of the race.

   i. Use a vector diagram to show how you could work out the **resultant** force acting. (*3 marks*)

   ii. If the resultant force was 200 N and the runner's mass was 50 kg, what would be his acceleration? (*2 marks*)

   iii. What would be the speed of the runner after 2 seconds, assuming that the acceleration is the same over that period of time? (*2 marks*)

   (*Total 25 marks*)

2. a. Figure 7.74 shows the elbow joint and the position of the triceps muscle in relation to it when supporting a load behind the head.

   i. Draw a simplified sketch to show the lever system, indicating the various forces that are operating. (*4 marks*)

ii. Using the values shown in Figure 7.74, calculate the load. Neglecting the mass of the ulna, estimate the effort needed to balance the system. (Take the gravitational force on 1 kg to be 10 N.) (*4 marks*)

iii. What anatomical factors would affect the value of the maximum load that this system could support, given that the angle between the long bones does not change? (*3 marks*)

iv. How would you expect the maximum load to change as the arm extends and briefly explain how this change of load affects the use of the arm in a sporting situation. (*2 marks*)

b. Sketch two other types of lever system within the body, labelling the effort, fulcrum and load in each case. (*6 marks*)

c. i. Briefly describe an experiment or investigation which would show the relationship between the forces exerted by different muscles and the muscle area of cross-section or girth. (*2 marks*)

   ii. Sketch a graph to show the relationship which might exist between cross-sectional area of muscle and muscular strength. (*2 marks*)

   iii. Relate the graph to muscle anatomy. (*2 marks*)

   (*Total 25 marks*)

3. a. Figure 7.75 shows a diagram of a sportsperson's foot pivoting at a point under the ball of the foot.

   i. Use your knowledge of the **principle of moments** applied to this lever to calculate the force F. Show **all** your working. (*4 marks*)

   ii. Sketch the lever system which would represent the action of the biceps muscle in **flexing** the arm. (*3 marks*)

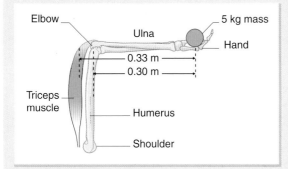

Fig. 7.74 The elbow joint and triceps muscle when supporting a load behind the head.

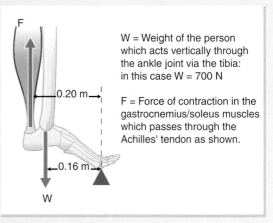

W = Weight of the person which acts vertically through the ankle joint via the tibia: in this case W = 700 N

F = Force of contraction in the gastrocnemius/soleus muscles which passes through the Achilles' tendon as shown.

Fig. 7.75 Sportsperson's foot pivoting at a point under the ball of the foot.

▶ **iii.** Explain why the biceps–radius lever system is much less efficient at exerting force on the surroundings than is the ankle–calf muscle lever system. (*3 marks*)

b. A high jumper firmly plants her foot on the ground before take-off. Figure 7.76 shows how the force of contact on the foot changes up to the point of take-off. *Note:* Positive forces are acting upwards. The weight of the jumper is 700 N.

  i. Sketch a **force diagram** to show all vertical forces acting on the jumper. (*2 marks*)

  ii. Explain why it is necessary for the foot contact force to be greater than 700 N. (*3 marks*)

  iii. Use your understanding of **Newton's Laws of Motion** to explain why it is necessary for the jumper to push her foot as firmly as possible into the ground just before take-off. (*3 marks*)

c. i. Briefly explain the meaning of **centre of mass** as applied to the human body and explain the effect if the line of action of the upwards force acting on the foot of the high jumper does not pass through her centre of mass. (*3 marks*)

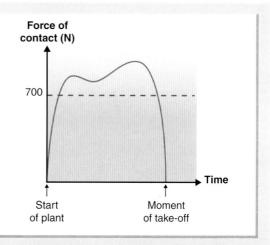

Fig. 7.76 Graph showing how the force of contact on a high jumper's foot changes up to the point of take-off.

  ii. Sketch a diagram and briefly explain how the centre of mass of the jumper can pass under the bar, while the jumper successfully clears it. (*4 marks*)

(*Total 25 marks*)

References

1. Wirhed R 1997 *Athletic ability and the anatomy of motion*, 2nd edn. Mosby, London
2. Hochmuth G et al 1984 *Biomechanics of athletic movements*, 4th edn. Sportverlag, Berlin
3. Hay J G, Reid J G 1988 *Anatomy mechanics and human motion*, 2nd edn. Prentice Hall, New Jersey
4. Watkins J 1983 *An introduction to mechanics of human movement*. MTP Press, Edinburgh

Rotating systems

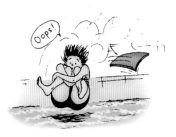

This final chapter on biomechanics deals with some examples of rotating systems in sport and the physical concepts involved.

Fig. 8.1

8.1 Angle and angular displacement

Learning objectives

On completion of this section, you will be able to:

1. Be familiar with the measurement of angles in **radians.**

2. Be aware of the use of a video system for the analysis of rotating human systems within a sporting activity.

3. Understand the concept of **angular velocity** as:

   angular velocity = angle turned through per second

4. Understand the concept of **moment of inertia** as applied to the human body when undertaking various spinning and rotating movements in a sports context.

5. Be aware of the concepts of **angular acceleration** and **rotational energy.**

6. Understand the concept of **angular momentum** as applied to sporting rotating human body situations, where:

   angular momentum = moment of inertia × angular velocity

7. Understand the **Law of Conservation of Angular Momentum** as applied to rotating human bodies and how this enables the sportsperson to vary his/her rate of spin.

Keywords

➤ angular acceleration
➤ angular displacement
➤ angular momentum
➤ angular velocity
➤ axis of rotation
➤ moment of inertia
➤ radian
➤ radius of gyration
➤ rotational energy
➤ rotational motion

Angle is a familiar concept to most people, so you readily understand what is meant by 30°, 90°, 180° and 360°. In scientific terms, angle is measured in **radians**. The radian as a unit of angle is defined in Investigation 8.1, Task 2, point 2; suffice it to say at this point that one radian is approximately 60°.

Angular displacement is defined similarly to displacement for linear systems and is the relative angle compared to some fixed position or line in space. For example, if a golfer starts his/her drive from the presentation position (i.e. with club just touching the ball) and backswings to the fully extended position with the club behind his/her back, the club shaft would have an angular displacement equal to the angle between the starting position and the fully extended position of the backswing. This would be a measure of the fluency and range of the swing and could be anywhere from 180° to 290° (or 3.142 to 5.06 radians!). Another example occurs in Investigation 8.1, where the angular displacement of the tumbling gymnast in Figure 8.2 between landing and starting is approximately 335° or 5.85 radians; it is less than 360° because he is leaning back as his feet touch the floor.

Investigation 8.1 Rate of turn of a tumbling gymnast

Aim: to examine the concepts of angle, angular velocity and the Law of Conservation of Angular Momentum in the context of a gymnast (or trampolinist) performing a somersault. Further study will enable the student to extend application of the concepts to other sporting situations.

Materials: a video camera with timer, together with a 360° protractor and a video playback machine with stop and slow controls and a turntable (for standing on – standard physics apparatus) or office swivel chair.

Task 1 – production of video film
1. The video camera is set up so that the field of view is at right angles to the tumble to be performed and far enough away for the student performing the action to fit within the field of view.

2. The student performs a variety of straight, piked and tucked forward or backward somersaults. If you have an expert student who can perform double somersaults, even better.

3. The student doing the filming will need to follow the action with the camera **with the on-screen timer running**.

Task 2 – information on angle
1. Although we are used to measuring angles in degrees, this is not adequate for scientific measurements.

2. To avoid adding to the complications of this investigation, we use a simple conversion factor from degrees into **radians**. The radian is the scientific unit of angle.

   1 radian = 57.2958 degrees
   1 degree = 0.017453 radians

3. Convert 30°, 60°, 105°, 360°, 47° into radians (use a calculator – some have automatic conversion).

Task 3 – analysis of video of motion
1. Locate the beginning of a suitable piece of film.

2. Using the pause and slow forward facility on the video machine, position the gymnast at the point at which his/her feet are just about to leave the floor (or trampoline bed). Note the time on the auto on-screen timer at which this occurs.

3. Measure the angle of the **gymnast's upper body** to the vertical at this time (Figure 8.2).

4. Record in Table 8.1 the angle (in degrees) against time (actually recorded on the film) and elapsed time (the difference between the film time and the answer to **2** above).
   Make your measurements with a protractor on the screen for every 30° of turn of the upper body of the gymnast. This is so that measurements are made at regular intervals of angle and the time is just sufficient to register a difference on the tenth of a second timer on the video film.
   Note: the first angle recorded, i.e. answer to **3** above, needs to be in the first row of the angle column. This will not necessarily be 0°, since at the instant the gymnast's feet leave the ground he/she may be leaning into the action of the tumble.
   (We are aware that the measurement of the upper body angle does not reflect the true averaged whole-body angle of the gymnast. However, this is an attempt to simplify the process without losing sight of the basic idea behind the investigation.)
   You will need a bigger chart if the gymnast does a double somersault!

5. Complete the fifth column of Table 8.1 by subtraction of successive times.

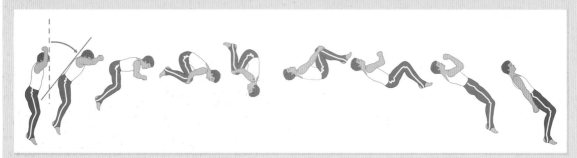

Fig. 8.2 A gymnast tumbling (after reference[2]).

Table 8.1 Angles against time

Angle (degrees)	Time (film) (s)	Elapsed time (s)	Angle (radians)	Time for previous 30° or 0.523 radians
30			0.5236	
60			1.0472	
90			1.5708	
120			2.0944	
150			2.6180	
180			3.1416	
210			3.6652	
240			4.1888	
270			4.7124	
300			5.2360	
330			5.7596	
360			6.2832	

Task 4 – calculation of angular velocities

1. Now comes the hard bit. Angular velocity is defined as 'angle moved through per second' and is measured in radians per second. A formula would be:

$$\text{angular velocity} = \frac{\text{angle turned through in radians}}{\text{time taken}}$$

2. Using your calculator and the data from Table 8.1, complete Table 8.2 of angular velocity against time for each segment of the somersault.

   Note: each segment of 30° is approximately 0.52 radians. Apart from the first calculation, this figure will appear on the top of the formula (the numerator).

3. Finally, compute an elapsed time halfway between the elapsed times for the beginning and end of each segment for column three of Table 8.2. For example, if at 30° the time is 0.2 seconds and at 60° 0.3 seconds, the average time at the middle of the segment will be 0.25 seconds.

Task 5 – graph of angular velocity against time

1. Plot a graph of angular velocity, from the second column of Table 8.2 (*y*-axis or vertical axis), against time, from the third column of Table 8.2 (*x*-axis or horizontal axis). Use as large a scale as possible so that the graph occupies as much of the paper as possible.

2. Draw a smooth curve through the points on the graph.

Table 8.2 Angular velocity against time

Segment of tumble	Angular velocity (rad s⁻¹)	Average time for segment
–30		
30–60		
60–90		
90–120		
120–150		
150–180		
180–210		
210–240		
240–270		
270–300		
300–330		
330–360		

Task 6 – interpretation of results

1. What does the graph drawn in Task 5 show? Angular velocity means rate of spin; can you relate the rate of spin to body shape? Examine again the video film from which the data were taken. The tucked or piked position adopted by the gymnast during the middle part of the somersault somehow made him/her spin faster. Why?

2. Examine a few textbooks[1-3] on spinning sporting systems. See if you can come up with a general rule that governs changes in rates of spin during a movement.

3. Sketch pin-men diagrams of body positions that lead to high rates of spin and compare them with similar diagrams for body positions within the **same** activity that lead to low rates of spin.

4. For example, with our tumbler the tightly tucked position seems to lead to a higher rate of spin than the open or straight position (see Figure 8.3). What happens with the spinning skater?

Task 7 – the spinning skater

1. Take a small turntable and stand on it with arms outstretched. (An alternative piece of apparatus would be an office swivel chair that can be rotated freely.) Another student should now spin you as quickly as possible.

2. You should now bring your arms to your sides – what happens?

3. The experiment can continue with various positions being adopted: hands overhead; one leg held out at right angles; body adopting a sideways 'V' shape (>) and so on (see Figure 8.4).

4. Each position should be drawn with a pin-man diagram and relative rates of spin mentioned.

5. What factor induces change of spin?

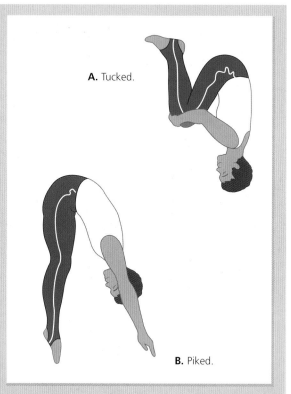

A. Tucked.

B. Piked.

Fig. 8.3 Styles of tumbling.

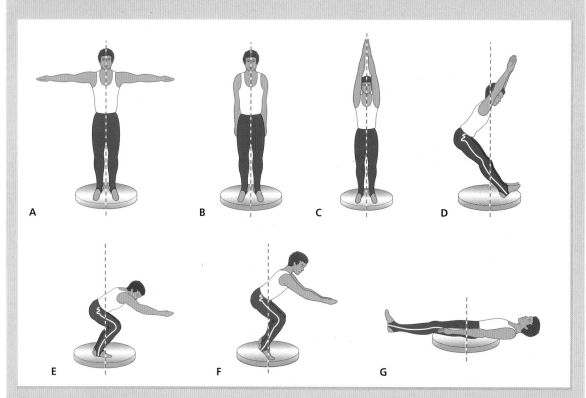

A   B   C   D

E   F   G

Fig. 8.4 Styles of spinning.

8.2 Moment of inertia

Definition of moment of inertia

Various texts have a lot of detail about this concept – see intermediate-level physics and mathematics books and references[1-7] for application of the idea to the sporting situation.

Basically, moment of inertia is the resistance to rotational motion (directly comparable with mass inertia for objects moving in straight lines – see p. 204 for an explanation of this).

The bigger the moment of inertia, the bigger the **moment of force** (or **couple** or **torque**) needed to provide the same **angular acceleration** in the body and vice versa. This is the same as in the linear situation only here, instead of moving in a straight line, the object spins about an **axis**; instead of acceleration (in m s^{-2}) we have **angular** acceleration (in radians s^{-2}); and instead of force we have **turning moment of force**.

Angular acceleration is the change of (increase of) angular velocity per second of the spinning body – see p. 252 for expansion of this idea and applications to sporting situations.

The concept of **moment of inertia** (**MI** – usually the symbol **I** is used) depends on the distribution of mass about the axis of rotation of a spinning system, i.e. the further away from the axis a mass is, the greater the moment of inertia and the harder it is to make it spin or stop it spinning if it is already doing so.

A simple example of this idea applied to a sport is that of the leg action during running. As the leg drives through at the moment of leaving contact with the ground, it is (or should be) as straight as possible to maximise the range of movement in the stride (see position 2 of Figure 8.5).

The next action that needs to be performed is to bring the leg through as rapidly as possible to the fully forward position (as in position 9 of Figure 8.5). The most efficient way of doing this would be to use the least possible force in the abdominal muscles, which would produce the least possible **moment of force** applied to the femur of the leg in question rotating about the hip joint. If the leg is as bent as possible and therefore has the **least possible moment of inertia** about the hip joint as an axis of rotation, then the least force would be required to rotate it. This is why the more efficient sprinter will have his/her heel as close to his/her backside as possible (as in position 7 of Figure 8.5) at this point in the stride pattern.

To relate to the tumbling gymnast in Investigation 8.1, the act of spinning in a straight position (as opposed to a tucked position) means that some of the gymnast's mass is further away from the axis of spin and therefore the **moment of inertia** is larger (Figure 8.6).

Similarly, for the skater, if the body is straight with no bits sticking out, the moment of inertia is low but as soon as a leg or arm is put out at right angles to the body, the moment of inertia increases, since more of the person's mass is further from the axis of spin (Figure 8.7).

Evaluation of moment of inertia

The definition of **MI** is:

> moment of inertia
> = the sum of [(mass of body part)
> × (its distance from the axis of rotation)^2]
> for all parts of the body

or

$$MI = \Sigma(m \times r^2)$$
(unit of MI – kgm^2)

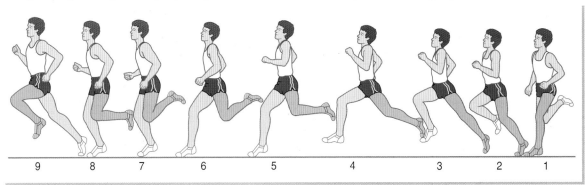

Fig. 8.5 Leg action during running.

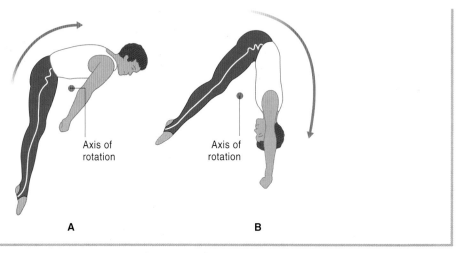

Fig. 8.6 Moment of inertia in tumbling. **A.** Straight position = large moment of inertia. **B.** Piked position = small moment of inertia.

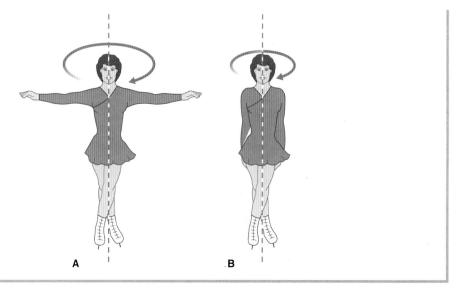

Fig. 8.7 Moment of inertia in ice skating. **A.** Wide arms = large moment of inertia. **B.** Arms held in = small moment of inertia.

It can be seen that the computation of **MI** is not simple for the complex shapes and variations that the human body can adopt in the sporting situation.

In Figure 8.8, a range of spinning body shapes is shown, the axis of spin is marked with a dotted or continuous line and the corresponding moment of inertia relative to the first example is shown (this first example has a nominal value I). I has a value of between 1.0 and 1.5 kgm^2 for a person of 60 kg mass.

Therefore, it can be seen that it is possible to double the moment of inertia by holding the arms out or one or more legs! The practicalities of the use of this idea are that the skilful sportsperson is able to vary his/her shape and hence the properties of the body insofar as spinning, tumbling, turning or twisting is concerned. This is done in a similar way to the variation of position of centre of mass of the body but in different situations.

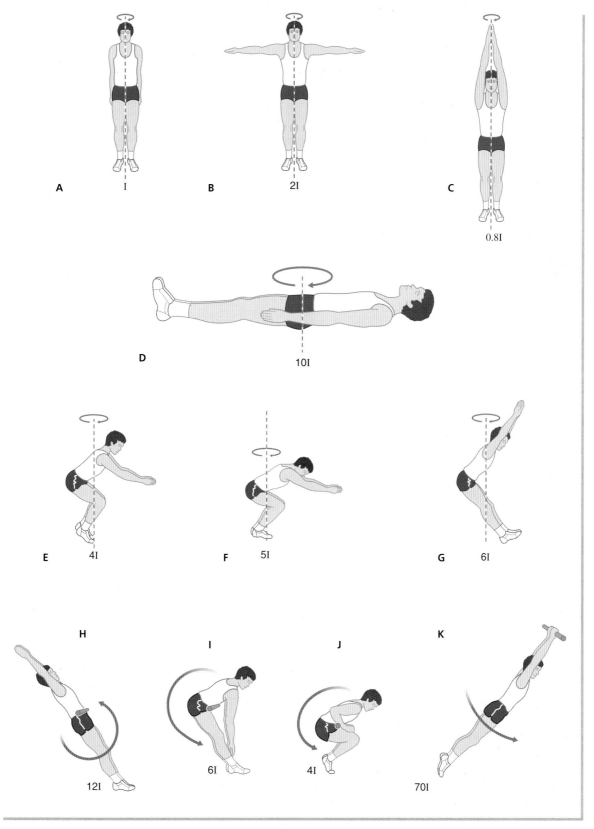

Fig. 8.8 Axes of spin and moments of inertia in spinning bodies.

Radius of gyration

This concept is related to the moment of inertia of a body and describes the **average** distance from the axis of rotation to the mass of the body. Radius of gyration can be expressed as **k** in the formula:

$$\text{moment of inertia} = MI = \Sigma(m \times r^2) = M\,k^2$$

Where   M = total mass of the body ($= \Sigma m$).

This is therefore as if **all** the mass of the body had been placed at a distance **k** (= radius of gyration) from the axis of rotation.

For example, the case of the spinning skater (whose mass of 60 kg is spread out over his whole body shape) in Figure 8.8A has radius of gyration k = 0.13 m. This would mean that the spinning skater adopting this shape would behave in the same way as a **single** mass of 60 kg spinning at a distance of 0.13 m from the axis of rotation. In Figure 8.8B, k would be 0.18 m, and in Figure 8.8E k would be 0.26 m. Hence the bigger the value of the radius of gyration, the bigger the value of moment of inertia, and the smaller the value of radius of gyration, the smaller the value of moment of inertia.

Rotational kinetic energy

This is defined by:

rotational energy
= ¹/₂ × moment of inertia × (angular velocity)²

It can therefore be seen that the spinning energy stored in a system depends on both the **moment of inertia** and the **angular velocity**.

Angular momentum

Angular momentum is defined as:

angular velocity × moment of inertia

This very difficult construct combines our two most difficult concepts in a slightly different way to the rotational energy concept outlined above. However, it enables us to explain why the rate of spin changes when the moment of inertia changes.

This is because **angular momentum of a system remains constant** throughout a movement provided nothing outside the system acts with a turning moment on it. This is known as the **Law of Conservation of** **Angular Momentum** and as far as is known, it is obeyed by all rotating systems. (There is a similar universal law in linear dynamics – see p. 224 – this is **not** the same law.)

In simple terms, this 'conservation law' means that if our gymnast or skater, **when already spinning**, changes his/her moment of inertia (by changing body shape), then the rate of spin will also change. So, if the skater spins rapidly with arms and legs held near the body and then the moment of inertia is **increased** (e.g. by sticking out an arm), the rate of spin will **decrease** (and, in fact, the angular momentum will remain the same; see Figure 8.9A).

Similarly the tumbler goes from an open shape with large moment of inertia into a tucked position with small moment of inertia and in doing so speeds up the rate of spin (see Figure 8.9B).

Other examples of this law applied to sporting situations are illustrated in Figures 8.10–8.13.

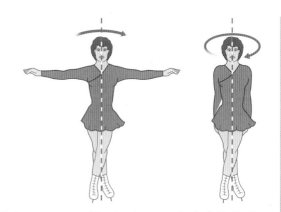

A. Large moment of inertia, slow rate of spin (left). Small moment of inertia, large rate of spin (right).

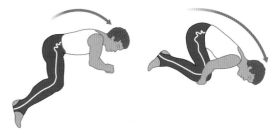

B. Large moment of inertia, slow rate of spin (left). Small moment of inertia, large rate of spin (right).

Fig. 8.9 Conservation of angular momentum.

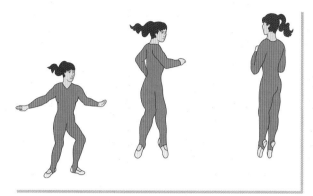

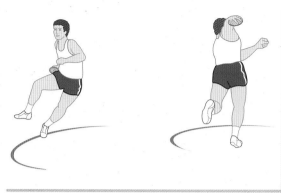

Fig. 8.10 The dancer begins her movement with arms wide and therefore a large moment of inertia. As she jumps and turns, she brings her arms to her side, reducing her moment of inertia and increasing the number of turns possible in the air before landing.

Fig. 8.11 The discus thrower kicks his leg wide at the start of the turn, thereby giving his lower body rotational momentum with a large moment of inertia. As he moves to the centre of the circle he brings his leg closer to the body, reducing his moment of inertia and increasing the rate of spin to the lower body so that it moves ahead of the upper body in the movement.

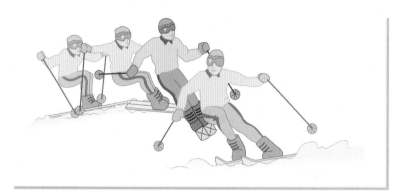

Fig. 8.12 The slalom skier begins his turn in a low, squat position with a high moment of inertia and, as he passes the gate, straightens his body into a shape with half the moment of inertia, doubling the rate of turn past the gate. After passing the gate, he reverts to the high moment of inertia position in order to slow down the rate of turn again.

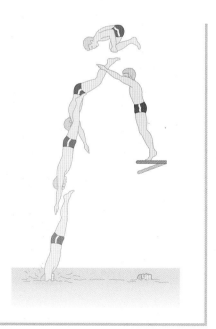

Fig. 8.13 Like the gymnast, the springboard diver varies his shape from straight (large moment of inertia, low rate of spin) to tucked (small moment of inertia, high rate of spin) and back to straight again before entering the water.

Review Questions

1. Figure 8.14 is incomplete. When complete, it should show three lines representing the relationships between:

   A – moment of inertia and time
   B – angular velocity and time
   C – angular momentum and time

   as a gymnast performs a back somersault. Only two of the three curves are shown and all labelling of the graphs has been omitted.
      Copy this graph and complete it by drawing in the missing line and labelling all three curves. Explain the shape of each of the three curves.

2. The angular momentum of a diver is recorded when attempting a one-and-a-half somersault rear dive and is found to be 78 kgm^3 s^{-1} at take-off. The moment of inertia of the diver at take-off was 12 kgm^2 and at entry to the water was 14 kgm^2. Calculate the angular velocity of the diver (in radians per second) at these two points in the dive.

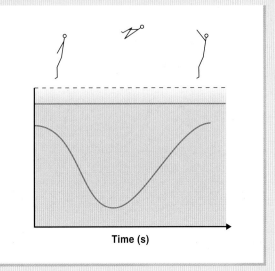

Time (s)

Fig. 8.14 To be completed by the student (see Review Question 1).

Angular acceleration

Angular velocity is defined in Investigation 8.1 as the rate of turning or spinning and:

$$\text{angular velocity} = \frac{\text{angle turned (in radians)}}{\text{time taken to turn}}$$

This is a similar definition to that for linear velocity in Section 6.1, except distance is replaced by angle in the formula. So, again in a similar way to linear systems, it is possible to define **angular acceleration** as:

$$\text{angular acceleration} = \frac{\text{change of angular velocity}}{\text{time taken to change}}$$

This concept applies to situations in which the rate of spin changes with time. Examples of this would be the hammer throw (in which the rate of spin increases throughout the movement up to the release of the hammer) and the tumbler, gymnast or diver (who speeds up the rate of rotation or slows it down by changing his/her body shape, as explained in Investigation 8.1 and Section 8.1).

Investigation 8.2   Spinning systems

1. Write in your own words a detailed explanation of why the rate of spin changes in the examples in Figures 8.10–8.13 or researched in Investigation 8.1.

2. a. Using the graph produced in Task 5 of Investigation 8.1, how would you expect the graph of moment of inertia against time to look?

   b. Sketch a graph of the moment of inertia of our gymnast against time. Estimate the values from the chart of moment of inertia in Figure 8.8 (don't worry about precise values – they aren't important at this stage).
      The graphs should have the properties shown in Figure 8.15. ▶

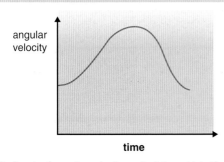

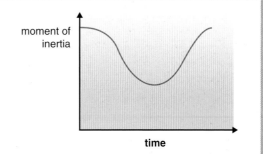

A. Graph of angular velocity against time. Note that the rate of spin increases in the middle of the movement to about double that at the start and finish of the movement.

B. Graph of moment of inertia against time. Here the moment of inertia falls in the middle of the movement to about half that at the start and finish of the movement, with the consequence that the product of moment of inertia and angular velocity remains the same throughout the movement.

Fig. 8.15 Properties of moments of inertia.

Exam-style questions

1. a. Define the terms angular velocity and moment of inertia. (*4 marks*)

   b. State the relationship between angular momentum, moment of inertia and angular velocity. (*2 marks*)

   c. Figure 8.16 shows a gymnast undertaking a forwards somersault following a run up.

      i. Sketch three traces on a single graph to represent any changes in angular momentum, moment of inertia and angular velocity for the period of activity between positions 2 and 9. (*3 marks*)

      ii. Explain the shapes of the traces that you have drawn. (*6 marks*)

   d. Just before take-off (position 1 of Figure 8.16), the gymnast must generate large forces to initiate the somersault.

      i. Sketch a pin man diagram of him just before take-off, showing all the forces acting. The forces must be clearly labelled and identified. (*2 marks*)

      ii. Explain why the vertical forces acting must be large in this case and how rotation is generated in the gymnast. (*3 marks*)

   e. i. During the landing (from position 10 onwards), what conditions must exist if the gymnast is to cancel out his existing forwards angular motion effectively? (*2 marks*)

      ii. Draw a diagram which shows the characteristics of the ground reaction force that you would expect to be present for position 10. (*3 marks*)

   (*Total 25 marks*)

2. A diver can make a number of different shapes in the air. Figure 8.17 shows three of these.

   a. Explain the meaning of **moment of inertia** in this context. (*4 marks*)

   b. During a dive a diver goes through the shapes shown in Table 8.3.

      i. Explain how the rate of spinning (angular velocity) would change through the dive. (*5 marks*)

      ii. Sketch a graph of this rate of spinning against time. Your sketch need only be approximate. (*4 marks*)

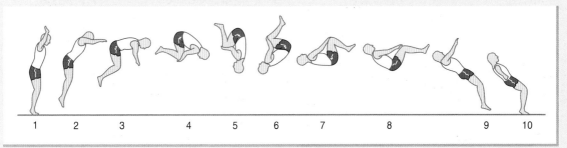

Fig. 8.16 Forwards somersault by a gymnast after a run-up (after reference[2]).

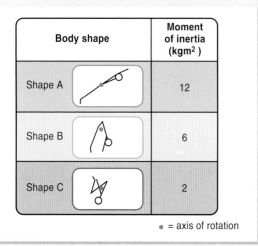

Fig. 8.17 Three shapes of a diver during a dive.

Body shape	Moment of inertia (kgm^2)
Shape A	12
Shape B	6
Shape C	2

● = axis of rotation

Table 8.3 Shapes of diver during dive

Phase of dive	Orientation	Shape	Time during dive (s)
1	Straight	A	0–0.5
2	Piked	B	0.5–0.7
3	Tucked	C	0.7–1.0
4 entry	Straight	A	1.0–1.1

c. i. Name the law of conservation which accounts for these variations in rate of spin. (*1 mark*)

ii. Explain and sketch the arc described by the centre of mass of the diver as he/she falls. (*3 marks*)

d. i. Describe in detail the body shape and movement within another sporting situation where rates of spin are affected by body shape. (*6 marks*)

ii. How would you stop the spinning in this situation? (*2 marks*)

(Total 25 marks)

3. a. i. Explain the concept of **moment of inertia**. (*2 marks*)

ii. Write down the formula for **angular momentum**. How can this quantity be used to explain the variations in motion of a high diver or a gymnast tumbler (diagrams optional)? (*4 marks*)

b. Figures 8.18A–D show a spinning skater in various positions. Under each diagram is an approximate value for the moment of inertia of the skater spinning about his/her central vertical axis. The **angular velocity** of the skater in Figure 8.18A is 3.0 revolutions per second.

i. What is the formula for calculating the skater's angular velocity? Calculate this quantity for the skater in Figure 8.18D. (*2 marks*)

ii. Sketch a figure showing a possible position which could cause the skater to attain an angular velocity of 4.0 revolutions per second and calculate what the moment of inertia of this shape must be. (*2 marks*)

c. Principles of angular momentum can be used to improve performance in a variety of sports. With the use of diagrams explain:

i. How a slalom skier turns through the gates at maximum speed. (*4 marks*)

ii. How a dancer manages to complete a triple spin in the air before touching the ground. (*4 marks*)

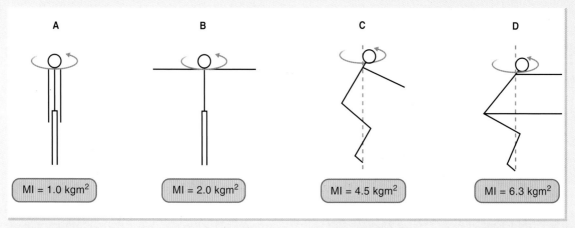

Fig. 8.18 Spinning skater in various positions. **A.** Moment of inertia = 1.0 kgm^2. **B.** Moment of inertia = 2.0 kgm^2. **C.** Moment of inertia = 4.5 kgm^2. **D.** Moment of inertia = 6.3 kgm^2.

iii. What process enables the dancer to stop spinning? (*2 marks*)

d. Figures 8.19A and B show a sportsperson's leg in two different positions. The values given are the moments of inertia of the leg as it rotates about the hip joint (shown as a large dot on each diagram). Explain the implications of these data for the efficiency of running style in a sprinter and in a long-distance runner. (*7 marks*)

(*Total 27 marks*)

4. Look again at Figure 8.16, which shows a diagram of a gymnast performing a single tucked forwards somersault. The numbers shown in the diagram are successive frames at 1/25 (0.04) seconds.

a. Explain the concept of the **moment of inertia** using examples from the diagram. (*5 marks*)

b. Table 8.4 sets out measurements of **angular velocities** (rates of spin) of the gymnast at successive times since the start of the somersault.

i. Plot a graph of angular velocity against time for the motion and estimate from your graph the **ratio** of angular velocities at times **A** and **B**. (*3 marks*)

ii. Use your understanding of **angular momentum** to explain why the angular velocity changes with time. (*4 marks*)

c. If the **moment of inertia** of the gymnast is 6 kgm^2 at time **A**, estimate the **moment of inertia** at time **B**, using data from the Table 8.4. (*2 marks*)

(*Total 14 marks*)

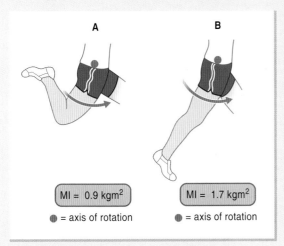

A B

MI = 0.9 kgm^2 MI = 1.7 kgm^2

● = axis of rotation   ● = axis of rotation

Fig. 8.19 Sportsperson's leg in two positions. **A.** Moment of inertia = 0.9 kgm^2. **B.** Moment of inertia = 1.7 kgm^2.

Table 8.4 Angular velocities at successive times after the start of a gymnast's somersault	
Time(s)	Angular velocity (degrees s^{-1})
0.00	600
A 0.04	700
0.08	750
0.12	1000
0.16	1300
0.20	1350
B 0.24	1400
0.28	550
0.32	200
0.36	150

REFERENCES

1. Wirhed R 1997 *Athletic ability and the anatomy of motion*, 2nd edn. Mosby, London
2. Watkins J 1983 *An introduction to mechanics of human movement*. MTP Press, Edinburgh
3. Walder P 1994 *Mechanics and sport performance*. Feltham Press, New Milton
4. Hochmuth G et al 1984 *Biomechanics of athletic movements*, 4th edn. Sportverlag, Berlin
5. Hay J G, Reid J G 1988 *Anatomy mechanics and human motion*, 2nd edn. Prentice Hall, New Jersey
6. Page R L 1978 *The physics of human movement*. Wheaton/Pergamon, Exeter
7. Bartlett R 1997 *Introduction to sports biomechanics*. Spon/Routledge, London

FURTHER READING

Biomechanics

Carr G 2004 *Sports mechanics for coaches,* 2nd edn. Human Kinetics, Champaign, Illinois
Dyson G 1980 *The mechanics of athletics*, 7th edn. ULP, London

Ecker T 1985 *Basic track and field biomechanics*. Tafnews Press, Los Altos, California
Roscoe D A, Roscoe J V, Honeybourne J, Davis R J, Galligan F 2003 *Physical education and sports studies AS/A2 level student revision guide*, 3rd edn. Jan Roscoe Publications, Widnes

Sprunt K 1996 *Sports mechanics,* 2nd edn. National Coaching Foundation (sportscoachingUK), Leeds

Walder P 1995 *Solutions and assignments for mechanics and sports performance.* Feltham Press, New Milton

Advanced biomechanics

Bartlett R 1999 *Sports biomechanics – reducing injury and improving performance.* Spon/Routledge, London

Bell F 1998 *Principles of mechanics and biomechanics.* Stanley Thornes, Cheltenham

Bloomfield J, Ackland T R, Elliott B C 1994 *Applied anatomy and biomechanics in sport.* Blackwell Scientific Publications, Oxford

Hall S J 2003 *Basic biomechanics,* 4th edn. McGraw Hill. Boston.

Hamill J, Knutzen K M 2003 *Biomechanical basis of human movement,* 2nd edn. Lippincott, Williams and Wilkins, Baltimore

Hay J G 1995 *The biomechanics of sports techniques,* 5th edn. Prentice Hall, New Jersey

Luttgens K, Deutsch H, Hamilton N 2001 *Kinesiology – scientific basis of human motion,* 10th edn. Brown and Benchmark, Madison, Wisconsin

McGinnis P 1999 *Biomechanics of sport and exercise.* Human Kinetics, Champaign, Illinois

Winter D 2004 *Biomechanics and motor control of human movement,* 3rd edn. John Wiley, Toronto

Zatsiorsky V 1998 *Kinematics of human motion.* Human Kinetics, Champaign, Illinois

MULTIMEDIA

CD-ROMs

Mentor Body Systems – Interactive Physical Education And Teacher's Manual. Department of Human Movement, University of Western Australia, Perth, 1996

Roscoe D A, Roscoe J V 2002 OCR/AQA/Edexcel Science and Sport Psychology Powerpoint Classroom Presentation CD-Rom. Jan Roscoe Publications, Widnes

Roscoe D A, Roscoe J V, Honeybourne J, Davis R J, Galligan F 2003 *Physical Education and Sports Studies AS/A2 Level Student Revision Guide,* 3rd edn. Jan Roscoe Publications, Widnes

Roscoe D A 2004 *Teacher's guide to physical education and the study of sport. Part I, the performer in action, biomechanics,* 5th edn. Jan Roscoe Publications, Widnes

Walder P 2003 *Mechanics and Sports Performance.* Feltham Press, New Milton

Walder P 2003 *Images for Biomechanics.* Feltham Press, New Milton

Video

Biomechanics – 2002 Video Education Australasia. UK supplier Boulton & Hawker Films Ltd

Notes

Synoptic movement analysis investigation

Consider Table 8.5 below in which a number of physical activities are listed in the left hand column. The student task is to research from Chapters 1 to 8 of this book the implications of the subsequent column headings. For example, for the first activity – pushing a hockey ball – in the action phase of the movement – and for the wrist joint, the joint type would be **condyloid**.

Note – not all sections of the table would need to be completed – the search for relevant answers would be part of the exercise.

Table 8.5

Physical activity	Movement phase	Joint used	Articulating bones	Joint type	Movement pattern	Plane of rotation	Axis of rotation	Agonist muscle
Pushing a hockey ball	Preparation	Spine						
	Action	Wrist						
Situp	Action	Spine						
	Action	Hip						
Vertical jump	Preparation	Knee						
	Action	Hip						
Kicking a ball	Preparation	Knee						
	Action	Ankle						

Remember that in the case of the slow press down and perparation for the vertical jump, the active muscles that are responsible for the changes in joint movement are muscles that are lengthening, but at the same time controlling (by resisting the lengthening of muscle) the joint angles.

Agonist type of contraction	Antagonist muscle	Antagonist type of contraction	Lever class	Type of motion linear/rotation	Type of motion constant velocity/acceleration	Forces applied	Newton's laws	Centre of mass applications

Table 8.5 *(Continued)*

Physical activity	Movement phase	Joint used	Articulating bones	Joint type	Movement pattern	Plane of rotation	Axis of rotation	Agonist muscle
Leg action in squat	Downward phase	Hip						
	Upward phase	ankle						
Over arm throw	Preparation	Elbow						
	Action	Shoulder						
Leg action in sprinting	Leg drive	Ankle						
	Recovery phase	Knee						
Set position sprint start	Position	Hip						
		Knee						
Push up	Action downward phase	Shoulder						
		Elbow						

	Agonist type of contraction	Antagonist muscle	Antagonist type of contraction	Lever class	Type of motion linear/ rotation	Type of motion constant velocity/ acceleration	Forces applied	Newton's laws	Centre of mass applications

Table 8.5 *(Continued)*

Physical activity	Movement phase	Joint used	Articulating bones	Joint type	Movement pattern	Plane of rotation	Axis of rotation	Agonist muscle
Push up (Cont)	Action upward phase	Shoulder						
		Elbow						
Upright row	Action	Shoulder						
		Elbow						
Putting the shot	Initial stance	Fingers						
	Travel	Spine						
	Throwing action	Hip						
	Release	Shoulder						
Tennis forehand stroke	Preparation	Shoulder						
	Action	Elbow						
	Follow through	Wrist						

Agonist type of contraction	Antagonist muscle	Antagonist type of contraction	Lever class	Type of motion linear/ rotation	Type of motion constant velocity/ acceleration	Forces applied	Newton's laws	Centre of mass applications

Glossary of terms

Part 1
Anatomy, physiology, exercise physiology, biomechanics

abduction movement pattern in which a body segment moves away from the midline of the body.

acceleration change of velocity per second, rate of change of velocity, includes change of direction, and both speeding up and slowing down. Measured in metres per second per second, m s^{-2}.

acclimatisation reversible physiological responses which occur through exposure to a climate such as high temperatures or altitude.

acetylcholine a major neurotransmitter that transmits nerve impulses across synapses and synaptic clefts.

acid–base balance the maintenance of a normal blood pH which ranges between 7.35 and 7.45 in arterial blood and 7.30 and 7.41 in venous blood.

action potential an electrical signal that propagates along the membrane of a neurone or muscle fibre. It involves depolarisation of the axon to a critical threshold point, which is temporarily positively charged in comparison to the outside of the membrane.

active mobility exercises used to improve joint mobility which are under the total control of the sports performer.

adaptation long-term changes produced in the human body which result from the training effects produced as a result of overload.

adduction movement pattern in which a body segment moves towards the midline of the body.

adenosine diphosphate (ADP) the product of the energy-producing reaction starting with ATP.

adenosine triphosphate (ATP) the fundamental molecule from which all energy is produced for biological functions. The reaction which produces the energy is ATP $\rightarrow$ ADP + P$_i$ + energy.

adrenaline otherwise known as epinephrine, this hormone is secreted by the adrenal medulla and has the effect of rapidly bringing into action the muscles, circulation and carbohydrate metabolism.

aerobic a biological process taking place in the **presence** of oxygen.

aerobic adaptations long-term changes produced in the human body by aerobic physical activity, which enable the body to cope better with endurance exercise.

aerobic power the maximum rate at which oxygen can be consumed during a progressive exercise test to exhaustion (also known as V̇O$_2$max). This can be equated to power in watts using the fact that each litre of oxygen consumed releases 22 kJ of energy.

aerobic system the series of chemical reactions in a tissue cell by which an abundance of ATP is regenerated (ready for energy release) in which oxygen is used freely.

agility the ability of a person to execute coordinated and smooth movements with balance and precision.

agonist/antagonist response the reaction to repetition of coordinated movements which enable control of an antagonist when the agonist is the prime mover in the activity involved.

agonist muscle a prime mover muscle which, as a result of active contraction, results in the desired movement at a specific joint.

air resistance drag force experienced when a body or object moves through air.

alactacid oxygen debt component the amount of oxygen needed to replenish phosphocreatine and ATP stores in tissue cells during the recovery process after exercise.

alactic anaerobic system the series of chemical reactions in a tissue cell in which ATP is regenerated (ready for energy release) using PC and ADP present in the cell. This occurs without oxygen.

all-or-none law a law that states that structures such as cardiac muscle and motor units either respond completely (all) or not at all (none) to a stimulus.

altitude training an exercise programme designed to produce reversible physiological adaptations which improve a person's tolerance to the reduction to oxygen partial pressures experienced at altitude.

alveolar duct a branch of a respiratory bronchiole around which alveoli are arranged.

alveolar oxygen tension represents the partial pressure of oxygen in the alveoli. This is the equivalent of 13 kPa at sea level (compared with atmospheric oxygen at 20 kPa).

alveolar ventilation the volume of air that enters the alveoli for gaseous exchange. A typical value at rest for a single breath is 350 ml. It can also be expressed as volume per minute, i.e. alveolar ventilation = (tidal volume – anatomical dead space) × respiratory frequency.

alveolus an air sac in the lungs through which gaseous exchange takes place.

anaerobic a biological process taking place in the **absence** of oxygen.

anaerobic adaptations long-term changes produced in the human body by anaerobic physical activity, which enable the body to cope better with powerful dynamic exercise.

anaerobic capacity the total energy available from work performed anaerobically (ability of ATP-PC and lactacid systems to regenerate the ATP used for energy release at tissue sites) during intense exercise to 60 seconds.

anaerobic power:
  mean anaerobic power (MP) the average or mean power achieved by someone exercising intensely over a period of 30 seconds
  minimum anaerobic power the least power rating achieved during a 30-second anaerobic power exercise test
  peak anaerobic power (PP) the maximum power rating achieved during an anaerobic power exercise test.

anaerobic threshold (AT) the highest level of exercise that can be performed without a significant change in blood pH.

anatomical dead space the volume of air that remains in the respiratory passages (such as the trachea and bronchi) during ventilation, which does not take part in gaseous exchange. A typical value is 150 ml.

angina severe constricting chest pains resulting from a reduced oxygen supply to heart muscle.

angular acceleration rate of change of angular velocity, change of angular velocity (rate of turning or spin) per second, increase in rate of spin. An example would be a hammer thrower whose rate of spin increases during the turning part of the throw.

angular displacement this is the net angle turned through by a rotating or turning object. Measured in degrees or radians.

angular momentum moment of inertia × angular velocity, this quantity is conserved (keeps the same value) for spinning systems which are isolated from the surroundings. This explains why the spinning skater spins faster or slower according to whether his or her arms are held in or out.

angular velocity the rate of spin or turning, angle turned through per second. Measured in radians per second and sometimes revolutions per second.

antagonist muscle the muscle which opposes the action of the agonist or prime mover muscle.

antagonistic muscle action the action of muscles working in pairs one of which opposes the action of the other. For example, the actions of biceps and triceps muscles on the elbow joint.

anticlockwise direction of rotation or spin – top of object turning to the left, in the opposite direction to a clock.

aorta the largest artery in the body, which carries oxygenated blood away from the left ventricle of the heart and into the systemic circulatory system.

aponeuroses a type of tendon that is flattened and ribbon-shaped.

appendicular skeleton the bones of the limbs and limb girdles that are attached to the axial skeleton.

arteriole a small artery (which branches from a larger artery) which supplies blood to capillaries.

arteriovenous oxygen difference (a-$\bar{v}O_2$ diff) the difference between the oxygen content of arterial and mixed venous blood and hence a measure of the ability of tissues to extract oxygen.

artery a thick-walled, elastic blood vessel that carries blood away from the heart to the smaller branching arterioles.

articular surface a surface of bone within a joint which moves against another such surface as the bones move.

asthma a condition characterised by increased constriction of the smooth muscle of the bronchioles in response to various stimuli. Symptoms include shortness of breath, wheezing and coughing. Exercise-induced asthma (EIA) occurs particularly in cold weather.

atherosclerosis the presence of irregularly distributed lipid deposits within the inner walls of large and medium-sized arteries.

atrioventricular (AV) node a specialist area of tissue located within the right atrium of the heart. Its job is to receive electrical (nerve) impulses from the SA node and to direct them towards the bundle of His located within the septum.

atrioventricular valves valves which are located between the atria and the ventricles of the heart which permit blood flow in one direction through the heart. The valve on the right side of the heart is called the tricuspid valve and on the left, the bicuspid valve.

atrium an upper (superior) chamber of the heart.

atrophy loss of size or mass of muscle tissue (or any body organ) due to lack of use.

axial skeleton part of the skeleton that forms the longitudinal axis of the body, i.e. skull, vertebral column and rib cage.

axis of rotation a line about which turning or spinning could occur.

balance the ability to retain the centre of mass of a sportsperson's body above the base of support.

balanced diet the combination and proportions of carbohydrates, fats, proteins, roughage, water and essential minerals and vitamins which best provides for a sportsperson's nutritional requirements.

ball and socket joint a joint in which a ball-shaped head of one bone fits a cup-shaped socket of a second bone, to permit movements along three axes.

barometric pressure the force per unit area exerted by the earth's atmosphere. At sea level it is 760 mm of mercury (mmHg) or 100 000 pascals = 100 kPa (1 pascal = 1 newton per square metre pressure).

baroreceptors sensory nerve endings found mainly in the aortic arch and carotid sinuses which are sensitive to stretching of the walls of these vessels due to increased blood pressure. If blood pressure increases, baroreceptors are activated and transmit sensory impulses to the cardiac centres, which causes decreased cardiac activity.

basal metabolic rate (BMR) the rate at which energy is used by basic bodily functions; this would be the metabolic rate when a person is at rest or sleeping.

base of support width of base of object within which the line of action of its weight must fall if the object is to avoid toppling or falling off-balance.

Bernoulli effect force produced by differential fluid flow across surfaces (enables aerofoils to fly); creates a pressure difference between the two surfaces. This effect creates downforce on racing car wings to increase friction when cornering.

bicarbonate ion (HCO$_3^-$) an ion which is formed as part of the formation of carbonic acid. Bicarbonate ions are the **main** way in which carbon dioxide is transported via the blood from tissue cell respiration sites to the lungs for expiration.

biological ageing a deterioration of body functions that results from long-term and permanent changes in a person's tissues.

blood acidity the normal blood pH which ranges between 7.35 and 7.45 in arterial blood and 7.30 and 7.41 in venous blood. If blood becomes more acid, there is a very small reduction of blood pH caused by increases in dissolved carbon dioxide and lactic acid produced during physical activity.

blood cholesterol a lipid-related compound which accumulates in the lumen of blood vessels and which can cause a narrowing of blood vessels (as in atherosclerosis). A high blood cholesterol level can be caused by eating a high-fat diet or it could be an inherited factor. Physical activity and a low-fat diet decrease blood cholesterol levels.

blood doping the removal and subsequent reinfusion of blood. This is an illegal practice and is undertaken to temporarily increase numbers of red blood cells and hence the oxygen-carrying capacity of the sportsperson's blood.

blood flow the volume of blood flowing through a vessel or organ per second.

blood pressure the pressure exerted by blood on the wall of a blood vessel ventricular systole and diastole. This is a function of cardiac output and peripheral resistance (the resistance to flow of blood mainly in arterioles). Clinically, blood pressure can be measured in arteries (such as the brachial artery).

body composition the relative proportions within a sportsperson's body of bone, muscle and fatty tissue.

Bohr effect the reduced effectiveness of haemoglobin to hold oxygen caused by an increase in acidity, temperature or carbon dioxide concentration. The net result is that the oxygen dissociation curve shifts significantly downwards and to the right.

bony features the rough shapes of bone surfaces that are classified as protrusions and depressions and which act to increase the surface area for attachment of tendons and ligaments.

bradycardia the enlarging and strengthening of the heart muscle (particularly the left ventricle) caused by repeated aerobic exercise. The heart muscle experiences hypertrophy under overload which produces bigger stroke volumes and lower heart rates (and therefore reduced cardiac distress) during endurance-based physical activity.

breathing the process by which air is drawn into and expelled from the alveoli within the lungs.

bronchiole a small air tubule which branches off a bronchus (as part of the air intake system to the lungs). Bronchiole walls consist of smooth muscle and elastic fibres.

bronchus one of the two larger branches of the trachea which is part of the airway from the throat to the lungs.

bundle of His specialised muscle heart fibres which conduct impulses from the atrioventricular node of the heart to the Purkinje fibres within the ventricular walls.

bursae capsule a closed sac containing synovial fluid, usually found in areas where friction occurs, e.g. within the knee joint.

cancellous bone or spongy bone is a type of bone which has a honeycomb appearance, located at the ends of long bones within the epiphysis and within flat and irregular and short bones.

capillarisation the tendency to increase the numbers and usage of blood capillaries through muscle tissue in response to the needs of the tissue for oxygenated blood. This is a long-term adaptation to repeated endurance exercise.

capillary the smallest of all blood vessels located close to tissue cells and whose function is to transport nutrients and waste products to and from tissue cell sites. Capillary walls are one cell thick and are permeable to oxygen, carbon dioxide, glucose and other nutrients and waste products.

carbaminohaemoglobin an organic compound resulting from the combination of carbon dioxide and haemoglobin and part of the means by which CO_2 is transported via the blood from tissue cell respiration sites to the lungs for expiration.

carbohydrates food fuels whose molecules consist of carbon/hydrogen/oxygen, which are hydrolysed to glucose in the digestive tract and then stored as glycogen in muscle and liver.

carbo-loading a method of increasing the glycogen stores in muscle and liver prior to major endurance exercise.

carbon dioxide produced as a waste product of aerobic respiration (within Krebs' cycle) and is transported as a bicarbonate ion to the lungs where it is exexcreted (breathed out). Inspired air contains about 0.04% CO_2, expired air at rest contains 4% CO_2 and this value increases during exercise. CO_2 is the **main** stimulus responsible for increasing the rate and depth of breathing via activation of the respiratory centre.

carbonic acid H_2CO_3, facilitates carbon dioxide transport via the blood from tissue cell respiration sites to the lungs for expiration. H_2CO_3 is formed in blood plasma by the combination of carbon dioxide and water under the action of the enzyme carbonic anhydrase and forms hydrogen ions (H^+) and bicarbonate ions (HCO_3^-) in solution.

cardiac related to the heart.

cardiac arrest otherwise known as a heart attack, when the heart stops beating.

cardiac cycle a complete heart beat that consists of a period of relaxation (known as diastole) followed by a period of contraction (known as systole).

cardiac impulse an electrical (nerve) impulse that originates from the sino-atrial node or pacemaker in the heart, which is responsible for initiating cardiac muscle contractions (systole).

cardiac output the volume of blood pumped from one ventricle in one minute. Cardiac output = stroke volume × heart rate (bpm).

cardiovascular disease non-transmissible disease of the heart and vascular systems.

cardiovascular endurance the ability of a person to sustain exercise without undue fatigue, heart distress or respiratory distress.

carotid artery a major artery which branches from the aorta and transports oxygenated blood to neck and head. It is a good artery to locate if you wish to measure pulse rate (heart rate).

cartilage a firm, smooth, stiffly elastic, non-vascular connective tissue. There are three main types of cartilage: yellow elastic, hyaline or articular and white fibro.

cartilaginous joint bones connected by cartilage, e.g. intervertebral discs.

central nervous system a major subdivision of the nervous system consisting of the brain and spinal cord.

centre of mass point at which the mass of an extended body appears to be – the body behaves as if the masses of all its spread-out components are a single total mass at this point. As a sportsperson bends and moves his or her arms or legs, the centre of mass moves and can lie outside the body shape.

cerebellum consists of the part of the brain behind the medulla and pons. It is important in maintaining muscle tone, balance and coordination of movement.

chemical energy energy produced from a chemical reaction. For example, the breakdown of ATP into ADP and P_i releases chemical energy which can be used to contract muscle tissue.

chemoreceptor a sensory receptor which detects the presence of chemicals. Central chemoreceptors (located in the respiratory centre in the brain) and peripheral chemoreceptors (located in blood vessels outside the brain) react to changes in concentrations of carbon dioxide and oxygen and changes in acidity (pH) within blood.

circuit training a type of interval training consisting of a group of exercises which are completed one after another as single sets with rest relief. The groups of exercises may then be repeated in sequence.

circulatory system vessels through which blood flows.

circumduction a body movement which consists of the angular movements flexion, abduction, extension and adduction so that the limb describes a cone in space. The joint, which forms the point of the cone, is relatively stationary.

clockwise direction of rotation or spin – top of object turning to the right, in the same direction as a clock.

compact bone a very hard connective tissue, which consists of tightly packed Haversian systems and provides the main structure of the skeleton. This is the tough outer shell of all bones.

component part of a vector; a vector can be split up into two components at right angles to one another, which represent the total properties of the vector.

concentric contraction occurs when a muscle is activated and shortens.

condyloid joint consists of a modified ball and socket joint which allows limited movement along two axes (circumduction).

constituents of blood blood consists of 55% plasma and 45% corpuscles.

construct validation a theory that accounts for any measure of an aspect of a physical or motor test which is not defined in the objectivity of the test.

continuous training training in which there are no rests or breaks (intensity may be varied), usually aerobic.

coordination the ability of a sportsperson to execute a sequence of movements correctly and with precision.

coronary thrombosis the formation of a blood clot that blocks a coronary artery.

corpuscles another name for any small cell. Normally associated with red blood cells, white blood cells and platelets which make up 45% of blood volume.

couple pair of forces equal and opposite in direction whose lines of action are offset, which cause an object to spin or rotate.

coupled reaction a series of two or more chemical reactions in which energy provided by the first reaction is used to initiate the second (and any subsequent reactions). An example is the regeneration of ATP using PC in

$$PC \rightarrow P_i + C + energy$$
$$\downarrow$$
$$energy + P_i + ADP \rightarrow ATP$$

which couple together to form:

$$PC + ADP \rightarrow ATP + C.$$

creatine a nitrogenous amine which occurs primarily in muscle tissue and which is found in abundance in fish and red meat. It is used as an ergogenic training aid to assist increase in PC stores required for highly explosive activity such as sprinting.

cross-bridges otherwise known as actin–myosin bonds, cross-bridges are a binding of myosin heads with the active sites in actin filaments.

cyclical loading periodic changes in exercise intensity and quality as part of a training programme.

deceleration change of velocity per second, negative acceleration, rate of slowing down.

delayed onset of muscle soreness (DOMS) muscle soreness occurring at least one day after exercise, possibly caused by structural damage within muscle membranes.

depolarisation the phase of the action potential in which the membrane potential moves towards the positive.

depression a downward movement of a part of the body.

depressions bony features that are dents on the surface of bones which provide extra surface area for attachments of muscle tendons and ligaments, e.g. bicipital groove.

development the process by which infants change into children and children change into adults.

diaphragm a dome-shaped sheet of muscle forming the floor of the thoracic cavity. When the diaphragm contracts during inspiration, the depth of the thoracic cavity increases, atmospheric pressure outside the body forces air into this cavity. When the diaphragm relaxes during expiration, this muscle ascends to its original position, the volume of the thoracic cavity reduces and air is forced out.

diaphysis the shaft of a long bone.

diastole the relaxation phase of the cardiac cycle.

diastolic blood pressure the pressure exerted by the blood on arterial walls during ventricular diastole, which will give the lowest pressure measured in a large artery, such as the brachial artery (a normal value is 80 mmHg).

dietary supplementation food supplements (above what is needed to ensure intake of a balanced diet) which act as an ergogenic aid to performance.

Examples include isotonic sports drinks, carbo-loading and creatine supplementation.

diffusion the net movement of the molecules of a liquid or gas, from a high concentration to a low concentration. In the human body diffusion takes place through very thin cell membranes with the rate of diffusion depending on the concentration gradient, size of molecule and diffusion distance (thickness of cell membrane).

direct energy measurement measurement of heat energy produced when food fuel is burnt in oxygen (by measuring the rise in temperature of 1 kg of water heated by the process).

displacement the direct distance from a starting point (as the crow flies), taking into account the direction.

distance the actual length of path taken from start to finish. For example, in a 10 000 m race taking place on a 400 m track, the distance covered is 25×400 m = 10 000 m. The displacement from start to finish would be zero because the start and finish are in the same place.

dorsiflexion an upward movement of the foot which brings the toes towards the tibia.

drag fluid friction force which tends to oppose motion through a fluid; this could be through air (a runner or cyclist) or through water (a swimmer or canoeist).

dynamic balance the ability of a sportsperson to perform a series of coordinated movements without loss of balance.

dynamic contraction a type of muscle contraction in which the muscle changes length and changes a joint angle.

dynamic strength maximal strength exerted during a movement or exercise in which muscle length changes. Most sports use this type of maximal strength.

eccentric contraction occurs when a muscle is activated and force produced but the muscle lengthens.

efficiency the ratio of energy output to energy input to a process, or the ratio of power output to power input. This is always less than 1 (100%) for living processes which means that some energy is wasted.

effort force exerted by a muscle (or group of muscles) acting on a joint as a lever.

elastic strength the ability to apply maximal force at a high speed of muscular contraction. This sort of strength is the most usual in sports situations, jumping, throwing, sprinting, most games or activities requiring flat out movements.

electrocardiogram (ECG) a recording of the heart's electrical changes that accompany the cardiac cycle. It consists of three components: the **P** wave, **QRS** complex and **T** wave.

electron transport chain the final series of chemical reactions in which oxygen is used and water created, which form part of the aerobic system for the regeneration of ATP (ready for energy release). This occurs

within the mitochondria of a tissue cell. Most of the ATP produced by the aerobic system is created in the electron transport chain.

elevation an upward movement of a part of the body.

endocardium the smooth inner lining of the heart chambers, which allows blood to move easily through the heart.

endochondral ossification bone formation that occurs as a result of bone replacing foetal cartilage.

endomysium a fine connective tissue sheath which surrounds a muscle fibre.

endothermic reactions those chemical reactions which in order to occur require energy from outside. For example, in the body the resynthesis of adenosine diphosphate (ADP) into adenosine triphosphate (ATP) requires energy :
energy + ADP + P_i = ATP

energy the ability to do mechanical work. Measured in joules or kilojoules:
1 kJ = 1000 J.

energy continuum the proportions of the different energy systems used in particular sports or games, the proportions of PC/lactic/aerobic systems used to regenerate ATP (which is then available for energy release) during the activity.

energy input energy taken in or ingested as food fuel.

energy output/expenditure energy expended by the body's functioning, including the functioning of all organs and by exercise.

epiglottis a semi-cartilaginous flap which serves as a valve over the glottis of the larynx, intended to prevent intake of food or drink into the lungs during swallowing.

epimysium the fibrous envelope surrounding a whole skeletal muscle.

epiphyseal plate a site at which bone growth in length occurs. Also called the growth plate.

epiphysis the prominent end of a long bone, separated from the diaphysis by the epiphyseal plate.

equilibrium a balance situation in which forces or moments cancel out; there would be no tendency to accelerate, decelerate or start or stop spinning.

ergogenic aids means by which performance at a physical activity can be enhanced. Such aids can be legal (within the rules of the sport) or illegal (against the rules of a sport) and can include mechanical, nutritional, pharmaceutical, hormonal and psychological methods.

erythropoietin (rEPO) a hormone produced by the kidney which stimulates the formation of red blood cells within bone marrow. Administration of rEPO (cloned throught genetic engineering) is an illegal sporting practice.

eversion the sideways movement of the foot that turns the foot outwards.

excess post-exercise oxygen consumption (EPOC) or **oxygen debt** or **oxygen recovery** during the recovery

process after exercise, this is the total amount of oxygen required to replace ATP, restore PC, remove lactic acid in the working tissue and return all body systems back to pre-exercise resting state.

exhaled air air which is removed from the lungs into the atmosphere during breathing.

exothermic reactions those chemical reactions which give out energy. For example, the breakdown of adenosine triphosphate (ATP) releases energy for muscular contraction: ATP = ADP + P_i + energy

expiration the process of breathing out.

expiratory reserve volume or **expiratory capacity** the volume that can be forcibly expired after a normal quiet breath. A typical value at rest is 1200 ml.

explosive strength the ability to apply maximal force at a high speed of muscular contraction. This sort of strength is the most usual in sports situations, jumping, throwing, sprinting, most games or activities requiring flat out movements.

extension a limb movement in which there is an increase in the angle between the two main bones which hinge at a joint.

external rotation a body or limb movement in which there is rotation away from the vertical body axis.

fartlek training fartlek meaning speed play; a method of training combining continuous and interval training, consisting of variation of speed from jogging to sprinting during the exercise session. This type of training stresses both aerobic and anaerobic systems of ATP regeneration.

fascia a general form of connective tissue which may be superficial or deep.

fatigue index (FI) is the power decline divided by the time interval between peak and minimum power in seconds, during an anaerobic power exercise test.

fats food fuels which should supply about 25% of the energy requirements of a sportsperson.

fatty acids and glycerol the resultant molecules produced by conversion of fats (lipids) in the digestive tract.

fibrous joint bones connected by fibrous tissue with no joint cavity, e.g. sutures of the skull.

filaments, actin and myosin form the basic protein structures within the sarcomere of muscle tissue cells.

fitness a general term referring to the ability of a person to perform a series of varied physical exercises.

fixator muscle a muscle which stabilises one or more joints crossed by the prime mover.

flat bone a bone which is smooth, flattened and usually slightly curved, consisting mainly of cancellous bone sandwiched between two thin outer layers of compact bone e.g. scapula, cranium.

flexibility the ability of a person to use his or her joints and musculature to the limits of their range of movement.

flexion a limb movement in which there is a decrease in the angle between the two main bones which hinge at a joint.

fluid friction drag force experienced when a body or object moves through a fluid, either liquid (water – boats, water skis, swimmers) or gas (air resistance – runners, cyclists, cars).

force push or pull; causes objects to change shape or move (accelerate), has a direction and is therefore a vector.

frequency of breaths (f) the number of breaths an individual takes in 1 minute. This value may change as a result of age, state of health, exercise and altitude.

friction forces forces which act between two surfaces which are sliding past one another or trying to slide past (feet slipping on muddy ground, tyres slipping on wet roads).

frontal axis a horizontal axis through the body passing from left to right, movements in the sagittal or median plane rotate about the frontal axis. Examples are kicking a ball or bending at the trunk.

frontal plane divides the body into front (anterior) and back (posterior) sections.

fulcrum (pivot) the point within a lever about which turning or rotation would occur.

functional residual capacity the sum of the expiratory reserve volume and the residual volume. A typical value in a healthy adult is between 2500 and 3000 ml.

fusiform muscle a spindle-shaped muscle such as the triceps brachii.

gaseous exchange the mechanism whereby gases, especially oxygen and carbon dioxide, are exchanged between atmosphere and blood vessels in the lungs and between blood vessel capillaries and respiring tissues in the body.

general motion a type of motion in which both linear and angular (rotational) motion are combined. This applies to most sports situations, for example, a cyclist who moves linearly along a road, but whose legs and wheels rotate and perform angular motion.

glandular malfunction production of hormones by the body's glands which are not in balance with the needs of the body. Such an imbalance could cause a person to utilise energy from food fuels too efficiently, and become overweight, or not efficiently enough, in which case the person would lose body mass.

gliding joint a joint in which two flat gliding surfaces on two adjacent bones allow a little movement in all directions.

glottis the true vocal cords.

gluconeogenesis during the recovery process after exercise, this is the process of converting non-carbohydrate sources (such as lactic acid and fats) into glycogen in the liver using ATP to provide the necessary energy.

glucose the sugar molecule which forms the starting point for the glycolysis process for the regeneration of ATP (ready for energy release) in muscle tissue during exercise.

glutamine an amino acid which is a constituent of skeletal muscle and T-lymphocytes, which form an essential part of the body's immune system. When skeletal muscle is under stress (after hard physical exercise, for example), available glutamine is used for tissue repair instead of the immune system. This means that a sportsperson is vulnerable to infection after training.

glycogen the sugar molecule which is stored as food fuel in muscle tissue and the liver. Glycogen is converted to glucose (a process called glycogenolysis) when there are energy demands by any respiring tissue.

glycolysis the first series of chemical reactions which form part of both the lactic and the aerobic system for regeneration of ATP (ready for energy release) using glucose as the starting molecule. This occurs within the sarcoplasm of tissue cells.

Golgi tendon organ a proprioceptive nerve ending located at the junction between a muscle and a tendon. Its function is to monitor tension in the muscle.

gradation of contraction neural activation of motor neurones in succession to enable muscle to produce graded muscle tension (from very weak to very strong).

gravitational field strength the force experienced per kilogram of mass when in a gravity field (9.81 newtons per kilogram at Earth's surface – usually abbreviated to 10 N kg^{-1}).

gravity field means of exerting force without touching due to the mass of objects.

growth increases in size and capacity of the individual when infants change into children and children change into adults.

haemoglobin (Hb) a substance found in red blood cells which consists of the protein globin and the iron-containing red pigment haem. Haemoglobin is responsible for the transportation of oxygen and carbon dioxide to and from tissue cell respiration sites.

haemoglobinic acid (HHb) produced as the end-product of chemical reactions in which a hydrogen ion (from carbonic acid) reacts with oxyhaemoglobin (HbO_2) to give HHb and oxygen, which is then available at tissue cell sites for tissue respiration. This reaction to the presence of carbon dioxide products in blood plasma increases the amount of oxygen available at tissue cell sites.

Haversian system the main structure of compact and cancellous bone, consisting of a single Haversian canal (containing blood vessels, nerves and lymphatics) and associated concentric lamellae and osteocytes or bone cells.

heart rate the number of heart beats per minute (bpm).

heart sounds sounds that can be heard using a stethoscope, which are the vibrations caused by the closing of the AV valves (**lub** sound) and the pulmonary and aortic valves (**dub** sound).

Hering–Breuer reflex an involuntary reflex involving muscle spindles located within the intercostal muscles, which prevent over-inflation of the lungs.

hinge joint a joint in which convex and concave surfaces fit together to allow movement around one axis (flexion and extension).

horizontal plane (transverse) divides the body into upper and lower sections.

HRmax represents the maximum heart rate value (measured in beats per minute) of an individual. Calculated as a function of age using the formula: HRmax = 220 – (age in years).

Huxley's sliding theory of muscle contraction a theory of muscle contraction in which thin actin filaments slide past thick myosin filaments to produce tensile force in the muscle cell.

hyaline or articular cartilage a smooth bluish-white, firm and yet toughly elastic type of cartilage that covers the end of bones that form synovial joints.

hyperpolarisation the part of the action potential curve in which the neural potential becomes slightly more negative than the resting value for a short period.

hypertension high blood pressure: normally systolic pressure exceeds 140 mmHg and diastolic pressure exceeds 90 mmHg.

hypertrophy an increase in size of a tissue (usually muscle tissue) as a response to overload training. Stress on the tissue causes a long-term increase in its ability to cope with the stressor; hence muscle tissue becomes bigger and stronger in response to repeated and frequent strength training.

impulse force × time (the area under a force time graph).

indirect energy measurement a way of computing energy used by measuring oxygen consumption of a person exercising. 22 kJ of energy is produced whenever 1 litre of oxygen is combined with food fuel.

inhaled air air brought into the lungs during breathing.

inhibition refers to the fact that sudden stretching of a muscle causes a reflex contraction in the muscle system to protect itself against injury. Training of the muscle (by stretching under force) will reduce inhibition and enable greater forces to be applied to a stretching system without reflex contraction and hence greater range of movement within a joint/muscle complex.

insertion the point of attachment of a muscle of a bone (the bone which tends to move during a concentric or eccentric muscle action, as opposed to the trunk or other body part to which the muscle is attached (the origin) which tends to remain relatively stationary).

inspiration the process of breathing air into the lungs.

inspiratory reserve volume or inspiratory reserve capacity the volume that can be forcibly inspired after a normal quiet breath. A typical value at rest is 3600 ml.

intercostal nerve innervates intercostal muscles and the skin over the thorax.

internal forces forces on the origins or insertions of a muscle exerted by the muscle itself within the body.

internal rotation rotation of a limb or body part towards the vertical body axis.

interval the time period between bouts of exercise during interval training.

interval training training characterised by sets, repetitions and rest relief; can be aerobic or anaerobic.

intramembranous ossification the process of bone formation in the developing foetus that occurs within fibrous connective tissue membranes.

inversion the sideways movement of the foot that turns the foot inwards.

irregular bone a bone that has no definite shape, consisting mainly of cancellous bone sandwiched between two thin outer layers of compact bone e.g. axis, patella.

isokinetic muscle contraction (mc) a dynamic contraction which occurs when the rate of movement of origin towards insertion of a muscle is constantly maintained throughout a specific range of motion even though maximal force may be exerted.

isometric muscle contraction (mc) a static contraction which occurs when a muscle develops tension but remains at the same length.

isotonic muscle contraction (mc) a dynamic contraction in which the speed of contraction is controlled by the sports performer.

joint capsule a sleeve of fibrous tissue surrounding a joint.

joule unit of energy. One joule is the energy produced when a force of one newton acts through a distance of one metre.
One kilojoule = 1000 joules.

Karvonen's Principle a method of calculating training heart rate by adding a given percentage of the maximum heart rate to the resting heart rate. This method gives a heart rate adjusted to the desired percentage of $\dot{V}O2max$.

kinetic energy energy a body possesses because of its motion, either linear (in a straight line – runners, cyclists, cars, boats) or rotational (spinning or turning – spinning skater, turning hammer thrower).

kinetic/ballistic mobility the use of quick, bouncing exercises which contract agonist muscles and force antagonist muscles to lengthen.

Krebs' cycle the part of the aerobic system (occurring in cell mitochondria) for the regeneration of limited amounts of ATP (ready for energy release), which incorporates a cyclic series of exothermic chemical reactions beginning with citric acid. Sometimes known as the citric acid cycle, its main function is to release carbon dioxide and hydrogen atoms (which then enter the electron transport chain).

lactacid oxygen debt component during the recovery process after intense exercise, this is the amount of oxygen needed to remove lactic acid which has accumulated in muscle tissue and blood during the exercise period.

lactate a salt formed from lactic acid.

lactate shuttle during the recovery process after intense exercise, a small proportion of the lactic acid produced is recycled back into glucose in the muscle cell (in the reverse process to glycolysis), requiring energy from ATP breakdown.

lactic acid the molecule produced as the endpoint of the glycolysis process for the regeneration of ATP (which is then available for energy release) when there is no oxygen present. The reason for muscle pain during intense exercise is the presence in muscle of large amounts of lactic acid and blood.

lactic acid anaerobic system the series of chemical reactions in tissue cell sarcoplasm by which a very limited supply of ATP is regenerated (ready for energy release), starting with glucose and finishing with lactic acid without oxygen being used.

laminar flow flow of a fluid past an object in which the fluid flows in continuous lines or layers.

larynx the voice box.

lever a bar or arm which would turn about an axis (fulcrum) under the action of forces.

ligament a sleeve of tough, fibrous connective tissue, which connects two or more bones.

linear motion a type of motion in which obects move in straight lines without spinning or turning

lipids fat molecules which form part of dietary fats.

load the force exerted on the surroundings by a joint acting as a lever.

local muscle endurance the ability of a person to sustain a physical activity relating to a muscle or particular group of muscles; for example, the number of press-ups possible in a minute would be a measure of the shoulder and upper arm local muscle endurance.

long bone consists of a hollow, cylindrical shaft, formed of compact bone, with cancellous bone located at the knobbly ends of the shaft e.g. femur.

lymph fluid flowing through lymphatic vessels. Lymph is formed when excess tissue fluid enters the lymphatic system and eventually returns to the vascular system via the left and right subclavian veins, thus supplying a constant blood volume.

macrocycle a period of training activity with definite and specific aims for skill learning and fitness, of between 4 and 6 weeks duration.

Magnus effect the Bernoulli effect applied to spinning balls in which air flow is faster across one side of the ball, creating a pressure difference between opposite sides of the ball, causing the ball to swerve, dip or soar.

mass fixed property of an object related to its inertia, the property of an object which creates and is acted on by a gravity field.

maximal strength the maximum force exerted by muscle groups during a **single maximal** muscle contraction.
This is the sort of strength power (weight) lifters use in competition.

median plane (sagittal) divides the body into left and right sections.

medulla oblongata inferior (lower) portion of brainstem that connects the spinal cord to the brain. Contains very important centres including the cardiac, respiratory and vasomotor centres.

menisci crescent-shaped structures or wedges of fibrocartilage which deepen and separate articular surfaces of joints, such as the knee joint. Their function is to increase joint stability and aid shock absorption.

mesocycle a period of training activity with definite and specific aims for skill learning and fitness, of about 2 weeks' duration.

metabolic rate the rate at which energy is used by all bodily functions including exercise.

metabolism the way in which energy is used and the rate of energy usage by the human body.

microcycle a period of training activity with definite and specific aims for skill learning and fitness, typically of 1 week duration.

minerals natural inorganic substances which need to be ingested as part of the nutrition process and which are necessary for normal metabolic functioning. For example, calcium is required for muscle contraction.

minute ventilation: $\dot{V}I$ or $\dot{V}E$ the volume of air inspired **or** expired in 1 minute. Minute ventilation is a combination of tidal volume and frequency of breaths ($\dot{V}E = TV \times f$).

mitochondria organelles (small distinct parts) within a tissue cell within which the chemical reactions occur which enable aerobic energy release by the cell.

mitral valve or bicuspid valve is situated between the left atrium and left ventricle. Its function is to direct blood flow through the heart.

mobility training an exercise programme designed to increase range of movement around joints.

moment of a force the turning effect of a force; moment = force × distance from force to fulcrum measured at right angles to the force.

moment of inertia the resistance to rotational motion, the effect of the spread-out nature of a body on its rotational inertia; $MI = \Sigma mr^2$.

momentum mass × velocity, has direction – a vector, is conserved in collisions.

motor end-plate a specialised structure that connects a motor neurone to the muscle fibres.

motor fitness the ability of a sportsperson to undertake coordinated activities skilfully and with precision.

motor neurone a neurone that innervates skeletal, smooth or cardiac muscle fibres.

motor neurone pool concentrated bundles of motor neurones (located within the grey matter of the spinal cord) which serve motor units in the same or related muscle.

motor skill coordination a pattern of behaviour or movements which can be learnt involving sensory, nervous and skeleto-muscular systems.

motor unit a single block of muscle fibres and its neurone

muscle fatigue a reduction in muscular performance or a failure to maintain muscle power output.

muscle fibre is another name for a muscle cell.

muscle fibre type I or slow twitch a muscle fibre characterised by relatively slow contraction time and high aerobic capacity, making it suited to long duration activities.

muscle fibre type IIa or fast oxidative glycolytic (FOG) a type of muscle fibre which, although it is classed as a fast-twitch fibre, shows some of the aerobic characteristics of slow-twitch muscle fibres.

muscle fibre type IIb or fast twitch glycolytic (FG) a muscle fibre characterised by a very fast contraction time and high anaerobic capacity, making it suited to high explosive work.

muscle fibre type FT type C a newly discovered type of muscle fibre that is thought to operate at the far end of the anaerobic metabolic continuum.

muscle glycogen stores the limited store of sugars/carbohydrate in muscle cells available for conversion into glucose (and hence available for glycolysis) during heavy exercise.

muscle group different muscles which contribute to the same action at a particular joint.

muscle pump the result of skeletal muscles contracting and relaxing and thereby squeezing veins to force blood flow (against gravity) back towards the heart.

muscle soreness the muscle pain felt during or after exercise caused mainly by reduced pH (caused by lactic acid accumulation) in the muscle tissue.

muscle spindle apparatus a sensory receptor located in muscle that senses the degree of muscle stretching.

muscle twitch a contraction of **all** the muscle fibres (belonging to a motor unit) in response to a stimulus.

myelination the process of increasing the fatty substance within the sheath which surrounds neurones.

myocardium middle layer of heart muscle consisting of branched striped cardiac tissue which is connected by intercalated discs. Hence the cardiac impulse spreads in all directions – this is an application of the 'all-or-none' law.

myofibril a fine longitudinal fibril within a muscle fibre composed of actin and myosin filaments.

myogenic involuntary neural control. For example, cardiac muscle is myogenic because it contracts automatically without the need for nervous stimulation.

myoglobin similar in structure to haemoglobin, myoglobin is found in large quantities in slow-twitch muscle fibre cells and is responsible for their red colour. Myoglobin has a stronger affinity for oxygen than haemoglobin and so acts as the agent for the transfer of oxygen from haemoglobin to the mitochondria in muscle cells. Oxymyoglobin acts as an emergency oxygen reserve to be made available to muscles when levels of oxygen in the blood supply are very low.

nasal cavity a mucus-lined cavity located on either side of the nasal septum (inner nose cavity).

negative energy balance the situation in which energy taken in as food fuels is less than the energy expended by all bodily functions including exercise.

nervous impulse the way in which information is transmitted in the nervous system.

net force the force produced when several forces acting in different directions are added together.

net oxygen cost oxygen consumed during exercise over and above that needed at rest.

neutral energy balance the situation in which energy taken in as food fuels exactly balances the energy expended by all bodily functions including exercise.

neutral equilibrium a state of balance in an object in which slight alteration in the position of the object does not change the state of balance – a new state of equilibrium would be created.

newton, the unit of force; 1 newton of force will cause a mass of 1 kilogram to accelerate at 1 metre per second per second.

nutritional balance the state of nutrition in which the combination and proportions of carbohydrates, fats, proteins, roughage, water and essential minerals and vitamins best provide for a sportsperson's health.

obesity a state of body health and nutrition in which excessive fat is stored as adipose tissue and within other body cells. It is generally agreed that body fat should not exceed 25% in males and 35% in females.

one repetition maximum (1 RM) the most force able to be applied in a single attempt at an exercise movement.

onset of blood lactate accumulation (OBLA) otherwise known as the 'lactate threshold', this is the point at which lactate levels in blood exceed resting values during the lactic acid build-up due to exercise.

origin the point of attachment of a muscle to bone that remains relatively fixed during the action of the muscle.

osteoarthritis a degenerative disease which affects joint cartilage. Affected joints become swollen and disfigured.

osteoblast a bone-forming cell.

osteoclast a bone-eating cell.

osteocyte a mature bone cell.

osteoporosis an age-related condition in which reduction in bone mass takes place due to reabsorption of minerals forming part of bone structure. This makes bones porous, brittle and liable to breakage. Commonly found in females following menopause. Limited by regular exercise and calcium intake.

overeating a state in which intake of food fuels exceeds the energy requirements of the body (for exercise or any other function).

oxidation of hydrogen atoms this occurs in the electron transport chain part of the aerobic regeneration of ATP in the mitochondria of tissue cells. Oxygen is taken into the chemical reactions and combined with hydrogen atoms to produce water and energy for the regeneration of ATP.

oxygen an odourless, colourless gas that makes up about 20% of atmospheric air at sea level and which is vital to all living creatures for tissue cell respiration. The partial pressure of oxygen in the atmosphere falls from its sea level value of 20 kPa as altitude increases, which can adversely affect the performances of athletes in endurance-based activities.

oxygen consumption an indirect way of measuring energy used during a period of exercise. Each litre of oxygen produces 22 kJ of energy when combined with food fuel.

oxygen deficit the difference between oxygen actually used and the oxygen required for an amount of exercise.

oxygen dissociation curve a graph which illustrates the relationship between the percentage saturation of haemoglobin with oxygen and the partial pressure (or tension) of oxygen in the blood plasma.

oxyhaemoglobin (HbO$_2$) haemoglobin which has formed a temporary affinity to oxygen (within red blood cells) to enable oxygen to be transported from the lung alveoli to respiring tissue cells. Each molecule of haemoglobin carries four molecules of oxygen.

oxymyoglobin a combination of oxygen with myoglobin abundantly located in slow-twitch red muscle tissue cells. A temporary store of oxygen which provides a small but vital supply of oxygen to cell mitochondria during intermittent exercise and following recovery from intense exercise.

pads of fat occupy gaps in and around a joint; help cushion the joint and act as shock absorbers.

parasympathetic nervous system (PNS) a subdivision of the autonomic nervous system which has many branches throughout the body and which works in opposition to the sympathetic nervous system (SNS). In terms of physical activity,

PNS responds by restoring bodily systems to rest; for example, the vagus (PNS) nerve acts on the pacemaker of the heart to slow down heart rate during the recovery period after exercise.

parietal membrane the outer membrane of the pulmonary pleura (general envelope surrounding the lungs).

partial pressure (p) the pressure a gas exerts within a mixture of gases. For example, the p of oxygen is 20 kPa and the p of carbon dioxide is 0.04 kPa within an overall atmospheric pressure of air of 100 kPa at sea level.

passive mobility exercises used to improve joint mobility which are assisted by an external force such as a partner who presses a joint into its end position.

pennate muscle a flat muscle in which the fibres are arranged around a central tendon.

perceptual ability the ability of an individual person to recognise and make sense of surrounding stimuli.

pericardium a double-layered membrane that surrounds the heart. It prevents over-extension of the heart during a heart beat and reduces friction with other contents of the thoracic cavity.

perimysium the fibrous connective sheath that surrounds large bundles of muscle fibres or fasciculi.

period a block of time within the method of organising training for sport in blocks or phases, each with its own definite and specific aims for skill learning and fitness.

periodisation the method of organising training for sport in blocks, periods or phases, each with its own definite and specific aims for skill learning and fitness.

periosteum a thick double layer of connective tissue sheath which covers the entire surface of bone, except the articular surfaces which are covered with cartilage.

peripheral nervous system the portion of the nervous system located outside the spinal cord and brain.

peripheral resistance the resistance to the flow of blood offered by blood vessel walls. Blood viscosity falls as temperature rises, so blood flows more easily when a sportsperson is warm, hence the peripheral resistance is less after warm-up.

pharynx a muscular tube, lined with a mucous membrane, which starts at the internal nares (inner nose cavity) and runs down the neck until it provides a joint opening to the oesophagus and trachea.

phosphagen restoration the process of replenishing PC and ATP within muscle tissue cells after a period of heavy exercise.

phosphocreatine (PC) a substance stored in the sarcoplasm of tissue cells and used in the alactic anaerobic system for the regeneration of ATP.

phrenic nerve innervates the diaphragm.

physical fitness the ability of a sportsperson to undertake a varied number of physical activities without distress.

pivot (fulcrum) the point within a lever about which turning or rotation would occur.

pivot joint a ring-shaped joint that allows uni-axial rotation of one bone around or against another bone (an example is the ulnar radius joint at the elbow).

plantarflexion a movement of the foot that results in the toes being pointed downwards.

plasma a straw-coloured, watery, non-cellular component of blood which consists of proteins such as fibrinogen (needed for blood clotting) and dissolved components such as salts, gases, waste products, hormones and enzymes.

platelets non-nucleated cell fragments which exist in blood, are made in red bone marrow and are involved in blood clotting.

pleural cavity the space between the visceral and parietal membranes of the pulmonary pleura (general envelope surrounding the lungs).

pleural fluid serous fluid found in the pleural cavity, which helps to reduce friction when the pleural membranes (part of the envelope surrounding the lungs) rub together.

plyometrics or depth jumping occurs during bounding exercises during which maximum effort is expended whilst a muscle group is working eccentrically (lengthening under tension).

pneumotaxic centre the portion of the respiratory centre in the pons varolii (part of the medulla oblongata), which has an inhibitory effect on the inspiratory centre.

pocket valve located in veins (except the venae cavae) that have diameters greater than 2 mm. Pocket valves allow blood flow towards the heart but not in the opposite direction.

position the location of a body measured as a grid reference or using coordinates measured from a fixed point or origin.

positive energy balance the situation in which energy taken in as food fuels is more than the energy expended by all bodily functions including exercise.

posture the position of the body as a whole.

potassium/sodium exchange pump the movement of potassium and sodium ions across the neural axon membrane which cause the action potential.

power the rate at which mechanical work can be done or the rate at which energy is given out in a physical process. Measured in joules per second or watts.

power decline (PD) during an anaerobic power exercise test, this is given by the formula:

$$PD = \frac{(\text{peak power} - \text{minimum power})}{\text{peak power}} \times 100$$

preadolescence the period of time just before the process in which a child matures into adulthood. Adolescence is the period of time during which secondary sexual characteristics develop in an individual human being.

precapillary sphincter a smooth, involuntary ring of muscle which controls blood flow from arterioles into the capillary bed.

principle of moments an object in balance must have all turning moments of forces cancelling out to zero: anticlockwise moment = clockwise moment.

pronation movement of the forearm so that the palm of the hand is facing downwards.

proprioceptive neuromuscular facilitation (PNF) a technique of passive mobility training in which a maximum static stretch is performed, followed by contracting and then further stretching, which will extend the range of stretch of the muscle.

proprioceptor an internal sensory receptor located within muscles, tendons and joints, which provides information about body position and movements.

proteins food fuels which provide the building molecules for tissue and enzymes within all body organs.

protrusions bony features that are uneven bumps on the surface of bones which provide extra surface area for attachments of muscle tendons and ligaments, e.g. the tibial tuberosity.

puberty the period of time during which secondary sexual characteristics develop in an individual human being.

pulmonary arteries blood vessels that carry deoxygenated blood from the right ventricle of the heart to the lungs.

pulmonary blood pressure the pressure exerted by blood on the walls of blood vessels supplying the lungs with deoxygenated blood. This pressure is significantly lower than systemic blood pressure.

pulmonary circulatory system a system of vessels which transport deoxygenated blood from the right ventricle of the heart, through the lung capillaries (where oxygenation takes place) and back to the left atrium of the heart.

pulmonary pleura a double-skin membrane (general envelope surrounding the lungs), which contains pleural fluid between the skins of the membrane.

pulmonary veins blood vessels that carry oxygenated blood from the lungs to the left atrium of the heart.

pulmonary ventilation the movement of air in and out of the lungs during inspiration and expiration.

pulse the rhythmic expansion and recoil of the arteries, resulting from a wave of pressure in the blood produced by contraction of the left ventricle of the heart. The pulse can be felt by applying pressure on arteries such as the carotid or radial arteries.

Purkinje fibres specialist cardiac muscle cells found beneath the endocardium of the ventricles. Their function is to conduct nerve impulses from the bundle of His to the ventricular myocardium (heart muscle).

PWC-170 test a submaximal physical fitness test which aims to measure aerobic power by evaluating data on work rate (in watts) or oxygen uptake ($\dot{V}O_2$max), at a given heart rate (namely 170 bpm).

pyruvic acid the substance produced as the end-product of the glycolysis process for the anaerobic regeneration of ATP in the sarcoplasm of tissue cells.

quiet breathing breathing which occurs when a person is in a resting state.

radial artery a branch of the brachial artery leading down the forearm, across the wrist and into the palm of the hand. This artery is a good site at which to measure heart rate.

radian scientific unit of angle; one radian = 57.3°.

radius of gyration the averaged distance of total mass of a body shape from an axis of rotation when the body is spinning. Related to moment of inertia by $MI = \Sigma(m \times r^2) = M\,k^2$, where k = radius of gyration and M = total mass of body.

ratchet mechanism the action within a muscle cell causing tension, in which cross-bridges (called actin–myosin bonds) attach, detach and reattach, thereby shortening the length of the muscle cell sarcomere.

reaction forces forces produced on a body when it exerts a force on another body or object; forces produced via Newton's third law of motion. For example, a jumper pushing hard down on the ground experiences an equal force upwards on his feet from the ground.

reaction time the time taken between a stimulus and its response. In sporting terms, an example would be the time between the gun being fired and the athlete beginning his or her drive into a sprint start.

red blood cells or erythrocytes are non-nucleated, biconcave discs consisting of cytoplasm bounded by a membrane. They are by far the most numerous cells in the blood and each red blood cell contains the respiratory pigment haemoglobin, a protein which is used to transport oxygen and carbon dioxide.

red muscle another name for muscle which mainly consists of slow-twitch fibres. The red colour is caused by the oxygen-carrying substance myoglobin.

reflexive movement an automatic response to a stimulus which occurs without conscious thought.

repetitions the number of times an exercise is attempted (within a set or part of a training programme).

repolarisation the restoration of an action potential (between the inside and outside of a neurone) towards its resting negative value.

residual volume or functional residual capacity the volume of air that remains in the lungs after maximal expiration which maintains inflation of the alveoli. A typical value is 1500 ml.

respiratory bronchiole the smallest bronchiole (part of the airway conducting air into and out of the lungs) that connects a bronchiole to alveoli ducts.

respiratory centre neurones within the brainstem which regulate the rate and depth of breathing.

respiratory exchange ratio (RER) or respiratory quotient (RQ) the ratio of the volume of carbon dioxide produced to volume of oxygen consumed during exercise. RER = 1.00 for carbohydrate consumption, 0.70 for fat consumption, 0.80 for protein consumption and >1.00 for anaerobic activity.

respiratory pump a mechanism which assists venous return due to changes in intrathoracic pressures.

rest relief the period of time after an exercise bout (or set or repetition) during which recovery occurs preparatory to a further exercise bout. A characteristic of interval training.

resultant force the result of an addition of two or more forces in different directions, found using the diagonal of a parallelogram for two forces.

rotating systems obejects which are spinning or turning as part of their motion

rotation limb movement around the axis down the centre of a long bone.

rotational energy energy a body possesses because of its spinning motion.

rotational motion a type of motion in which a body or object is spnning or turning.

saddle joint two saddle-shaped articulating surfaces positioned at right angles to each other, permitting movements along two axes, with circumduction (an example is the thumb joint).

sagittal axis a horizontal axis through the body passing from front to back; movements in the frontal plane rotate about this axis. An example is a cartwheel.

sagittal plane (median) divides the body into left and right sections.

saltatory conduction the way in which a nerve impulse jumps from one node of Ranvier to the next along a motor neurone.

sarcolemma is the plasma membrane of a muscle fibre.

sarcomere the basic structural unit of a muscle cell consisting of that part of the myofibril between adjacent Z lines.

sarcoplasm the jelly-like material outside the nucleus which forms the main body of a tissue cell.

scalar a quantity having size only and no direction (mass, temperature, volume, speed, energy, etc.).

semilunar valves also known as the aortic and pulmonary valves. Situated at the exits of the left ventricle to the aortic arch and the right ventricle to the pulmonary arteries in the heart. Each valve consists of three semilunar cusps and prevents backflow of blood into the ventricles.

sensory neurone a nerve that transmits nerve impulses towards the central nervous system (afferent).

set a block of excercise or exercises consisting of a number of repetitions of the exercise. A characteristic of interval training.

short bone a small, roughly cube-shaped bone, consisting mainly of cancellous or spongy bone, surrounded by a thin layer of compact bone, e.g. carpals.

single muscle fibre block a group of muscle fibres which are connected to a single motor unit.

sino-atrial (SA) node or **pacemaker** a mass of specialist cardiac muscle fibres located in the right atrium of the heart. It generates action potentials that are conducted across the wall of the right atrium to the atrioventricular node.

skeletal muscle voluntary muscle which is attached to the skeleton and contracts to produce major body movements.

skeleton any structure in any organism that maintains the shape, provides support and assists movement of the living organism.

skinfold measurements measurements of the thickness of skin (and hence adipose tissue), which measure the proportion of body fat in a sportsperson.

smooth muscle consists of involuntary spindle-shaped muscle cells that line the walls of hollow organs such as the oesophagus and blood vessels. This type of muscle is adapted for slow involuntary contractions.

somatotype a method of classifying body shape. There are three extreme body shapes:

ectomorph lean linear build with long limbs and a low proportion of body fat and muscle. For example, a high jumper.

endomorph a rounded appearance, often pear shaped, with a high percentage of body fat. For example, a sumo wrestler.

mesomorph a shape with broad shoulders, narrow hips and a higher proportion of muscle mass. For example, a male gymnast.

spatial summation the staggered stimulation of many motor units such that different blocks of muscle fibres (each block controlled by a motor neurone) contract in succession. This spreads out the energy use (and fatigue) among all the muscle fibre blocks in a muscle.

specific dynamic action (SDA) the energy used by a person to convert food fuels into the molecular form required for tissue cell use.

speed distance travelled per second (not taking account of the direction – speed is a scalar). Measured in metres per second.

sphygmomanometer a medical instrument which measures blood pressure.

spirometer a machine which measures lung volumes during ventilation.

stability a constant state of balance.

stable equilibrium a state of balance of an object in which an alteration of the position of the object results in its return to the original balance position.

stage training a method of circuit training in which sets of each exercise are repeated several times before moving on to the next exercise in the circuit sequence. This method creates greater overload than conventional circuit training.

Starling's Law of the Heart the greater the length of stretched cardiac muscle fibres, the stronger the contraction.

static balance the ability of a person to sustain a position of balance without moving.

static contraction another name for an isometric contraction in which a muscle develops tension but remains the same length.

static strength maximal strength exerted without change of muscle length, for example holding a weight at arms length, or pushing hard in a stationary rugby scrum.

steady state represented by a plateau reached at a constant heart rate, oxygen consumption or minute ventilation during submaximal exercise. This plateau indicates that oxygen tissue demands are being met by the heart supplying sufficient quantities of oxygenated blood.

streamlining method of reducing fluid friction or drag by shaping the object so that lines of flow are continuous and laminar as opposed to creating vortices. The use of Lycra sports clothing is an example of this.

strength the ability of a sportsperson to exert maximum force within the context of a movement or exercise.

strength endurance the ability of muscles to undertake intense effort in order to repeat movements in spite of apparent fatigue. Examples of this sort of strength include doing a maximum number of chin-ups, or performing shuttle runs flat out to failure.

maximal strength the maximum force exerted by muscle groups during a **single maximal** muscle contraction. This is the sort of strength power (weight) lifters use in competition.

static strength strength exerted without change of muscle length (see Chapter 1, p. 27), for example holding a weight at arms length, or pushing hard in a stationary rugby scrum.

dynamic strength maximal strength exerted during a movement or exercise in which muscle length changes. Most sports use this type of maximal strength.

explosive/elastic strength the ability to apply maximal force at a high speed of muscular contraction. This sort of strength is the most usual in sports situations, jumping, throwing, sprinting, most games or activities requiring flat out movements.

striated muscle another way of describing skeletal muscle. This refers to the lined appearance of muscle sarcomeres due to longitudinal protein filaments.

striped cardiac tissue (myocardium) middle layer of heart muscle consisting of branched striped cardiac tissue which is connected by intercalated discs. Hence the cardiac impulse spreads in all directions. This is an application of the 'all-or-none' law.

stroke volume the volume of blood pumped out of the left ventricle per heart beat. A typical resting value for an untrained subject is 75 cm^3 and for an aerobically trained subject is 105 cm^3.

supination movement of the forearm so that the palm of the hand is facing upwards.

sympathetic nervous system (SNS) a subdivision of the autonomic nervous system which has many branches throughout the body and which works in opposition to the parasympathetic nervous system (PNS). In terms of physical activity, the SNS prepares the body for action; for example, transmitting impulses from the cardiac centre to the pacemaker (hence increasing heart rate) in response to the body's increased demands for oxygen.

synapse a junction between two neurones.

synergist muscles which work together to enable the agonist muscle to operate.

synovial fluid fluid found inside synovial joints and bursae, which lubricates the joint and helps maintain joint stability.

synovial joint a freely moving joint characterised by the presence of a joint capsule and cavity.

synovial membrane a connective tissue lining the inside of a joint capsule.

systemic circulatory system a system of vessels which transports oxygenated blood from the left ventricle of the heart, through the body's capillaries (where some of the oxygen is released for tissue cell respiration) and back to the right atrium of the heart.

systole the phase of the cardiac cycle during which the cardiac muscle contracts. It consists of atrial systole, during which blood left in the atria is forced into the ventricles, followed by ventricular systole, when the ventricles contract to pump blood into the two circulatory systems.

systolic blood pressure the pressure exerted by the blood on arterial walls during ventricular systole, which will give the highest pressure measured in a large artery, such as the brachial artery (a normal value is 120 mmHg or 16 kPa).

target zone using ranges of heart rate to indicate an intensity of effort to be undertaken during exercise. Otherwise known as a training zone developed from Karvonen's Principle.

tendon strong, mainly inelastic dense connective tissue which connects a muscle to a bone.

tetanic contraction uncontrolled contraction of skeletal muscle during maximum stimulus (this happens during cramp).

thresholds times after the beginning of an exercise when one energy system takes over from another as the predominant way in which ATP is regenerated (ready for energy release). For example, after about 7 seconds of flat-out effort, the ATP-PC system would be exhausted and then the lactacid system takes over as the predominant method of ATP regeneration.

tidal volume (TV) the volume of air inspired **or** expired in one breath (about 500 ml during quiet quiet resting conditions).

tissue fluid a fluid that surrounds and bathes tissue cells which allows the transport of oxygen and nutrients to and waste products away from the body's tissue cells. Tissue fluid is produced by the ultrafiltration of blood plasma.

tissue respiration the process by which oxygen combines with food fuel within a tissue cell to produce carbon dioxide, water and energy.

torque turning effect of a force; moment of a force.

total lung capacity the total volume of air in the lungs following maximal inspiration which equals the sum of residual volume and vital capacity. A typical value for a healthy adult is 6000 ml.

total metabolic rate the rate at which energy is used by all bodily functions including exercise.

trachea also called the windpipe, this air tube extends from the larynx into the thorax where it divides into two bronchi. It consists of incomplete rings of hyaline cartilage.

training principles

cool-down the process of gentle exercise and stretching which keep capillaries open and flush away waste products as part of the recovery after intense exercise.

duration the (long-term) time over which a training regime is undertaken.

frequency the number of times per week (or per cycle of training) in which elements of a training programme are planned.

individual response a training programme should be adapted to the needs of individuals, since each sportsperson will have different strengths and weaknesses.

intensity the difficulty and quantity of training undertaken.

moderation the notion that some training need not be too physically exacting in the interests of prevention of injury.

overload training activities which are harder, more intense and/or lengthier than the normal exercise undertaken for the sport or activity. Stress on biological tissue causes a long-term increase in its ability to cope with the stressor; hence overload increases the capability of the sportsperson's body to cope with the demands of his or her sport.

progression the notion that a training programme should increase its demands on the sportsperson in a systematic and organised manner.

regression or reversibility the notion that long-term training produces long-term adaptations in the sportsperson's body which enable him or her to perform better at the sport and that if training stops, the adaptations will return to the untrained state.

repetition the notion that a training activity should be done many times in order to apply suitable stress (overload) and to learn skills to a suitable level.

specificity the way in which training is directed towards a definite skill or sport, with all elements of the training relevant to the needs of the sport.

variance the element of a training programme by which type of exercise, skills learnt and the quantity and intensity of exercise are **changed** in order to help improve performance.

warm-up the method of preparing the body for exercise involving light exercise, stretching and practice at the skill-related movement patterns involved in the sporting activity about to begin.

transfer the way in which efforts at one activity can have an effect on performance at another, possibly unrelated activity. Transfer can be positive or negative and, if positive, can be used to enhance sports performance.

transverse plane (horizontal) divides the body into upper and lower sections.

triad vesicle a sac located within a muscle fibre that contains cellular secretions such as calcium.

tricuspid valve is the right atrioventricular valve located between the right atrium and right ventricle of the heart. Its function is to prevent backflow of blood into the right atrium.

triglycerides fat molecules created by the fat metabolic system which form the bulk of body fat or adipose tissue.

tropomyosin a tube-shaped protein found in muscle cells which twists around actin strands.

troponin a complex protein found in muscle cells which is attached at regular intervals to actin strands and tropomyosin.

underwater weighing the process by which a sportsperson would be weighed in water and in air, the difference being a measure of the person's proportion of body fat. This method relies on the fact that the density of fatty tissue is less than that of muscle and bone tissues.

unstable equilibrium a state of balance of an object in which a slight change of its position causes toppling (out of balance). An example of this would be a gymnast holding a handstand.

vascular shunt the automatic opening up of blood vessels (arterioles) to active muscle tissue and the constriction of blood vessels (arterioles) to non-active tissue as a response to an increase in exercise. This allows blood to flow freely and in large quantities to muscle tissue where the demand for oxygen and energy is high and reduces the flow of blood to inactive tissue (such as the kidneys, stomach and liver) where the demand for energy is relatively low during exercise.

vasoconstriction the reduction in the diameter of a blood vessel. This would be caused by the vasomotor centre or by local conditions such as temperature, blood pressure or chemical factors such as K^+, H^+, lactate, adenosine or nitric oxide concentrations in the blood. Such factors combine to constrict blood vessels (arterioles) to non-active tissue during the vascular shunt, as a response to an increase in exercise.

vasodilation the increase in the diameter of a blood vessel. This would be caused by the vasomotor centre or by local conditions such as temperature, blood pressure or chemical factors such as K^+, H^+, lactate, adenosine or nitric oxide concentrations in the blood. Such factors combine to open up blood vessels (arterioles) to active muscle tissue during the vascular shunt, as a response to an increase in exercise.

vasomotor centre part of the medulla oblongata which contains neurones which regulate blood vessel diameter as a response to adrenaline. This is so that the vascular shunt can redistribute blood to active muscle tissue (by increasing the diameter of arterioles to muscle tissue) and restrict blood flow to non-active tissue (by reducing the diameter of arterioles to this tissue).

vasomotor control the neural regulation of the smooth muscle of arteries (and particularly arterioles) which controls changes in blood vessel diameter as a result of vasoconstriction and vasodilation.

vector a quantity which has direction as well as size (force, velocity, displacement, acceleration, etc.).

vein a thin-walled elastic blood vessel which transports blood away from tissue sites (via a venule, then a vein) towards the right atrium of the heart.

velocity distance travelled per second taking into account the direction of travel, a vector. Measured in metres per second.

venae cavae two major veins that return deoxygenated blood to the right atrium of the heart. The superior (upper) vena cava returns blood from the head and arms and thorax and the inferior (lower) vena cava returns blood from all body parts that are lower than the heart's position in the (upright) body.

venoconstriction the limited ability of veins to reduce the diameter of the lumen (or the central space) in veins. The net effect is to increase venous return by reducing the volume/capacity of veins to store blood.

venomotor control the neural regulation of the smooth muscle of veins which produces changes in the shape of veins and therefore changes the velocity of venous blood flow.

venomotor tone the degree of tension in the muscular coat of a vein that determines the shape of the lumen. Venomotor tone is controlled by the autonomic nervous system so when stimulated by the SNS, limited venoconstriction (of the muscular coat of the vein) occurs, blood velocity increases and hence venous return increases.

venous return mechanism the mechanism by which blood returns to the right atrium of the heart, which is dependent on pocket valves sited in most veins (which prevent backflow of blood), the limited action of venomotor tone and the actions of the muscle and respiratory pumps.

ventricle one of a pair of chambers which lie below the atria in the heart. The right ventricle receives deoxygenated blood from the right atrium and pumps this blood to the lungs. The left ventricle receives oxygenated blood from the left atrium and pumps this blood into the aorta for general distribution to the rest of the body.

venule a small thin-walled vein that transports blood from the exit side of the capillary bed to a vein.

vertical axis axis through the body from top of head to between the feet. Movements which rotate about this axis take place in the horizontal or transverse plane. The spinning skater has this movement pattern.

visceral membrane the inner membrane of the pulmonary pleura (general envelope surrounding the lungs).

viscosity a term which describes the resistance to flow of any fluid. One of the benefits of warm-up is to reduce blood viscosity and hence increase blood flow.

vital capacity the maximum volume of air that can be forcibly expired from the lungs following maximal inspiration. A typical value in a healthy adult is 4500 ml. This value decreases during exercise.

vitamins micro-organic substances which need to be ingested as part of the nutrition process and which contain complex organic molecules required for the synthesis of molecules that participate in life processes. Classified as fat soluble or water soluble.

$\dot{V}O_2max$ the maximum rate at which oxygen is consumed during a progressive exercise test to exhaustion. Measured in litres per minute per kilogram of body mass. This is an indirect measure of aerobic power.

voluntary movement movement under conscious control.

watt unit of power. One watt is the power rating when 1 joule is used per second.

wave summation the build-up of tension in a single muscle fibre block (controlled by a single motor neurone) caused by rapid repeated stimulation of the same neurone. The time interval between stimuli is not enough for relaxation of the muscle fibre block to occur and so the tension in the muscle block rises.

weight force due to gravity; acts towards the centre of the Earth (downwards); has a value of 10 newtons per kilogram of mass at the Earth's surface.

white blood cells otherwise known as leucocytes, they originate in the red marrow of bone tissue. There are three main types of white blood cell (granulocytes, lymphocytes and monocytes) and all are concerned with protecting the body against infection and disease.

white fibrocartilage a tough, slightly flexible cartilage consisting of a dense mass of white fibres in a solid matrix, with cells spread thinly among the fibres. Intervertebral discs are an example.

white muscle another name for skeletal muscle that predominantly consists of fast-twitch muscle fibres.

Wingate anaerobic power test a 30-second all-out cycling exercise test from which anaerobic power is computed.

work mechanical energy produced when a force acts through a distance. Work = force × distance moved in the direction of the force.

yellow elastic cartilage yellow elastic fibres running through a solid matrix, with cells lying between the fibres, e.g. the external ear structure.

Part 2

The performer as a person

Ros Bull

9. The nature and classification of skill
10. Information processing in perceptual-motor performance
11. Principles of learning and teaching
12. Psychology of sport performance: individual differences and performance enhancement
13. Psychology of sport: social influences on performance and mental preparation

Glossary of terms

So far in this book we have considered the way in which the body works when we perform physical tasks. In physical education the body is central to what we do; if it is not trained and functioning properly we cannot achieve our intentions. But we must not ignore the mind in our studies because in complex skills and movements, such as those we employ in physical education and sport, body and mind work together. Next time you hear a sportsperson interviewed on television or radio, note how he or she talks about the mental aspects of preparation and performance as well as the physical aspect.

The science which studies how people's minds work, and how they behave, is called psychology. Behaviour is a result of how people think and feel in a situation and may or may not be an 'automatic reaction'. So when we are interested in what sportspeople do to prepare for competition and how they react in the competition itself or when we study dancers as they perform and choreograph or when we observe and analyse what motivates the water sportsperson or mountaineer, then we use psychological theories and methods. You will be introduced to some of these aspects as you work through this section.

People have a number of different motives for participating in sport: to stay fit, to meet the challenge of competition and prove themselves, to share an enthusiasm with friends. But research has shown that what people tend to put high on their list of reasons for involvement in sports is the desire to improve skill and achieve excellence. So it is important for students of sport to understand how we become skilful in physical activities; in other words, how we learn or acquire skill and the factors which make this process easy or difficult. Chapters 9–11 deal with this topic, which is referred to in the literature as skill acquisition. They introduce you to the nature of skill, to some ways in which skills may be classified and to a consideration of the way in which people learn to become skilful in an activity. A theoretical model is presented which sets out to analyse performance and learning in terms of the way in which information is processed and we also look at learning from the teacher's or coach's point of view.

Chapters 12 and 13 consider how sportspeople prepare themselves for performance or competition; we look at some of the things that could go wrong and what coaches, teachers and the performers themselves can do

277

to optimise their performance. We look at the performance itself, how people behave, how they achieve success (or failure) and what factors influence their performance in physical activities. Although we tend to focus our attention on sport and most of the additional reading you do will be about sport, you should remember that the ideas apply equally to any form of physical activity – dance or outdoor pursuits, for example. They apply when anyone is learning and trying to do something to the best of her or his ability.

Associated with each section of work are suggestions for practical activities, which either illustrate the theory presented or form the basis for investigations. At the end of each section are review questions and some examples of questions typical of those you will find in GCE 'AS/A2'-level examinations. Additional reading is suggested and the ideas contained therein might prove useful when you discuss your practical work, its results and your observations or prepare answers to the questions. This reading will also help to extend your knowledge and understanding of the key concepts and issues. It will be particularly useful to those who choose to carry out an investigation in skill acquisition or sport psychology.

The nature and classification of skill

9.1 Skill defined

Keywords

- cognitive skills
- consistency
- economy of effort
- efficiency
- fluency
- learning
- motor skills
- perceptual skills
- perceptual–motor skills
- performance
- predetermined results
- psychomotor skills
- skill
- technique

The concept of '**skill**' is used in several different ways.

- We use the word to mean an element of a game or sport, a **technique** – for example, passing, volleying or somersaulting.
- Later in this section we refer to sports themselves as 'skills', for example, diving, archery or tennis.
- Also, we use the word 'skill' to imply a quality which a sportsperson possesses.

We use the word 'skilful' in the same way. In using the concept of skill in this way we must ensure also that we are differentiating 'skill' from 'ability', for in the literature on motor learning and skill acquisition these mean different things.

Let us first identify three different types of skill.

1. When you do arithmetic in your head (for example, when you are computing a darts score) you are employing intellectual (cognitive) skill. **Cognitive skill** is the ability to solve problems by thinking.

2. If you look at Figure 9.1 you can probably see two different images. With practice you will be able to switch between these two images at will. You are employing **perceptual skill**. Perception is the process by which you sense things and interpret them. In sport, you use this skill, for example, to determine where and when to pass the ball or in judging the type of shot to play in golf.

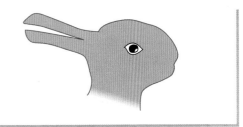

Fig. 9.1 Perceptual skill.

3. As you write your name, your hand is moving across the page and you are thus using essentially motor skill. You could probably do this with your eyes closed. **Motor skills** are those in which voluntary movement is predominant and perception plays a less important role.

The skills we employ in PE and sport usually incorporate elements of all three types and certainly include perception and movement. They are thus called **perceptual–motor** or **psychomotor skills** but often this is shortened to **motor skill**; the perceptual element is usually implied, however.

Investigation 9.1   To identify the characteristics of skill

Task 1
Work in pairs. One person demonstrates a perceptual–motor skill, which can be performed very well; for example, a badminton serve. If you are short of space or equipment, throw and catch one or two tennis balls.

Observations: Note down all the things about the performance that enable you to describe it as 'skilful'. In other words, what is it about the performance that suggests that 'skill' is being demonstrated? You may find it helpful to contrast this performance with one where lack of skill is evident; for example, you might ask your partner to try to juggle two or three tennis balls with one or two hands (Figure 9.2).

Task 2
If possible, watch a video of experienced performers in action. What is it about their performances that tells us they are top class?

Discussion
From your observations, outline the characteristics of skilled performance.

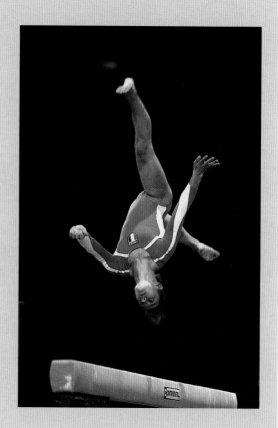

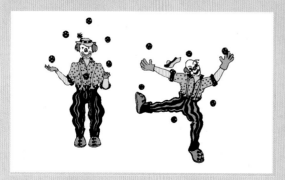

Fig. 9.2 Skilled performance.

The characteristics of skilled performance (Investigation 9.1), summarised in the 'key points', lead us to definitions of skill, of which there are several. One useful one states that skill is 'the learned ability to bring about predetermined results with maximum certainty, often with the minimum outlay of time or energy or both'.[1,2]

Notice that two terms keep occurring in this description: **learning** and **performance**. You will come to a clearer understanding of these concepts as you

KEY POINTS

● **Skill is learned**. It requires practice and results from experience. Learning is usually defined as a relatively permanent change in behaviour and/or performance that persists over time. We recognise this idea when we refer to an early success as a 'fluke' (accidental or not the usual performance) and when we acknowledge a skilful gymnast as one who can reproduce, for example, a vault successfully time after time.

- **Skill has an end result**. We refer to it as 'goal directed'. It is obviously important that the learner is aware, before the skill is attempted, of what this goal is and the reasons for aiming to achieve it. These are the 'predetermined results'. There is usually a 'best way' to achieve these results and the skill will thus be based on a technically sound model.

- Skilled performers achieve their goals **consistently**. There is much more likelihood that a skilful racket sports player will place shots exactly as intended; there is 'maximum certainty'.

- Skill results in **economic and efficient movement**, which is well coordinated and precise. A skilled performer can vary the timing of the movement, performing it quickly or slowly according to the demands of the moment. A beginner may use a lot of energy and still not succeed but an experienced performer is able to fit the energy required to the demands of the task. The movement is efficient. It therefore appears fluent, controlled and in many instances aesthetically pleasing.

- A skilled performer makes accurate analyses of the demands of a sport situation and **appropriate decisions** about how to deal with these. Skill is not just about being a good technician but about being able to use techniques at the right moment

progress through Part 2 (in particular, Chapter 11), but we need to be able to distinguish between these terms at this stage.

Performance is a demonstration of the solving of a problem or task at a given moment in time. Learning is shown by relatively permanent incremental improvements in performance over time.

Learning is a process, a life-long process. Even top-class sportspeople claim that they are still learning about their sport and aiming to improve. But a sport has definable elements or stages of learning associated with it and so a gymnast, for example, can be said to have learned to perform a back somersault. What we mean is that her early performances were unsuccessful (or that she was reliant on her coach for support) but that with practice she became able to produce a well-formed somersault that would achieve good marks in a competition and was able to produce this performance consistently. A good coach or teacher defines stages of learning (i.e. intermediate goals) within a learning process so that the gymnast knows which elements of the skill have been mastered and which need further refinement. Learning is thus shown by improvements in performance – we have learned a skill when we can show a relatively permanent improvement. Of course, what we mean by 'relatively permanent improvement' depends to some extent on the accuracy requirements of the task. We do not say that a professional golfer had not learned to putt just because she or he occasionally misses! This subject is dealt with further in Chapter 11.

9.2 Skill classified

Keywords

- ➤ balance
- ➤ body (muscular) involvement
- ➤ classification of skill
- ➤ closed skills
- ➤ coactive skills
- ➤ complexity
- ➤ continuity
- ➤ continuous skills
- ➤ continuum
- ➤ coordination
- ➤ discrete skills
- ➤ environmental requirements
- ➤ externally paced skills
- ➤ fine skills
- ➤ gross skills
- ➤ individual skills
- ➤ interaction
- ➤ learning
- ➤ open skills
- ➤ organisation
- ➤ pacing
- ➤ self-paced skills
- ➤ serial skills

Let us return to the idea of skills being activities, such as climbing, dancing or playing a shot in badminton. Clearly, these are very different and may well have to be learned in different ways. Teachers, coaches and performers themselves therefore find it useful to be able to classify skills so that differing characteristics can be taken into account. **Classification** is the process of grouping similar skills together and giving them a generic label. You are already familiar with the 'cognitive– perceptual–motor' classification (see Section 9.1). As you complete your further reading, see how many different classifications you can find.

For example, Singer[3] classifies skills in terms of:

- bodily involvement
- duration of movement
- pacing conditions
- cognitive involvement
- feedback availability.

Stallings[4] has a slightly different list:

- continuity
- coherence
- pacing
- environmental conditions
- intrinsic feedback.

The classifications that sport psychologists or coaches choose to use depend on what aspect of learning or performance they want to analyse.

We consider here a classification system with seven elements: muscular involvement, environmental requirements, continuity, pacing, difficulty, organisation and interaction.

Each of these elements can be thought of as a **continuum**. This means that two ends of the continuum are opposites and there is a gradual change in characteristics from one end to the other.

Muscular involvement continuum

Fine skills are those that involve small movements of specific body parts. Rifle shooting, for example, involves the movement of just the trigger finger (though considerable perceptual ability and steady posture are needed) and is an example of a fine skill.

Gross skills involve large muscle groups and movement of the whole body; an example of this would be the high jump.

In between these two extremes are skills with either greater or lesser body involvement, for example a basketball or netball free shot (Figure 9.3). Coaches and players must also consider that within a gross skill, such as bowling in cricket, there may be very important fine movements that must be analysed and

practised. In the bowling example, it might be the use of the fingers across the seam to produce a particular kind of spin.

Continuity continuum

Continuous skills are those that have no obvious beginning or end (Figure 9.4); in theory they can be continued for as long as the performer wishes. The end of one cycle of the skill becomes the beginning of the next.

Discrete skills, on the other hand, have a clear beginning and end; the skill can be repeated but the performer 'starts again'.

Serial skills are composed of several discrete elements, strung together to produce an integrated movement. The order in which the elements are performed is important; for example, in a high jump or a triple jump, the run up, take-off and the components of the jumping phase happen in a particular order. Note that whereas we refer to these as serial skills, they are also clearly discrete, so the two terms are not mutually exclusive.

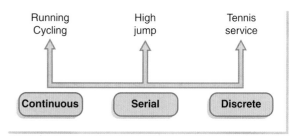

Fig. 9.4 The continuous/discrete continuum.

Pacing continuum

The **pacing** continuum (Figure 9.5) is concerned with the extent to which the performer has control over the timing of the action. Actions are said to be 'self-paced' or 'externally paced' (or somewhere between these two extremes) according to the extent to which the performer can decide when to start the action.

Self-paced skills are those in which the performer has control over the rate at which the action takes place. Some examples are: a tennis player determines the timing of the action of the serve; some floorwork moves in men's gymnastics may be done slowly or quickly, depending on the effect required; a climber may move up a pitch slowly and carefully, savouring the technical problems posed, or may decide that the weather is closing in and it would be better to hurry.

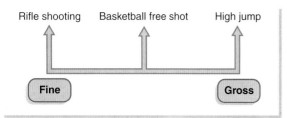

Fig. 9.3 The body involvement continuum.

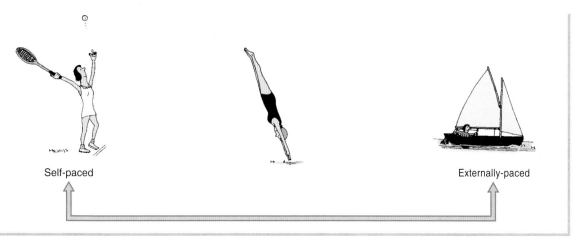

Fig. 9.5 The pacing continuum.

In others, the start of the action can be controlled but thereafter the movement takes place at a given rate; for example, a diver decides when to start his dive but once he has left the board he cannot slow down his rate of progress to the water!

Externally paced skills are those in which timing and form are determined by what is happening elsewhere in the environment; for example, a sailor adjusts the trim of the sails and the direction to be taken according to the wind.

Environmental requirements continuum

The pacing continuum leads us to an important classification proposed by Poulton and developed in relation to sport skills by Knapp.[2] The continuum is based on the extent to which environmental conditions affect the performance (Figure 9.6). Note that by 'environment' we do not only mean the weather conditions but everything surrounding the player including, importantly, the actions of other players.

Open skills are those in which the form of action is constantly being varied according to what is happening around the performer. The environment is unpredictable.

Closed skills are prelearned patterns of movements that can be followed without (or with little) reference to the environment that is essentially predictable.

At first sight this seems to be a fairly straightforward idea but as one tries to identify skills as more or less open or closed, complexities arise. For example, one might identify soccer as essentially an open skill because players are constantly reacting to other players but within the game there are skills that are clearly closed, for example taking a penalty. We call these 'closed skills in open situations'. It is very important

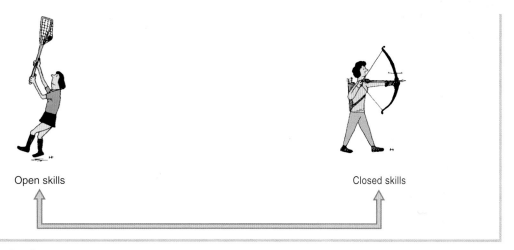

Fig. 9.6 The open/closed continuum.

that performers, teachers and coaches recognise where on the continuum a skill lies, because open skills need to be practised differently from closed skills.

When learning and practising a closed skill, such as in trampolining or athletics, the performer and coach have a model of the required movement pattern in mind and the task of the performer is to make the performance conform as closely as possible to that model. Practice therefore entails gradually refining performance and, once the movement pattern has been established, repeating it until it becomes habitual and the performer can reproduce the movement consistently without having to pay too much attention to it.

Open skills, on the other hand, require practice that takes into account the many different ways in which the techniques are to be used. For example, a fielder in cricket, rounders or baseball must be able to throw an infinite variety of distances to ensure the ball reaches the receiver at just the right height.

Interaction continuum (Figure 9.7)

In preparing a performer for competition, coaches might need to consider the nature of the interactions between competitors and the extent to which the opposition can affect their player's performance.

Individual skills are those that the competitor performs alone, without the physical presence of the opposition. Can you think of an example in which the opposition is not even present? Figure skating is an example of a sport in which competitors can, if they wish, largely distance themselves from each other, even before and after performance. In a high jump event, other competitors are in the area but they do not perform at the same time and cannot physically affect performance, though they may exert psychological pressure. Performance in individual activities is the least likely to be affected by the opposition.

Coactive skills are those in which competitors are performing at *the same time* but where they are physically separated and in which one competitor

cannot physically inhibit the performance of another. Examples would be 100 m sprint events in athletics or swimming. As in the case of individual activities, however, the good or bad performance of one may have a psychological effect on another. For example, you are more likely to produce a personal best in a 100 m sprint event if you are in competition with people who are as fast as, or a little bit faster than, yourself.

Interactive skills are those in which performance can be controlled by the opposition. In most games, how well you play is dependent on how well your opponent allows you to play. Highly interactive activities are those in which space is shared and in which body contact is allowed, for example rugby or American football. There is potentially less interaction as less body contact is allowed, for example in basketball, and less interaction still when areas of play are segregated, for example in tennis or volleyball. In theory, the greater the level of interaction, the greater the potential for opponents to affect each others' performance. Thus maintaining possession and avoiding being tackled or intercepted are important tactics in invasion games.

Difficulty (complexity) continuum (Figure 9.8)

The term 'complexity' is usually used in this context in preference to 'difficulty' because it relates to the skill itself whereas 'difficulty' also relates to the stage of learning of the performer. A skill which is difficult to perform as it is being learned is not as difficult when it is well practised but it remains as complex. A number of factors contribute to the complexity of a task:

- amount of information to be processed
- number of decisions to be made
- speed at which information processing and decision making have to occur
- number of subroutines and the extent of coordination required
- speed/power required

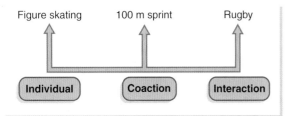

Fig. 9.7 The interaction continuum.

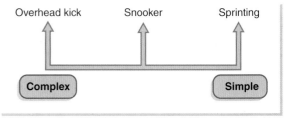

Fig. 9.8 The complexity continuum.

- accuracy needed
- type and timing of feedback available.

A highly **complex task** will require high levels of all or most of these components; a simple task will need lower levels in each or in some nothing at all. Thus an overhead kick in a crowded goalmouth requires high levels of all except feedback and is complex, whereas potting a snooker ball is a simpler skill, since it needs only high levels of visual perception, accuracy and control, with fewer decisions and more time to make them in. In very **simple skills** such as sprinting, competitive success derives from very high levels of only one or two of the components, in this case speed and power. This is not to say that running 100 m in 10 seconds is easy, just that it is a simple skill.

Organisation continuum (Figure 9.9)

Most skills comprise a number of parts, known as 'subroutines' (see Chapter 10). For example, a tennis serve consists of the initial stance, the throw-up, the racket swing, the strike and the follow-through.

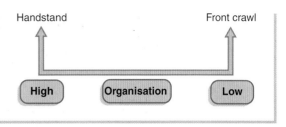

Fig. 9.9 The organisation continuum.

In **highly organised skills**, these subroutines are closely integrated and difficult to separate in practice without destroying the movement dynamics of the skill. They are thus best practised as a whole (unless there is danger in so doing or they are too complex: see Chapter 11). Many gymnastic skills are examples of high organisation.

Low-organisation skills are made up of subroutines that tend to be discrete and may be practised separately and then integrated into the whole skill without too many problems. Swimming strokes, particularly front or back crawl, are examples of this.

KEY POINTS

	BODY INVOLVEMENT	
Fine Small movements Importance of accuracy, e.g. rifle shooting		Gross Large muscle groups Power/endurance, e.g. high jump
Continuous No clear beginning/end, e.g. cycling	CONTINUITY Serial, e.g. high jump	Discrete Clear beginning/end, e.g. tennis serve
Self Performer controls start and pace, e.g. floorwork sequence	PACING	External Environment/others control start and pace, e.g. sailing
Open Perceptual Environment unpredictable, e.g. passing in basketball	ENVIRONMENTAL REQUIREMENTS	Closed Habitual Environment predictable, e.g. archery
Individual Performance alone, e.g. figure skating	INTERACTION Coaction Competitors perform together, e.g. sprinting	Interaction Competitors affect performance Shared or separate space, e.g. games
Complex High levels of a number of factors, e.g. overhead soccer kick	COMPLEXITY	Simple Low levels of a number of factors or high levels of only a few factors, e.g. snooker
High Subroutines closely integrated, e.g. handstand/somersault	ORGANISATION	Low Subroutines discrete, e.g. front crawl

Investigation 9.2 To explore the classification system

Method: Work in pairs. Each makes a list of physical education skills. Exchange the lists and place the activities you have been given onto each of the seven continua we have studied so far.

Observations: As you think about these classifications, you will realise that to assign a particular activity a place on a continuum can be a complex task. Much depends on the circumstances. For example, skiing could be open or closed depending on the state and gradient of the piste. And one could argue that whereas a game such as tennis clearly demands open skills, once a player has decided what sort of shot to make, has positioned him/herself correctly and read the pace and spin of the ball, the resulting stroke is closed, hence the idea of 'closed skills in open situations'.

Discussion: Try to come to some agreement with your partner about the placing of the various activities. Suggest what some of the implications of this classification for sportspeople might be. In spite of the difficulties you may have identified, the idea of classifying skill is an interesting one and gives us food for thought when deciding how a skill should be practised. We return to this in Chapter 11.

Review questions

1. Give a definition of skill.
2. Define and give an example of (a) a perceptual skill and (b) a motor skill. Why are sport skills referred to as 'psychomotor' skills?
3. Give an example of a sport skill that is both discrete and closed.
4. How are open skills different from closed skills?
5. What is 'a closed skill in an open situation'?
6. Place a forehand tennis drive in open play on each of the seven continua and justify your placing.
7. Why is it useful to be able to classify skills?

9.3 Skill and ability

Keywords

- ability
- dynamic precision
- dynamic strength
- explosive strength
- extent flexibility
- gross motor ability
- motor ability
- perceptual ability
- psychomotor ability
- speed
- stamina
- static precision
- static strength
- trunk strength

We need at this stage to distinguish between two terms, **skill** and **ability**, which are often used in everyday language to mean the same thing but to sport psychologists these are technical terms that mean two different things.

Skill is acquired. Skills must be learned and the process of this learning is considered in Chapter 11.

Ability (for example, to react quickly) is a stable, enduring, mainly genetically determined characteristic (or trait) that underlies skilled performance and can be used in a variety of skills.[5] Abilities develop through maturation; they are modified by experience but are generally considered to be innate and enduring (though some psychologists question this). As with skills, abilities can be essentially perceptual, essentially motor or a combination of the two. Since most abilities to do with action are a combination, they are referred to as **psychomotor abilities**. The term is often shortened to 'motor abilities'.

Abilities underpin and contribute to skills. For example, someone with good natural balance, shoulder flexibility, upper body and wrist strength has the pre-requisites to perform a handstand. The handstand is a skill and the gymnast has to learn to use and coordinate these abilities effectively to learn to do a handstand.

Maturation, the result of growth and development, varies with individuals and causes differences in the rate at which individuals learn. A second factor that leads to individual differences in rate of learning is psychomotor ability; this may also set limits on the level of performance in any one skill that an individual is capable of achieving. For example, if you have not inherited enough fast-twitch muscle you will never make a top-class sprinter, no matter how hard you train.

It is important to remember that there is as yet no definitive list of psychomotor abilities. Different researchers categorise ability in different ways and even the terms used to describe the abilities vary slightly.

Stallings,[4] for example, selects her list on the following grounds: each ability has been identified in a number of studies; they can be developed and assessed; and they are relevant to physical educators (Figure 9.10).

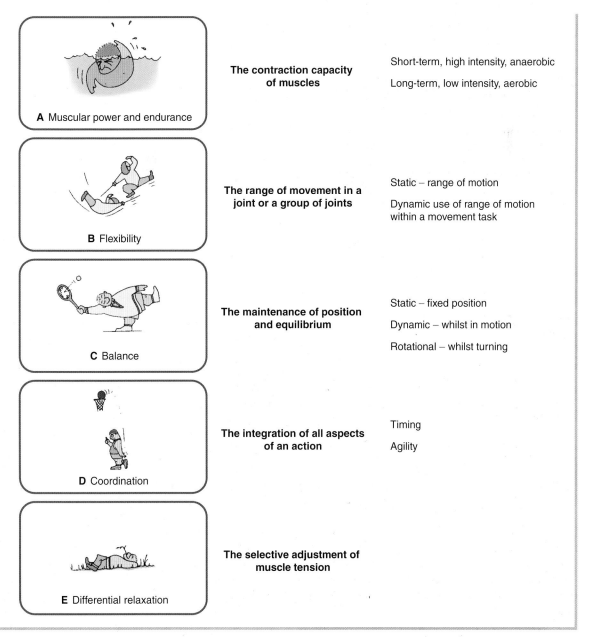

A Muscular power and endurance — The contraction capacity of muscles — Short-term, high intensity, anaerobic / Long-term, low intensity, aerobic

B Flexibility — The range of movement in a joint or a group of joints — Static – range of motion / Dynamic use of range of motion within a movement task

C Balance — The maintenance of position and equilibrium — Static – fixed position / Dynamic – whilst in motion / Rotational – whilst turning

D Coordination — The integration of all aspects of an action — Timing / Agility

E Differential relaxation — The selective adjustment of muscle tension

Fig. 9.10 Stallings' motor abilities.[4]

Fleishman[6] identified the characteristics of motor performance in a major research programme that involved over 200 tasks and many thousands of subjects, as follows.

1. A series of **psychomotor abilities** derived from limb coordination tasks:
   - reaction time
   - response orientation (i.e. choice reaction time)
   - speed of movement
   - finger dexterity
   - manual dexterity
   - response integration (i.e. making sense of a variety of sources of information, as in interactive games).

2. Nine 'physical proficiency abilities', referred to later as **gross motor abilities** (see Figure 9.11).

EXTENT FLEXIBILITY:	flexing or stretching the trunk and back muscles as far as possible in any direction.
DYNAMIC FLEXIBILITY:	making repeated rapid movements in which the ability of the muscles to recover is critical.
EXPLOSIVE STRENGTH:	expending a maximum amount of energy in one or a series of strong, sudden movements.
STATIC STRENGTH:	the maximum force which can be exerted for a brief period.
DYNAMIC STRENGTH:	exerting muscular force repeatedly or over a period of time.
TRUNK STRENGTH:	dynamic strength specific to the abdominal muscles.
GROSS BODY COORDINATION:	coordinating the similtaneous movements of different body parts whilst involved in whole body action.
GROSS BODY EQUILIBRIUM:	maintaining balance whilst blindfolded.
STAMINA:	continuing to exert maximum effort over time.

Fig. 9.11 Fleishman's gross motor abilities.[6]

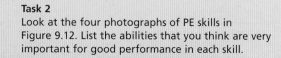

Investigation 9.3 To consider the abilities required for particular skills

Task 1
Discuss Fleishman's inventory of abilities with a friend. Check up on the meanings of the terms if you are not sure.

Task 2
Look at the four photographs of PE skills in Figure 9.12. List the abilities that you think are very important for good performance in each skill.

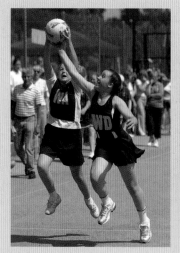

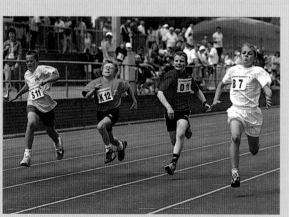

Fig. 9.12 Physical education activities.

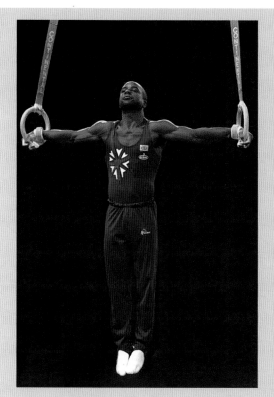 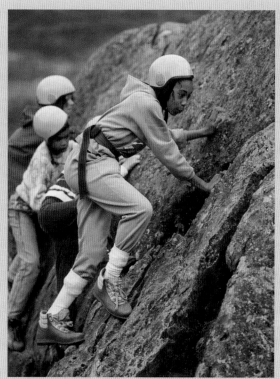

Fig. 9.12 Physical education activities.

You have probably found that several abilities keep being mentioned over and over again. Strength, speed and coordination seem to be requirements for most motor skills and this led early researchers to argue for the idea of an inherited general motor ability. We hint at this when we say that someone is a 'natural' games player, meaning that they are good at most sports. But more recent research suggests no evidence for such a general ability, arguing that specific skills require specific abilities. The coordination required to kick a ball, for example, is not the same as that required to execute a complex dance step. There are more than 100 motor abilities, so when we talk about a 'natural' sportsperson we mean someone who has inherited and developed a large number of the abilities that underpin skill in sport, including the ability to learn motor skills efficiently. This implies that, in addition to motor abilities, we could also argue that there are perceptual abilities that are important in sport, concerning the way in which we notice significant things that are happening around us and how quickly and effectively we make decisions about how to deal with them. These abilities, which Stallings[4] identifies as visual, auditory, tactile and kinaesthetic, are discussed in more detail in Chapter 10.

However, research in this area goes on[7,8] and you will find reference to 'superability' and the 'modular

> **KEY POINTS**
>
> - Skill = Ability + Technique
>
> - Skills must be learned.
>
> - Abilities are usually thought of as stable and enduring traits that underpin skills and contribute to the speed with which individuals learn psychomotor skills and to the quality of their performance.
>
> - There is no such thing as general psychomotor ability. Specific skills require specific abilities and individuals vary in the range of abilities they possess. The 'natural', all-round athlete possesses a number of abilities appropriate to sport.

view' of abilities but these ideas have not yet replaced the 'specificity hypothesis'.

The measurement of psychomotor abilities

If psychomotor abilities are fundamental to the learning and performance of skills then it is useful for us to be able to measure ability in sportspeople for research purposes, to add to our knowledge of how skill works or to find out our own personal ability make-up. You will be doing some investigations of motor abilities in your work on training and fitness in Chapter 4. Arnot & Gaines,[9] in their book *Sports-talent*, show how a knowledge of the specific tasks of an activity such as windsurfing or tennis can allow participants, with simple 'home-made' tests, to measure the strengths and weaknesses of relevant abilities in their profile. They can then choose activities they have the potential to be good at or to compensate for, say, lack of strength with good coordination.

Investigation 9.4   Measurement of psychomotor skills

In the three tasks below, work in pairs. The scorer has a stopwatch.

Task 1 – to measure static balance (gross body equilibrium)

Method: This test measures the ability to balance using the inner ear mechanism only; that is, not using the considerable positional information provided by the eyes. It is quite difficult and not suitable for young children. If you find difficulty in scoring, perform the test with eyes open.

The subject stands as in Figure 9.13. It is best to wear trainers and to be standing on a hard surface. Stand on your preferred leg; keep your bent knee well out to the side. The experimenter starts timing as soon as you close your eyes (don't cheat!). The watch is stopped when you open your eyes, move your hands, take your foot off your knee or move your standing foot from the spot. Wobbling is permissible as long as you don't do any of the above. Take the test three times (with rests in between) and record your best time.

Results: Use Table 9.1 to find your score in points; record your points score.

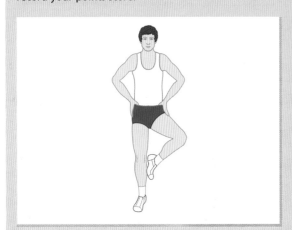

Fig. 9.13 Stork balance.

Table 9.1 Blind stork balance (from reference[9])

Men		Women	
Best time (s)	*Points*	*Best time (s)*	*Points*
60	20	35	20
55	18	30	17
50	16	25	14
45	14	20	11
40	12	15	8
35	10	10	4
30	8	5	2
25	6		
20	4		
15	3		
10	2		

The conversion of points in Tables 9.1–9.3 enables men's and women's scores to be compared directly, given that standardised mean times of men and women on the tasks are different.

Task 2 – to measure coordination (agility)

Method: Measure out a 66 cm-per-side hexagon on the floor as shown in Figure 9.14. Cover the lines with masking or plastic tape so that the outside edge of the tape becomes the outside of the hexagon.

Stand in the middle of the hexagon, facing side A; face this way throughout the test. On the command 'go', when the watch is started, jump with both feet across line B and immediately back into the hexagon (remember to keep facing front). Then jump over side C and back and continue until you are back in the hexagon, having jumped over side A. This is one complete circuit; do three circuits altogether. The watch is stopped when you have completed the third circuit. Record your time. If you make a mistake, by treading on a line or jumping over the wrong line, start the trial again. Count the times for successful trials only. Have three goes with rests in between and note your best time.

Results: Use Table 9.2 to record your points score. ▶

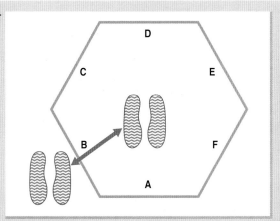

Fig. 9.14 The hexagon.

Table 9.2 Hexagonal obstacle (from reference[9])		
Best time without sides (s)		*Points*
Men	*Women*	
9.0	9.0	10.0
10.1	10.6	9.0
11.2	12.2	8.0
12.3	13.8	7.0
13.4	15.4	6.0
14.5	17.0	5.0
15.6	18.6	4.0
16.7	20.2	3.0
17.8	21.8	2.0
18.9	23.4	1.0
20.0	25.0	0.0

Task 3 – to measure the endurance strength of the quadriceps

Method: The subject stands with his/her back against a smooth wall. Do the test barefoot or in trainers that do not slip, as your feet will tend to slide. When you are ready, gently slide your back down the wall until you are in the position shown in Figure 9.15. Your feet should be comfortably apart. There should be angles of 90° at the hip and knee.

Lift one foot about 5 cm off the ground. Your partner should start timing now. The watch is stopped when you put your foot back down on the floor. Stand up

by putting your hands against the wall by your hips and pushing forwards slowly. Stand up gently. Record your time. Take a rest and then repeat the test with the other leg supporting. Again record your time.

Results: Taking the lower of the two times, record your points score using Table 9.3.

Discussion

Look at your profile of points for the three tests. Which is your highest points score? Is this what you would have expected?

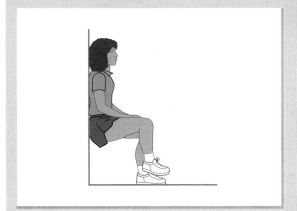

Fig. 9.15 The wall squat.

Table 9.3 Wall squat (from reference[9])		
Time (s)		*Points*
Men	*Women*	
120	70	8.0
111	65	7.6
102	60	7.2
93	55	6.8
84	50	6.4
75	45	5.6
66	40	4.8
57	35	4.0
48	30	3.2
39	25	2.4
30	20	1.6
21	15	0.8

As you read further you will find many examples of psychomotor ability tests other than those in Investigation 9.4. Sometimes you will recognise that these measure more than one ability, for it is often difficult to isolate abilities in simple tests. The three tests in Investigation 9.4 measure the motor aspect of ability, i.e. the work that the muscles are doing. In your further reading you will find tests that measure the perceptual aspects of ability.

Ability testing is a useful addition to fitness testing but because of the complex interaction of abilities in sports skills, such testing is inappropriate for predicting how good an athlete will become.

Review questions

1. List four differences between abilities and skills.
2. Why is there 'no such thing as a general motor ability'?
3. What do we mean when we say someone is a 'natural' sportsperson?
4. Why is it important to distinguish between ability and skill?
5. To what extent do abilities limit the level of acquisition of skills?
6. What are the advantages and difficulties of measuring motor abilities?
7. Place Fleishman's six psychomotor abilities in order of importance to (i) an archer; (ii) a gymnast; (iii) a rugby player; (iv) a weightlifter.

Exam-style questions

1. If you were watching a number of performers in sport, what characteristics would you expect the movements of a skilled performer to have? (*4 marks*)

2. Use practical examples to explain each of these characteristics of skill:
   • Consistent
   • Efficient
   • Goal directed (*3 marks*)

3. Figure 9.16 shows a profile for the racing start in swimming scaled across five continua that represent certain characteristics of skilled movements.
   a. With reference to the profile, briefly describe the swimming racing start in terms of each of the five characteristics of skilled movement. (*5 marks*)
   b. i. Using the same five continua, sketch a profile to describe the characteristics of a tennis serve. (*3 marks*)
      ii. Justify your choice of position on the continua for **coherence** and **environmental conditions**. (*5 marks*)
      iii. Explain briefly how your profile of the tennis serve might help a coach decide how to organise practices for players learning this skill. (*7 marks*)
   (*Total 20 marks*)

4. By using examples from physical education, explain what is meant by fundamental motor skills and why they are so important. (*4 marks*)

5. a. You are observing a number of tennis players being coached. There is a mixture of abilities. What is meant by ability? (*3 marks*)
   b. Give two types of abilities that are important to playing tennis effectively. (*2 marks*)

6. a. Why is the tennis serve often regarded as a closed skill? (*2 marks*)
   b. Using passing skills in a team game, explain what is meant by an open skill. (*4 marks*)
   c. Give one example from sport of each of the following and state why you have chosen your example: continuous skills; serial skills; discrete skills. (*3 marks*)

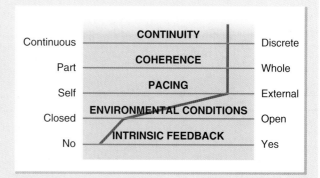

Fig. 9.16 Profile for the racing start in swimming (adapted from reference[4]).

References

1. Guthrie E R 1952 *The psychology of learning*. Harper and Row, New York
2. Knapp B 1977 *Skill in sport*. Routledge and Kegan Paul, London
3. Singer R N 1982 *The learning of motor skills*. Macmillan, New York
4. Stallings L M 1982 *Motor learning from theory to practice*. Mosby, St. Louis
5. Schmidt R A 1991 *Motor learning and performance: from principles to practice*. Human Kinetics, Champaign, Illinois
6. Fleishman E A 1972 *The structure and measurement of psychomotor abilities*. In: Singer R N (ed) The psychomotor domain: movement behavior. Lea and Febiger, Philadelphia
7. Beashel P, Taylor J (eds) 1996 *Advanced studies in physical education and sport*. Nelson, Walton on Thames
8. Schmidt R A, Lee T D 1999 *Motor control and learning: a behavioral emphasis*, 3rd edn. Human Kinetics, Champaign, Illinois
9. Arnot R, Gaines C 1984 *Sportstalent*. Penguin, Harmondsworth

Further reading

*Particularly useful for students

*Honeybourne J et al 2004 *Advanced physical education and sport for A Level*, 3rd edn. Stanley Thornes, Cheltenham

*James R et al 2003 *Complete A–Z physical education,* 2nd edn. Hodder and Stoughton, London

Magill R A 2003 *Motor learning: concepts and applications*, 7th edn. McGraw Hill, Massachusetts

McMorris T 2004 *The acquisition and performance of sports skills*. John Wiley, Chichester

*Roscoe D Roscoe J V, Honeybourne J, Davis R, Galligan F 2003 *Physical education and sport studies AS/A2 level student revision guide*. Jan Roscoe Publications, Widnes

Schmidt R A, Lee T D 1999 *Motor control and learning: a behavioural emphasis*, 3rd edn. Human Kinetics, Champaign, Illinois

Schmidt R A, Wrisberg C A 2004 *Motor learning and performance: a problem-based learning approach*, 3rd edn. Human Kinetics, Champaign, Illinois

Sharp B 2004 *Acquiring skill in sport*. 2nd edn. Sports Dynamics, Cheltenham

*Webster S 2002 *AS/A2 sport psychology guide*. Jan Roscoe Publications, Widnes

*Wesson K et al 2004 *Sport and PE: a complete guide to advanced level study*, 3rd edn. Hodder and Stoughton, London

*Woods B 1998 *Applying psychology to sport*. Hodder and Stoughton, London

Multimedia

Videos

The Fitness Series, Video Education, Australia 1996. *Analysing physical activity – the learning of skills*. UK suppliers Boulton and Hawker Films Ltd

Video Education Australia 2003 *Acquiring skills*. UK suppliers Boulton and Hawker Films Ltd

CD-ROMs

*Particularly useful for students

Roscoe D A Teacher's guide to physical education and the study of sport. Part 2 The Performer as a Person, skills acquisition 5th edn. Jan Roscoe Publications, Widnes

Roscoe D A, Roscoe J V 2002 OCR/AQA/Edexcel Science and Sport Psychology Powerpoint Classroom Presentations. Jan Roscoe Publications, Widnes

*Roscoe D A, Roscoe J V, Honeybourne J, Davis R, Galligan F 2003 Physical Education and Sport Studies AS/A2 Level Student Revision Guide 3rd edn. Jan Roscoe Publications, Widnes

Information processing in perceptual-motor performance

So far we have defined skill by describing it. Knapp's approach is thus a 'descriptive definition'. Let us now consider a different form of definition – one which analyses **how** the skill is performed. This is known as an 'operational definition' and we will build it around a theoretical model known as the **information-processing** approach.

Learning objectives

On completion of this section, you will be able to:

1. Understand how information is transmitted through the central and peripheral nervous systems.

2. Use an information-processing model to analyse sport performance (self and others).

3. Understand the relationship between sensory input, perception, decision making, memory and motor output in the performance of skilled actions and in the learning process.

4. Measure reaction time and test hypotheses using reaction time data.

5. Understand the difference between open and closed modes of motor control.

6. Define and apply to physical education activities the keywords listed at the beginning of each section.

10.1 Introduction to information processing

Keywords

- central nervous system (CNS)
- cognitive system
- decision making
- decision mechanism
- display
- effector mechanism
- extrinsic feedback
- information processing
- input
- intrinsic feedback
- memory
- muscular system
- output
- perception
- perceptual mechanism
- peripheral nervous system
- physiological system
- receptor system
- response programming
- sensory system
- stimulus identification
- translatory mechanism

The information-processing approach is so called because it is a theory or, more accurately, a series of theories which seek to explain human action by showing how we take information from our surroundings and make decisions about what to do next on the basis of our interpretation of that information. Investigation 10.1 shows you how to begin to use the information-processing approach in a sport/PE context.

Method: Watch a video (preferably played in 'slow motion') of a player receiving or catching and making a pass or shot (net or invasion game). Alternatively, while playing a game concentrate on what you are doing while you yourself are receiving and sending.

1. Note down everything that you do (or the player does), from first picking out where the ball is as it approaches to assessing the effectiveness of the shot or pass. Be really detailed about this, e.g. 'as the ball was coming towards me I tried to decide how much it was bouncing'. Include things you are thinking about.

2. Group the thoughts or actions you have identified into:
   a. those concerned with identifying what is happening to the ball. Head this list **'Input'**
   b. those concerned with making decisions about where to move and what to do. Head this list **'Decision making'**
   c. those concerned with making an appropriate movement as a result of the decision. Head this list **'Output'**.

You will go through this process twice – one set of activities is concerned with receiving and one with sending.

Arrange your three lists as in Figure 10.1.

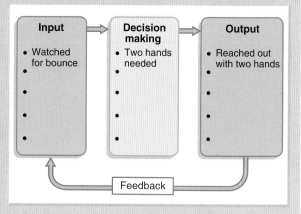

Fig. 10.1 A simple information-processing model.

In Investigation 10.1 you constructed a simple information-processing model, based on your own analysis of a sport skill. This model suggests that there are three main stages in the production of any conscious movement:

1. taking in and analysing information about what is happening
2. making decisions about what to do on the basis of this information

3. programming the muscles to produce the movement required.

There are many such models, some of which you will come across in your further reading, but they all contain these three basic elements. You should remember that these models are only representations of what psychologists think is going on within a player's **central nervous system (CNS)**. We can assess what is entering the system and we can observe what the player does to respond but we can only hypothesise about the processes in between.

The definitions given in Key Points suggest that we need to expand the model further. Schmidt's[1] model (Figure 10.2) shows what is happening in more detail.

- **Stimulus identification (perception).** As the player receives information from the environment he/she needs to make sense of it, i.e. to perceive it, interpret it and identify elements in it which are important, for example whether the ball is spinning or not, what the flight path of the shuttle is, whether there is a gap in the defence which can be exploited.
- **Response selection.** Once the player has interpreted what they are seeing (other senses are used also) they must decide what to do, i.e. 'my opponent has come up to the net; I'm going to lob'.

KEY POINTS

- **Input** is the information from the environment which the player is aware of and uses to decide on a response to the situation.

- **Decision making** refers to the combination of recognition, perception and memory processes used to select an appropriate response to the demands of the situation.

- **Output** is the response which the player makes. In sport this is usually in the form of a movement of some kind. Output becomes a form of input (**feedback**) in that the player perceives the outcome of his/her response and this in turn becomes the basis for further decision making.

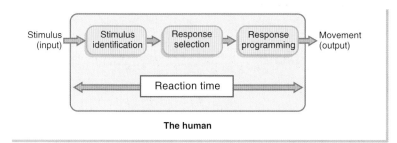

Fig. 10.2 Schmidt's information-processing model.

- **Response programming**. Following decision making about what to do, the muscles needed to carry out the required movement must be identified and activated. In skilled players this becomes almost automatic.

Look carefully at Figures 10.1 and 10.2. They look very similar but there's an important difference. Schmidt's 'three boxes' are all concerned with what the brain does, i.e. they are subsumed in the 'decision making' box of Figure 10.1. If we combine the two models we arrive at Figure 10.3, Whiting's[2] information-processing model, which gives us more detail still.

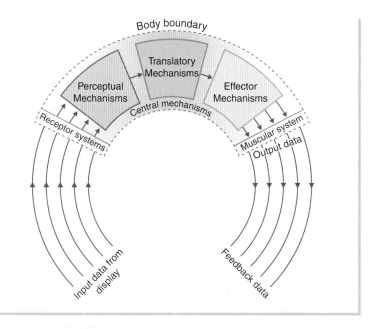

Fig. 10.3 Whiting's model of information processing.[2]

Investigation 10.2   To use an information-processing model to analyse a skill

Method: Work in pairs. Use your knowledge of a striking skill (tennis, badminton, hockey, football, etc.) to analyse the action of striking using either Whiting's[2] model (see Figure 10.3) or Welford's[3] model (Figure 10.28).

1. Define and explain all the terms in Figure 10.3. Use Figure 10.2 as a reference to help you with this.
2. Give a practical example of what is happening in each of the processes identified in the model.
3. Compare your examples with those of a colleague to check your analysis.

KEY POINTS

- **Display** – the surroundings or environment.

- **Stimuli** – the aspects of the display which the player is attending to.

- **Sensory and receptor system** – the part of the CNS which passes information from the sense organs to the brain.

- **Perceptual mechanism** – the process by which the interpretation of stimuli takes place.

- **Decision and translatory mechanism** – the process which deals with receiving the interpretation of the input and using the memory of previous similar situations to decide upon a response.

- **Effector mechanism** – on the basis of the decision made, a motor plan or programme is constructed which informs the muscles of the movement requirements.

- **Muscular system** – the nerves and muscles which are involved in the particular movement.

- **Response** – the movement which results from the whole information-processing sequence.

- **Intrinsic feedback** – information about the movement provided by proprioception (see Section 10.2).

- **Extrinsic feedback** – information about the outcome of the response.

Skilled movement thus relies on the transmission of information through the nervous system. The nervous system has two elements:

1. the **CNS** – the brain and the spinal cord
2. the **peripheral nervous system** – the nerves that connect the spinal cord with all parts of the body, radiating from and returning to the CNS.

Review questions

1. Why are information-processing models useful?
2. Draw Schmidt's information-processing model and define each of the terms used.
3. What does Whiting mean by the 'translatory mechanism'? How does it relate to decision making?

Exam-style questions

1. **a.** The items in the boxes in Figure 10.4 represent the elements of a simple information-processing model of skill. Arrange the boxes and add lines and arrow heads to represent the flow of information during the execution of an **open** skill (see Chapter 9). (*3 marks*)

   b. With reference to open passing skills, what difficulties might a beginner expect to experience with each of the elements of the model? (*8 marks*)

   (*Total 11 marks*)

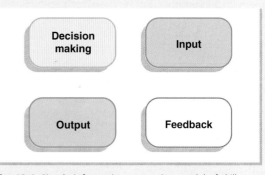

Fig. 10.4 Simple information-processing model of skill.

The following sections take the elements of the information-processing model and consider them in detail. In so doing we will build up Welford's[3] model which includes the important elements of memory and attention. If you wish to see what this model looks like before you start studying these sections, turn to Figure 10.28.

10.2 Sensory input: the receptor mechanism

Keywords

➤ audition
➤ equilibrium
➤ internal sensors
➤ kinaesthesis
➤ proprioception
➤ touch
➤ vision

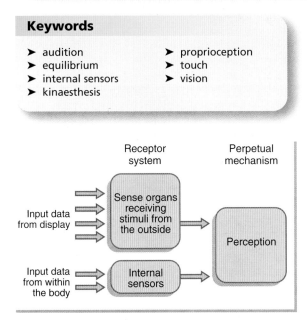

Fig. 10.5 Sensory input in information processing.

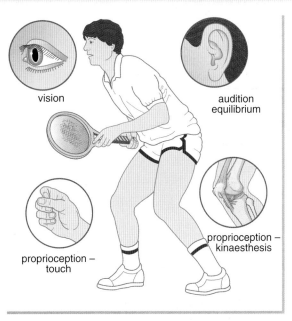

Fig. 10.6 Major sensory input systems in games.

When we are doing any physical activity we are aware of our surroundings. We use all our senses to locate ourselves in space and decide on the requirements of the task, whether it is to pass a ball or perform a gymnastic or dance movement. Taste and smell are not used to any great extent in physical activity but vision, hearing and proprioception are (Figure 10.6). Information is passed to and from the brain by the nervous system. This consists of two elements: (i) the brain and the spinal cord which together form the central nervous system (CNS) and (ii) the peripheral nervous system, which comprises the nerves that connect the spinal cord with all parts of the body, radiating from (the efferent system) and returning to (the afferent system) the CNS. Both efferent and afferent nerves transmit information by electrochemical conduction. The afferent system transmits information to the CNS about events and processes that are happening both inside and outside the body. For example, if you are running a marathon on a warm day, you can both see the sunlight and feel yourself getting hot. The efferent system transmits information from the CNS to the muscles. Full details of this process are given in Section 1.6.

Vision and hearing (audition) deal with information from the external environment. As light falls upon the retina at the back of the eye, it is converted into electrical impulses and so transmitted to the brain, which allows us to see the image through visual perception. Hearing works in a similar way; in this case, sound waves cause the eardrum to vibrate and this is converted into electrical impulses and transmitted in a similar way to visual images, though dealt with in a different part of the brain.

Proprioception is the means by which we know how our body is oriented in space and the extent to which muscles are contracted or joints extended; it allows us to feel the racket or ball. The three components of proprioception are **touch, equilibrium and kinaesthesis**.

Touch (or the tactile sense) enables us to feel pain, pressure and temperature. In sports and dance we are mostly concerned with the pressure sense to tell us how firmly we are gripping a racket, for example, or whether our climbing partner is on a tight rope or whether we struck the ball hard or 'stroked' it. If we are sensible we take heed of any pain warnings we receive.

Equilibrium is the sense that tells you when your body is balanced and when it is tipping, turning or inverting. It is obviously important for divers, gymnasts and trampolinists, as well as dancers, to be able to orientate themselves in space. This is done by means of the sense organs in the vestibular apparatus of the middle ear.

Kinaesthesis is the sense that informs the brain of the movement or state of contraction of the muscles, tendons and joints. A skilled performer knows whether a movement has been performed correctly or not not only from seeing its effect but also from sensing how the movement felt to perform. This is known as **intrinsic feedback**. It is implied in Whiting's model but is explicit in Welford's. You may have experienced a foot or a limb 'going to sleep' and you will know how difficult it is not only to move the limb but also to know what is happening to it. The messages to and from the muscles have been interrupted and kinaesthetic sense impaired. Investigation 10.4 illustrates how we use our kinaesthetic sense.

Investigation 10.3   To investigate the effects of sensory deprivation on performance

1. Vision

Task 1

Method: Play a game of five-a-side soccer or basketball (or any passing or striking game). One team plays as normal. Players in the other team have one eye covered with a medical eye patch. Do not continue this activity for too long.

Observations: What are the effects on the visually deprived players? What does it feel like to play like this?

Task 2

Method: Reverse team roles so that the other team is visually deprived. This time restrict peripheral vision (your ability to see 'out of the corner of your eye' things which you are not looking at directly). You can do this by cutting a strip of card (8 cm × 60 cm), stapling the narrow ends to form goggles and attaching it around your eyes with elastic or string (Figure 10.7).

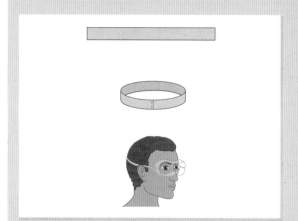

Fig. 10.7 Goggles to restrict peripheral vision.

Observations: What is the effect of the goggles? What does it feel like to play like this?

Task 3

Method: Try a gymnastic or dance sequence with which you are familiar, using the same vision restrictors.

Observations: What are the problems? What does the sequence feel like?

We use vision a great deal in physical activities. Imagine the difficulties for a blind or partially sighted person. Discuss with a partner any knowledge you have of visually handicapped people participating in sport or physical activity. How do they compensate?

2. Audition

Task 4

Method: Select an activity in which sound is an integral part (for example, the sound of the ball against the racket in tennis or the bed in trampolining). Try this activity when wearing headphones or ear plugs to block out the sound.

Observations: How does this affect your performance? To what extent do we use sound in these activities?

3. Proprioception

Task 5

Method: Play a ball-handling game such as basketball, netball or softball in thick gloves. Perform a gymnastic or dance sequence with which you are familiar in stiff trainers.

Observations: It will obviously feel strange, but what are the particular problems?

Discussion: Explain the difficulties in terms of your loss of some tactile sense.

Investigation 10.4   To illustrate kinaesthesis

Method: Make a loop of fairly strong elastic and loop it round your fingers, as in Figure 10.8. Your partner holds a ruler horizontally and you stretch the elastic to a length specified by your partner. You relax the elastic, your partner removes the ruler and you try to repeat the exact stretch again but this time with your eyes closed. Repeat this several times, each time with a different length to reproduce.

Observations: How accurate were you? Calculate your percentage error each time.

Discussion: Discuss with your partner how kinaesthesis is being used.

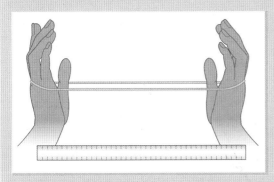

Fig. 10.8 Equipment to illustrate kinaesthesis.

We take our sense organs very much for granted in sport and recreation and do not always appreciate that our ability to make appropriate decisions is based on receiving the right information. Whether or not we get the right information depends on:

- the efficiency of our sense organs
- the intensity of the stimulus
- our ability to interpret the stimulus correctly, i.e. our perceptual capability.

Exam-style questions

1. The **information-processing** theory sheds light on the actual processes that take place during the learning of motor skills. Whiting's model,[2] shown in Figure 10.3, is a well-known illustration of the information-processing theory.

   a. i. Input data comes from the display. What is meant by the term **display**? (*1 mark*)

   ii. Identify the **three** main receptor systems used by performer in a **named** motor skill. (*3 marks*)

   b. Explain why kinaesthetic feedback is so important to gymnasts. (*6 marks*)

   (*Total 10 marks*)

10.3 Perception: the DCR process

Keywords

- ➤ comparison
- ➤ detection
- ➤ memory
- ➤ noise
- ➤ recognition
- ➤ stimulus
- ➤ stimulus identification

Perception (Figure 10.9) is the process by which the brain interprets and makes sense of the information it is receiving from the sensory organs. Consider all the information available to you at the present moment: sights, sounds, smells, the feel of the book and your pen, your feet on the floor, whether you are relaxed or tense, tired or hungry. Imagine yourself competing in your favourite sport and all the additional stimuli you have to deal with to be successful, not all of which are helpful to you.

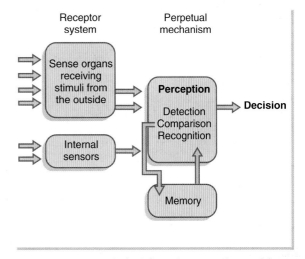

Fig. 10.9 Perception in the information-processing model.

Perception consists of three elements:

- detection
- comparison
- recognition.

Detection is the process by which the brain identifies that a stimulus is present. The brain detects many more stimuli than we are aware of. It registers everything that the sense organs are capable of detecting for a brief moment. If we attend to that information, even briefly, then it is passed on for further processing but if we do not attend to it then it quickly fades out of the system. For example, when playing an invasion game, all the players within our range of vision are detected but if you concentrate on the player you are closely marking, you will not be aware, in detail, of what the others are doing.

Comparison is what happens when we attend to something we have sensed. The coded message that represents the stimulus is passed through the memory and compared with similar codes that have been stored in memory. There are two levels of comparative analysis within the perceptual process:

- **preattentive** – before we have become conscious of the stimulus (the 'cocktail-party syndrome'); to identify those stimuli we need to be attending to
- **postattentive** – after we have become aware of a stimulus; to interpret the important aspects of the environment in order to produce an appropriate response.

Recognition occurs when the code of the incoming information matches a code stored in memory and the stimulus is then perceived, i.e. identified and recognised. As before, this occurs in two phases, preattentive and postattentive.

This process is considered in more detail in the next section, which is about memory, and in Chapter 11, which deals with the learning of skills. Why do you think memory is such an important part of the DCR process?

Each of the factors you noted in Investigation 10.5 is a **stimulus**: the spin of a ball, the flight path of a shuttle, the size of a hold on a climb. The word 'stimulus' is used here to mean any item of information that stands out from background information and to which the player pays more attention. The 'background' is those aspects of the display that are not directly relevant to the task in hand but which nevertheless enter our sensory system. Examples of 'background' are the surroundings of the court or the audience. Psychologists refer to this background information as 'noise'. Noise used in this sense is information that is present and that we might be aware of but it is not directly relevant to the task in hand. We usually try, therefore, to ignore it and concentrate on the important stimuli such as the flight and bounce of a cricket ball and ignore the pigeons in the outfield. We study in Chapter 12 how the ability to differentiate background from stimuli is partly learned but partly a personality trait and also that noise can be a problem in decision making.

We are more likely to detect a stimulus if it is intense, i.e. loud, bright, large, contrasting, fast-moving, unusual. Hence the referee's whistle is shrill, team strip is distinctive and sight screens are used in cricket to help the batsman pick out the ball.

Investigation 10.5   To investigate perception in physical activities

Method: Participate in (or imagine you are participating in) any open skill. Remember that an open skill is one in which the important aspects of the environment are constantly changing. As you participate, be aware of those aspects of your surroundings to which you pay particular attention.

Observations: List all the things that you take notice of in order to perform well. In a ball game you need to note the flight of the ball as it comes towards you; as you climb a rock or wall, you attend to the changes in the surface; as you canoe, you watch for waves, rocks and currents.

Discussion: Talk these over in detail with a colleague.

Investigation 10.6   To investigate the effect of background and ball colour in tennis

Method: Play two games of short tennis, one with balls that contrast with the surroundings and one with balls which blend with the court and wall colour. (Dye a few tennis balls to find a colour that blends with your particular sports hall.)

Observations: How did the colour of the balls affect your game?

10.4 Perception: selective attention and memory

Keywords

➤ long-term memory
➤ memory
➤ selective attention
➤ short-term memory
➤ short-term sensory store

Perception depends on three processes:

- **detection**
- **comparison**
- **recognition**

which were introduced in the previous section. Each of these processes relies on memory to function and provide information to the player.

Detection: the short-term sensory stores

All the senses feed a vast amount of information into the CNS. Think for a moment of all the aspects of your surroundings and your body on which you can focus your attention if you choose. The games player can switch attention from the opponent to the ball to the grip on the stick or bat (for example) very quickly. She/he is able to do this because all the information that enters the sensory system is held for a very short time in a section of the memory known as the **short-term sensory stores** (Figure 10.10). Evidence suggests that there is a separate store for each sense. In these stores, the coded message for each stimulus is compared with all the information held in the long-term memory to allow it to be identified/recognised. This

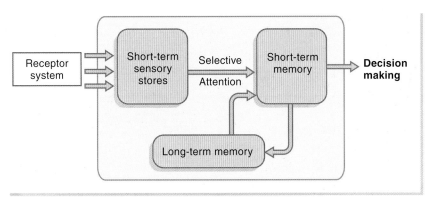

Fig. 10.10 Memory and selective attention in the information-processing model.

has to be done very quickly because the short-term stores have a large capacity but retain each stimulus for less than a second. If the perceptual mechanism decides that the stimulus is not relevant or important, the sensory memory held in the short-term sensory store fades and is lost. All this happens before we are conscious of it. The short-term sensory store has a very large capacity for information but a minimal storage time; its purpose is to filter out irrelevant information so the system is not overloaded.

Selective attention and processing capacity

If we are looking out for some particular stimulus (intentional attention) or if a particular happening catches our attention (involuntary attention), then we focus on that by the process of **selective attention**. This focusing of attention passes the selected information into the **short-term memory** and allows more detailed

processing. The short-term memory holds the information for several seconds and allows it to be consciously analysed.

> ### KEY POINTS
>
> - Selective attention (SA) is the process by which information important for performance is 'filtered out' for further processing.
>
> - It is very important in sport when accuracy or fast responses require concentration on the goal of the action without letting other aspects distract, e.g. the full-back catching a high ball in rugby needs to ignore the on-rushing forwards.
>
> - SA is an instinctive process but its effectiveness can be improved through learning from past experience.

Investigation 10.8 To investigate selective attention

Task 1

Method: Listen through stereo headphones to an audiotape that has been recorded with two separate passages of prose on the two tracks of the tape.

Alternatively use two tape/CD players at the same volume. If this is not available, work in threes. A and B simultaneously read out loud (at the same volume) two different passages from a book or magazine. C tries to listen to and remember the details of both readings.

Observations: Can you listen to them both simultaneously? What strategies did you adopt to make as much sense as you could of both passages? What aspects of the passages made you switch your attention?

Task 2 – to investigate the effect of selective attention on the performance of a motor skill

Method: You need five yellow tennis balls and one of a contrasting colour. A catcher stands 2 m from a line of six throwers, each of whom has a tennis ball held so that it cannot be seen.

1. On the command 'throw', given either by one of the throwers or by the scorer, the throwers throw simultaneously and gently to the catcher, who attempts to catch the contrasting ball. Score successful catches out of 10 trials.

2. The instructor gives the command 'throw' and the name of one of the throwers. All throw; the catcher is to catch the ball thrown by the nominee. Score successful catches out of 10.

3. The instructor gives the command as in 2 above but only the nominee throws. Score successful catches out of 10.

Results: Draw a bar chart to illustrate the mean scores for the whole class on each of the three tests (an example is given in Figure 10.11). Note that a bar chart, with spaces between the bars, is used because the horizontal axis shows three separate trials: it does not represent a scale, as it would if a histogram was drawn.

Discussion: In which of the three tests is selective attention easiest? Suggest reasons.

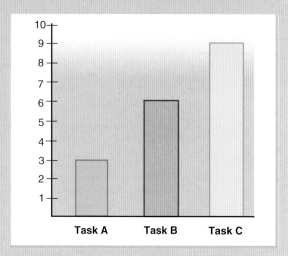

Fig. 10.11 Hypothetical group mean scores on three tests to illustrate selective attention.

For the sportsperson, selective attention has advantages and disadvantages. On the one hand, it ensures that unimportant information is filtered out so that it doesn't disrupt the decision-making process. Thus a cricket fielder concentrating on catching a 'skied' ball is oblivious to almost everything else around him. On the other hand, there are times when we would like to be able to concentrate on several things at once but find it difficult or impossible. A youngster learning to trampoline tries to listen to what the coach is saying but can't because just staying on the bed requires total concentration (maybe there is a lesson for the coach here).

These examples and Investigation 10.8 suggest that our capacity to process information has limitations and an automatic process of selectivity occurs at an early stage in processing.

In Task 1 (Investigation 10.8), you probably managed to get an idea of what both passages were about only by listening to sections alternately, i.e. one after the other, or **in series**. This represents one theory: attention is a single resource, which is directed as it is required but which is limited in capacity and we must deal with one source of information before we can deal with another.[3] Yet when you play a game, you are clearly able to do several things at once. The lacrosse player keeps the ball in the stick, manoeuvres away from an opponent, reads the movement of other players, hears a call for the pass, spots the moment to pass and does so, almost simultaneously. The theory that explains this suggests that the player is processing information **in parallel**. How can we reconcile the two examples?

Current theory suggests that there is an overall limitation on our capacity to attend to a range of stimuli.

As we learned earlier, intensity of the stimulus may attract our attention – for example, loudness, brightness, colour contrast, speed of movement – but we are also attracted to unusual stimuli (we try to make sense of them) or to stimuli in which we are particularly interested, as in Task 2 of Investigation 10.8.

Comparison: the short-term memory

Stimuli are passed from the short-term sensory stores to the **short-term memory** (see Figure 10.10), the 'workplace' of the information-processing system. Here the characteristics of the incoming stimulus are **compared** with those of similar stimuli which have been previously learned and stored in the long-term memory. For example, you are a hockey defender, given the task of marking a talented forward. You've watched them on video and you've learned that you can judge which way they will try to go round you by the pattern of their footwork. That information is stored in your **long-term memory**. In the game, as you move in to tackle, you watch the player's footwork carefully. Each move is stored for a short time in your short-term memory. When the footwork you are seeing matches the memory of what you saw on the video, you recognise the dodge your opponent is about to try and can counter it.

Investigation 10.9 To investigate the capacity of the short-term memory

Method: Play 'Kim's Game'. About 15 everyday items are placed on a tray and all the subjects given about 15 seconds to study them. The tray is removed and the subjects write down as many of the items as possible.

Results: Record the total number of correct items recalled.

Discussion: If a group played the game, what was the mean score and what was the range? What strategies did people use to memorise the items? Which were the items that most people remembered and which were the 'problem' items? Why? What have you learned about visual memory from playing this game?

People's short-term memory capacity varies but the norm is between five and nine items. If you have a longer period to study the contents of the tray or if you have mastered memory skills, you can remember more than this because you are able to extend retention in the short-term memory by a process of rehearsal or practice, i.e. by using the long-term memory.

Investigation 10.10   To investigate the implications of the characteristics of short-term memory

Task 1

Method: Work in pairs. One composes two lists of five three-letter sequences. Five are meaningful words, e.g. cup, dog; five are nonsense, e.g. frz, xvu. Present one list to your partner for a period of 10 seconds and then ask him/her to repeat the list. If a mistake is made, return the list for another 10-second viewing and repeat until your partner can reproduce the list accurately to you. Repeat the exercise with the other list.

Results: Score the number of attempts before a correct list is reproduced. Which list took fewer attempts to remember?

Discussion: What strategies did you adopt to try and memorise the 'nonsense' list? Assuming you found that the meaningful list was easier to remember, there are two reasons for your answer. Can you suggest what they are?

Included in your suggestions should have been:

- the short-term memory is better at storing information that is meaningful

- since its capacity would seem to be about seven items, it is more efficient to 'chunk' items together if this can be done. So the letters C-A-T, instead of being three items, become one, CAT, which also has a meaning (a visual image) attached to it.

Task 2

Method: Change roles and repeat the task but as the memoriser is studying the list (the primary task), the partner asks questions for which answers are demanded – anything to distract (a secondary task).

Discussion: What are the effects on the memory task? What are the implications of your findings for learning in physical education? If you were helping a friend to master a particular skill in your favourite activity, how would you present the information?

Task 3 – to try out coaching strategies based on an understanding of memory processes

Method: Think up a discrete sports hall skill that you can coach, but with which your partner is not very familiar. It could be a game or gymnastic skill, a particular set of moves on a climbing wall, a dance step to a complex rhythm or similar. Work out how you are going to introduce and coach the skill, bearing in mind the principles we have just identified. Teach your partner the skill you have devised. As you coach, be aware of your own teaching points and also analyse your partner's performance. If possible, video the session.

Observations: Afterwards, analyse the recording and/or discuss with the learner (i) when your comments were helpful and (ii) when your comments were not helpful and why. Remember we are focusing on the extent to which you helped your partner to remember what you wanted them to do.

'Attention', 'relevance', 'meaning', 'chunking', 'brevity' are the key words (Figure 10.12). Did you use 'demonstration'?

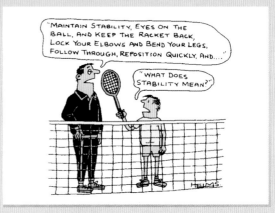

Fig. 10.12 (Adapted from reference[10])

KEY POINTS

The short-term memory:

- acts as the 'workplace' of the processing system

- receives coded stimuli from both the short-term sensory stores via selective attention and the long-term memory (retrieval)

- sends information to the long-term memory for future reference (rehearsal)

- makes information available for decision making.

Recognition: the long-term memory

Recognition is the process of retrieving from the long-term memory (LTM) an image (or a sound, sensation, etc.) which is identical with or very similar to the stimulus, comparing it with the stimulus and deciding that it is close enough to something that you already know to be able to recognise it. This process operates as you play 'Kim's Game'. As you first perceive the objects on the tray, you go through the following process: you detect the object and compare what you see with a memory of it from earlier experiences stored in the LTM. This allows you to identify it, name it and recall its characteristics and how to use it. This is the DCR process.

For example, you might have learned from past experience that when your opponent in tennis or badminton 'shapes up' to serve in a particular way, then he/she is going to produce a particular type of serve. You see this happening; you detect, compare and recognise. We monitor our surroundings in this way all the time; our brain is constantly operating the DCR process, even when we are not consciously aware of it.

Recall

Long-term memory is also the store for information that we constantly need to refer to or which has been so well learned or practised that it remains in permanent store. It has an almost limitless capacity, as long as information is stored effectively and the memory is not interfered with. It is beyond the scope of this book to consider the form in which skills are memorised but in a later section we consider the concept of motor programmes, which takes us some way to an understanding of this. Some continuous motor skills seem to be stored particularly well – we never forget how to ride a bicycle. This may be because there is a motor memory store within the muscles and tendons (see Martenuik's[9] model of closed-loop control, Figure 10.27).

Being able to quickly and efficiently retrieve information from the long-term memory is one of the qualities of a skilled performer. It allows appropriate selection of response and technically good, well co-ordinated movement. Research[4] suggests that expert players in open skills also have a superior ability to recall patterns of play and players' positions. You will notice this when you hear professional football players describing, during television interviews, the game they have just been involved in. This is an important factor in their ability to anticipate.

Strategies for improving retention and retrieval

Our knowledge of the capacities of the short- and long-term memories is important to us when we are learning, practising or coaching skills.

Knowing 'that' and knowing 'how'

Memory for skills has both a cognitive component and a motor component. Coaches should explain what the learner is learning as well as showing how to do it. It sometimes helps when learning a new skill to say action words to yourself as you are practising, to get both the action and the rhythm ('reach, glide, pull' in breaststroke arm action).

Brevity

Remember the small capacity of the short-term memory. When first hearing or seeing something, we can only process a little at a time. 'Three coaching points, then practise' is a good rule for a coach or teacher.

Clarity

Keep it simple to start with; greater complexity and refinement can be added later. Avoid trying to learn or teach two similar but distinct items in the same session, as the memory of one may **interfere** with the memory of the other. For example, in a 'skills circus' session, it is not a good idea to move straight from badminton to tennis; the strokes have similarities but important differences.

Chunking

Learners can hold more in the short-term memory if the information is 'chunked', instead of being presented as individual items. In the breaststroke example given earlier, the three actions of 'reach, glide and pull' are better memorised and practised as one movement. This then allows space in the memory to add the leg action. Experts also use chunking; they can take in more information in a single glance than can learners because their superior knowledge of the activity allows them to group information into larger, more meaningful units. This allows them to recognise a developing pattern of play early and helps them to anticipate.

Organisation

We remember more easily if we organise the way in which we are to learn and ensure that the information is meaningful. Coaches often use imagery to aid organisation.

Association

Good coaches and teachers always ensure that new learning is linked to what players already know. Passing in lacrosse is often introduced by reminding learners what it is like to throw a ball by hand, for example. This helps to organise the skill in the learner's mind. In skills which involve complex sequences of movements, it is helpful, as well as teaching the individual components of the sequence, to allow plenty of practice which links the end of one movement with the beginning of the next, so that end and beginning patterns of movement are associated in the memory. Trampoline, gymnastic and skating sequences are examples of skills where this technique is important.

Practice

No skill is learned without practice (rehearsal). Practice shuttles the image of the skill backwards and forwards between the short- and long-term memory and in doing so establishes what is known as a 'memory trace' or pathway. The more this occurs, the more permanent becomes the memory and the more readily it is recalled.

Exam-style questions

1. A generalised model of the memory process is shown in Figure 10.13.

   a. Explain 'selective attention' using an example from physical education or sport to illustrate your explanation. (*3 marks*)

   b. As a teacher or coach, how would you plan your coaching to ensure that the information you give would be retained in the performer's long-term memory? (*3 marks*)

   (*Total 6 marks*)

2. a. Using Figure 10.13, state what is meant by short-term memory and long-term memory. (*2 marks*)

   b. How can information be retained in the long-term memory? (*4 marks*)

3. a. Using the example of a table tennis player receiving a serve, what information would be held in the short-term sensory store and for how long? (*2 marks*)

   b. Name and describe the purpose of the process by which information is transferred from the short-term sensory store to the short-term memory. (*4 marks*)

   (*Total 12 marks*)

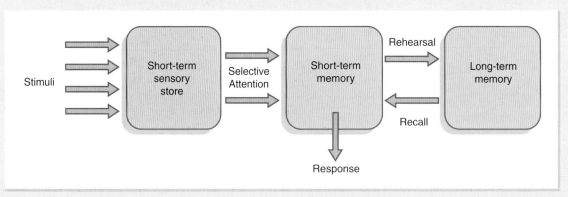

Fig. 10.13 A model of memory processes.

10.5 Decision making

Keywords

➤ anticipate
➤ attend
➤ choice reaction time
➤ initiations
➤ movement time
➤ psychological refractory period
➤ reaction time
➤ response time
➤ simple reaction time

Our perceptual ability provides us with the information we need to make decisions about what to do next in a physical task. This might be intrinsic to the skill itself ('I can feel my body is vertical – now is the moment to push against the box-top to complete the vault') or it might be extrinsic ('my opponent has pushed the ball a little too far ahead – now is the moment to tackle').

Reaction time

The speed at which we make decisions, or **reaction time**, is of great interest in this area of study. This is partly because in many sports and activities, being able to react quickly allows the performer to be in greater control: the quicker you respond to the gun and are away from your blocks in a 100-metre track event, the more you can dominate the race; the more quickly you can respond to an unexpected eddy in white water, the less likely you are to capsize. The study of reaction time is also important because it tells us a lot about the process of making decisions (Figure 10.14).

Figure 10.15 shows the whole sequence of responding to a stimulus in the context of a sprint. As you can see, this is a complex business. Study the diagram carefully and ensure that you understand all the terms and the processes. Check in the glossary if you are not sure. Also notice that:

Response time = reaction time + movement time

It is important to use the above terms correctly. Broadcasting commentators often talk about a player's fast reactions when they mean 'responses'. In the normal course of observing sport it is difficult to differentiate reaction from movement.

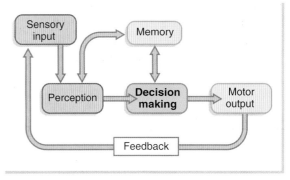

Fig. 10.14 Decision making in the information-processing model.

Studying Figure 10.15 also reminds us that there is always a period of stimulus transmission through the nervous system before any response is started, i.e. reaction time. Organisers of international athletic sprint events now use the notion of there being a minimum reaction time (100 ms for men) below which any start must have anticipated the gun. Each athlete's reaction time is measured electronically and if any fall below the set minimum, a false start is declared and the offending athlete penalised.

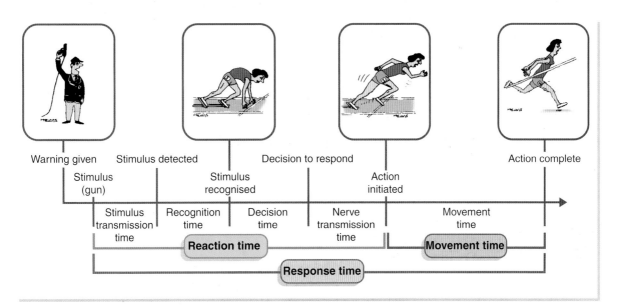

Fig. 10.15 The components of response time.

Task 1

Study Figure 10.16 – the pitcher delivers the ball at a velocity of 32 m s^{-1}. The reaction time of the batter is 0.18 s and the time to swing from back to contact is 0.2 s. How far out of the pitcher's hand can the batsman afford to let the ball travel before he starts to swing?

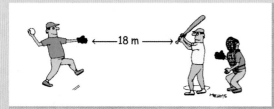

Fig. 10.16 (Adapted from reference[11])

Did you get an answer of 5.8 m? Obviously, when we are playing striking games we do not consciously make this kind of calculation each time we play the ball but the faster we react, the more time we have to make a decision about the kind of shot to play. A fast reaction or response time is more important in some skills than in others. Refer back to the section on classification of skill in Chapter 9.

Task 2

Method: Work in pairs. Make a list of skills. Decide, for each skill, the importance of a fast reaction time (or the disadvantage of a slow reaction time) for effective performance.

Discuss the extent to which fast reaction times contribute to performance in (i) self and externally paced skills; (ii) open and closed skills.

Reaction time is an ability; it varies between individuals. Research suggests that the following individual characteristics are likely to affect reaction time:

- age and sex (Figure 10.17)
- health – ill health slows reactions
- body temperature – the colder, the slower the reaction
- personality – extroverts tend to have faster reactions than do introverts
- length of neural pathways – the further information has to travel, the slower the reaction and also the slower the response time
- state of alertness, arousal and/or motivation.

The demands of the task and the nature of the stimulus also influence reaction time. Some of these influences are:

- the intensity of the stimulus
- the probability of the stimulus occurring
- the existence of warning signals and the extent to which the stimulus is expected
- the sense being used for detection – Figure 10.18 shows how reaction time varies with the sense being used.

So far we have considered time of reaction as if it is to one stimulus only. At the start of a track event, this is so – there is one gun and the athlete is expecting it – but in other events there may be several stimuli and the performer has to choose which one to respond to or which of several possible responses (for example, shots in a racket game) to make for a given stimulus. These two forms of reaction time are known as **simple** and **choice** reaction time (SRT and CRT).

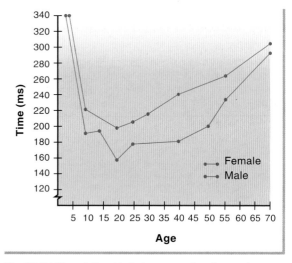

Fig. 10.17 The relationship between reaction time and age for each sex.

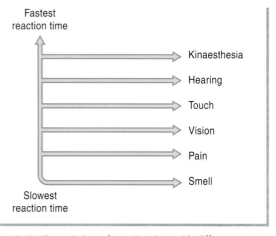

Fig. 10.18 The variation of reaction time with different senses.

Investigation 10.12 To measure reaction time

There are a variety of ways in which reaction time can be measured in the laboratory or classroom. Choose the one(s) for which you have the appropriate equipment. Most are more accurately measures of response time, because it is not possible to identify the point at which reaction is complete and movement starts.

Methods

1. Use a computer program to measure eye–hand or possibly ear–hand SRT and CRT.

   a. Compare SRTs and CRTs.

   b. Explain why CRTs are longer.

   c. Devise an experimental hypothesis that compares RTs with another variable, for example dominant–non-dominant eye or preferred–non-preferred hand. Collect appropriate data and test out this hypothesis.

2. Use reaction time apparatus (described in many motor learning text books) to investigate:

   a. SRT, CRT and movement time; preferred and non-preferred hand reaction to auditory and visual stimuli; foot reaction as above (if the apparatus includes footpads).

   b. Devise a hypothesis that predicts association between two of the variables you have measured and test this.

3. Use the 'ruler drop' test to measure SRT and CRT. The only apparatus you will need for this test are two metre rulers. Convert the distance the ruler drops into a response time using the formula:

$$d = ut + 1/2\, at^2$$

   where *d* is the distance the ruler falls (cm); *u* is the initial velocity of the ruler which in this instance is 0 cm s⁻¹; *t* is the response time(s); *a* is the

acceleration of the ruler due to gravity (constant at 981 cm s⁻²).

   You will need to use some simple algebra to arrive at an expression for *t*. Compare your score on this test with your score on a comparable version of one of the other tests, if possible. Explain any differences in the scores in terms of:

   a. reaction and movement time

   b. experimental procedure.

4. Work in pairs. You will need a stopwatch and a set of playing cards. The task is to sort the shuffled pack. Your partner will give a start signal, time you to completion of the sort and note the time.

   a. Separate red cards from black (two groups).

   b. Separate the four suits (four groups).

   c. Separate four suits of court cards and four suits of non-court cards (eight groups).

   d. Calculate the mean time for the whole class on each of the three tasks.

   e. Plot a graph of time against the number of possible alternative placements for each card (two, four or eight).

Discussion

Note that the type of stimulus (colour, suit) determines the movement response required (which pile to place the card on). What does this graph tell you about the relationship between response time and the number of stimulus–response alternatives available? Explain this relationship in information-processing terms. Identify some sport situations in which choice response time is an important part of the activity.

Explain why short reaction times are important in sprinting, football and table tennis. List some sports in which short reaction times are *not* particularly important and explain why not.

Your answer to **4** in Investigation 10.12 should lead you to an important principle for the learning of motor skills. This is known as Hick's Law and is shown graphically in Figure 10.19.

The more choices that are available to us, i.e. the greater the number of stimulus–response alternatives, the longer we take to react. So when we are in the early stages of skill learning, when we need to concentrate on the production of effective movement as well as choose an appropriate response, it is best if we are not presented with too many choices. This allows the learner more time to operate the DCR process and

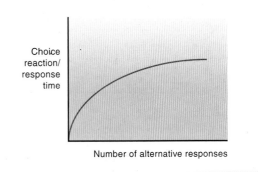

Fig. 10.19 Hick's Law.

relate recognition of the stimulus to the production of the appropriate movement. Hence, not only should instructions be simple and brief (as discussed earlier) but also the task should not involve too much decision making. Two against two or three against three games induce better learning than a premature introduction to the full seven, 11- or 15-a-side game.

Psychological refractory period

When we are involved in physical education activities we have to respond to a constant stream of stimuli. If these are well spaced and we have time to respond to each in turn, reaction time seems to be unaffected. But often a second stimulus arrives before we have a chance to complete, or even initiate, our response to the first.

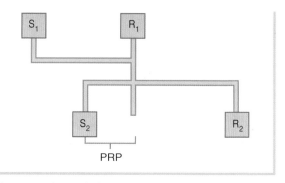

Fig. 10.21 The psychological refractory period.

Opponents often do this to us on purpose by disguising a shot or 'selling a dummy', for example. In slalom canoeing a wave may hit just as the canoeist is negotiating a gate. This principle is illustrated in Figure 10.21.

S_1 and S_2 are two stimuli and R_1 and R_2 are the initiations of the responses to these stimuli; thus the distances S_1–R_1 and S_2–R_2 represent reaction time. This is not easy to demonstrate with simple equipment, but Investigation 10.13 illustrates what happens. You can see from Figure 10.21 that the reaction to the second stimulus is longer. The time between S_2 and R_1 is known as the psychological refractory period (PRP).

It would appear that when a performer detects a stimulus and starts to select a plan of action and response, he must devote his attention to the process. Research summarised in Figure 10.21 suggests that while he is doing this he is unable to deal with any other decision that requires attention. This is where 'faking' or 'selling a dummy' comes in. The attacker makes a fake move and then uses the defender's PRP to move the other way or play a different shot. Martenuik[9] suggests that this strategy 'is effective even if the player does not usually begin to move in response to the fake. All that is necessary is to have him begin the search for an action, since he cannot amend this process until the search is completed'.

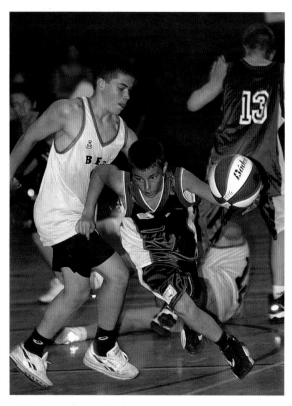

Fig. 10.20 'Selling a dummy.'

Investigation 10.13 To illustrate the psychological refractory period

Task 1
Work in pairs – one person acts as 'catcher', the other as 'feeder'. The feeder needs to be able to throw underarm consistently with both hands. Stand approximately 5 m apart, with the feeder holding a tennis ball in each hand.

There are 20 trials. Each trial consists of the thrower saying a warning 'ready!' and then throwing gently to the catcher who attempts to catch with two hands. The throws should be consistent and accurately placed into the catcher's hands. In 10 of the trials one ball only is thrown, sometimes from the feeder's left and sometimes from the right hand. In the other 10 trials (which should be mixed in with the former trials at random), one ball is thrown immediately followed by the other – not both together (this takes some practice by the feeder!). One point is scored by the catcher **(i)** if he catches the **only** ball thrown or **(ii)** if he catches the **second** thrown (no points for catching the first). Note the scores out of 10 for when one ball is thrown and for when two balls are thrown.

Which score do you think will be the highest and why?

Task 2
Play a game in which to fake or dummy is a realistic strategy. When attacking make the most of opportunities to do this. Practise the timing necessary. Remember that if your second move occurs more than one normal reaction time (200 ms) after the first, then your opponent can read it (unless he/she has actually been 'wrong-footed', in which case your opponent must recover and you have gained even more time).

Task 3
If you have the appropriate equipment (a film camera and frame analysis equipment or a video camera and playback machine with a freeze-frame facility) experiment with analysing reaction time and PRP by film. Select a variety of activities in which reaction time is an important aspect of the skill and film them, making sure that the initial stimulus as well as the response can be identified.

Improving response time

Reaction time itself is an inherent ability, but overall response time can be improved by practice. Coach and sportsperson need to analyse the type of skill and the requirements of the sport and decide where in the overall response gains can be made. There may be scope for improvement in the following.

- **Detecting the cue** in simple reaction time situations, e.g. in a sprint start, focusing on the starter's voice and the sound of the gun and separating this from background crowd noise and negative thoughts.
- **Detecting relevant cues** in choice reaction time situations and practising appropriate responses, e.g. a goalkeeper learning to analyse body language at penalties.
- **Decision making** in open skills by working on set pieces and game situations as well as plenty of practice in the game itself.
- **Change in attentional focus** (see Chapter 12), e.g. being able to switch quickly from concentration on the opponent or the ball to concentration on the field of play in invasion games.
- **Controlling anxiety** which slows reaction times by adding competing neural activity to the information-processing system.

- **Creating optimum levels of motivation**, e.g. 'psyching up'.
- **Warm-up** to ensure the sense organs and nervous system are ready to transmit information and the muscles to act upon it.

Anticipation

Anticipation is a strategy used by sportspeople to reduce the time they take to respond to a stimulus. Two examples illustrate two types of anticipation:

- the sprinter who attempts to anticipate when the gun will go off (temporal anticipation)
- the tennis player who anticipates the type of serve the opponent will use (spatial or event anticipation). In this case the player has learnt to detect certain cues early in the serving sequence which predict the type of serve. This means that she can start to position herself for the return earlier in the sequence than usual and thus give herself more time to play the shot when the ball arrives.

Obviously there are dangers for both the sprinter and the tennis player in anticipating in this way. They will look very foolish if they are wrong but the advantages of getting it right are great.

Review questions

1. Define reaction time, response time and movement time.
2. List two skills in which fast response times are important and two skills in which fast response times are unimportant. Justify your choice.
3. State Hick's Law and give an example of its relevance in sport.
4. Draw a diagram of the psychological refractory period and label S_1, S_2, R_1 and R_2 with a specific sport event, e.g. a feint dodge.
5. How can coaches/players improve response times?

Exam-style questions

1. The time it takes for a sportsperson to react to stimuli can affect the resultant performance.
   a. Define **reaction time, movement time** and **response time**. (*3 marks*)
   b. If you were the **receiver** of a server in tennis, give three factors which could affect your response time. (*3 marks*)
   c. How would you cut down the time it takes for you to respond to the server? (*3 marks*)
   d. Sketch a graph to illustrate the relationship between reaction time and the number of possible responses. (*2 marks*)
   (*Total 11 marks*)

2. If the ball hits the top of the net during a rally in tennis, the receiver has to adjust the response. There is a delay between processing the first stimulus and the final response. What is this delay called and explain why this delay might occur? (*3 marks*)

3. a. Give the three main receptor systems used by a performer in sport. (*3 marks*)
   b. Where is the filtering mechanism found in an information processing model? Explain what happens with information as it passes through this mechanism. (*2 marks*)
   (*Total 5 marks*)

4. a. What is the difference between reaction time, movement time and response time? What advice would you give to a sprinter to cut down on reaction time at the start of a race? (*4 marks*)

   b. Sketch and label a graph to illustrate Hick's Law. (*2 marks*)
   c. How does the number of choices available to a performer affect his/her performance? (*1 mark*)
   d. When taking part in a badminton game, the shuttle occasionally hits the netcord during a rally and the receiver has to adjust his/her return shot. This causes a delay before the final response can be made. What is this delay called? Explain why it occurs. (*4 marks*)
   (*Total 11 marks*)

5. a. Improvement in performance of a skill can be better understood by reference to the processes involved. Figure 10.3 shows Whiting's information processing model. Other models may use different terms to describe the various stages involved. Explain the meanings of the terms: **response selection, stimulus identification** and **response programming** and relate these terms to stages in the Whiting model. (*3 marks*)
   b. Figure 10.3 also shows five arrows entering the perceptual mechanism and only one leaving. What is the name given to this process and why is it necessary? (*4 marks*)
   c. Identify three factors which might help a performer with this process. (*3 marks*)
   (*Total 10 marks*)

6. Name the three main stages in information processing and use a practical example to illustrate what happens in each stage. (*6 marks*)

Teachers and coaches can develop appropriate anticipation strategies with learners by identifying significant cues to look out for in opponents' play and by giving players practice in observing these cues and timing their responses. For example, netball and basketball shooters are coached to judge when and where the marker is going to jump to intercept the shot and then to time the shot when the marker is on the way down.

10.6 Motor output and feedback

Keywords

- ballistic skills
- closed loop control
- concurrent feedback
- delayed feedback
- effector mechanism
- executive programme
- external feedback
- hierarchical
- immediate feedback
- internal feedback
- intrinsic feedback
- knowledge of performance
- knowledge of results
- motor programmes
- new skills
- open loop control
- phase theory
- plan of action
- recall schema
- recognition schema
- schema
- sequential programming
- subroutines
- supplementary feedback
- terminal feedback

This section is concerned with how the performer learns to produce the movements required for a skilled action. This part of the process is controlled by the effector mechanism (see Figure 10.3), which consists of the nerves and muscles that serve the limbs involved in the movement. As a learner practises a skill, representations of the movements required are built up in the long-term memory. Gradually, less effective aspects of the movement are eliminated and successful actions are reinforced. With repetition this becomes stored as a **plan of action** associated with the set of stimuli which normally precedes it. So the hockey goalkeeper knows that as the ball arrives at her feet, the plan required is a long, low kick to the side.

Motor programmes

Before we consider how this process works, let us look in more detail at these plans of action or **motor programmes**. Note that different writers give different definitions of the term 'motor programme'. In this text we define a motor programme as a set of movements stored as a whole in the memory, regardless of whether or not feedback is used in their execution.

The motor programme specifies what movements the skill is composed of and in what order these occur. It can be seen from Figure 10.23 that a skill such as a tennis serve (which is known as the executive programme) is made up of shorter movements, known as subroutines, which in turn operate at several levels. In open skills the executive programme has to be adaptable and flexible in order to cope with the variety of environmental requirements. Each pass or shot that you make has a different trajectory, pace and distance programmed in. The subroutines are short fixed sequences which, when fully learned, can be run off automatically, without conscious control.

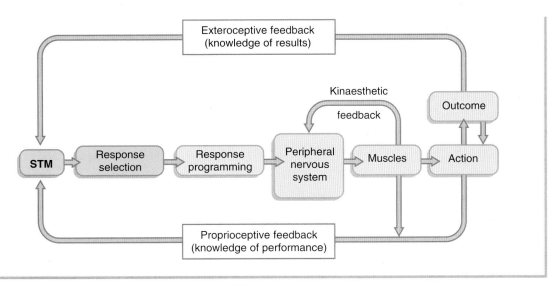

Fig. 10.22 Motor output in the information-processing model.

KEY POINTS

A motor programme is:

- a series of movements

- stored in the LTM

- retrieved from memory as a whole

- put into action by the effector mechanism

- operated under open or closed loop control
(see pp. 320–321).

Investigation 10.14 To identify executive programmes and subroutines

Method: Work in pairs. Each selects a skill which can be well demonstrated repeatedly and the partner observes and analyses the skill to produce a model similar to that in Figure 10.23.

Analysis: Compare your analysis with others in the class – are some subroutines common to several skills?

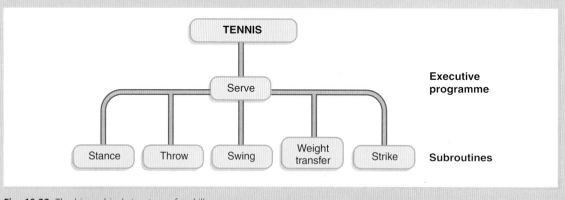

Fig. 10.23 The hierarchical structure of a skill.

Motor learning in early childhood is about the establishment of these subroutines; the youngster learns to run, jump, turn, grip, strike, etc. These are **fundamental motor** skills and they contribute to more complex skills developed later. To children these are executive programmes but as they develop more complex activities, these become the subroutines for their new skills. As they become more versatile, learners become adept at transferring subroutines already learned into new executive programmes.

The importance of this hierarchical organisation of motor programmes is that it allows parts of the skill, or indeed the whole skill, to be stored in the LTM as a complete programme and recalled for use automatically, leaving the performer to concentrate on the perceptual or interpretative aspects. Speaking of Torvill and Dean's strategy of always running through

their whole ice dance at final rehearsals (rather than isolating sections for practice), Christopher Dean commented:

> *Every time you do the programme in full you're adding to your store of experience and self-confidence. The more you can drill yourself into automatic mastery on the ice, the more you can give yourself to presentation when the big moment comes.*[5]

Let us look in more detail at how this 'automatic mastery' works.

Motor control

Open loop theory

This theory suggests that when a skill is being learned, an overall plan or programme of that skill is built up

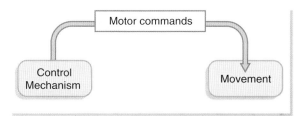

Fig. 10.24 Open loop control.

in long-term memory. This is called the **executive programme**, which consists of **subroutines**. The whole programme is organised **hierarchically**, i.e. the executive programme is made up of a number of subroutines which in turn consist of small subroutine units.

ACTIVITY 10.1

Executive programmes and subroutines

- Identify the executive programmes and the subroutines in Figure 10.25.

- Which smaller subroutines would make up the skill?

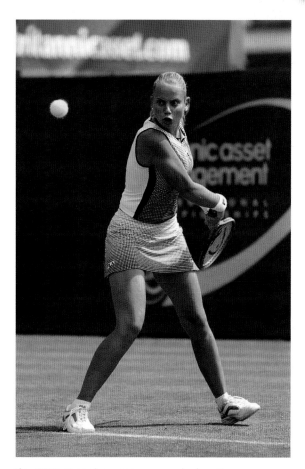

Fig. 10.25 Executive programmes and subroutines.

The programme is also ordered **sequentially**, i.e. it is able to tell the muscles in what order to produce the appropriate subroutines.

Learning the tennis backhand means practising the skill so that the subroutines are properly sequenced and coordinated and also become increasingly automated until the whole executive programme is also automatic. By 'automatic' we mean that the performer does not have to think about the performance. Once the programme has been put into operation, the motor programme commands the entire movement.

In teaching a backhand, a teacher therefore needs to ensure that the subroutines are well established and then that the whole skill is practised, emphasising the timing and coordination of the subroutines.

Once the skill is learned, open loop theory suggests that it can be put into action without feedback being used **to control the movement**. Knowledge of results is used only at the end of the movement to give the learner feedback on the outcome. For example, as the team's penalty taker you will have practised shooting for a considerable amount of time, so that once you have decided on a particular shot it will be performed

under open loop control (Figure 10.24). The outcome feedback will be very apparent (to everyone!).

Another example of open loops is the case of **ballistic** skills, in which the limbs swing fast and move temporarily under their own momentum, e.g. in a fast cartwheel. Golf is a difficult game partly because the golf swing is ballistic and not controllable once it has started.

Closed loop theory

If a skill is under closed loop control (Figure 10.26), then the motor programme is structured in the same way but its commands can be countermanded by the need to correct errors. Kinaesthetic feedback is used to do this.

If, for example, a gymnast is learning a slow, controlled cartwheel, it is possible to sense that the body is not properly aligned and to make adjustments while the skill is being performed. Of course, this can only happen once the gymnast has learnt enough to know what the correct body alignment feels like.

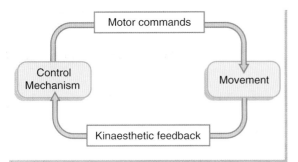

Fig. 10.26 Closed loop control.

Adams,[6] in discussing closed loop theory, suggested that as a particular movement is reinforced during learning, it is stored in the long-term memory as a memory trace. It is strong if:

- the movement has been extensively rehearsed
- the information has been stored in 'chunks' so that relationships between individual subroutines are well established
- the movement or stimulus has strong emotional intensity, i.e. it is important to the learner
- the kinaesthetic image of the movement is reinforced by visual imagery (mind pictures).

This memory trace includes both the subroutines and the executive programme of the movement. For example, a gymnast learning a cartwheel on the beam has a memory trace of the whole movement and the various elements of it – the leg extension, the hand positions, the landing, the timing, etc. As the cartwheel is performed, a **perceptual trace** is recorded in the short-term memory and compared with the memory trace. If the match is good, the movement continues; if there is a mismatch, the learner tries to correct the error (for example, by adjusting the foot position as it lands to achieve a better balance). Adams[6] suggests that the closed feedback loop operates throughout the movement and thus allows correction during the movement.

Some sports psychologists are dissatisfied with the either/or view of motor control; they believe that performance involves both open and closed loop processes. Schmidt[7] suggests that both are used at different points in an action. Consider a serve in tennis – which elements do you think might be under closed loop control and which under open loop control? Evidence from experiments involving continuous tracking movements (e.g. using a joystick to play a computer game) indicates that short bursts of activity may be programmed centrally and the outcome checked (peripherally) for error and correction before the next burst of activity is initiated.[7]

Schema theory

A second theoretical alternative to the 'open loop versus closed loop' perspective is schema theory. One of the problems with open and closed loop theories is that they require movements to be stored as separate units. When you think of how many separate memory traces this requires, memory capacity would seem to be a problem. Also, they do not adequately account for how open skills can be infinitely varied to fit the demands of the situation. Schema theory[8] claims that what is stored in memory is not a fixed pattern of movement (programme) but a set of relationships or rules that determine the performance of the skill. This is the **schema**. This 'set of relationships' could be thought of as a programme of sorts but a generalised one, which can be run differently according to the demands of the situation.

A schema is made up of two elements – recall and recognition. The **recall schema** is the schema responsible for the production of the movement. It is made up of information stored in the long-term memory about:

- the initial conditions under which the movement is to be produced, e.g. 'where am I in relation to the ball?'
- the required response specifications, i.e. the movement requirements, e.g. 'what have I got to do and how do I do it?'.

The **recognition schema** is the schema responsible for evaluating the movement response. Initially this information is stored in the short-term memory for comparison with the recall schema. The two elements of information are:

- the sensory consequences, i.e. the kinaesthetic feel of the movement
- the response outcomes, i.e. what happened as a result of the movement.

When a movement is completed, all these elements are stored in long-term memory for use in future movements which may be the same or similar.

You may have noticed similarities with Adams' theory of memory and perceptual traces, but you should note the important differences.

In order to develop a schema for kicking or throwing (for example) a player practises to establish the rules for a relationship between the distance the ball is to be sent and such variables as muscular force, limb speed, angle or direction of release, etc. This

---

> **ACTIVITY 10.3**
>
> **Comparison of the schema and the open loop and closed loop theories**
>
> Discuss how **(i)** open and closed loop theory and **(ii)** schema theory analyse how a cricketer or baseball player learns to throw a ball into the wicket or base from 30 m out. Which theory do you think best explains this learning?

---

schema is adapted to his/her perception of the specific requirements of the task.

Schema can apply at any part of the skill hierarchy. Thus, you developed a schema for throwing a ball as a youngster, which is then refined to throw, for example, a basketball; it can also be generalised to help you learn a new throwing action, for example, the javelin. Schema theory sees learning as the generation of increasingly more comprehensive general programmes. You should be realising that schema theory fits in with several ideas we discussed earlier, for example the need to teach open skills by stressing variety of practice and decision making. Schmidt[8] developed some important implications of his schema theory for the learning of motor skills.

- **People learn from errors**. Where appropriate, errors could even be included in practice to update and strengthen the schema. For example, how far can you 'lean' on your paddle before capsizing your kayak? There's only one way to find out!
- **Terminal feedback is important** in learning, because it strengthens the schema in memory.
- **Practice must be varied and relevant** to the game or competition. In open skills, in particular, do not spend too long practising a specific move or stroke over the same distance and in the same direction. The learner must have plenty of opportunity to establish rules such that a strong schema is developed, which takes into account all the possible situations. This is known as 'variability of practice'.

Motor control is an aspect of skill acquisition, the theory of which is still developing, so it is important to view the various theories as hypotheses still to be tested. Whereas these can be usefully applied to the practical problems of learning skill, equally we need to be aware of their limitations.

> **KEY POINTS**
>
> - In open or closed loop theory, the motor programme is stored as an **exact model** of the movement to be produced in the future.
> - In schema theory the motor programme is stored as a **generalised model** or set of rules about how a skill is to be produced given the conditions at the time.

Feedback

The final element of the information-processing model to consider is the feedback loop. Feedback, in motor control terms, is information about performance and the outcomes of that performance which the sportsperson uses to evaluate the effectiveness of the skill. Study Figure 10.22 (p. 311) and you will see that there are three loops.

- **Exteroceptive feedback** from the outcome of the skill (e.g. the shot on goal) back to the performer through the senses and the short-term memory. This may come directly from observation of the outcome by the performer ('great, the smash was in') or it may come from team mates, coach or a video recording (augmented feedback). It is also called **extrinsic feedback** or **knowledge of results**.
- **Proprioceptive feedback** from the proprioceptors in the muscles and tendons, and the balance sensors, giving information to the short-term memory about the 'feel' of the movement. Skilled performers are able to make good use of this loop to correct errors as movement is being performed, because they have a well-defined memory trace to compare with. This loop also allows them to know the likely outcome of a movement before they see the result, from the 'feel' of the rhythm and coordination feedback.
- **Kinaesthetic feedback** is the information fed directly into the spinal cord from the muscles,

tendons and joints to give information that can be responded to without conscious control. This occurs, for example, when we are running on an uneven surface and our ankles and knees automatically adjust to this whilst we are concentrating on the strategic elements of the activity.

A combination of proprioceptive feedback and kinaesthetic feedback is also called **intrinsic feedback** or **knowledge of performance**.

Each of these loops plays an important role in the production of skilled movement but at different stages of learning and with different types of action. Martenuik's[9] model of motor control demonstrates this.

Levels of motor control

Martenuik[9] suggests there are three levels at which movement is controlled, with feedback playing a different role in each (see Figure 10.27).

Level 1

Some movements seem to be produced without reference to any feedback, because they happen too quickly for feedback to have any effect. Fast typing would be an example of this kind of skill, which is known as **open loop control**. It happens at a subconscious level and does not make any attention demands on the system.

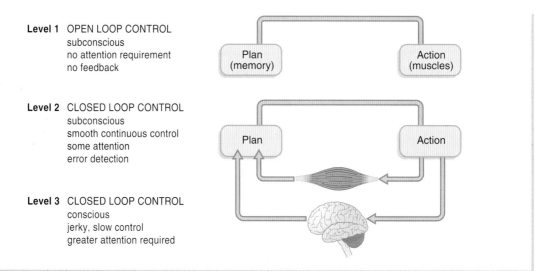

Level 1	OPEN LOOP CONTROL
	subconscious
	no attention requirement
	no feedback

Level 2	CLOSED LOOP CONTROL
	subconscious
	smooth continuous control
	some attention
	error detection

Level 3	CLOSED LOOP CONTROL
	conscious
	jerky, slow control
	greater attention required

Fig. 10.27 Levels of motor control.

Level 2

At Level 2, feedback does operate but the loop is a short one. As you know from your work in exercise physiology, the muscle spindles have sensory receptors, which can act as error detectors. If a muscle contraction during a movement is not what was prescribed by the motor programme (for example, if a skier hits a patch of ice when expecting soft snow), then a message is sent directly to the muscle to correct the error (with a copy to the brain to tell it about the ice!). This allows the correction to take place quickly (within 50 ms), because the important part of the message did not have to be brought to the level of consciousness. You can experience this kind of control if you try balance-walking along a narrow beam. This is known as **closed loop control**. It is essentially subconscious but because feedback is operating, it demands some of the attention channel. Its function is to provide smooth continuous movement while allowing for error detection. Since it relies on comparing what is actually happening with the demands of the motor programme, it develops as expertise develops, i.e. when the programme is well established.

Level 3

Level 3 is also an example of closed loop control in that it, too, relies on feedback. In this case visual and kinaesthetic feedback is used and thus the control is conscious and voluntary. The performer checks on the outcome of the first part of the skill before moving on to the next and thus there may be delays between successive movements; the whole appears jerky and uncoordinated. As we learned earlier, perceptual anticipation can speed things up but even then a considerable amount of the attention channel is being used up, so the performer does not have much capacity left to focus on the environmental demands of the task. This type of control is characteristic of beginners. It also applies to experts who suddenly experience a problem, for example a skater whose triple jump has gone wrong and so has to concentrate very hard on regaining balance and getting back into the routine.

There is more discussion of feedback in relation to learning in Chapter 11.

This chapter has given you the theory underpinning our knowledge of how people learn and perform skills. It has presented models of what psychologists think is happening. The models we have studied in each section can be combined into Welford's[3] model of information processing shown in Figure 10.28.

At each point in the model we have considered practical examples, but the real test of the usefulness of a theory (theory doesn't need to be useful) is whether practitioners can apply it in their work. The next chapter studies how coaches and teachers have used theory to plan and implement coaching strategies based on an understanding of how people learn.

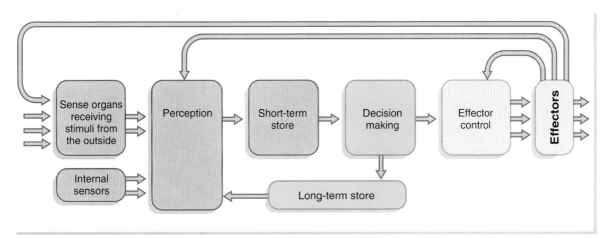

Fig. 10.28 (Adapted from Welford's[3] model of information processing)

Review questions

1. What is a motor programme?
2. Analyse a high jump in terms of the executive programme and the subroutines.
3. What are the differences between open loop theory and closed loop theory?
4. What does schema theory tell us about how open skills should be learned and practised?
5. Define exteroceptive, proprioceptive and kinaesthetic feedback.
6. What are the differences between Level 2 and Level 3 closed loop control?

Exam-style questions

1. Having interpreted information, a performer of a motor skill then formulates a plan of action. Some theorists state that an **executive motor programme** will be used by the performer.

   a. Using an example from **one** physical education activity, explain what is meant by an executive motor programme and identify the subroutines of that programme. (*3 marks*)

   b. Use the same example to show how an executive motor programme can become a subroutine. (*2 marks*)

   c. How can the performance of a skill be refined using **closed loop** theory? (*4 marks*)

   (*Total 9 marks*)

2. How is closed loop control used to make a movement more skilful? (*3 marks*)

3. a. Using Figure 10.29, list six major subroutines of the executive programme for throwing. (*6 marks*)

   b. Using examples from sport, identify four items of information stored as schema. (*4 marks*)

   c. Comparing the skills of throwing the javelin and taking a free throw at basketball, explain how the skills are related using schema theory. (*4 marks*)

   d. Briefly explain how the analysis of skills will influence a coach in organising training for javelin throwing as compared with basketball free throw. (*4 marks*)

   (*18 marks*)

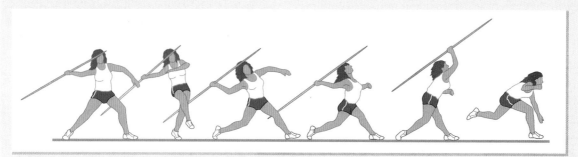

Fig. 10.29 Major subroutines of throwing.

References

1. Schmidt R A 1991 *Motor learning and performance: from principles to practice*. Human Kinetics, Champaign, Illinois
2. Whiting H T A 1969 *Acquiring ball skill*. Bell, London
3. Welford A 1968 *Fundamentals of skill*. Methuen, London
4. Williams A M, Davids K, Williams J G 1999 *Visual perception and action in sport*. E and FN Spon, London
5. Hennessy J 1984 Torvill and Dean. David and Charles, London
6. Adams J A 1971 *A closed loop theory of motor learning*. Journal of Motor Behavior 3:111–150
7. Schmidt R A 1988 *Motor control and learning: a behavioral emphasis*, 2nd edn. Human Kinetics, Champaign, Illinois
8. Schmidt R A 1975 *A schema theory of discrete motor skill learning*. Psychological Review 82:225–260
9. Martenuik R G 1976 *Information processing in motor skills*. Holt, Rinehart and Winston, New York
10. Singer R N 1968 *The learning of motor skills*. Collier Macmillan, New York
11. Davis D et al 1986 *Physical education: theory and practice*. Macmillan, Basingstoke

Further reading

*Particularly useful for students
*Honeybourne J et al 2004 *Advanced physical education and sport for A Level*, 3rd edn. Stanley Thornes, Cheltenham
*James R et al 2003 *Complete A–Z physical education*, 2nd edn. Hodder and Stoughton, London
Magill R A 2003 *Motor learning: concepts and applications*, 7th edn. McGraw-Hill, Massachusetts
McMorris T 2004 *The acquisition and performance of sports skills*. John Wiley and Sons, Chichester
*Roscoe D et al 2003 *Physical education and sport studies AS/A2 Level student revision guide*. Jan Roscoe Publications, Widnes
Sharp B 2004 *Acquiring skill in sport*. 2nd edn. Sports Dynamics, Cheltenham
Schmidt R A, Wrisberg C A 2004 *Motor learning and performance: a problem-based learning approach*, 3rd edn. Human Kinetics, Champaign, Illinois
Schmidt R A, Lee T D 1999 *Motor control and learning: a behavioural emphasis*, 3rd edn. Human Kinetics, Champaign, Illinois
*Webster S 2002 *AS/A2 sport psychology guide*. Jan Roscoe Publications, Widnes
*Wesson K et al 2004 *Sport and PE: a complete guide to advanced level study*, 3rd edn. Hodder and Stoughton, London

*Woods B 1998 *Applying psychology to sport*. Hodder and Stoughton, London

Multimedia

Video

The Fitness Series, Video Education, Australia 1996. *Analysing physical activity – the learning of skills*. UK supplier Boulton and Hawker Films, Ipswich
Video Education, Australia 2003. *Acquiring skills*. UK supplier Boulton and Hawker Films, Ipswich

CD-ROMs

Roscoe D A 2004 Teachers guide to physical education and the study of sport. Part 2 The performer as a person, skills acquisition 5th edn. Jan Roscoe Publications, Widnes
Roscoe D A, Roscoe J V, Honeybourne J, Davis R, Galligan F 2003 Physical education and sport studies AS/A2 level student revision guide, 3rd edn. Jan Roscoe Publications, Widnes
Roscoe D A, Roscoe J V 2002 OCR/AQA/Edexcel Science and Sport Psychology Powerpoint Classroom Presentations. Jan Roscoe Publications, Widnes

Principles of learning and teaching

11.1 Introduction: learning, performance and learning curves

Keywords

- cognitive strategy
- decreasing errors graph
- learning
- learning curve
- linear graph
- negative acceleration curve
- performance
- plateau
- positive acceleration curve

In Chapter 9 we defined learning in general terms and contrasted it with performance. Let us look again at the definitions of learning and performance.

Learning may then be considered to be a more or less permanent change in performance associated with experiences but excluding changes which occur through maturation and degeneration, or through alterations in the receptor or effector organs.[1]

Performance may be thought of as a temporary occurrence ... fluctuating from time to time because of many potentially operating variables. We usually use performance to represent the amount of learning that has occurred, for the process of learning must be inferred on the basis of observations of change in performance.[2]

ACTIVITY 11.1

Meaning of learning and performance

Work in groups of two or three. Discuss the meaning of the two definitions given in the text to make sure you understand them. In particular, explain:

- permanent change in performance
- associated with experiences
- maturation and degeneration
- alterations in the receptor or effector organs
- potentially operating variables
- inferred on the basis of observations of change in performance over time.

Investigation 11.1 To distinguish between learning and performance

Method: Work with a partner. One is the pupil, the other his/her instructor. The instructor, out of sight of the pupil, composes a sequence of movements, chosen at random. Keep the movements simple and 'nonsense'. About 10 separate movements are sufficient. The instructor practises this sequence so that it can be demonstrated fluently to the pupil. The sequence is then taught to the pupil by demonstrating it in full once only; the pupil then performs it as best he/she can. This performance will probably contain some errors or omissions. Without any explanation or correction, the instructor shows the sequence again and requests another demonstration. Repeat this procedure, without verbal coaching, until a completely correct sequence is produced.

Results: Note how many mistakes of movement pattern or sequencing are made at each performance. Draw a graph as in Figure 11.1.

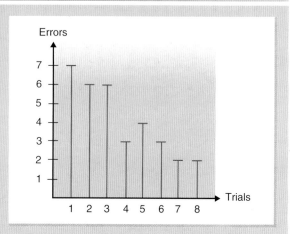

Fig. 11.1 A graph of decreasing errors to demonstrate learning.

The graph you drew in Investigation 11.1 is one of **decreasing errors** – one way of measuring learning and showing that it has occurred. Another way would be to measure how much better your partner was getting at an activity by measuring increases in performance, i.e. the number of successful catches in a juggling task. The graph might then look like that in Figure 11.2.

Each attempt at the task is a **performance**, a demonstration of the learner's ability in that task at that time. While a person is learning, each performance is likely to be different from (and hopefully better than) the last. As the skill is learned, performance becomes more consistent. So learning is the process by which performance is refined in such a way that it represents a permanent change of behaviour. As we shall see later in the chapter, however, we have to be careful about making too many assumptions about learning based on performance measures at any given moment.

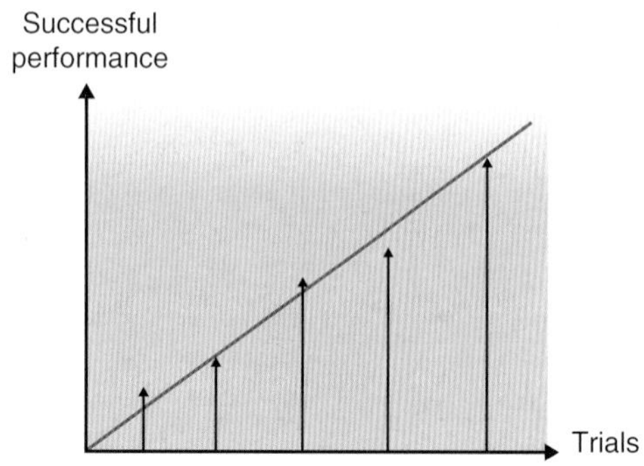

Learning curves

If you smooth out the fluctuations in performance shown in Figure 11.1, as has been done in Figure 11.2, you obtain a **linear** representation of the rate of learning in which learning (improvement in performance) is directly related to the number of trials (performances). Graphs of real learning experiences are seldom, if ever, as simple and symmetrical as this. People differ in the rate at which they learn. Some skills can be learned quickly, which produces a very 'steep' graph; others take more practice, so the graph is flatter.

Usually, however, the rate of learning changes throughout the learning of the skill and so plotting a graph over a period of practice time usually produces not a straight line but a series of **learning curves**. Figure 11.3 shows two such curves for two different skills.

Causes of plateaux (Activity 11.2)
Your graph should look 'S-shaped' and indeed, this is what it is called. The point where the curve is 'flat' for a period of time or number of trials is called a **plateau**. Plateaux usually indicate a period of transition in the learning or development of the skill or changes in the motivation or lifestyle of the athlete.

Fig. 11.2 A graph of increasing gains in learning.

ACTIVITY 11.2

A learning curve

Draw a hypothetical (not based on reality, but on your imagination) learning curve to represent the efforts of a learner who initially finds it hard to make progress, starts to learn quickly, but then faces a learning 'block' or **plateau** in which he/she maintains the standard of performance but makes no further improvement.

Why do you think the plateau might have occurred? What could the teacher or coach do about it?

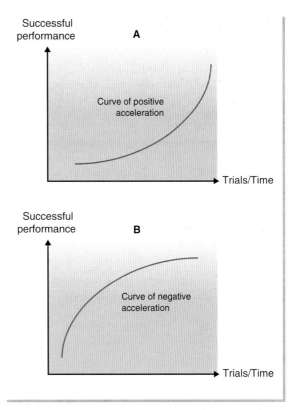

Fig. 11.3 Curves of **A.** positive and **B.** negative acceleration.

Christina & Corcos[3] categorise causes of plateaux as follows.

- **Psychological factors** – anxiety, lack of motivation, boredom, emotional problems.
- **Physical fitness deficiencies** – inadequate or inappropriate training, fatigue, lack of physical ability.
- **Changes in technique** – as a learner focuses on a new aspect of the technique or tactic, established routines may deteriorate temporarily or the skill as a whole may not progress. For example, as a discus thrower introduces the turn (after first learning a static throw) his/her distances may not improve for a while or may even get worse, but once the new technique is incorporated into the action, performance will start to improve again, often at an increased rate.
- **Changes in cognitive strategy** – the way in which the athlete thinks about the skill, both before and during performance, affects learning. If this is changed, performance is affected. For example, if the coach introduces the athlete to a new

visualisation technique, the athlete needs time to learn and adapt to this and progress may be delayed in the short term while this adjustment is made. Similarly, if a teacher asks a beginner breaststroke swimmer to think about swimming through a narrow tube (in order to make the stroke more streamlined), concentrating on this may temporarily disrupt coordination and the swimmer may feel he/she is not making progress.

The teacher/coach can help the learner overcome these difficulties by:

- explaining that plateaux are a normal part of the learning process
- explaining the cause of the plateau and reassuring the learner that it can be overcome
- planning appropriate goals to ensure continued progress
- structuring training and practice appropriately
- providing psychological support and not putting the learner under pressure if stress is a possible cause of the plateau.

Review questions

1. Define 'learning' and 'performance' and show how they are related.
2. Draw a series of learning curves that show positive acceleration, negative acceleration and S-shaped curves.
3. What causes plateaux and what can teachers or coaches do to help the learner overcome these?

Exam-style questions

1. You see a novice complete a number of tennis serves over a period of 20 minutes of **massed practice**.

   a. Sketch a graph, with time in minutes on the horizontal *x*-axis and success rate on the vertical *y*-axis, showing the possible changes **in performance** of the novice over the practice period. (*3 marks*)

   b. Explain the shape of the performance curve on your graph. (*4 marks*)

   c. What **strategies** might the teacher employ to help improve the performance of any closed skill by a novice during a 20-minute practice session? (*4 marks*)

   (*Total 11 marks*)

11.2 Learning: principles and theories

Keywords

- association theory
- classical conditioning
- cognitive map
- cognitive theories
- conditioned response
- conditioned stimulus
- connectionist theory
- drive theory
- executive programme
- feedback
- gestalt
- habit
- instrumental conditioning
- law of effect
- law of exercise
- law of readiness
- modelling
- motivation
- negative reinforcement
- neutral stimulus
- observational learning
- operant conditioning
- positive reinforcement
- punishment
- reflex
- reinforcement
- response
- reward
- shaping
- social learning theory
- stimulus
- stimulus–response (S–R) subroutine
- transfer
- unconditonal response
- unconditional stimulus

In Chapter 10 we considered learning to be the commitment of skills and knowledge to memory. We discussed 'input', which can also be termed 'stimulus', and how this is processed to produce an appropriate 'output' or 'response'. We saw that this process requires that we view what is to be learned as relevant, that we are attentive to what we are doing and that we are prepared to practise so that the information or movement becomes 'grooved' in memory.

In this section we will consider three important general theories of learning:

- associationist (stimulus–response) theory
- cognitive theory (including the gestalt approach)
- social learning theory.

Firstly, however, a word of warning. Much of what we know about motor learning derives from laboratory experiments. They have (mostly) been well constructed and the methods used are reliable and valid, because experimenters are able to control variables that cannot be easily controlled in a 'real-life' situation. What is often not clear, however, is (i) how permanent the observed improvements in performance are and (ii) whether observed learning in the laboratory can be transferred to sport situations. Bear this in mind when your further reading introduces you to actual experiments and in particular if you devise your own for a project.

Another thing to remember as you read this section is that the most important factor to influence learning is the amount of practice the player has. To maximise learning and performance, maximise practice. But there are two kinds of practice: (i) that which occurs through participation in the sport or activity, the game, the tournament, the dance performance, the expedition; (ii) what Ericsson[4] calls 'deliberate practice', i.e. activities designed by the coach to improve specific aspects of performance. We all know that this kind of practice requires effort and isn't always enjoyable so throughout all the advice given to coaches and teachers about how to structure motor learning runs the underlying maxim that motivation must be maintained and practice, if not always enjoyable, must be satisfying.

Before moving to the main learning theories, we will study a model of learning which links closely with the information-processing approach (see Chapter 10).

Phases of motor learning (Figure 11.4)

We know that people learn at different rates and have different preferred ways of learning; good coaching takes account of these differences. It is clear also that the coaching needs of an expert are different from those of a novice. Fitts & Posner[5] suggest that this progression from novice to expert can be modelled using information-processing concepts (in particular cue selection memory, rehearsal and feedback). Their model helps coaches to analyse what stage of learning their athletes are at and structure practice accordingly. Fitts & Posner's model is shown in Figure 11.4 and identifies three phases or stages of learning. You should also consider this model in relation to 'forms of guidance' in Section 11.5.

Cognitive (early) phase
The learner tries to get to grips with the nature of the activity to be learned, to 'figure out what to do'. Demonstrations are important, but so are verbal explanations to highlight the important cues. Problem solving also seems to work in the pre-practice stage ('Did you see how I really got my body behind the ball, even though it was an easy take? Why do you think I did that?). The learner tries to memorise sequences of movements and it often helps to verbalise these (e.g. 'bend, kick, together' for the breaststroke leg action). Teachers must be aware that information

Fitts and Posner (1967)	
Cognitive (early) phase	Understanding of the nature of activity.
	Analysis of techniques.
	Establishment of 'models'.
Associative (intermediate) phase	Focus on movement.
	Comparison of action with model.
	Error detection and correction.
	Movement is variable and inconsistent.
Autonomous (final) phase	Action has become automatic.
	Attention can be given to environmental aspects of game/activity.
	Strategy can be focused on.

Fig. 11.4 Phases of motor learning.

overload is a danger at this stage, because the learners have to think about almost every element of the action as they practise it and may have to visually focus on the movement as well as the area of play or performance. Teachers should also bear in mind that many learners want to 'get on with it and have a go'. Feedback should focus on the reinforcement of correct responses and on 'shaping'. Performance is full of errors and movement is inconsistent and lacks fluency. 'Trial and error' learning interspersed with feedback and instruction will fulfil most learners' needs.

Associative (intermediate) phase
The learner now understands the aim of the activity. Movement patterns are now more fluent and integrated. Simple aspects of the skill are becoming well learned and there is scope to refine the more complex aspects. The aim of the learner is to begin to associate the 'feel' of the movements with the end results. Feedback should be specific and focus on both knowledge of performance and knowledge of results to allow the association of kinaesthetic feedback with outcomes.

Autonomous (final) phase
Movement patterns are now well integrated and automatic; they can be performed without the performer giving conscious attention to the movement, unless

it is required. The performer can concentrate on the external demands of the environment and give a lot of attention to subtle cues. For example, a tennis player can use the opponent's wrist and racket action to judge what kind of spin is being put on to the ball, a task impossible for a novice because there is too much else to think about. There is less need for feedback from the teacher, because the performers are able to judge their own performances, but any information feedback can now be very detailed and specific.

The rate at which a learner progresses through the phases is determined by practice, effectiveness of information processing and the nature and extent of the reinforcement, guidance and feedback available.

Association (stimulus–response) theories

This group of theories (also referred to as 'behaviourist' theories) are all about the relationship between a stimulus (the task or problem) and the response (the performance). Learning is said to have occurred when the presentation of the **stimulus** (e.g. the presentation of the baton in a track relay) usually produces an appropriate **response** (e.g. the outgoing runner takes the baton cleanly and at maximum speed). The more stimulus and response occur close together in practice, the more the **S–R bond** is established in the memory and strengthened.

Early psychologists focused on the automatic nature of this bond.

Classical conditioning

This is a basic form of S–R learning. It was studied by Pavlov, an eminent Russian physiologist, who used dogs as his subjects. In a controlled experiment, he presented food to a hungry dog, first ringing a bell a few seconds before giving the food (Figure 11.5). The smell and/or sight of food causes dogs to salivate automatically, as a reflex. At first, the bell had no effect on the dog (neutral stimulus), but within a few trials the dog started to associate the sound of the bell with food and began to salivate as soon as the bell sounded, even before the food was produced.

It is important to recognise what has been learned in this example – not new behaviour but to behave in the same way to a new stimulus through association of the first stimulus with the second.

> ### KEY POINTS
>
> - **Classical conditioning** is the pairing of a neutral stimulus with an unconditional stimulus so that an association is formed between them and the original unconditional response becomes a conditioned response.
>
> - The important point to remember about classical conditioning is that for it to be termed 'classical', the response must be a reflex (or unconditional response).
>
> - **A reflex** is an involuntary, unlearned response to a particular stimulus not controlled by any conscious thought and has an evolutionary basis and purpose in helping the animal to adapt to the environment or be protected.[6]

> ### ACTIVITY 11.3
>
> **Reflexes**
>
> - Write down at least three human reflexes – make sure they really are reflexes.
>
> - What are the purposes of these reflexes in evolutionary or protective terms?
>
> - Which are particularly important to us in physical activity?

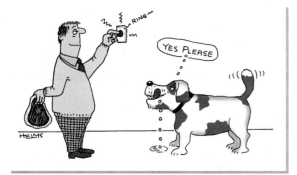

Fig. 11.5

Humans can learn through classical conditioning. For example, if a puff of air is blown into someone's eye to make them blink and this stimulus is paired with a bell, the person soon learns to blink when they hear the bell. But human reflexes are limited in number. Most of our learning depends on developing new responses and skills, not on association with innate, unconscious reflexes.

Some writers[7] refer to 'learned reflexes', i.e. movements which have been learned but which are not under conscious control. Withdrawing your hand from a hot surface or ducking if something is thrown near your head are two examples. If we accept this notion (not all psychologists do), we can extend the range of behaviours which we could claim to be 'classically conditioned'. We could learn irrational fear responses by this form of conditioning. This might explain some children's (and adults') fear in a swimming pool. But it is still an association between two stimuli which is being conditioned, not the behaviour. As physical educationalists or sport scientists, it is the behaviour we are interested in. So where do completely new skills, for example performing a somersault, come from?

Operant (instrumental) conditioning

Skinner[8] suggests that, even though much of our behaviour is not reflexive, it can still be conditioned, but not by classic methods. Naturally occurring, learned behaviour is called **operant** behaviour. If this behaviour is rewarded in some way, then there is an increased likelihood of it occurring again; we seem to be programmed to seek reward or satisfaction.

A young swimmer is learning a tumble turn. The first attempts at the somersault (the operant behaviour, already learned) are not successful but sooner or later, perhaps accidentally, his/her feet touch the wall and the push-off is effective. This is a good feeling, particularly if the coach gives praise and encouragement. This satisfaction acts as a **positive reinforcer**. It strengthens the connection between the stimulus and the response (Figure 11.6).

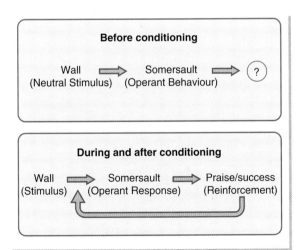

Fig. 11.6 Operant conditioning: learning the tumble turn in swimming.

> **KEY POINTS**
>
> - **Operant conditioning** – process by which the desired response (selected from a range of naturally occurring responses) is reinforced and so developed. Note that in operant conditioning the focus is on the relationship between the response and the reward; the stimulus is less important. It is the environment that is manipulated to produce new behaviour.
>
> - **Reinforcement** – the process of increasing the desired behaviour by giving satisfaction to the learner.
>
> - **Positive reinforcement** – providing a feeling of satisfaction to increase the likelihood of the desired response being repeated.
>
> - **Negative reinforcement** – removing an unpleasant experience in order to increase the likelihood of the desired response being repeated.

Positive reinforcement is a relatively straightforward concept. Feelings of satisfaction can be generated by the outcome of the response, as illustrated in the tumble turn example given above, or can be given by the teacher in the form of praise (bear in mind that praise only acts as a reinforcer if it gives satisfaction to the learner).

Negative reinforcement is rather more difficult to understand. Look again at the definition; an example may help. The coach has been working with the soccer team on some defensive drills. The team has been working hard but is keen to put the drills into a 'real game'. The coach is trying to set up a conditioned game but the players are anticipating the excitement of competition and are not paying attention. The coach wants them to listen (desired response). He stops the explanation, waits for attention and says, 'Until you stand still and listen to what we are going to do, we are not going to start. It's your playing time we are wasting'. Not allowing the coaching session to continue is the negative reinforcement; it's unpleasant because the team are keen to play. Paying attention to the coach is the required response. Once the team are doing so, the negative reinforcement is removed, i.e. the coach stops holding up the game. Hopefully the players learn that if they want to have plenty of time in the game they must listen to the coach.

It is important not to confuse negative reinforcement with punishment. Punishment is given as a **consequence** of a response and to prevent the response occurring again. To extend the example, if one of the team continued to 'mess about' the coach might say, 'Sam, I've warned you once. You're still not doing what I asked, so you're not going to play for the first 10 minutes. Go and get your tracksuit on.' The punishment of not playing is designed to stop Sam misbehaving in future.

Skinner extended his theory of operant conditioning to include the concept of **shaping**. He recognised that with complex skills, for example a tennis serve, you cannot immediately reinforce the whole action because it is unlikely to be produced in the first trial. So the coach might:

- break the skill down into small, easily learned parts and progressively reinforce these, building the whole skill up; this is sometimes called **chaining**
- or introduce the whole skill, but 'shape' it by reinforcing actions which are along the right lines, even if not quite right. By reinforcing actions which are closer and closer approximations to the desired end result, the overall correct movement is gradually learned.

Operant conditioning facilitates the initial learning of the skill. Once a skill is learned, there is no need to continue reinforcement and so it can be gradually withdrawn and transferred to the learning of a more advanced skill. As long as this withdrawal does not happen before the skill is learned, the S–R bond will not be weakened.

Thorndike's laws of learning

Thorndike[9] was an extremely influential S–R theorist. He established three laws of learning (of readiness, of effect and of exercise) which are particularly important in skill development.

Law of readiness

Learning can only take place when the nervous system is sufficiently mature to allow the appropriate S–R connections. Basic body management skills, such as jumping, running, skipping, should be developed before the implementation of striking and catching skills. This concept of nervous system readiness is in addition to issues of muscle strength and skeletal maturity, which are also very important considerations.

We can extend this idea to cover the idea of **mental readiness**. We learn best when we:

- really want to acquire the knowledge/skill
- have a clear understanding of the requirements of the task
- know and accept why we are practising the task.

Law of effect

Learning occurs when a particular response has an effect on the person, i.e. when the response is reinforced. Satisfying reinforcers increase the strength of the S–R bond and increase the likelihood of the response being repeated. Thus, to enable early success it is important for a coach or teacher to use positive feedback to reinforce correct attempts.

Failure in a task can also act as reinforcement because it produces the opposite of satisfaction: annoyance. This is generally less effective than positive reinforcement.

If the learner knows what he/she is trying to achieve, then observed success can serve as a positive reinforcer and failure as a punishment, without a teacher or coach being there to provide supplementary reinforcement. This process has become known as 'trial and error' learning. It depends on the learner being able to recognise success and to feel satisfaction with the response or alternatively to be annoyed that a response is not appropriate and to try another. The problem of this approach to skill learning is that it can allow learners to establish 'bad habits', i.e. responses that are immediately successful at the beginner stage but that do not allow further development.

Law of exercise

Repetition strengthens the S–R bond, hence the importance of practice. Even though a skill may have

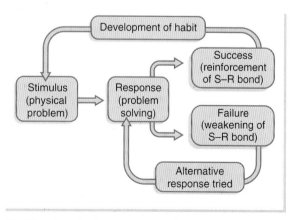

Fig. 11.7 The stimulus–response bond.

apparently been learned effectively, practice beyond this point leads to 'mastery learning'. Mastery learning ensures that a skill is not easily forgotten and can be performed under varied and difficult circumstances.

Cognitive theories

S–R theory has been very influential in helping us to understand how people become skilful but many psychologists, particularly today, do not believe it is the whole answer. They argue that the extent, variety and richness of human learning cannot be explained solely by S–R bonding. A number of alternative theories, known as **cognitive** theories, have been put forward. These are called cognitive because they place a greater emphasis on thought processes and on understanding how concepts relate to one another than is evident in S–R theory.

Tolman[10] believed that behaviour is driven by purpose and expectation, so learners are motivated to work towards goals of which they are aware. In sport and PE these are the skills and understandings which make up the particular activity. Learners progress towards the goal (for example, being able to intercept a pass in football) by recognising cues, using past experience and forming what Tolman referred to as a **cognitive map** of the activity, which becomes more complex and sophisticated as the learner becomes more skilful.

A group of psychologists (Koehler, Koffka, Lewin), known as the **Gestaltists** (*Gestalt* is German for 'form' or 'shape'), proposed two principles of learning.

- Learning can be accelerated by using 'insight' or 'intuition' to solve a problem. For example, a gymnast and her coach might want to link two moves in a floor sequence but are not sure how to do it. The gymnast may experiment with several ideas (trial and error) which help to clarify the problems and possibilities and might then suddenly say, 'I know, how about . . .' and produce the movement solution – a moment of insight.

- Learning is most effective when a problem is seen as a whole or when the whole pattern of a movement can be practised. This enables the learner to understand all the issues and relationships which need to be considered. Gestaltists therefore advocate that learners practise a tennis serve as a whole, without breaking it down into parts.

Social (observational) learning theory

Social learning theory explains how our behaviour is influenced by the behaviour of other people. Coaches and teachers are using this theory when they employ demonstration as a learning tool. Demonstration is a powerful teaching tool in skill acquisition. Youngsters are involved in observational learning when they copy sporting heroes.

Demonstration is the application of 'modelling' or 'observational learning'. This theory maintains that much social behaviour is learned through observation of models. Skilled behaviour is no exception to this. One problem of observational learning is that teachers and coaches cannot always control what players are learning. A youngster might learn a lot about skill from watching his football hero but he may also pick up some bad habits too!

Bandura[11] suggests that there are four processes in observational learning:

- **attention** and **retention**, which relate to the acquisition of the skill
- **motor reproduction** and **motivation**, determining performance (see Figure 11.8).

Coaches and teachers use this model when they demand that players **attend** to instructions or provide cues about how best to perform ('Don't watch where the ball goes, watch how my racket swings through at waist level and where it finishes').

Retention is the process of remembering the modelled behaviour. Good coaches help this process by repetition, by making learning interesting, by encouraging mental imaging of the skill and by 'catchphrases': 'step-step-step-lift' helps the hurdle step in springboard diving.

Motor reproduction refers to the attempt by the learner at the modelled skill. It is important that the coach has demonstrated correctly and also that the learner has the physical make-up to be able to do the task. Further guidance is usually helpful at this stage.

People tend to imitate what they are interested in and be **motivated** to achieve. Good coaches understand what motivates their players and use this as an important coaching tool. They use reinforcement to enhance motivation.

Review questions

1. Explain the difference between classical and operant conditioning. Give some sport-related examples of each.

2. What is meant by 'shaping'? Select a closed skill and explain how a coach might 'shape' the learning of it.

3. Why are Thorndike's three laws of learning important in skill acquisition?

4. Explain the difference between negative reinforcement and punishment.

5. How might coaches encourage the use of 'insight' in their players and why might they wish to do it?

Exam-style questions

1. Discuss the advantages of the **whole and part** methods of learning and comment on any general factors the coach should consider when determining the appropriate way of coaching a new skill. Illustrate your answer with examples of sports skills. (*20 marks*)

2. We use demonstrations a great deal in physical education and Bandura[11] has suggested that we learn many of our behaviours through the observation of others. The model in Figure 11.8 illustrates this.

   a. Explain this model and apply it to the coaching of an individual skill. (*6 marks*)

   b. Give an example of a specific video you might watch to try to motivate yourself in a particular game. Would you always use the same video for instilling confidence in skill development? (*5 marks*)

   (*Total 11 marks*)

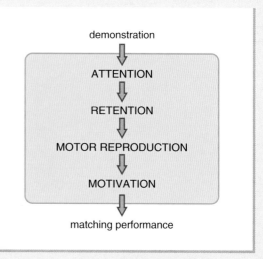

Fig. 11.8 Model of Bandura's observational learning.

3. a. Referring to Figure 11.7 and using examples from sport, explain what is meant by the S–R bond. (*3 marks*)

   b. Explain how a teacher of a sports skill could ensure that a correct response follows a particular stimulus. (*5 marks*)

   (*Total 8 marks*)

4. a. What is meant by operant conditioning? Show how you would use operant conditioning to teach a named sports skill. (*5 marks*)

   b. State what is meant by reinforcement and give examples of different types. (*4 marks*)

   c. Explain what is meant by classical conditioning and give an example from sport. (*4 marks*)

   (*Total 13 marks*)

5. a. In racquet sports, coaches give demonstrations to aid skill development. Identify the stages of

Bandura's model of observational learning, giving an appropriate example of each stage to illustrate your understanding. (*4 marks*)

   b. Explain the cognitive theory of learning as proposed by Gestaltists and apply this to a practical situation. (*4 marks*)

   (*Total 8 marks*)

6. a. Name the three phases of learning and explain their significance to a performer. (*3 marks*)

   b. Identify two characteristics of a performer in the final phase. (*4 marks*)

   c. How might the type of mental practice change in the last phase of learning? (*2 marks*)

   (*Total 9 marks*)

7. Explain how feedback differs through the associative and autonomous phases of learning as a performer makes progress. (*4 marks*)

11.3 Motivation and feedback

Motivation and drive theory

The topic of motivation occurs throughout the theory and practice of teaching and learning. To achieve anything at all, we need to be motivated. In Chapter 12 we refer to it as 'the drive to strive'. Hull[12] defines learning in terms of motivation; he suggests that whenever we have a need to learn, this sets up a psychological drive to satisfy that need. This in turn leads to an action or response. If this is successful, then the drive is reduced and motivation will only be maintained if a new need to learn arises or is presented to us (Figure 11.9).

This is a very complex theory in its totality but stated simply and applied to physical activity, it suggests that as a movement problem arises, for example in dance choreography or the performance of a particular skill in a game, this generates a need for competence, a

need to solve that problem. This need in turn develops a drive and an incentive to learn to solve the problem and also a habit (the way of performing the skill). So we start to practise. At first the performance is not effective but as success comes it is perceived as a **reward** and thus acts as **reinforcement**. As a result a memory bond is forged between the stimulus (the problem) and the **response** (the effective performance). The two become associated in the memory and a 'habit' (a successful performance) is developed (see Figure 11.7).

As our performance improves, so the habit is strengthened and the drive to go on learning reduced. At this point the teacher or coach needs to extend the problem or present a new one to maintain interest and motivation. The coach also needs to be aware of what Hull called **inhibition**. This is a phenomenon we have probably all noticed, that during a long practice session our performance may be less good at the end than it was earlier in the session. This does not mean, however, that we are not learning throughout the session; what is evident at the end of practice may not be what is retained or what is transferred into the competitive or performance environment.

Developing motivational strategies as a teacher or learner can be complex; we all know how difficult it is to motivate ourselves to do something we are not too keen on. To be successful, coaches need to be aware

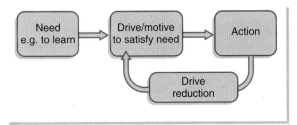

Fig. 11.9 Drive reduction theory.

of just what motivates their players and how to get the best out of them. Schmidt[13] states the problem very simply; to him motivation consists of:

- making the task seem important
- goal setting.

Would you wish to add anything else?

We shall consider these in more detail in Chapter 12 and also 'feedback as motivation' next.

Feedback

Feedback is sensory information that results from movement. You will find several different terms used to define it. In Chapter 10, for example, we identified exteroceptive feedback, proprioceptive feedback and kinaesthetic feedback. These were used within the context of a model of motor control.

We can simplify matters if we focus on feedback as it is consciously used by the learner and coach as motivation and information giving.

Schmidt[13] names two forms: **inherent feedback and augmented feedback** (see Figure 11.10).

- **Inherent (intrinsic) feedback** derives from the performance of the skill itself. It is information about the muscles involved, the coordination and timing of the movement, the effectiveness and the outcome. It is used for error detection as the movement is in progress, by the comparison of movement as it progresses with the model stored in memory. It is also used for reinforcement: a javelin thrower might know that the throw 'felt good' but waits in anticipation of the javelin coming back to earth to see if the throw is as long as he feels it is. Both are examples of inherent feedback.

- **Augmented (extrinsic) feedback** is information provided about the task which is in addition (or supplemental) to that provided as a direct result of the movement (inherent feedback). It might be provided by an official, a coach, a video, a results board or team mate. There are several dimensions to augmented feedback. Figure 11.11 lists and defines these.

Immediate	Presented immediately after the action
Delayed	Some time after the action
Concurrent	Presented during the movement
Terminal	Presented after the movement
Verbal	Presented in a form that is spoken or capable of being spoken
Non-Verbal	Presented in a form that is not capable of being spoken
Accumulated	Feedback that represents an accumulation of past performance
Distinct	Feedback that represents each performance separately

Knowledge of results and knowledge of performance

Fig. 11.11 Dimensions of augmented feedback.[13]

These dimensions should not be thought of as independent of each other. For example, terminal feedback (given at the end of a performance) can either be verbal or non-verbal and in addition could be either delayed or immediate, etc. The dimensions define most forms of feedback used. Being aware of them helps the coach to decide how best to provide feedback in a particular set of circumstances.

Functions of feedback

Feedback has four functions.[3]

- Information about performance or outcome
- Reinforcement (either positive or negative)
- Punishment
- Motivation

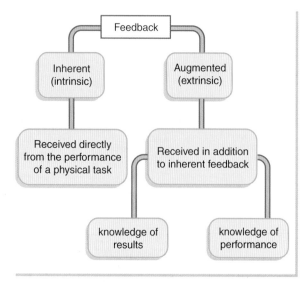

Fig. 11.10 Forms of feedback.

Feedback for information

Information feedback can be either inherent or augmented. Augmented feedback should be structured by the teacher or coach such that it gives (i) reinforcement of correct performance and (ii) help with correcting errors. It should include:

- the outcome of the performance (if not clear to the learner)
- correct and incorrect aspects
- what the correct movement response should feel like
- explanation of the cause of errors
- changes in technique or tactics to correct the errors
- why these changes are suggested.

The good coach gives positive information feedback first, followed by error correction (Figure 11.12) and finally some motivational comment. Before giving feedback, the coach also gives the learner a moment or two to evaluate and come to conclusions about his/her own performance. Sometimes questions can be used: 'What did that feel like?', 'Why do you think that happened?'. This gives control to the learner, identifies to the coach the ability of the learner to analyse his/her own performance and ensures the coach does not tell the learner what he/she already knows.

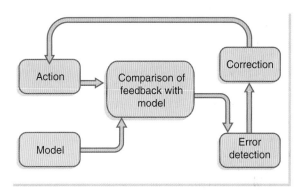

Fig. 11.12 Feedback as error detection.

Investigation 11.2 The effects of knowledge of performance on learning

Method: Work in two groups of subjects with one person acting as the experimenter. Ideally, once the task has been decided upon, the subjects should both be aware of the details of the experiment. Devise a closed skill motor task which is unfamiliar to all members of both groups and which is likely to show some learning over a short period of time. Aiming at a target with the non-dominant hand might be an example, but you can probably think of a better one. Organise about 10 blocks of practice which can be scored. At the end of this phase, give a 5-minute break and then about five 'performance' blocks. Group A is given both knowledge of performance and knowledge of results after each of the first 10 blocks of practice; Group B is given knowledge of results and social reinforcement (encouragement without reference to either knowledge of performance or knowledge of results).

If you have the opportunity, repeat the test after a week and plot these results on the same graph.

Results: Record your data for each member of the group and obtain a mean score for each group, for each block of practice. If your data are appropriate, plot a learning curve as in Figure 11.13.

Discussion: What do your results, or the hypothetical results in Figure 11.13, suggest about the importance of knowledge of performance to learning?

What is the effect on the results of the test taken one week later? How would you explain any change you see in the shape of the graph?

How would you adapt the methodology to investigate other forms of feedback?

Can you suggest any improvements to the methodology to improve the reliability and validity of your results?

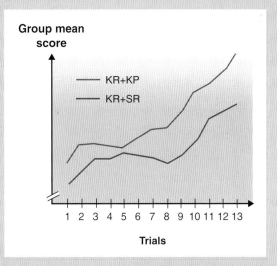

Fig. 11.13 A hypothetical learning curve to show the effects of different forms of feedback on learning. (Adapted from reference[21])

For beginners, information feedback should be simple and concise. It should focus on sequence and timing so that the motor programme can be developed effectively. It should be given as frequently as possible, after each trial if feasible; it should help the learner identify important cues; it should rely on visual and verbal input.

For intermediate learners, feedback can be given less frequently; the learner needs opportunity to link the feel of the movement with the outcomes, so information feedback should focus on this. The feedback can be more detailed.

Advanced performers require much less augmented information feedback; what is given should be detailed and technical.

Feedback for reinforcement

We discussed reinforcement in Section 11.2 – you should refer back to this if you are not sure about the concept. Reinforcement is used a great deal in the early learning stages and through all the phases for open skills. It can be intrinsic or augmented. Positive reinforcement is given to strengthen the desired technique. It can be used to 'shape' responses. In sports contexts positive reinforcement usually takes the form of praise and encouragement. Augmented negative reinforcement requires the removal of an unpleasant consequence of the error. For example, there is a device which a golfer may attach to his/her club that gives a loud click if the golfer 'snatches' the swing. Negative reinforcement is the avoidance of the click by swinging smoothly. Practising allows negative reinforcement to eliminate the error and reinforce the correct swing. Reinforcement must be given immediately following the response if it is to be effective.

Feedback as punishment

Coaches and teachers ideally should not need to punish, but players are not angels and occasionally misbehave or refuse to accept a coach's or teacher's advice. Punishment carries risks and should be used sparingly and only if all other forms of feedback appear to be ineffective. An example of punishment is to demote a player to 'the bench' for a game for missing a practice.

Punishment **should not**:

- be physical or involve physical activity
- demean the learner or damage their self-esteem
- be given in frustration or anger.

Punishment **should**:

- be perceived as such by the learner
- be given after warning
- be used consistently and fairly
- be used against the undesirable behaviour, not the person
- be supplemented by positive reinforcement and motivational feedback.

Feedback as motivation

Learners are motivated when they have clear goals and want to achieve them. Goal setting in sport is an important element in learning and the good teacher or coach ensures that learners have clear, achievable structured goals to which they are committed.

Motivational feedback gives learners information about their progress towards these goals. It helps them to understand the difference between their present performance level and that needed to achieve their goal. It is important that it also gives them self-belief and the confidence to continue to practise through the ups and downs of learning. Breaking down long-term goals, for example to reach the national championships, into more immediate goals (perhaps in terms of personal bests or league position) is a helpful motivational strategy. Progress charts and training or competition diaries are useful in this respect, because they help the learner to see improvement. But often the most satisfying motivational feedback comes as acknowledgement of progress from the teacher or coach. Goal setting is considered in more detail in Chapter 13.

KEY POINTS

- Different forms of feedback seem to be appropriate at different stages of learning.
- Individuals differ in the form of feedback they prefer and respond to best.
- One form of feedback may be more appropriate for a particular sport or activity than another.
- A common generalisation is that the sooner augmented feedback occurs after an action, the better; but information-processing theory suggests the performer needs time to process inherent and concurrent feedback before dealing with any further information. In any case, immediate augmented feedback is not always practical.
- Augmented feedback should not delay the next attempt at the skill too long, otherwise forgetting occurs.

- Similarly, augmented feedback should not be given after every attempt. The learner, once he/she understands the task and has an idea of what it feels like to perform, should be allowed to concentrate on the internal feedback available.
- The amount of feedback which should be given is difficult to gauge. The teacher or coach should focus on the critical components of the skill, i.e. those subroutines which are essential to early mastery. But too much concentration on detail in the early stages can impede effective learning.
- The specificity of the augmented feedback required depends on the age and stage of the learner and his/her capacity to process information.

Review questions

1. Give four functions of feedback.
2. What points should a coach consider when giving feedback?
3. Define motivation and explain drive theory.

Exam-style questions

1. **a.** Define the term feedback and briefly describe three functions of feedback. (*4 marks*)
   b. Figure 11.14 illustrates two ways of classifying sources of feedback. Where possible, explain the kinds of feedback available to a performer that would be classified as A, B, C and D respectively. (*4 marks*) (Note: see Figure 11.11 for help with this)

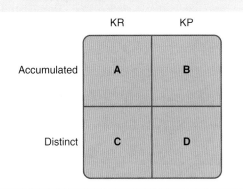

Fig. 11.14 Classifying sources of feedback.

2. **a.** What is meant by intrinsic and extrinsic motivation? Give practical examples to illustrate your answer. (*4 marks*)

   b. How can extrinsic motives affect intrinsic motivation? (*2 marks*)
   (*Total 6 marks*)

3. **a.** What sort of motivation methods would you use to motivate a beginner in gymnastics? (*4 marks*)
   b. How would the motivation methods used for a skilled performer differ from those used for a beginner? (*3 marks*)
   (*Total 7 marks*)

4. **a.** A number of PE students are attending trials at their chosen sport. Describe the Inverted U theory and explain how it might affect a student's performance at the trials. (*5 marks*)
   b. Rewards may be used to improve the motivation of a performer. What are the problems if rewards are given excessively? (*3 marks*)
   (*Total 8 marks*)

5. **a.** A coach reinforces good performances in training with praise. Why does this reinforcement work rather than punishing poor performance? Explain what is meant by reinforcement and punishment in this case. (*5 marks*)

6. Discuss the idea that improvement in skill performance is dependent upon the nature and frequency of the feedback provided by the coach. (*7 marks*)

11.4 Transfer of learning

Keywords

➤ negative transfer
➤ proactive transfer
➤ positive transfer
➤ retroactive transfer
➤ zero transfer

Schema theory (see Chapter 10) seems to imply that certain aspects of a skill learned in one situation can determine performance in another similar situation. For example, the motor programme for throwing a ball over-arm can be adapted for use in a variety of similar throwing actions, e.g. the javelin or a lacrosse ball. This is named **transfer** in the skill acquisition literature.

Transfer is defined as the effect of the learning and performance of one skill on the learning and performance of another.

If skill A is learned first and then has an effect on skill B which is learned later, this is known as **proactive transfer**. For example, the stride pattern of running over low canes (skill A) is learned first and then transferred to running over hurdles (skill B).

If skill B is learned first and subsequently modified by practising skill A, this is known as **retroactive transfer**. An example of retroactive transfer: a dancer practises a dance step but finds the dynamics difficult (skill B); s/he works on the dynamics in a different exercise (skill A) and then transfers this learning into the original step pattern (skill B), improving it.

Note that both retroactive and proactive transfer can be positive or negative. See the Key Points box below for descriptions of positive and negative transfer.

Transfer is a complex concept and is not easy to apply in the learning–teaching situation. What can we learn from the research literature?

- The greater the actual similarity between skills, the greater the possibility of positive transfer.
- The greater the dissimilarity, the less likelihood exists of positive transfer.
- Where skills share some similarities but have important differences, there is the danger of negative transfer.
- Athletes learn new techniques and tactics more effectively if new learning builds on and is related to skills already learned.

- Coaches or teachers should emphasise the similarity between skills when teaching for transfer (e.g. by letting players practise throwing the ball by hand before attempting an overhead pass in lacrosse).
- Tactical understanding can be transferred (e.g. zone defending in basketball and netball).
- General principles of attack and defence play can be transferred in invasion games.
- The more thoroughly the first skill has been learned, the more effective is the transfer.
- In activities where bilateral transfer is encouraged (e.g. basketball dribbling, soccer kicking), it is important that the skill is well learned on the preferred limb before transfer is attempted to the other.

KEY POINTS

- **Positive transfer** occurs when learning in one task is promoted by previous learning in another; for example, you may initially be better able to throw a ball with a lacrosse stick if you have a good basic throwing action with your hand.

- **Zero transfer** (no transfer at all) may occur, even between skills which appear on the surface to be similar.

- **Negative transfer** occurs when the learning of a new task is interfered with by knowledge of a similar activity; for example, the flexible use of the wrist in a squash or badminton shot may interfere with learning the firm wrist needed for a tennis drive or vice versa.

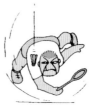

Fig. 11.15 Negative transfer.

- Virtual reality – reality transfer: does playing a computer-based game of soccer, for example, improve skill in 'the real thing'? Research[19,20] indicates that knowledge of the procedures of the skill may be enhanced but there is little evidence of transfer of the perceptual and motor elements. Results from an experiment with a table tennis game were more positive.

ACTIVITY 11.5

Examples of transfer types

Put the following pairs of skills into one of the categories: (i) very similar; (ii) likely to cause interference; (iii) dissimilar.

- Tennis serve and volleyball serve
- Long and short serve in badminton
- Golf drive and ten-pin bowling
- Straight arm pull and bent arm pull in back crawl
- Rugby League and Rugby Union
- Dismounts from the high bar and the rings in men's gymnastics
- Scottish and Irish folk dancing
- Ice hockey and field hockey.

Let us consider transfer of learning in a broader context by taking the example of a good gymnast who goes to college and follows a beginners' dance course as part of his or her A-level or undergraduate studies. To what extent does successful experience in gymnastics aid learning in dance? Using Figure 11.16 to analyse the situation, consider the following.

- The **student's attitude** to the new activity contributes considerably to early learning. Our gymnast will be confident about his/her body image in a movement task and will enjoy showing a competent individual performance. In this respect there is likely to be positive transfer. On the other hand, a gymnast is used to having performance choreographed by a coach or trainer and may approach the creative element of dance with trepidation. The rule- and technique-governed nature of competitive gymnastics may even cause negative transfer initially.
- In **skill-transfer terms**, evidence suggests that the actions he/she has learned as a gymnast do not transfer readily to dance unless the choreography is particularly gymnastic in style. In this respect there is no obvious transfer effect.
- In terms of **ability–skill transfer**, there is much more likely to be some positive effect. Balance, coordination, flexibility and many other abilities developed in gymnastics can be used very effectively in dance. The rhythmic ability so necessary for dance may or may not be present.
- **Practice-to-performance** transfer depends on how well the gymnast has learned to use later practice

1. Skill-to-skill	Between two skills. Evidence suggests little long-term positive transfer.	
2. Practice-to-performance	Positive transfer likely only to occur if environmental conditions are similar in both situations. Practices should simulate the stimuli and cues which occur in performance.	
3. Abilities-to-skill	Abilities do not transfer totally to the performance of skills which they underpin, but contribute significantly.	
4. Limb-to-limb (bi-lateral)	Positive transfer of learning and training occurs between limbs (hand–hand; leg–leg). Effect most obvious in transfer from preferred to non-preferred limb.	
5. Principles-to-skill	Under particular learning conditions knowledge of a skill principle, e.g. body shape/speed of rotation, will enhance the learning and performance of the skill.	
6. Stage-to-stage	Motor skill development depends on building each new skill upon those learned previously.	

Fig. 11.16 Categories of transfer. (Adapted from reference[14])

sessions as a rehearsal for the 'real thing'. If this strategy is also used in preparation for dance performances, then positive transfer could occur.

- **Repetition and variation** are two important dance choreography principles. One way of both repeating and varying the movement is to use both sides of the body in a dance phase. If the gymnast has developed this skill, then positive transfer to dance occurs; however, gymnasts tend to be 'one-sided', for example, always using the same foot for take-off, which may be a difficulty in dance work.

- **Movement principles** are universal, although they are analysed and expressed differently. The gymnast's knowledge of, for example, biomechanics transfers directly to the production of good technique in dance. Research does, however, show that we must have reservations about the extent to which the performance of an action is aided by knowledge of the principles of that action.

Investigation 11.3 Positive transfer effects in skill learning

Method: Select one form of transfer from categories 1–5 in Figure 11.16. Select two groups of subjects, Group 1 and Group 2, matched for motor learning ability as far as possible. Devise two novel tasks (A and B) by which you might expect learning in task A to transfer positively to learning in task B. Make your tasks relevant to the category of transfer you have chosen. Ensure that the tasks are 'learnable' in the time you have available, but they should present some degree of difficulty.

Decide on the criteria to use to determine that learning has taken place; for example, you might decide that seven accurate shots out of 10 in a novel aiming task constitutes learning.

Group 1 learns task A and then task B; Group 2 learns only task B.

Results: Determine which group learned task B more quickly.

Discussion: Assuming all other variables have been controlled (a dangerous assumption under the circumstances of a class experiment), what do your results tell you about the possibility of transfer between task A and task B for Group 1? How might you improve the experiment so that you could be more confident of your results?

For teachers and coaches to undertake transfer work positively, they must make a careful analysis of the relevant tasks and the teaching environment, to ensure that all the potential points of transfer are stressed.

To summarise our work on learning, use Investigation 11.4 to study the relationship between stage of learning and appropriate feedback.

Investigation 11.4 Stages of learning and feedback

Method: Work in threes, with roles of 'learner', 'teacher' and 'observer'. Before the start of the investigation, each member of the trio selects a simple, novel psychomotor skill to teach; a short sequence of hopping and stepping would be appropriate or a mirror-tracing task if such a task has not been used before. Exchange roles for each of the following learning episodes (if videoing the episodes is possible, this will aid your analysis and discussion).

Method A. The teacher demonstrates the skill to the learner, who practises it. No feedback is given, but the skill is demonstrated by the teacher at intervals. The observer attempts to identify when learning changes from 'cognitive' to 'associative' to 'autonomous'. A video of the learning allows review.

Method B. The teacher demonstrates the skill to the learner, who practises it. The teacher focuses on giving

instructions appropriate to the phase of learning, i.e. demonstration and general verbal guidance in the cognitive stage, error detection and specific guidance in the associative stage and a focus on style and/or speed in the autonomous stage. The observer checks the appropriateness of the instruction given.

Method C. The teacher demonstrates the skill to the learner, who practises it. The teacher has identified beforehand examples of supplementary feedback which give (a) knowledge of results and (b) knowledge of performance and uses these during the learning episode. The observer notes these and attempts to identify which are intended as knowledge of results and which as knowledge of performance.

Discussion
- Were the skills essentially open or closed?
- How does instruction in the different stages differ between open and closed skills?

- What evidence did the observer use to identify the different stages of learning?
- How effective was the teacher in giving appropriate instructions?
- Do teacher and observer agree about the examples of knowledge of results and knowledge of performance?
- How helpful did the learner find the instruction and the feedback in terms of amount, timing and specificity?

Review questions

1. Give a sport-related example of (a) positive transfer and (b) negative transfer.
2. List the six categories of transfer and give an example of each.
3. List four requirements for positive transfer to occur.
4. Give an example of a coach using positive transfer to develop a technique.

Exam-style questions

1. **a.** Using a practical example, explain what is meant by the term **transfer** in skill learning. (*3 marks*)

   b. How can transfer be detrimental to performance? Give a practical example. (*3 marks*)

   c. How can a teacher or a coach ensure that as much positive transfer takes place as possible in a training session? (*5 marks*)

   (*Total 11 marks*)

2. **a.** Define the terms positive transfer and negative transfer in the context of someone learning a sport skill. (*2 marks*)

   b. Figure 11.17 shows different amounts of transfer in different situations labelled X, Y and Z. For each of these situations, give examples of one pair of games-type skills which illustrate the kinds of transfer indicated. (*4 marks*)

   c. Explain the reasons for your choices of skills. (*6 marks*)

   (*Total 12 marks*)

3. Describe and evaluate the use of video playback in the **learning** of sport skills. (*10 marks*)

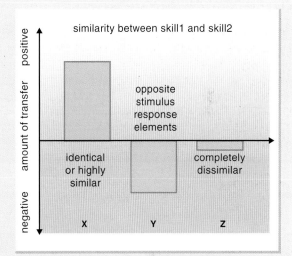

Fig. 11.17 Extents of transfer in various situations.

11.5 Teaching

Keywords

- command style
- discovery style
- distributed practice
- fixed practice
- guidance
- manual guidance
- massed practice
- mechanical guidance
- mental rehearsal
- modification of display
- negative transfer
- organisation
- part practice
- practice style
- problem solving
- progressive part practice
- progressive part presentation
- pure part presentation
- reciprocal style
- spectrum of teaching styles
- task analysis
- trial and error
- variable practice
- verbal guidance
- visual guidance
- whole method
- whole–part–whole method
- whole–part–whole practice
- whole practice

So far in this chapter we have considered some elements of the learning process. This section focuses on how learning may be structured so that it is achieved efficiently. You should bear these points in mind when planning your own practice or training or when helping others with theirs. We have referred to teaching and coaching as if they are the same activity. Whereas some would argue that they have different aims and purposes, current approaches suggest that teaching physical education and coaching sport share much common ground, so we treat them as one process.

The teaching process

Most learning is achieved by being taught in one way or another, although 'trial and error' learning or 'learning by experience' also occur. Teaching others is a process we are all involved in, even though we may not consider ourselves to be teachers. Teaching is about giving experiences or advice which aids learning.

The teaching process can be summarised as in Figure 11.18, which echoes an old Chinese proverb about learning, attributed to the philosopher Confucius:

> *I hear and I forget;*
> *I see and I remember;*
> *I do and I understand.*

Current theory suggests there are **four** elements of the teaching process – instructing, demonstrating, applying and confirming – and good teaching progresses through each in turn.

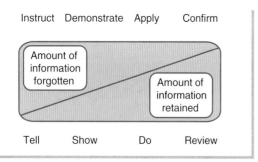

Fig. 11.18 The teaching process. (Adapted from reference[18])

Instructing

In the instructing (telling) phase, teachers make sure that learners understand the task and have enough information to allow them to start practising. Usually this is done verbally, though written practice schedules or worksheets are sometimes used. The danger in this phase is that the teachers give too much information (in their eagerness to ensure that the learners completely understand). Unless the information given is clear and concise, most of it is quickly forgotten.

Demonstrating

As we have seen, demonstrating (showing) is an important aspect of skill learning because of the need for the learner to establish a model of the skill in memory. It needs to be carefully planned so that both teacher and learner are clear about the purpose of the demonstration and what exactly is to be learned from it. A bad demonstration may be worse than no demonstration at all.

Applying

Applying (doing) is the opportunity for the learner to practise the skill; without plenty of time for this, effective learning is unlikely to take place. The teacher's role is to structure this practice effectively and by appropriate guidance to help learners to apply what they have learned from instruction and demonstration to the activity itself.

Confirming

Confirming (reviewing) is the feedback process, which is covered in detail in Section 11.3. It is an essential part of the learning process but is sometimes omitted by teachers, to the detriment of learning. An important part of reviewing is to question the learner about what he/she has learned and the progress made. This not only helps the teacher to confirm what has been learned, but also encourages the learner to be self-evaluative and reinforces learning.

Styles of teaching

Within the four elements of the teaching process described above there are many different ways to teach. These are known as **styles** and have been analysed and classified in much the same way that we have classified skill, that is, by observing action, noting the characteristics of that action and devising a theoretical framework to fit the observations.

Mosston & Ashworth[15] produced a classification (based on observations of physical education but applicable to all teaching) which they have labelled the 'spectrum of teaching styles' (Figure 11.19). They suggest that teaching and learning are essentially about making decisions: what to teach–learn; when to teach–learn; how to present and acquire the ideas and skills, etc. Their model suggests that at one end of

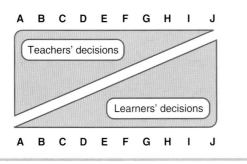

Fig. 11.19 The spectrum of teaching styles.

the spectrum the teacher makes all these decisions and at the other end the learner makes them all. In between are a range of styles in which the teacher and learner are both involved in decision making. The styles are distinct and Mosston & Ashworth give them letter labels and names (for example, style A = command style).

The teacher in Investigation 11.5 is probably nearer to **command style**, the one in which the teacher makes all the decisions. It is very difficult to teach for long in this style and it is not advisable to do so, because we usually want to hand some of the decisions to the learner, e.g. 'start when you're ready'. Command style is used when a teacher wants tight control over what the learner is doing or wants uniformity in a class. A lot of aerobics and keep-fit teaching is done in command style. Style B is **practice style** – the teacher sets the task but the students work on it in their own time.

Style C is known as **reciprocal style**. Pupils work in pairs – one is the 'doer' and the other the 'observer'. In this style the teacher hands over all contact with the learners (the 'doers') to fellow pupils (the 'observers'). The teacher makes sure, either by a worksheet or by very explicit instructions, that all the pupils understand the task and the criteria for successful completion of it. It is then up to the observer to help the doer; the teacher helps the observers with their teaching. It is a useful style with large groups because it allows each learner a lot of immediate feedback. Look back to p. 336 to remind yourself of the advantages of this. No doubt you can think of some disadvantages, however.

Investigation 11.5 Decision making in teaching and learning

Method: Work in pairs – one is the teacher and one the learner. The teacher devises a simple task to teach the learner. It may be something the learner can already do and wishes to improve. It can be classroom or sports hall based but it should have a motor component. Spend some time teaching and practising the task. This period of time is known as an 'episode'.

Discussion: When the episode is over, discuss with each other and list all the decisions which were made by both the teacher and the learner:

- before the episode
- during the episode
- when the episode was over.

1. Who made each decision?

2. What was the ratio of teacher decisions to learner decisions?

3. Do you think the teacher was nearer to style A or style J?

In both styles A and C the teacher is concerned not only with what the learners learn but also with how they learn it; a specific product and process. At other times the teacher may focus on 'how to learn' and adopt a problem-solving style. A task or problem is set which the pupils have to solve in their own ways. The problem may be defined by a single solution which the teacher wishes the pupils to **discover** (style F) or there may be several possible solutions (not all of which the teacher may have thought of) and the pupils' task is to investigate these and select the one which most interests them (style H). Teachers of creative dance and educational approaches to gymnastics use these styles a lot; so, in a different way, do teachers of outdoor pursuits.

There is not the space here to discuss the whole spectrum of styles, nor to go into much detail about each, but it is important that you begin to grasp that there are many ways of learning and therefore of teaching and the skilful teacher selects appropriately from the range. So when you are next helping a friend or group of juniors with an activity, consider ways in which you can vary your approach.

Modes of presentation

Teaching style is concerned with the way in which a teacher opts to deal with the range of decisions that the teaching process imposes. One of these decisions is, 'How do I present this new information or skill to

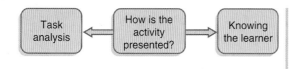

Fig. 11.20 Deciding on presentation.

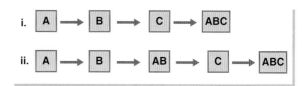

Fig. 11.21 'Part' methods of presentation.

my pupils?'. The answer to this question depends on the teacher's analysis of two important factors, which is illustrated in Figure 11.20.

Task analysis involves deciding what the important elements of the task are. Information-processing theory helps here.

- What are the perceptual requirements?
- What are the decision-making requirements?
- What techniques does the performer need?
- What feedback is available?

Answers to these questions indicate the complexity of the task. Note that complexity relates to the nature of the task; whether a task is simple or difficult depends upon the amount of attention/processing space that needs to be given to it and the experience of the learner.

Analysis should also indicate the extent to which the skill is organised. Skills which are not easily broken down into constituent parts are said to be highly organised. Swimming strokes are examples of low organisation, because the leg, arm and breathing actions are all different and separate, although obviously they need to be well coordinated for effective performance.

This **task analysis** should be compared with an analysis of the state of readiness and the capabilities of the learner. The good teacher and coach consider age, previous experience, physical abilities, preferred learning style, motivation and goals.

Whole practice

Ideally, a skill should be taught as a whole. The learner can then appreciate the end product and can develop a feeling for the flow of movement necessary for a smooth, efficient production of the skill; he/she can see the relationship between the movements which constitute the whole action.

Part practice

However, for some skills it is not appropriate or sensible to teach the whole all at once, such as:

- when the skill is too complex and/or difficult for the learner, i.e. a lot of information processing is required
- when there is an element of danger.

In these cases the skill is broken down into its constituent parts (subroutines); these parts are taught as separate actions and then put together, which can be done in a variety of ways (Figure 11.21).

Part methods of teaching are useful when the skill is complex and/or difficult, not highly organised and the mechanics of the movement are important. Closed skills, such as those in gymnastics, diving and trampolining, are usually taught in this way. It lessens fear and risk in dangerous skills and allows the teacher to focus on key elements of the skill. It may help motivation, as the teacher can structure the teaching of the parts as 'mini wholes', thus giving the learner a feeling of success and progress. The main problem is one of transfer, for it is essential that the separately taught elements be practised in the same way as they are performed within the whole skill, which is not easy to achieve. It is also important that the whole skill be demonstrated to the learner initially so that the end product can be appreciated in terms of its purpose, pace, flow and organisation.

> **Investigation 11.6** The effectiveness of whole and part methods of teaching a novel sequence of movement
>
> *Method:* The class is divided into four groups; four group leaders are appointed. The class teacher has previously devised and taught to the group leaders a sequence of movements which flow into one another and which contains some complex (but not impossible) moves. The constituent parts of the sequence are agreed.
> - Group A learns the sequence by the 'pure part' method (Figure 11.21i).
> - Group B learns the sequence by the 'progressive part' method (Figure 11.21ii).
> - Group C learns the sequence as a whole.
> - Group D learns by the whole–part–whole method.
>
> *Discussion*
> 1. Which group takes the longest to learn?
> 2. Which group performs the sequence best?

3. What seems to be the best method of teaching for this particular skill?
4. You have been investigating teaching methods, but what are the 'confounding variables' in this experiment, i.e. factors other than teaching method which may have affected the result?

Whole–part–whole practice

Many skills can be taught by the **whole–part–whole method**, whereby the learner first tries out the whole skill to get the feel of its performance requirements and to identify the easy and difficult elements. These may be different for each individual. By careful observation the teacher can isolate the difficult elements and teach them as parts, finally integrating them into the whole again.

Whole and part methods assume that the parts of the skill are taught as if they were being performed within the whole and they rely on positive transfer. If, however, the whole is complex but not easily broken down into parts that are meaningful, then the task itself may be simplified. A good example of this is the current focus on the 'mini-game' for youngsters. Short tennis and pop lacrosse have many of the elements of the full adult game but are played with modified rules and equipment.

If simplification of this kind is inappropriate, the idea of shaping the performance may be used. This is an aspect of operant conditioning as described earlier. The coach or teacher rewards aspects of the performance as the correct technique is approached and so the performer gradually acquires the skill. This is also known as **gradual metamorphosis** of the skill.

Forms of guidance

When we practise or experience a skill or activity, some learning inevitably takes place but we learn most efficiently by a combination of experience and guidance. Sharp[16] differentiates between 'practice' (which is **without** guidance) and 'training' (which is practice **with** guidance), but not all writers make this distinction.

ACTIVITY 11.9

Practice and training

Using Sharp's distinction between practice and training, which do you think is the most efficient way to learn? Discuss and justify your conclusion.

KEY POINTS

- Practising for long periods without guidance may be demotivating; it also allows errors to creep into the skill that may be difficult to eradicate.

- Learners need time to practise without feeling under pressure from the teacher or coach, so that they can work out their own solutions to problems.

- Guidance should be given before and after, but rarely during an attempt at the skill or task.

Bearing the key points in mind, a second set of decisions a teacher must make is about the type of guidance to give. There are three basic forms of guidance or methods a teacher may use to transmit information about performance:

- visual
- verbal
- manual or mechanical.

Guidance is received by the learner through the senses; because we have several of these, information can be communicated to us in a variety of ways. Two points are important here:

- the senses interact, so a combination of forms of guidance can be effective
- people differ as to the type of guidance they prefer.

Visual guidance (Figure 11.22)

This is used at all stages of teaching and learning but is particularly valuable in the early (cognitive) phase to introduce the task and set the scene.

Demonstration

Demonstration relies on imitative learning and/or modelling[11] and is a powerful tool. It is efficient, 'on the spot' and interesting to learners but it must be accurate and relate to their age, experience and gender. It must show the activity as it occurs in real life. Teachers should avoid talking too much as a demonstration is taking place but it is necessary to focus the learners' attention on important performance cues.

Visual aids

Visual aids can be of value if constructed and presented thoughtfully. Photographs, charts and models are cheap and readily available; they can be tailored to the exact requirements of the particular situation but they are static and thus limited. Video is generally agreed to be more beneficial, particularly if action can be slowed down, but playback equipment is expensive. Video can be used either in place of demonstration or to provide information feedback on the learners' performances. Computer analysis is increasingly being used in elite athlete research and training centres to provide detailed information about performance.

There is now a great deal of opportunity for off-air recording of top-level sport performances which can be used in the coaching or teaching situation. Camcorders have extended the usefulness of video to record learners' progress, but it is time consuming to video and analyse large groups.

Investigation 11.7 To produce a visual aid

Method: Select a skill or aspect of an activity with which you are especially familiar. Decide on a particular aspect which you might focus upon when helping a friend to learn the activity. Produce a visual aid to support your proposed coaching. Try making a video if you wish, but this is a time-consuming task so you are probably better advised to avoid the technicalities of filming and concentrate on producing a good chart or model. Think about:

* simplicity
* clarity
* use of colour
* highlighting the important performance cues.

Try out your visual aid on a friend and invite constructive criticism of it.

Modifying the display

Sometimes it is appropriate to give assistance by enhancing perception of the important aspects of the surroundings. We discussed signal detection in Section 10.3 and the way, for example, the colour of tennis balls might affect play. Areas of space might be highlighted; for example, a coach might mark a target on a court for serving practice or chalk the points on a gymnastic mat where the hands should be placed for a cartwheel. Coloured bibs or different strips not only help the referee, they help player identification in a team game.

Manual or mechanical guidance

This form of assistance involves physical contact, for example by the coach supporting and guiding the movement (as in the practice of a gymnastic vault) or by the support of a device such as a swimming armband, a trampoline belt or a 'tight rope' in climbing. It allows the learner to discover the timing and spatial aspects of the movement but does not help her acquire knowledge of the forces that act on the body or of the movement cues. The aim is to reduce error and fear – important when there are safety considerations. Such support is therefore generally used with youngsters and people with special needs. Two forms of manual guidance have been identified.

* **Physical restriction** – a person or an object confines the moving body of the performer to movements which are safe, e.g. a trampoline belt.
* **Forced response** – the learner is guided through the movement, e.g. a coach may physically guide a player through a forehand drive in tennis.

Verbal guidance

A great deal of teaching and coaching is done using verbal guidance. A good coach is able not only to set the task clearly and unambiguously and to describe the actions; he/she is able to highlight the important performance cues. With advanced learners these cues are detailed and technical. With beginners it may be more appropriate to express the cues in ways that may not be entirely accurate but that will convey the feel of the movement to the learner: 'Climb with your eyes!'; 'Stretch your toes to the ceiling!'. The advantages of using verbal guidance are that it is 'on the spot' and,

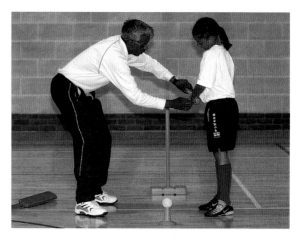

Fig. 11.22 A coach modifies the display and gives mechanical guidance to help a beginner.

when used by a knowledgeable and perceptive teacher, is directly relevant to the problems and capabilities of the individual learner.

There are some difficulties which a teacher must work to overcome.

- Does the learner understand the instructions?
- Can the learner remember what has been said (remember the capacity of the short-term memory)?
- Can the learner translate from the spoken word to movement?

Types of practice

The concept of open and closed skills also gives the teacher guidance in deciding how to structure the practice of a particular activity. We saw, in Section 11.2, how, as a general rule, open skills should be practised with as much variety as feasible (**variable practice**) to allow a general schema to be developed; whereas in closed skills (in which the replication of a specific movement pattern is the aim), **fixed practice**, with repetition to allow the movements to be overlearned, is appropriate.

A third decision about practice which the teacher needs to make concerns the length of the practice periods and the extent to which the learners need rest during practice. For teachers, these decisions relate to how they structure practice within a lesson, how long each episode should be and how to change the focus of practice while maintaining the pace of learning. For a coach, the decision also includes how many times a week the athlete should train and how long the training period should be, as well as what the training should consist of.

If learners need rest during a practice or training session, how long should the rest periods be and what should the learners do in them? This is an important question for, as you probably know from your own experience, if fatigue or boredom sets in, learning decreases markedly.

What is the best form of practice organisation? There is not a straightforward answer. **Massed practice** appears to be most suitable for activities in which:

- the skill is simple
- motivation for learning is high
- the purpose of the practice is to simulate fatiguing conditions that might be experienced in competition or performance
- available practice time is very short
- the learners are experienced, able and fit.

> **KEY POINTS**
>
> - **Variable practice** – practising a skill in a variety of different contexts and experiencing the full range of situations in which the technique or tactic might be used in competition.
>
> - **Fixed practice** – a specific movement pattern is practised repeatedly. Often known as 'drills'.
>
> - **Massed practice** – the skill is practised until learned without taking any breaks.
>
> - **Distributed practice** – practice is interspersed with breaks which can either be rest or the practice of another skill.

Thus if the performers are highly skilled, fit and well motivated, massed practice may be the most appropriate form of organisation. This means that the learners work continuously at an activity without any breaks until the skill is mastered or time runs out. Massed practice is efficient and allows concentration and overlearning.

Distributed (spaced) practice should be used for activities in which:

- the skill to be learned is new and/or complex
- there is a danger of injury if fatigue sets in
- attention spans are short, i.e. with young learners
- motivation is low
- learners are not fit enough
- weather conditions are adverse.

In distributed practice organisation, the total practice session is split into several shorter periods with intervals between. These intervals may be rest periods or the teacher may set alternative tasks. From what you now know about **negative transfer**, what must the teacher be careful about in organising alternative tasks in the intervals?

In general, both researchers and teachers agree that distributed practice is the most effective in the majority of cases. One of the advantages of distributed practice is that the rest intervals can be used for **mental rehearsal**. This is the process whereby the performer, without moving, runs through the performance in his/her mind. The learner can do this in several ways:

- by watching a demonstration or film
- by reading or listening to instructions
- by mental imagery, if the skill is established.

Obviously, this is a useful strategy for experienced performers and many use it in preparation for competition but interestingly it also appears to enhance the learning process. Research[17] suggests that when mental rehearsal occurs, the muscular neurones fire as if the muscle is actually active. Because of this, it is suggested, mental rehearsal has a real learning effect. Though few sports psychologists would claim that a skill can be learned entirely by mental rehearsal, evidence suggests that a combination of physical and mental practice is beneficial. Mental rehearsal is dealt with as a cognitive preparation strategy in Chapter 13.

Whatever methods of practice are used by coaches, an indisputable fact is the amount of practice needed to produce top-level performers. Research evidence indicates a close relationship between the level of skill and the total number of hours of practice. It has been suggested that by the time a professional quarterback reaches his peak he will have made 1.4 million passes; a 10-year-old female gymnast needs about 8 years of daily practice to reach an Olympic final (some countries start serious training of their gymnasts a lot younger than this). This suggests that Olympians may not so much be supermen and -women as people who are prepared to devote a considerable proportion of their life to training for their sport.

Review questions

1. Draw Priest & Hammerman's[18] model of the teaching process. What constitutes confirming and reviewing?
2. What are the essential differences between teaching by command and teaching by discovery?
3. Under what conditions would you teach (a) a whole skill and (b) by the progressive parts method?
4. Briefly describe four types of guidance.
5. Why is variable practice of open skills important?
6. Give an example of the use of mental practice.

Exam-style questions

1. a. What must be taken into account before any decision can be made about how to teach a skill? (*6 marks*)
   b. Generally a skill should be taught as a whole as far as possible. Give reasons for this. (*3 marks*)
   (*Total 9 marks*)

2. Some skills need to be split up into subroutines to be taught effectively. What are the advantages and disadvantages of this type of skill presentation? (*6 marks*)

3. a. Define massed and distributed practice. (*2 marks*)
   b. Justify the choice of practice conditions for a training session of a sport of your choice. (*8 marks*)
   (*Total 10 marks*)

4. In a test set up to investigate the effects of distributed and massed practice on the learning of a new skill, students were asked to complete a mini assault course consisting of a balancing, a climbing and a crawling task. They repeated the experiment 10 times (trials).
   The distributed group were given 60 seconds rest between trials, and the massed group no rest.
   Figure 11.23 shows the results of the test – mean times for the two groups to complete the course over trials.
   a. Use the chart to describe the results of the test, giving two possible explanations of the results. (*4 marks*)

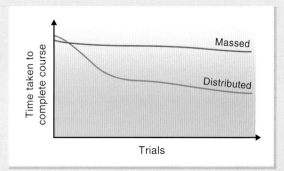

Fig. 11.23

   b. Name two characteristics of the task and two attributes of the learner which might lead you to decide which method of practice (massed or distributed) to use. (*4 marks*)
   (*Total 8 marks*)

5. a. Figure 11.19 shows Mosston & Ashworth's spectrum of teaching styles in terms of decision making in the learning process. Identify the teaching style at A and explain its consequences for teaching method. (*2 marks*)
   b. What are the advantages and disadvantages of this style in teaching physical education? (*6 marks*)
   (*Total 8 marks*)

► **6. a.** What is meant by the reciprocal teaching style and what are its drawbacks? (*3 marks*)

   b. What are the main advantages of the discovery method of teaching? (*4 marks*)

   (*Total 7 marks*)

7. a. Other than visual guidance, what other main methods of guidance are there? Give a practical example for each. (*6 marks*)

   b. How would you optimise the use of visual guidance in teaching motor skills? What are the drawbacks of this method? (*4 marks*)

   (*Total 10 marks*)

References

1. Knapp B 1973 *Skill in sport*. Routledge and Kegan Paul, London
2. Singer R N 1982 *Motor learning and human performance*. Macmillan, New York
3. Christina R W, Corcos D M 1988 *Coaches' guide to teaching sport skills*. Human Kinetics, Champaign, Illinois
4. Ericsson K A et al 1993 *The role of deliberate practice in the acquisition of expert performance*. Psychological Review 100: 363–406
5. Fitts P M, Posner M I 1967 *Human performance*. Brooks Cole, Belmont, California
6. Miller G A 1972 *Psychology: the science of mental life*. Penguin, Harmondsworth
7. Davis D et al. 1986 *Physical education: theory and practice*. Macmillan, Melbourne
8. Skinner B F 1974 *About behaviorism*. Vintage Books, New York
9. Thorndike E L 1932 *Fundamentals of learning*. Columbia University Press, Columbia
10. Tolman E C 1946 *Studies in spatial learning*. Journal of Experimental Psychology 36: 221–229
11. Bandura A 1977 *Social learning theory*. Prentice-Hall, Englewood Cliffs, New Jersey
12. Hull C L 1943 *Principles of behavior*. Appleton Century Crofts, Norwalk, Connecticut
13. Schmidt R A, Lee T D 1999 *Motor control and learning: a behavioral emphasis*, 3rd edn. Human Kinetics, Champaign, Illinois
14. Stallings L M 1982 *Motor learning*. Mosby, St Louis
15. Mosston M, Ashworth S 1986 *Teaching physical education*. Merrill, Columbus, Ohio
16. Sharp B 2004 *Acquiring skill in sport*. 2nd edn. Sports Dynamics, Eastbourne
17. Heuer H 1996 *Coordination*. In: Heuer H, Keele S W (eds) Handbook of perception and action. Volume 2: Motor skills. Academic Press, San Diego, pp.121–180
18. Priest S, Hammerman D 1989 *Teaching outdoor adventure skills*. Journal of Physical Education, Recreation and Dance 63(1): 64–67
19. Wickens C D, Baker P 1995 *Cognitive issues in virtual reality*. In: Barfield W, Furness TA (eds) Virtual environments and advanced interface designs. Oxford, New York
20. Todorov E et al 1997 *Augmented feedback presented in a virtual environment accelerates learning of a difficult motor task*. Journal of Motor Behavior 29: 147–158
21. Wallace S A, Hagler R W 1979 *Knowledge of performance and the learning of a closed motor skill*. Research Quarterly 50: 265–271

Further reading

*Particularly useful for students

*Honeybourne J et al 2004 *Advanced physical education and sport for A Level*, 3rd edn. Stanley Thornes, Cheltenham

*James R et al 2003 *Complete A–Z physical education,* 2nd edn. Hodder and Stoughton, London

Magill R A 2003 *Motor learning: concepts and applications*, 7th edn. McGraw-Hill, Massachusetts

McMorris T 2004 *The acquisition and performance of sports skills*. John Wiley and Sons, Chichester

*Roscoe D, Roscoe J V, Honeybourne J, Davis R, Galligan F 2003 *Physical education and sport studies AS/A2 Level student revision guide*. Jan Roscoe Publications, Widnes

Sharp B 1992 *Acquiring skill in sport*. Sports Dynamics, Cheltenham

Schmidt R A, Wrisberg C A 2004 *Motor learning and performance: a problem-based learning approach*, 3rd edn. Human Kinetics, Champaign, Illinois

Schmidt R A, Lee T D 1999 *Motor control and learning: a behavioral emphasis*, 3rd edn. Human Kinetics, Champaign, Illinois

*Webster S 2002 *AS/A2 sport psychology guide*. Jan Roscoe Publications, Widnes

*Wesson K et al 2004 *Sport and PE: a complete guide to advanced level study*, 3rd edn. Hodder and Stoughton, London

*Woods B 1998 *Applying psychology to sport*. Hodder and Stoughton, London

Multimedia

Video

The Fitness Series, Video Education, Australia 1996. *Analysing physical activity – the learning of skills*. UK supplier, Boulton and Hawker Films, Ipswich

Video Education, Australia 2003. *Acquiring skills*. UK supplier, Boulton Hawker Films, Ipswich

CD-ROMs

Roscoe D A 2004 Teachers' guide to physical education and the study of sport. Part 2 The performer as a person, psychology of sport, 5th edn

Roscoe D A, Roscoe J V, Honeybourne J, Davis R, Galligan F 2002 OCR/AQA/Edexcel Science and Sport Psychology Powerpoint Classroom Presentations. Jan Roscoe Publications, Widnes

Roscoe D A, Roscoe J V, Honeybourne J, Davis R, Galligan F 2003 Physical Education and Sport Studies AS/A2 Level Student Revision Guide, 3rd edn. Jan Roscoe Publications, Widnes

Psychology of sport performance: individual differences and performance enhancement

12.1 The nature of sport psychology

In Chapters 9–11 we considered the processes by which people become skilful and the factors which influence motor skill learning. We now turn our attention to performance and study what is happening while people who have become relatively proficient take part in physical activity for recreation and competition.

We call this study the psychology of sport; it is also referred to as sport psychology. Currently, sport psychologists are extending their field of study to encompass fitness, exercise and activities such as dance and outdoor pursuits, so the subject is now usually entitled 'sport and exercise psychology'. Psychology in general is the scientific study of the minds and behaviours of individuals. There are many different fields, each with its experts, e.g. psychoanalysis, psychotherapy, social psychology. Sport psychology has, in the past, derived much of its theory from mainstream psychology, but as it develops as a discipline in its own right, it is beginning to generate theory specific to its own interests, e.g. hypotheses about 'home advantage'. Sport psychology, therefore, deals with the behaviour of people in sport and exercise contexts. There are two branches, which are distinct but related.

- Academic sport psychologists work in or with university departments on research questions such as the use of imagery by athletes or the effectiveness of certain anxiety regulation strategies. They also teach undergraduate students of sport psychology and physical education,

supervise postgraduate research and offer courses for coaches and teachers. Their work is largely theoretical but intended to be applied to real-life sport situations. Sport psychology laboratories are often used by performers in their preparation for competition.

- Applied sport psychologists act as consultants and work directly with performers and their coaches, offering advice and assisting in the management of training programmes. They use the theory generated by the academics where they find it helpful; they often discover strategies that seem to work with performers and which the academics then test out and seek to explain. A sport psychologist may be both an academic and a consultant.

Coaches and teachers are increasingly using the ideas and theories generated by sport psychologists in planning their programmes and in getting the best out of the young people with whom they work. They recognise that as more and more people have access to sophisticated training methods and aids, it is a performer's mental approach that gives him or her the 'winning edge'. Sally Gunnell (Olympic 400 m hurdler) said, 'Once you've got your technique right and your training is going well, it's your own control of your thoughts that makes the difference between success and failure'.

Chapters 12 and 13 introduce you, as a student of sport psychology, to these theories and show you how they have been applied in real-life sport settings.

In this chapter, we consider how psychologists have attempted to identify what makes up personality and whether the kind of person you are affects your performance in sport (or whether the activities you participate in affect your personality). This leads us to consider attitudes in and to sport: how they arise and what their impact is on sport, players and spectators.

We take our study of motivation further and consider the effects of such factors as attribution, confidence and achievement motivation. Chapter 13 deals with how being a part of an activity group or team affects people and the extent to which competition itself and the spectators (including the media) are a factor in success.

12.2 A brief history of sport psychology

Sport psychology emerged at the end of the 19th century, as mainstream psychology was beginning to make an impact. The first psychological essays on athletic behaviour and sport appeared in France, Germany and Russia in 1897.[1] At the same time in the USA, Triplett, a university psychologist and cycling enthusiast, became interested in why he tended to ride faster when out cycling with his friends than he did when he was alone.[2]

This is not to say that there was no interest in, or knowledge of, the relationship between activity and behaviour before this time. The Platonic ideal of 'a healthy mind in a healthy body', the mediaeval concept of chivalry, muscular Christianity and the English public school association of athleticism and character building all reflect an awareness of the relationship between and the implications of activity, thought and morality. These are psychological as well as sociological concepts and they have sport, recreation or action as their focus. You will find information about these ideas elsewhere in this book.

Sport psychology is defined, however, as the scientific study of behaviour in sport contexts. For a study to be 'scientific', it must be, amongst other criteria, systematic; it was not until the early years of the 20th century that sport began to be studied in a systematic, academic manner. Coleman Griffith is credited as being the 'father' of sport psychology. Like Triplett, he was an academic psychologist but during the 1920s and early 1930s he also taught in the Physical Welfare Department of the University of Illinois, USA, where he founded the first sport psychology laboratory and acted as a consultant to a number of baseball and American football clubs. He also published some of the first books and scientific research articles on sport psychology.

Griffith's work, though carried out largely in professional isolation, opened the way for the development of departments of sport psychology and motor development in universities in Britain, Europe and the USA in the immediate postwar period (1945–65). Initially the work focused on the science of motor skill development, through the work of people such as Henry in the USA and Whiting and Welford in Britain, and this continues to be an important branch of the discipline.

But sport psychology was still very much in its infancy. In the USA and Australia there was not yet any universal recognition of its application to and usefulness for competitive performers. In Britain the continuation of the amateur ethic in sport bred a scepticism on the part of most performers and coaches about 'all this psychological stuff' and academics were not really taken seriously by their colleagues. But elsewhere national sport teams were beginning to effectively apply psychology to their training and support. As early as 1956, the Brazilian soccer squad at the World Cup finals included a sport psychologist.[3] In some cases the sports schools of the then USSR and Eastern bloc countries employed sport psychology specialists and in these countries, sport psychology became a regular part of national team training methods during the 1960s. Not unexpectedly, in the political climate of the cold war period, they kept the secrets of their success to themselves. When people began to analyse the overwhelming success of the Eastern bloc nations in the 1960s, it was recognised that psychology played a part in this.

This, together with the growing number of research studies, led the USA, Western Europe and later Britain to begin to take the subject seriously within academic circles and to apply it in sport. In 1965 the International Society of Sport Psychology (ISSP) was established with Italian sport psychologist Ferruccio Antonelli as its first president. National and continental associations were formed in 1967 in the

USA (the North American Society for the Psychology of Sport and Physical Activity (NASPSPA)) and in Europe in 1969 (the Federation Europe de Psychologie des Sports et des Activites Corporelles (FEPSEC)). Later, the Asian-South Pacific Association of Sport Psychology (ASPASP) came into being. These associations initiated conferences and the publication of research journals, which spread ideas, theories and information and opened up networks and communication across political boundaries and between academics and those coaches who realised the significance of the developments for their performers. From the mid-1970s sport psychology has continued to develop along five main lines.

- National Olympic Committees have recognised the importance of sport psychology in the preparation of national teams.
- In 1986 the applied branch of the subject was established with the formation of the Association for the Advancement of Applied Sport Psychology (AAASP) and the publication of the journal *The Sport Psychologist*.
- Coach development programmes (e.g. sports coach UK, formerly the National Coaching Foundation, in Britain and the Masters Coaching Program in America) have included sport psychology in their courses.
- Research programmes and undergraduate courses in the subject have proliferated, particularly in Britain with the expansion of higher education in the 1980s.
- Openings for consultant sport psychologists have emerged to work directly with individual performers and teams and to advise coaches on aspects such as how to deal with competitive anxiety, how to develop self-confidence, how to eliminate negative thoughts, the setting of SMART goals, working together as a team.

As the number of practising sport psychologists grew during the 1980s, it became clear that there was a need to ensure the quality of the advice that was being offered. National associations therefore developed processes of registration and accreditation whereby only those practitioners who satisfy professional criteria (such as their qualifications, experience and publications record) can be recommended by the association. Britain took the lead in this in 1988 when the then British Association of Sport Sciences (BASS), now the British Association of Sport and Exercise Science (BASES), developed a register of accredited sport psychologists. These days, only sport and exercise psychologists on this register (or those accredited as chartered psychologists by the British Psychological Society) are recommended to work with performers by sports coach UK or the British Olympic Association (BOA). The BOA now has a Psychology Steering Group and registration process and BASES has a Code of Conduct for Sport and Exercise Psychologists.

Where does sport and exercise psychology go from here? A number of trends seem to be emerging, some or all of which may become the focus for the students of today. It is important for you to know where the discipline has come from and to be familiar with the theories and data that have formed its basis to date. These you will find in the following two chapters. But as you read about current research, you will find people discussing ideas of the future such as:

- the psychological benefits of exercise and the use of exercise to enhance psychological well-being
- the development of more valid and reliable measures of psychological variables in sport, such as thought processes during competition
- the use of IT, not just to analyse data but to generate it also, perhaps in such areas as attitudes and patterns of play in games
- action theory, which recognises that people are complex organisms and the things that control their behaviour (such as personality, attitude, motivation, interpersonal skills) all act together and not in isolation, which is how we have tended to study them in the past
- the need to work with people in other disciplines such as sport sociologists, exercise physiologists and IT and to view sport and exercise synoptically.[4]

12.3 Personality

Keywords

➤ body image
➤ character
➤ EPI/Q
➤ extroversion
➤ intellect
➤ interactionist approach
➤ introversion
➤ models
➤ neuroticism
➤ psychoanalytic theory
➤ psychodynamic theory
➤ psychometric methods
➤ physique
➤ roles
➤ significant others
➤ social learning theory
➤ stability
➤ state measures
➤ STEN score
➤ self-concept
➤ self-esteem
➤ self-report questionnaires
➤ 16PF
➤ source traits
➤ surface traits
➤ temperament
➤ trait
➤ trait theories

What is personality and why is it important that we understand it? As a player, captain, teacher or coach, you need to be aware of how different people are and how they react differently to the same situation. Some people train with single-minded determination; others are easily distracted or 'put off' by difficulties. Some players react badly to defeat or apparent unfairness; others seem to take it all in their stride. Knowing and understanding yourself and the people you train and play with is likely to help you get the best out of yourself and others.

> **KEY POINTS**
>
> • Personality has been defined as the combination of a person's characteristics which makes him/her unique.
>
> • Eysenck[5] suggests that personality is the 'more or less stable and enduring organisation of a person's character, temperament, intellect and physique which determines the unique adjustment to the environment'.

Investigation 12.1 To derive a common-sense definition of personality

Method: Work in groups of three or four. Think of a televised sport with which you are all familiar. Select two 'personalities' within that sport who contrast in the way they behave as they play.

Discussion: What is it about them that differs? What characteristics do they show through their responses to things that happen in the game or competition?

You have been talking about a pattern of characteristics which makes these two people different. You have begun to define their personalities.

Note the use of the term 'unique' in both the definitions in Key Points and the range of attributes which Eysenck says contributes to personality. Did the list of characteristics that you produced in Investigation 12.1 include examples from each of these headings? Note, also, that Eysenck claims that personality determines how people react to their surroundings.

The structure of personality

There are many different theories about what personality is and how it develops. A good review, which considers those theories most applicable to sport and physical activity, can be found in Cox.[6] Most current theories view personality as being structured in 'levels' or 'layers'. These levels refer to how deeply rooted a particular personality trait is in our psyche. Figure 12.1 illustrates this structure. It represents an individual who, as part of his/her psychological core is highly achievement oriented, wants to succeed in everything. As a games player this gives him/her a tendency to show aggressiveness when under pressure. This is known as the typical response. When made captain, however, this drive to achieve remains (it is stable and enduring) but becomes transferred to the need for the team to have a good model, so the aggressiveness disappears (role-related behaviour). This level is the least stable of the three; you can probably think of instances when a sportsperson has acted 'out of character' or reverted to previous habits.

Theories of personality

There are a number of different theories of personality, which relate to the different levels of Figure 12.1. They each take a somewhat different approach because (a) personality is a complex, multifaceted concept and (b) psychologists have studied it using different methods. It is useful to understand them all and then to decide

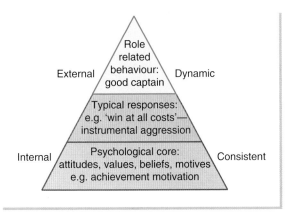

Fig. 12.1 The structure of personality.

KEY POINTS

- Personality can only be inferred from behaviour or from what a person tells us about him/herself.

- In Figure 12.1, we can see evidence of the aggressiveness and the good behaviour model, but the underlying achievement motivation is abstract.

which you think best describes and explains the particular event or behaviour that you are interested in.

Psychodynamic/psychoanalytic theories

The term 'psychodynamic' has two main meanings in psychology:

1. a theory that emphasises that people are dynamic and subject to change
2. any theory where the central concept is drive.

Psychodynamic theories are based on the idea that subconscious processes affect behaviour. Though it has been very influential in mainstream psychology, this group of theories has, to date, been little used in sport psychology, except in Scandinavia. There are three possible reasons for this:

1. the theories deal largely with unconscious drives, which are difficult to positively identify
2. therefore experienced, qualified, clinical psychoanalysts are needed to work with performers and
3. most of the recent studies are reported in Scandinavia and therefore not read by British and North American sport psychologists.[7]

The best known of the psychodynamic theories is Freudian psychoanalytic theory. Freud suggests that the personality is made up of three interacting systems (Figure 12.2).

The **id** is innate and consists of our basic instincts to seek pleasure and avoid pain. It is constantly trying to assert itself. The **superego** is the moral part of our personality, developed through socialisation. It consists of our conscience, which distinguishes right from wrong, and our ego ideal (the high standards we aspire to). The **ego** is the mediator between the id and the superego. It deals with the reality of living in a social world where we cannot always have what we want, but in trying to control the id, internal conflicts are often set up. Sometimes these conflicts are dealt with by the person setting up defence mechanisms. A defence mechanism is an unconscious strategy that protects our conscious mind from anxiety. Freud suggests that defence mechanisms act by distorting our perception of reality so that we are better able to cope with the situation (Figure 12.3).

Everyone uses defence mechanisms. They act like the body's white blood cells, resisting the infection of anxiety. But as with white blood cells, they can sometimes turn against the individual and themselves become harmful.[7] This is known as adaption and

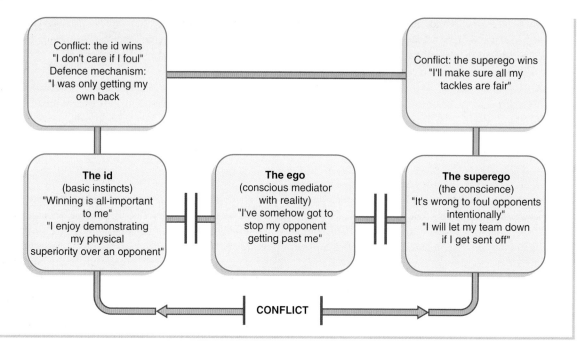

Fig. 12.2 Freudian psychoanalytic theory.

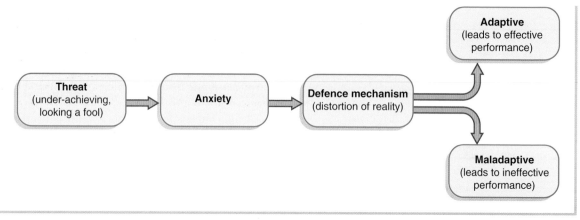

Fig. 12.3 Defence mechanisms in sport.

maladaption and is shown in Figure 12.3. For example, a gymnast is worried about her beamwork; there's a move in the routine that is difficult and she sometimes falls in attempting it. Her subconscious defence mechanism is to repress the fear. If this allows her to focus on important cues in the routine and to remember her coach's advice she is likely to give a good performance (adaptive defence). If the repression leads her to avoid practising the move sufficiently or to refuse to attend to the build-up of the move in the sequence, the move is likely to continue to pose problems (maladaptive defence).

A number of defence mechanisms have been identified and related to sport contexts by Apitzsch & Berggren.[8] Since competitive sport often presents anxiety-producing situations, the concept of defence mechanisms may prove to be useful. It is therefore important for coaches to realise that not all performer behaviour is under conscious control and can be managed by rational motivational strategies. We see this, for example, when a highly trained professional footballer who has already received a yellow card commits a second serious foul at a crucial stage in the game and is sent off. 'Why did he do that?' ask his manager, his teammates and the crowd. Psychodynamic theory suggests that at that moment, his basic instincts were stronger than any conscious knowledge of the implications of what he was doing.

Trait theories

A **trait** is a general, underlying, enduring predisposition to behave in a particular way each time a given situation occurs. For example, if we always feel nervous before a competition we could be said to possess the trait of 'competitive anxiety'. Trait theories assume that our personality is made up of many traits. Two theorists in particular, Eysenck and Cattell, suggested that these traits are organised in a hierarchical way (Figure 12.4). Their research led to a model of personality in which those traits that seem to cluster together are given a label that summarises a group of behaviours. For example, think of a sportsperson whom you would label as 'extrovert'. Now list some words which describe his/her behaviour and which define the term 'extrovert' in this case. Did you think of words like outgoing, confident, talkative, publicity seeking?

Cattell[9] identified 171 behaviours, which he believed we all exhibit to a greater or lesser extent. He grouped these into 16 clusters, which he labelled source traits or first-order (primary) factors. Certain of these primary traits then form further clusters, e.g. high anxiety–low anxiety, as shown in Figure 12.5. Cattell called these surface traits or second-order (secondary) factors. It was these that Eysenck[10] was most interested in.

Eysenck identifies second-order factors or types; the two most usually referred to are extroversion and neuroticism (Figure 12.6). **Neuroticism** is associated with emotionality and is characterised by a tendency to worry, to exhibit physical symptoms associated with anxiety and to experience unstable mood states. Its opposite construct is **stability**. **Extroversion** is a tendency to be outgoing, sociable and to enjoy physical action; **introversion** is its opposite.

Type A and Type B personality theory is a more recent addition to the trait approach. This contrasts two personality types. The Type A personality is characterised by impatience, competitiveness, anger and hostility and a sense of always working against the clock. The Type B personality is characterised by a relaxed approach to life, tolerance and a lack of competitiveness. These types were developed in relation to health research and it was found that Type A people were more prone to stress-related heart disease. Research that has been done in relation to sport and these two types has been largely inconclusive, though common sense would lead one to think that successful contact sport participants would be more likely to be Type A than Type B. However, the findings of previous trait research lead us to be wary of stereotyping in terms of sport personalities.

Trait theory was very important in the early years of sport personality research, largely because it provided a straightforward way of assessing personality (by means of self-report questionnaires) which sport

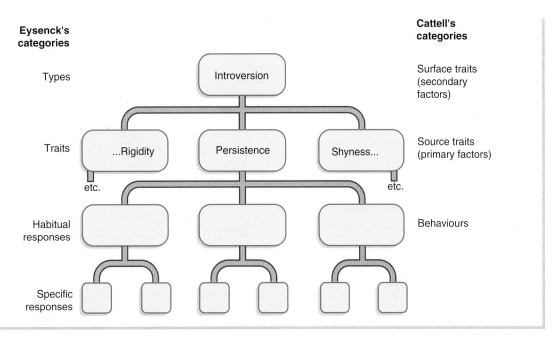

Fig. 12.4 Eysenck's and Cattell's hierarchical models of personality.

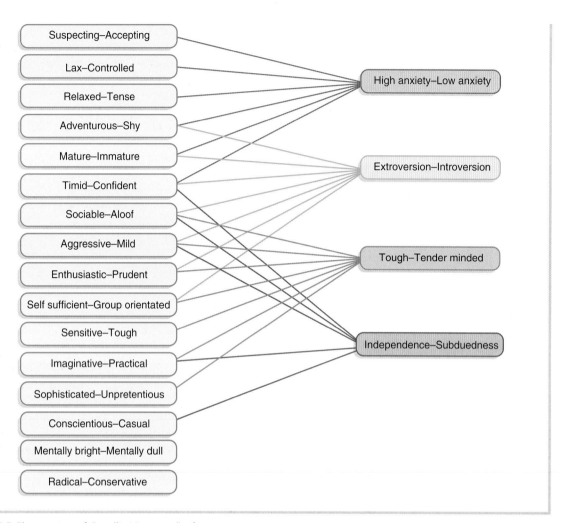

Fig. 12.5 The structure of Cattell's 16 personality factors.

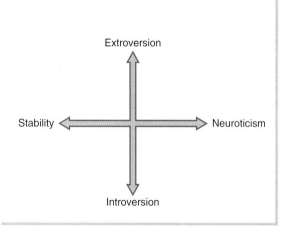

Fig. 12.6 Personality dimensions: extroversion and neuroticism.

psychologists and coaches could use with their athletes. However, although the tests themselves have been shown to be valid and reliable, they do not appear to predict behaviour consistently. For example, a young swimmer might be confident and sociable within his sport and with his friends in the club, but shy and lacking in confidence when required to make a speech at a club function. His core personality is probably somewhere between shy and confident, depending on how he views himself. Because psychologists like to use measures of personality to try and predict behaviour, this lack of predictive validity is a problem. Another problem with trait theory is that it tends to suggest that personality is innate, i.e. we inherit a predisposition to develop certain traits, which largely determine our behaviour. Eysenck's evidence for this comes from research that relates introversion and extroversion with physiological functioning. Critics of trait theory refute this and claim that we learn our behaviour from how we interact with our environment.

Interactionist approaches

Most sport psychologists today acknowledge the existence of traits and the fact that traits to some extent determine behaviour, but recognise that their effects can be modified by particular situations. They take an interactionist approach (Figure 12.7). This can be summarised as saying that behaviour (B) is a function (f) of both the person (Personality, P) and the environment (e): $B = f(Pe)$.

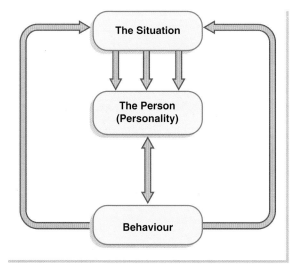

Fig. 12.7 Personality, behaviour and the situation: an interactionist model.

Social learning theory

Social learning theory explains behaviour in terms of our reactions to specific situations. An extreme view of this is stimulus–response (S–R) theory, which we studied in Chapter 11. S–R theory suggests that our behaviour is controlled by reinforcement alone; personality plays no part in the process. Bandura's social learning theory[11] is not so extreme and acknowledges the role of personality in behaviour, in so far as a person comes to a situation with certain preconceptions. Bandura claims that we learn to deal with situations by observing others (or by observing the results of our own behaviour on others) and by modelling our own behaviour on what we have seen. Social approval or disapproval reinforces our responses. Thus behaviour is determined largely by the situation and the role of personality is played down. You should note, therefore, that social learning theory is not a theory of personality but a theory about behaviour.

Humanist theories

Humanist theories of personality arose as a reaction to the mechanistic and deterministic view of people and their behaviour offered by the psychoanalysts and the behaviourists (see Chapter 11). Humanism deals with the person as a whole and is interested in the **self-concept** and **self-esteem** (see p. 365). Humanists believe that people are innately loving, creative, ready to learn and in control of their own destinies. It recognises that the environment in which people live may frustrate these innate tendencies and thus the theories are also interactionist.

One of the most influential humanist psychologists was Carl Rogers. He developed client-centred therapy, the basis of which is that people should establish their own goals rather than having these imposed on them. This approach has been widely adopted in counselling. Coaches and teachers who believe their role is to help young people make their own decisions (e.g. about performance goals or training programmes), rather than dictating to them, are using a humanistic approach to their work.

A second important concept within humanistic psychology is that of subjective experience. Subjective experience is the way in which each individual perceives and interprets what is happening to them; this may or may not reflect reality. A good coach or team manager will recognise and take into account the existence of subjective experience, for example by acknowledging that watching a game or event will not be the same as participating in it. What looks possible to achieve from the bench may not appear so straightforward to those on the field.

How is personality assessed?

Just as there are many theories of personality, so there are several distinct ways in which personality can be assessed. The most widely used in coaching, of course,

---

ACTIVITY 12.1 INTERACTIONIST THEORY

A young tennis player shows promise, but worries about playing in important tournaments and underperforms in these situations. Her coach works with her on anxiety management strategies and in her next tournament she wins. How would you explain this, using interactionist theory?

is **observation** – 'getting to know you'. Good coaches and teachers observe their athletes carefully, noting when they are consistent in their behaviour and when the situation seems to affect what they do, i.e. taking into account both traits and situations. Good coaches or teachers are good communicators and, particularly, good listeners and so they get an all-round understanding of their athletes.

Sport research, on the other hand, mostly uses **psychometric methods** which set out to quantify personality; to say, for example, just how extrovert someone is. This is normally done by means of self-report questionnaires.

Trait measures

Trait measures assess a person's general disposition to behave in a particular way. Some of these measures focus on a complete personality profile, e.g. Cattell's Sixteen Personality Factor Questionnaire (known as the **16PF**), which has been widely used in sport

research. This questionnaire, after considerable preliminary work, proved to be a valid and reliable measure of these 16 surface traits. The scoring system allows, if the researcher wishes, further grouping of the source traits into four surface traits or second-order (secondary) factors.

There are 141 statements in the 16PF questionnaire, each assessing a particular trait. The statements are similar to the following example.

I feel the need every now and then to engage in tough physical activity:

a) Yes
b) In between
c) No.

When the scoring of the questionnaire is completed, the subject has a standardised score out of 10 (known as a **STEN score**) on each of the 16 factors and his/her profile might look like that in Figure 12.8.

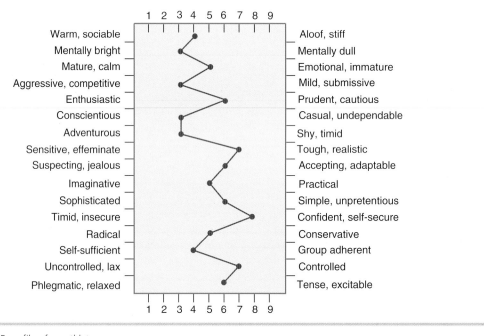

Fig. 12.8 The 16PF profile of an athlete.

Investigation 12.2   To analyse a 16PF profile

Method: Imagine you have collected data on an athlete's personality using the 16PF questionnaire and have constructed a profile as in Figure 12.8.

Observations: Analyse the profile, noting particularly those traits in which the athlete's scores fall outside the range 3.5–6.5. We consider the implications of scores such as these later in the section.

Eysenck developed a similar self-report questionnaire, shorter and with a 'Yes/No' answering format, in contrast to Cattell's three-point scale. This is known as the Eysenck Personality Inventory (or Questionnaire), the **EPI** or the EPQ. There is also a version for children. This measures the three traits continua of extroversion–introversion, neuroticism–stability and psychoticism.

Other trait measures which you may come across in your reading and which have been used in sport are the Profile of Mood States (POMS),[12] Nideffer's Test of Attentional and Interpersonal Style (TAIS),[13] Spielberger et al's State-Trait Anxiety Inventory (STAI)[14] and Martens' Sport Competition Anxiety Test (SCAT).[15] Examples of these kinds of tests can be found in the Teacher's Guide which accompanies this book.

State measures

As the interest in interactionist theory grew, there developed a number of situation-specific measures, designed to assess a person's state of mind at a particular moment in time and in a particular sport context. These are useful for sport psychologists who want to plot changes in an athlete's mental approach to competition, for example. Some such tests that you may come across in your further reading are the Competitive State Anxiety Inventory (CSAI-II)[16] and the Tennis Test of Attentional and Interpersonal Style (TTAIS).[17]

KEY POINTS

- Trait measures give information about an athlete's typical way of behaving in general. They are likely to reflect the 'psychological core' (see Figure 12.1).

- State measures give information about an athlete's state of mind at a particular moment and in a specific situation, i.e. 24 hours before the final of a major table tennis tournament.

The use of personality measures in sport

As in other walks of life, personality assessment can provide useful information to both the coach and the performer but psychological testing is an invasive process and must be subject to ethical guidelines.

ACTIVITY 12.2

Identifying confidence problems

You are a golf coach and an accredited sport psychologist (ASP). You are concerned about a young golfer whose putting goes well in practice but who becomes inconsistent in competition. You think you know him well; he is normally a confident, relaxed person and appears to enjoy competitions but you suspect he may lose confidence or concentration at crucial times in his game. Discuss how you might use (a) observation, (b) trait measures and/or (c) state measures to help identify the problem.

Note that the coach in Activity 12.2 is an accredited sport psychologist (ASP) and therefore has had training in the administration of tests. If coaches wish to make use of such tests they should always seek the advice of an ASP and be aware of the following:

- the limitations of the test being used
- how to interpret the results appropriately
- the ethical guidelines for test administration
- results of tests should always be used for the benefit of the performer and not for purposes of team selection
- the need to use both state and trait measures
- the advisability of using sport-specific tests whenever possible
- the importance of fully briefing the performer on the reasons for the test, the use of the results and the results themselves.

Further information about psychological measurement, including discussion about the validity and reliability of testing, is given in the chapter dealing with the project on the CD-ROM.

What does the research tell us about personality?

During the 1960s and 1970s a great deal of research was carried out, using mostly Cattell's and Eysenck's inventories, into the relationship between personality and sport. Sport scientists were interested in answers to three questions.

1. Is there an athletic 'type'?
2. Can success in sport be predicted from measures of personality?

3. Does personality change as a result of participation in sport?

Is there an athletic type?

Do certain groups of sportspeople, performers or recreationists differ from the norm in terms of their personalities (for example, do they have scores which fall outside the 3.5–6.5 range in the 16PF)? The results of research into these questions are very unclear, largely because of theoretical and methodological problems associated with the research itself. The most clearcut evidence seems to emerge when second-order factors are considered. A good review of the great wealth and variety of data is given in Butt.[18] When studying research data we must remember that it is mean scores that are reported and within any group of athletes, there is a wide variety of personalities. However, what does seem to emerge is that both male and female sportspeople show traits of extroversion, dominance, enthusiasm, confidence, assertiveness and high activity levels.[18]

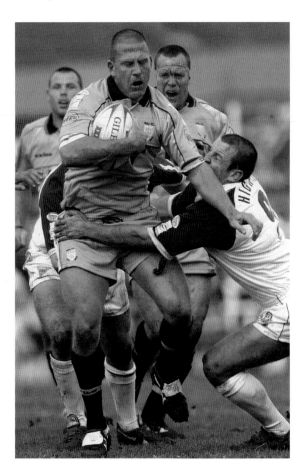

Fig. 12.9 Sportspeople show traits of dominance, confidence, assertiveness and high activity levels.

Is a particular personality profile necessary for performance at the top level?

In some countries psychological testing is used, in addition to measures of performance and body composition, to identify children who are suitable for intensive training in a sport. You may be aware of the increasing use of personality testing in the selection of people for executive positions in industry and commerce in the UK. Evidence to support such selection processes is not conclusive, however; there is no consistent personality profile that discriminates athletes from non-athletes.[19] Morgan,[20] using the Profile of Mood States (POMS) inventory, identified a relationship between athletic success and mental health, suggesting that successful athletes have a significantly more positive mental health profile than either less successful athletes or the general population (Figure 12.10). Morgan's work has been used to justify the use of POMS to identify potential champions but as with other personality measures, this would be inappropriate since (a) it was developed to identify mood changes and (b) there is some uncertainty about the generalisability of Morgan's findings.[21]

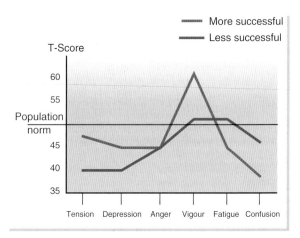

Fig. 12.10 The 'iceberg profile'.

Does personality change as a result of participating in sport?

Morgan's research[20] begs the question as to whether athletes are successful because they have a particular personality profile or whether their success has given them this profile. As with other questions, research has not yet given us an adequate answer. Traditionally, sport and tough physical activity have been associated with the development of 'character' and 'team spirit'.

Recent research into exercise participation (jogging, aerobics, swim-fit programmes, etc.) does suggest beneficial effects of regular exercise on psychological well-being as well as for physical improvement. Girdano et al[22] claim that personality characteristics associated with stress, tension and cardiovascular disease can be modified by exercise programmes, with resulting improvements in health; Sonstroem[23] has shown that improvements in self-esteem have been associated with exercise. Self-esteem as a particular aspect of personality is discussed in the next section. Willis & Campbell[24] offer a useful review of exercise participation research in much more detail than can be given here.

On the whole, the traditional research relating personality and performance has been inconclusive and recently, sport psychologists have turned their attention to the mental strategies which successful performers use. These strategies are more a function of skills and training than of personality and are dealt with in Chapter 13 in the section on mental preparation for performance.

The self concept

An interesting element of personality, and one that certainly affects the way in which we participate, learn and perform in physical activities, is the self concept. This is a particularly important aspect of **humanist theories** of personality. As you read you will find many different terms and definitions in this area. We confine ourselves to two: self concept and self-esteem.

- The self concept is the descriptive picture we have of ourselves. It includes physical attributes,

> **KEY POINTS**
>
> - Research has had little success in predicting achievement in sport from personality profiles.
>
> - There is some evidence of particular personality profiles being associated with specific sports, but this is inconclusive.
>
> - There is stronger evidence that successful athletes have a more positive mental health profile than less successful athletes or the general population.
>
> - There is evidence of a relationship between psychological well-being and regular exercise participation.

attitudes, abilities, roles and emotions. It is important to remember that it represents how we see ourselves, which may not reflect reality or the way others see us.

- Self-esteem is the extent to which we value ourselves. Again, this may or may not match up to the expectations of others. For example, a player may take pride in an ability to tackle hard, whereas the referee and the coach may see it as unnecessary aggression.

Several theories that describe the structure of the self concept exist, summarised in Fox.[25] In this text we assume that the self concept is built in levels, as illustrated in Figure 12.11.

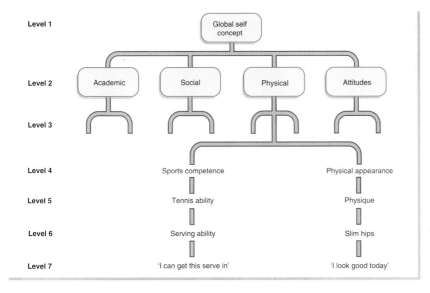

Fig. 12.11 The structure of the physical self concept.

The development of the self concept

Developmental psychology tells us that the newly born child cannot distinguish between itself and its environment. Growth and maturation bring an increasing awareness of self, of other people and of control over the surroundings and events. At this point the self concept comes into existence. Some aspects of the self concept are enduring; others change as our experiences, our roles and our position in society change.

Factors which influence the self concept

Figure 12.12 represents the internal and external factors that give rise to a particular self concept and self-esteem. Some are objective – they are aspects of yourself which can be measured or readily agreed upon. But others are socially developed and depend upon how you and other people view or value the objective characteristics.

Let us consider in a little more detail the social or interactional view of the development of the self concept, referred to in Figure 12.12. We are interested in how other people see us and we take note of their reactions to things we do and say. In this sense other people act as a mirror to reflect us and we internalise what we perceive. If you have received praise and encouragement as you learned to participate in physical activity, then you are likely to have begun to think of yourself as good at sport, dance or gymnastics.

As this picture of self begins to clarify we ask ourselves, 'Well, how good am I?'. We start to compare ourselves with others to see how we 'measure up'. Interestingly, we appear to be sensible about this and in order to obtain a reasonable evaluation, we do not compare ourselves with others who are 'out of our league'. For example, if you are a good college tennis player you will, for the moment, compare yourself with your teammates and those above you in the club ladder, not the Wimbledon champion!

Roles

Our roles in society determine very much how others see and react to us. A role is a set of behaviours associated with our position in a family, group or organisation. The longer and more fully we play a particular role, the more we internalise it. You are interested in sport or dance or other forms of physical activity. Others begin to think of you as a sportsperson, dancer or climber. You may like the idea of being seen in this role and reinforce it by, for example, wearing clothes that identify you with it and adopting the associated role behaviours.

Part of learning to play a particular role is the way in which we identify with others who we see to be playing the role successfully (this is assuming that we want to). Sports heroes act as models in this respect, which is partly why sports authorities believe it to be

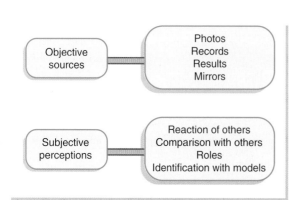

Fig. 12.12 Factors affecting the self concept and self-esteem.

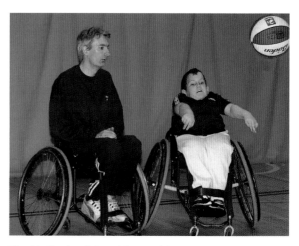

Fig. 12.13 Identifying with a model is important in developing a sport self concept.

important that players at the top of a sport behave in a way which 'sets a good example' to youngsters.

Investigation 12.3 To identify aspects of role

Method: Each member of the group makes a list of the roles they play; examples might be sister, team captain, student. Select six or so, which are common to all members of the group. Each person then writes down the behaviours that are inherent in that role. In groups of two or three, devise a 'role play' to illustrate one of the roles but which does not directly name it. Other members of the group have to identify the role being acted out.

Discussion: What were the behaviours and attitudes that most obviously characterised each role?

	Perceived competence	Perceived importance	Self-esteem
Basketball	L	L	O
Fitness	L	H	L
Gymnastics	H	L	O
Dance	H	H	H

Key:
L = Low rating
H = High rating
O = Little effect

Fig. 12.14 The effects of perceived competence and perceived importance on self-esteem.

The establishment of self-esteem

The process described above allows us to develop a particular view of ourselves and also to place a value on that view. If the majority of our experiences with people and of events are enjoyable and satisfying we develop a positive self concept and high self-esteem. If we often feel 'put down' and incompetent, we may have a correspondingly negative self concept and/or low self-esteem. In fact, it is not quite as simple as this for two reasons.

- Self-esteem is a reflection of how significant others value us. We do not seem to be so interested in the evaluations of people who are not important to us. So if parents, teachers or coaches treat our efforts with respect and support, self-esteem rises independently of how competent we actually are or even perceive ourselves to be. People are significant at different periods of our life; early on, it is parents but later the evaluations of our peers become much more important to us.
- Self-esteem in relation to a particular activity or attribute is a reflection of how important we see it to be. So friends laughing at you for being 'hopeless' at soccer when you are not very interested in it does not have as much effect on your self-esteem as it would if you really wanted to be seen as a good player. This is illustrated in Figure 12.14.

The effects of levels of self-esteem on learning

Research has shown that differing levels of self-esteem give rise to differing personality profiles. People with

high self-esteem tend to be optimistic, resilient, adventurous and to enjoy challenge. People with low self-esteem tend to lack confidence, to be self-protective and to be critical of others. It must be remembered that self-esteem can be specific to one particular activity or area of life or it can be global, but high or low global self-esteem colours all our ideas about ourselves.

Once self-esteem is established, it predisposes us to view new experiences in particular ways. This is known as attribution and is considered in more detail in Section 12.6, but we should note the contribution of the self concept to this process. This is shown in Figure 12.15. This relationship, together with the personality factors we know to be associated with high and low self-esteem, suggests that self-esteem is an important variable in learning and that self concept is important in the avoidance of or adherence to physical activity. It seems to be a cyclical relationship (Figure 12.16).

	Existing positive self concept	Existing negative self concept
Positive experience of PE	Self concept enhanced	Self concept may become positive
Negative experience of PE	Self concept may become negative	Self concept reinforced

Fig. 12.15 The relationship between experiences and the self concept.

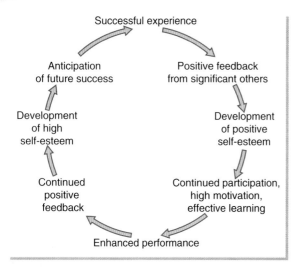

Fig. 12.16 The self concept wheel.

KEY POINTS

- A significant way in which individuals differ in how they learn and perform is in their personalities and the way they view themselves.
- Research into personality and sport has tended, in the past, to focus on finding an 'athletic type', but more recently sport psychologists have been trying to find ways of using sportspeople's self-knowledge to help them get the best out of themselves.
- The extent to which we value ourselves seems to play a large part in effective learning and a satisfying performance.

If this is the case and if we believe that physical activity is something which everyone should have the opportunity of enjoying and being successful in, then what are the implications for the way in which we present, teach and coach physical activity?

Discuss this question in terms of the:

- range and type of activities offered to young people
- teaching and coaching styles used
- place of competition in physical education
- place of fitness training in physical education
- role of dance and adventure activities in physical education
- use of award schemes, e.g. Royal Life Saving Society.

Review questions

1. Define the term 'personality' and outline the trait and social learning approaches to personality theory.
2. Why has it been difficult to obtain consistent information from research about the relationship between personality and sports participation?
3. Name one sport-specific and one general personality questionnaire. Which might a coach find most useful and why?
4. List six ways in which a coach might use personality theory to help an athlete during training and competition.
5. Define the terms 'self concept' and 'self-esteem'. How does exercise participation affect self concept and self-esteem?

Exam-style questions

1. **a.** What do we mean by the term personality? Why is it important for sports psychologists to know about personality? (*3 marks*)
   b. Eysenck identified two dimensions of personality as in Figure 12.17.
      i. Describe the trait approach to personality. (*2 marks*)
      ii. What do the traits extroversion and stability mean? (*2 marks*)
   c. From Figure 12.17 describe the characteristics of players A and B. (*4 marks*)
   d. By using an example from sport, outline the social learning approach to personality. (*3 marks*)
   e. What do we mean by the interactionist approach to personality? (*2 marks*)
   (*Total 16 marks*)

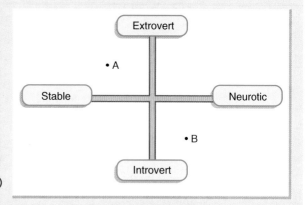

Fig.12.17 Adapted from *Trait theory* by Eysenck, 1975.

2. Hollander[67] viewed personality as a structure with layers of influence. Using examples from sport, explain Hollander's structure of personality. (*8 marks*)

3. What is the iceberg profile and how does it relate to the personalities of elite athletes? (*4 marks*)

4. A rowing coach wants to improve the performance of his squad. In doing so he would want to consider psychological and physiological factors. The coach wants to identify the personality types of the squad members.

a. What are the limitations of using personality tests? (*2 marks*)
b. Some rowers behave differently between competition and training. Explain this pattern of behaviour, in terms of the interactionist theory of personality. (*2 marks*)
c. What do you understand by the term **motivation**? Explain the different types. (*3 marks*)
d. How could a coach use the different types of motivation with a group of beginners? (*2 marks*)

(*Total 9 marks*)

12.4 Attitudes in sport

Learning objectives

On completion of this section, you will be able to:

1. Define the term 'attitude' and describe how attitudes are measured; state the three components of attitude and indicate how attitudes are developed.

2. Understand how prejudice and stereotyping can arise in sport contexts.

3. Show how attitudes in sport might be changed by means of persuasion and cognitive dissonance techniques.

Keywords

➤ affective component
➤ attitude
➤ attitude object
➤ behavioural component
➤ cognitive component
➤ cognitive dissonance
➤ persuasive communication
➤ scale
➤ stereotype

We saw in Section 12.3 how our 'core' personality is made up of a combination of attitudes, beliefs, values and motives. The study of attitudes in and to sport and physical education is important because of the way in which attitudes seem to influence our behaviour. Thus, if I feel angry about being constantly fouled by my opponent I may well behave aggressively towards her. More positively, if you believe it to be important to keep fit and enjoy exercise, and particularly if you intend to keep fit, then you are likely to participate in sport or an exercise programme regularly.

Definition of 'attitude'

Attitudes are a combination of the beliefs and feelings we have about **attitude objects**, which predispose us to behave in a certain way towards them. An attitude object might be an object (for example, a new team strip) or it might be a person/people, a situation, a place or a concept (for example, sportsmanship). The attitude we have towards a particular object usually leads us to be judgemental about it. We have a positive attitude or a negative attitude, i.e. we like something (or think it's good) or we dislike it. If we do not know very much about something, we are likely to have a neutral attitude towards it.

The three components of attitude: the triadic model

Some theorists (e.g. Triandis[26]) suggest that an attitude consists of three elements (Figure 12.18). The implication of this model is that an attitude consists of:

- a **cognitive** component – the knowledge and beliefs held about the attitude object, i.e. fitness training
- an **affective** component – the positive or negative feelings and emotions towards the attitude object, i.e. enjoyment of training
- a **behavioural** component – the intended behaviour towards the attitude object, i.e. attending training sessions regularly.

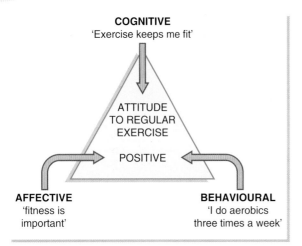

Fig. 12.18 The three components of attitude.

Development of attitudes

Attitudes are learned. They are 'organised through experience'.[27] They arise through direct experience or from other people or from a combination of the two. Fishbein & Ajzen[28] stress that attitudes form as soon as knowledge and beliefs about an object are present. As a variety of beliefs about an object are acquired, these often reinforce each other but sometimes conflict. For example, a young swimmer may be ambitious and believe that it is important to train hard, but friends may lead her to believe that training is getting in the way of her social life. Her experience of training is that it is unpleasant and tiring; thus her attitude to training is complex. The dominant attitude is dependent on the strength of the individual beliefs and the balance of positive and negative in the belief structure.

Socialisation is also an important determinant of attitude. We acquire many of our most deeply rooted attitudes when young from listening to and copying significant others such as parents/carers and peers. In order to become part of a particular society or group, it is important to us to hold and demonstrate the normal attitudes of that group, so there is a lot of pressure on people to acquire attitudes which correspond to those of the group. This is discussed later when considering prejudice and stereotyping in sport. However, attitudes can change or be changed, as knowledge and beliefs change or if the individual joins a group with different norms.

The interrelationship between beliefs, emotions and intended behaviour is usually quite strong. Thus, if you value physical fitness and you enjoy activity, then you intend to keep yourself fit. The relationship

between attitudes and actual behaviour is not as strong, though research does indicate that if you intend to do something, there is a likelihood that you will do it. Can you think of any examples from your own experience when having a particular attitude about something (a) means you usually act out that attitude and (b) does not necessarily mean you do anything about it?

Attitudes to sport and participation

Research into attitudes to and in sport (see[29]) has traditionally focused on establishing the views of particular groups about issues or situations. Some examples are:

- children – attitudes to their school PE programmes
- women – views on the availability of sport opportunities in their area
- athletes – attitudes to training
- teachers – attitudes to the physical and intellectual abilities of black children
- general attitudes to women in sport.

The results of this research show no general patterns of attitude to sport, i.e. it is not straightforward to predict attitudes to sport from other variables such as gender or age. Neither is it easy to predict participation or behaviour in sport from attitude. Recent research focuses on the relationship between attitudes to and participation in exercise and fitness programmes[30,31] but tends to show that it is practical issues, such as time and facilities, which affect 'staying with' or 'dropping out' of a fitness programme, as much as attitude or intention. Problems of consistency in research results may, however, be due to difficulties in attitude measurement; for example, some studies only focus on the cognitive element of an attitude or on the fact that research into the value of physical education in schools has shown generally positive attitudes of teachers, parents and pupils, though pupils are somewhat more critical of the content of the programme. Society seems to be becoming more egalitarian in its view of women in sport, though evidence of gender stereotyping still exists, as does racial stereotyping.

People with positive attitudes to sport and physical activity:

- have had some success in or satisfaction from participating
- believe in the value of the activity in promoting health and well-being
- have been encouraged by 'significant others'
- have opportunities to continue participation
- are likely to participate in physical activity regularly
- are likely to be willing to try new activities
- have a positive physical self concept.

People with negative attitudes to sport and physical activity:

- may have had negative experiences in sport or PE
- find sport frustrating or boring
- do not believe in its value for health and well-being
- lack encouragement or have been discouraged

- are unlikely to participate regularly, if at all
- have lifestyles that make regular physical activity difficult
- may have a negative physical self concept.

Sport stereotypes and prejudice

A stereotypical attitude is one that leads the holder to expect people characterised as belonging to a particular group to behave in a certain way. In sport this usually leads to expectations about what people are or are not able to achieve. Although stereotypes can be positive, negative stereotyping has been instrumental in holding back particular groups by limiting opportunity or access. This happens either because provision is not made for such groups or because the public (including coaches and teachers) have stereotypic attitudes which encourage low expectations. Examples of such negative stereotyping are or have been:

- women in contact, strength or endurance sports
- participation of the disabled in physical activity
- older age groups' interest and ability in sport
- participation of particular ethnic groups in specific sports or positions within teams.

Prejudice arises from stereotyping. A prejudice is an attitude based on inadequate knowledge and inflexible beliefs. It can be positive or negative. Can you think of some examples of positive and negative prejudice in sport?

Measurement of attitudes

Research into attitudes to sport is based on measurement of attitudes. This may be done in a variety of ways. Since attitude tends to be linked to behaviour, we can observe, record and analyse people's behaviour in situations that are likely to reflect their attitudes and then infer their attitudes from that behaviour. Can you think of some sport and non-sport examples of how you might do this? For example, how might you collect information about students' attitudes to the meals provided in your school or college canteen?

There are problems of validity with such methods, however, so the most usual form of attitude measurement is a scale. A scale is a questionnaire which has been carefully constructed to be valid and reliable and to give a score for an individual on a particular attitude. There are three major types of scales, named after their authors: **Thurstone scales**, **Likert scales** and **Osgood semantic differential scales**. They differ slightly in their construction but all consist of asking

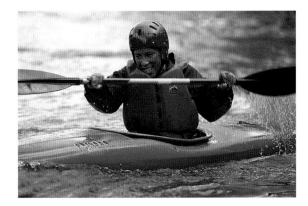

Fig. 12.19 People with positive attitudes to sport are likely to be willing to try new activities.

Investigation 12.4 To measure schoolchildren's attitudes to PE

Method: Obtain permission to gather data from a mixed class of school pupils (boys and girls) of any age, from your own school or a neighbouring one. Use the Likert scale below or construct your own. If you construct your own you should do a pilot study initially to choose those items which best differentiate the sample, i.e. produce both high and low scores. Do not include the scores on the questionnaire.

Make sure you understand how the scoring works; you must take the minus signs into account. The higher a positive score, the more positive is the pupil's attitude to PE.

Calculate each pupil's total attitude score and then calculate: (i) a whole group mean score; (ii) a boys' mean score and (iii) a girls' mean score.

1. What do you notice about the differences (if any) between these three means?
2. How might you explain them?
3. How could you improve the scale?

Attitudes to PE Questionnaire

For each statement, tick the extent to which you agree.

1. Most PE lessons are enjoyable
   - strongly agree (+2)
   - agree (+1)
   - don't know/neutral (0)
   - disagree (–1)
   - strongly disagree (–2)

2. I miss PE lessons whenever I can
   - strongly agree (–2)
   - agree (–1)
   - neutral (0)
   - disagree (+1)
   - strongly disagree (+2)

3. I want to get a good report in PE
   - strongly agree (+2)
   - agree (+1)
   - don't know/neutral (0)
   - disagree (–1)
   - strongly disagree (–2)

4. PE doesn't really teach you anything important
   - strongly agree (–2)
   - agree (–1)
   - don't know/neutral (0)
   - disagree (+1)
   - strongly disagree (+2)

---

respondents to indicate the extent to which they agree or disagree with a particular statement.

Osgood's semantic differential scale asks respondents to rate the attitude object on a series of continua between bipolar constructs, such as:

Gymnastics lessons are:

boring	7	6	5	4	3	2	1	*fun*
easy	1	2	3	4	5	6	7	*hard*

(scoring not included in questionnaire)

Gill[32] gives a useful comparison of the different types. Investigation 12.4 contains an informal example of a Likert scale.

As with personality scales, the most useful published scales for researchers interested in attitudes to sport are those that have been constructed with a sport-specific attitude object. Examples of these are:

- Kenyon's Attitudes towards Physical Activity[33]
- Sonstroem's Physical Estimation and Attraction Scale[34]
- Smoll & Schutz's Children' Attitudes to Physical Activity.[35]

There are two important points to remember about attitude scales.

- They appear simple to construct, but in fact it is very difficult to ensure that you have composed a valid and reliable measure. If you wish to use an attitude scale in an investigation it is sensible to use one that has already been constructed and validated for the attitude which you are interested in.
- Although scales are composed of a number of questions, each scale represents the same attitude (though you may have more than one scale in a questionnaire). Ensuring that you are only dealing with one attitude, with the questions you have constructed, is one of the problems that affects validity.

Changing attitudes

PE teachers are familiar with the need to change negative attitudes towards physical activity into positive ones. For coaches and activity leaders, this is less of a problem but they may find it necessary to work on changing attitudes, for example to winning and losing or to aggressive behaviour.

Persuasive communication

Persuasive communication theory suggests that for an attitude to change, the person must attend to, understand, accept and retain the message.[36] Persuasion to change an attitude in sport works best when:

- The coach/teacher or significant other is perceived as:
  - expert
  - trustworthy
- and the message is:
  - clear
  - unambiguous
  - appropriately balanced between emotion and logic, pros and cons.

Cognitive dissonance theory

Cognitive dissonance theory[37] claims that people need to be consistent not only in the three components of attitude (knowledge, feelings and behaviour) but also *within* the knowledge element. If any elements conflict, then dissonance is set up. For example, you might reject the need for instrumental aggression in your sport (belief 1) but think that in order to win against a particular team, you must physically intimidate your opponent (belief 2). The two beliefs conflict; they are **dissonant**. You resolve the dissonance by telling yourself that it's all right to play hard against these particular opponents because they play that way too, so that is what you do (modification of belief 1).

In this situation a coach might use cognitive dissonance theory by recreating the conflict: 'Skilful players don't need to resort to that sort of behaviour – they can win the ball without it. You're a skilful player, so why are you playing like a thug?' The coach is trying to persuade the player to resolve the dissonance by changing belief 2 and thus the behavioural outcome. Changing attitudes in this way is not always easy because humans have a tendency to maintain attitudes once they are formed.

KEY POINTS

Gill[32] specifies two methods of attitude change:

- persuasive communication
- cognitive dissonance theory.

ACTIVITY 12.3 CHANGING ATTITUDES TO TRAINING

You are a swimming coach. Your squad believe that the only way they will be successful is to train in the pool for longer and longer periods. You believe that it is the quality of training that counts and you want them to cut down on their pool time and do more general conditioning and cognitive strategy work. Discuss how you would use persuasion theory and cognitive dissonance theory to change their attitude to training.

Review questions

1. Define the term 'attitude'. How are attitudes measured?

2. Describe the three components of attitudes.

3. What is meant by the terms 'stereotype' and 'prejudice' in attitude terms? Give some examples from sport.

4. Describe the 'persuasion' and 'cognitive dissonance' methods of attitude change.

Exam-style questions

1. a. What do we mean by the term attitude? (*1 mark*)
   b. We often refer to someone as having a positive attitude in sport. Using the triadic model, describe the characteristics of a positive attitude. (*3 marks*)
   c. What factors influence our attitudes? (*4 marks*)
   (*Total 8 marks*)

2. a. If you wished to change a young person's negative attitude to sport into a positive one, what strategies would you employ? Use psychological theory to back up your answer. (*4 marks*)
   b. What do we mean by the term prejudice and how does it manifest itself in sport? (*4 marks*)
   (*Total 8 marks*)

3. Observing behaviour is one method of measuring attitudes. What are the advantages and disadvantages of such a method? (*4 marks*)

12.5 Aggression in sport

Learning objectives

On completion of this section, you will be able to:

1. Define aggression and differentiate it from assertion.

2. Discuss theories of aggression: instinct, frustration-aggression and social learning.

3. Describe the antecedents of aggression in sport contexts and discuss ways in which aggression can be eliminated from sport.

Keywords

- aggression
- aggressive cue hypothesis
- assertiveness
- bracketed morality
- catharsis
- drive theory
- frustration–aggression theory
- hostile aggression
- instinct theory
- instrumental aggression
- interactional theory
- moral reasoning
- social learning theory

Violent behaviour in and associated with sport is currently attracting particular attention. As the rewards of winning become increasingly more substantial, at both professional and amateur levels, so emotions tend to run high and some players (and coaches) seem to believe that almost any means can justify the end – that of winning. That is not to say that this is a modern phenomenon (look at some of the photographs of mob games in the 'history' section of this book!) but the organisation and codification of games during the 19th century was designed to bring a spirit of control and 'fair play' to potentially violent activities.

Definitions of aggression

One of the main difficulties in studying this area from a psychological viewpoint is that there can be confusion in defining the term, since we use the word extensively in everyday life. A good starting point for your study of aggression would be to video a game and then identify, and discuss as a group, all the incidents of aggressive behaviour you find. This will raise some interesting questions.

- Is a strong but fair tackle aggressive?
- Is it aggressive to shout at the referee?
- What about throwing your racket to the ground after a bad line call?
- Are some soccer fans' chants aggressive?

The answers you arrive at will depend on how you define 'aggression'.

As sport psychologists, it is very important that we agree about what is an aggressive act and what is not, otherwise we find ourselves using the same words to study and talk about different phenomena. Sport psychology theorists are very clear.

Aggression is 'any form of behaviour directed toward the goal of harming or injuring another living being who is motivated to avoid such treatment'.[38] If we look carefully at this definition (which is universally accepted in sport psychology), we must conclude that any form of aggression in sport is wrong and not to be tolerated (assuming we believe that harming or injuring people is wrong). In only one official sport, boxing, is it a requirement that opponents hurt each other and in this case one could argue that by stepping into the ring, boxers are not 'seeking to avoid such treatment' and thus not behaving aggressively. This is a debatable point, however.

Because of the 'intention to harm' criterion, most people agree that aggressive behaviour in sport is wrong. This idea presents coaches, players and commentators with a problem; it also gives rise to some inconsistencies in the literature. Few coaches advocate or condone aggression, but they certainly *do* want players, particularly of contact invasion games, to play with commitment, effort and energy and to dominate the opposition by physical presence and forceful play. Different words are needed to describe this type of play. Husman & Silva[39] provide these by adapting an earlier psychological theory to sport. They differentiate between hostile aggression, instrumental aggression and assertiveness (see Figure 12.20).

Assertiveness is the use of legitimate force, energy and effort to achieve the purpose, with no intent to cause harm. If injury results, this is of course very regrettable but the act is not aggressive because there was no intent to injure. **Hostile (reactive/angry) aggression** is an act in which the main purpose is to hurt or harm the other person, purely for the satisfaction gained from inflicting hurt. **Instrumental (channelled) aggression** is an act that also intends to cause harm but in which the main aim is not to cause suffering but to achieve dominance or a point/goal.

Taking this view of aggression, we can see that the frequency of hostile aggressive acts between participants in sport is less than we might have at first thought. There may well be players who set out with the intent to injure, because their coach has told them to or because they have a score to settle or perhaps because they enjoy hurting others. But it is likely that

these are very much a minority. What is probably more worrying to governing bodies of sport, and to those who value the socialising potential of sport, is the apparent increase in **instrumental aggression**. Invasion games and contact sports offer plenty of scope for this kind of behaviour. The difficulty is that the boundaries between hostile aggression, instrumental aggression and assertiveness are not easy to distinguish. For example, you commit yourself to a sliding tackle in soccer: time it correctly and you have saved a certain goal and are applauded by all, even the opposition; a fraction of a second late and you have broken your opponent's leg. Only you really know whether you intended to hurt or not. For this reason, most contact sports penalise careless assertive play, i.e. where there is no apparent intention to hurt, but where assertive behaviour causes danger to others.

During play the task of sorting all this out falls to referees and officials; it becomes more difficult as cynical coaches (particularly in professional sport) train players in how to be aggressive without it being noticed and how to pretend to be a victim of aggression (e.g. feigning injury after 'diving' in soccer). Coaches and teachers must take as their main concern the task of encouraging non-aggressive behaviour in players and the control of anger and frustration which, as we shall see later, can lead to aggression. Sports commentators and interviewers should use unambiguous language when they are applauding assertive play, for there is no escaping the fact that, using the definitions of aggression that we have described, aggressive behaviour is wrong and should not be condoned under any circumstances.

Theories of aggression

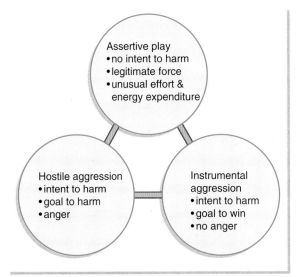

Fig. 12.20 Aggression and assertion from the player's perspective.

Instinct theories

Instinct theories[40] are based on the belief that aggression is innate and instinctive, developed through evolution to help us survive as a species. According to this assumption, we all from time to time experience a build-up of aggressive energy, which must be released in some way. Instinct theorists see sport as an appropriate way of dissipating pent-up aggression; it acts as a **catharsis**. The word 'catharsis' derives from psychoanalytic theory (see Section 12.3) and means the expression of repressed feelings (aggressive energy) through an acceptable medium (sport), leading to a release of tension and a feeling of well-being. This is an interesting idea but it does not have general recognition, either in theory or in terms of evidence. From your own experience, what flaws can you see in it or do you agree with the idea of 'sport as catharsis'?

Frustration–aggression theory

The frustration–aggression hypothesis[41] is one of the 'drive' theories (see Section 12.6). It suggests that frustration (being blocked in the achievement of a goal) causes a drive to be aggressive towards the source of the frustration. As frustration mounts, so does the drive to remove the block to achievement. If this is an opponent and she/he is consistently beating you, then aggression automatically follows. This aggression is usually directed towards the source of the frustration. Where this is not possible (for example, if you are a soccer fan who has been physically restrained from getting anywhere near the referee), aggression may be directed elsewhere.

Whereas the frustration–aggression hypothesis idea makes sense in some examples, there are problems with it as a general theory. Can you suggest what these problems may be? In discussing this you should focus on the theory's claim that aggression automatically follows frustration.

Social learning theory

Social learning theory[42] claims that aggression is learned, in the same way that much other behaviour is learned. Bandura's experiments[42] suggest that aggression is learnt by observation and social reinforcement. This means that if players (and spectators) are frequently exposed to the aggressive behaviour of others, and particularly if they are praised or rewarded (either directly or indirectly) for their own aggression, then they are likely to develop aggressive responses to some situations in sport. However, this theory also indicates a positive factor; an individual can also learn non-aggressive ways of dealing with the same situations; hence the importance of teachers and coaches establishing clear, unambiguous behavioural codes for themselves and their players, so helping players to deal positively with sources of frustration. This theory continues to generate scientific support and is readily applied in sport contexts.

Revised frustration–aggression theory: the agressive cue hypothesis

Berkowitz[43] combined the original frustration–aggression theory with social learning theory to formulate an aggressive cue hypothesis. This theory is represented in Figure 12.21. This suggests that frustration increases the likelihood of anger, which in turn creates a 'readiness' for aggression. This readiness is mediated, however, by social learning. The important point here is that anger is not a drive (which

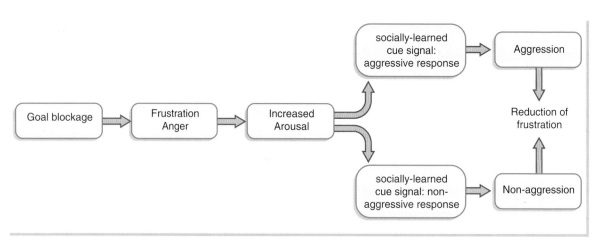

Fig. 12.21 The aggressive cue hypothesis.

has to be resolved), but an emotion which people can learn to deal with. Thus aggression only occurs as a response to frustration if that is the response which has been observed, reinforced and socially learned. If alternative responses have been learned (for example, changing tactics or using stress management strategies), then aggression is not the automatic outcome.

ACTIVITY 12.4 AGGRESSION

View a video of aggressive and/or assertive behaviour in a sport context. Using the four theories described in the text, speculate on the causes of the behaviour that you have seen. Did you judge the behaviour to be assertive, hostile aggression or instrumental aggression?

Causes of aggression in sport

Cox[6] cites two main causes of aggression.

- **Physiological arousal**. Research has shown that to feel anger towards another person, the individual must be highly motivated and thus physiologically aroused and ready for action. There is thus an increased danger of aggression in sports where high pre-game arousal is encouraged, such as invasion team games.
- **Underdeveloped moral reasoning**.[44] This theory suggests that players with low levels of moral reasoning are more likely to be aggressive than players with well-developed morality. Bredemeier[44] concludes that participation in sport in which aggressive behaviour is tacitly condoned may retard players' moral development because it teaches a confusing double standard ('aggression is wrong in real life, but OK in sport'), known as **bracketed morality**.

More specific causes of aggressive behaviour amongst players have been listed by Cox[6] and Weinberg & Gould[19] and are summarised below.

- High environmental temperature
- Home or away
- Embarrassment
- Losing
- Pain
- Unfair officiating

- Playing below capability
- Large score difference
- Low league standing
- Later stage of play
- Reputation of opposition ('get your retaliation in first'!)

Eliminating or preventing aggressive behaviour

Coaches, teachers, officials, parents and players themselves have a responsibility to help prevent and eliminate aggression in sport, while maintaining a healthy 'will to win'. It is important that young players are taught that aggression as we have defined it is wrong; there should be no 'mixed messages'. Equally, coaching should include plenty of opportunity to learn to be forcefully assertive in the game; this is a skill, to be developed alongside all other game skills. Young players should be taught anger management strategies.

Coaches may need to talk to colleagues and parents to ensure that they understand how to respond appropriately. Professionals who appear frequently in the media have a particular responsibility because they are the models whom young players seek to emulate; they set the standard. Spectator aggression, particularly in large, partisan crowds, is a broad issue and has its roots in social issues that may be only indirectly associated with the game itself. However, evidence shows that spectators are more likely to demonstrate physical and extreme verbal aggression if:

- players are aggressive to each other
- the officiating is perceived as poor or biased
- alcohol is available prior to and during the game
- spectator accommodation is overcrowded
- there is opportunity for racial or national abuse
- the crowd is composed largely of adult males.

The International Society of Sport Psychology (ISSP) has recently produced the following recommendations to combat aggression and violence in sport.

1. Management should make fundamental penalty revisions so that rule-violating behaviour results in punishments that have greater punitive value than potential reinforcement.
2. Management must ensure proper coaching of teams, particularly at junior levels, which emphasises a fair-play code of conduct among participants.
3. Management should ban the use of alcoholic beverages at sporting events.

4. Management must make sure facilities are adequate regarding catering and spacing needs and the provision of modern amenities.

5. The media must place in proper perspective the isolated incidents of aggression that occur in sport, rather than making them 'highlights'.

6. The media should promote a campaign to decrease violence and hostile aggression in sport, which should also involve the participation and commitment of athletes, coaches, management, officials and spectators.

7. Coaches, managers, athletes, media, officials and authority figures (i.e. police) should take part in workshops on aggression and violence to ensure they understand the topic of aggression, why it occurs, the cost of aggressive acts and how aggressive behaviour can be controlled.

8. Coaches, managers, officials and the media should encourage athletes to engage in prosocial behaviour and punish those who perform acts of hostility.

9. Athletes should take part in programmes aimed at helping them reduce behavioural tendencies towards aggression. The tightening of rules, imposing of harsher penalties and changing reinforcement patterns are only parts of the answer to inhibiting aggression in sport. Ultimately the athlete must assume responsibility.[45]

ACTIVITY 12.5 DEALING WITH AGGRESSION

- Critically review the ISSP recommendations. What amendments would you make?

- Role play. A junior league team has experienced poor coaching for several years and has become frustrated by their lack of success and aggressive in their play. This aggression is being reinforced by a group of enthusiastic parents who are vocally aggressive themselves. A new young coach and assistant are appointed who deplore the behaviour of the players and parents. They start to work effectively with the players on dealing with frustration non-aggressively. The players start to respond well (though they are not entirely convinced). The coaches decide that they need to talk to the parents. A small group of students each take the role of coach or player or parent (there can be more than one of each). Role play the ensuing meeting, whereby the coaches try to persuade the parents to modify their own behaviour and not to reinforce aggression in the players.

Review questions

1. Give a definition of 'aggression'.

2. Differentiate between hostile aggression, instrumental aggression and assertiveness, using examples from sport.

3. Briefly outline the frustration–aggression (drive) theory of aggression and show how it has been modified by social learning theory.

4. How can coaches reduce the likelihood of aggression being shown by their athletes?

Exam-style questions

1. a. What do we mean by the term aggression in sports psychology? Give an example from a sport or game which would illustrate your answer. (*2 marks*)

   b. How would you distinguish between aggression and assertion? (*2 marks*)

   c. Some team players display unwarranted aggression. What are the possible causes of such aggression? (*4 marks*)

   (*Total 8 marks*)

2. a. Explain in more detail what is meant by social learning when applied to aggression. (*4 marks*)

   b. How can aggressive tendencies be eliminated in a sports situation? (*4 marks*)

   (*Total 8 marks*)

3. a. Using examples from sport, briefly describe the difference between **aggression** and **assertion**. (*2 marks*)

   b. Using examples from sport, explain the **frustration–aggression** hypothesis. (*4 marks*)

   (*Total 6 marks*)

4. Discuss how theories of aggression can be applied to sport. (*4 marks*)

12.6 Motivation

Keywords

- ability
- achievement motivation
- attribution
- avoidance
- competence
- confidence
- continuity
- control
- direction
- effort
- emotional arousal
- expectancy
- extrinsic motivation
- extrinsic reward
- intensity
- intrinsic motivation
- law of effect
- learned helplessness
- locus of causality
- luck
- modelling
- motives
- need to achieve
- need to avoid failure
- pace
- performance
- performance accomplishments
- persistence
- personality
- play
- risk taking
- self-confidence
- self-efficacy
- self-fulfilling prophecy
- situational factors
- stability
- task difficulty
- verbal persuasion
- vicarious experience

Motives and motivation

In Chapter 11 we briefly considered motivation as a factor in the learning process. In this section we study it as a factor in performance, particularly in terms of the role it plays in people's continuing participation in physical activity. Motivation is considered briefly as a drive, but primarily in terms of personality/social perception variables, i.e. need to achieve, competitiveness and attribution processes.

Early ideas about motivation were based on drive theory. This was discussed in relation to stimulus-response learning theory in Section 11.3 and we will return to it again in considering arousal in Chapter 13. In this sense motivation can be defined as a psychological drive to fulfil a particular need. At a basic level, if we are hungry (need food) we experience a desire (drive/motivation) to find something to eat (fulfil the need). You will recognise that there is a strong instinctive emphasis in drive theory. Recent thinking about motivation focuses on why people think and behave as they do and thus personality factors and goal orientation (ambition) become important. Motivation has five components.[46]

- **Direction**. Acts of seeking out or avoiding situations. For example, an ambitious athlete might be motivated to attend additional training sessions, whereas a demotivated, burnt-out player might start to skip practices.
- **Intensity**. The amount of effort and energy expended. Highly motivated people put in a lot of effort.
- **Persistence**. The extent to which a performer concentrates on a task.
- **Continuity**. The extent to which a performer returns to a task, e.g. attends training sessions on a regular basis.
- **Performance**. Although motivation does not directly determine how well you perform, we can assume that if someone consistently performs at a high level then they have been motivated to achieve and maintain that level.

KEY POINTS

- Motivators are the reasons why sportspeople think and behave as they do.

- Motivation has five components: direction, intensity, persistence, continuity and performance.

- Early theories focused on the notion of 'drive'. Current theories are based on social perception and goal orientation.

Participation motives

ACTIVITY 12.6 PARTICIPATION MOTIVES

Individually, write down the reasons why you enjoy participating in sport or other physical activity. As a group, pool these reasons and then put them into categories, e.g. all those to do with fitness. List these categories (not the individual reasons) and ask all members of the group to rank them in order of personal importance: for example, if the main reason you play sport is because it is important for you to stay fit, rank this as '1'. Combine these ranks to see which are the most important participation motives for your group. Compare your results with Table 12.1; analyse the similarities and differences. Can you account for any differences?

Youth sport participation	Adult exercise participation
improving skills	health factors
having fun	weight loss
being with friends	fitness
experiencing thrills	self-challenge and excitement
achieving success	feeling better
fitness	socialising

Table 12.1 Major motives[19]

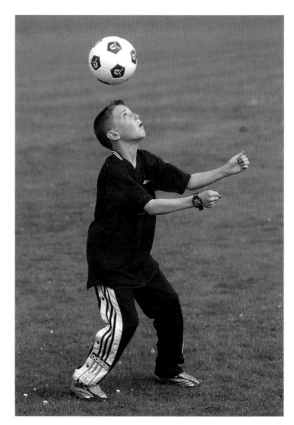

Fig. 12.22 Sport mastery motives are strong in youngsters.

Table 12.1 is only a broad generalisation of the results of a growing number of research studies into why children, young people and adults participate in sport and exercise. For example, the table does not differentiate between males and females. It also groups together participation motives for competitive sport and health-related exercise (e.g. aerobics, 'step', line dancing, gym training) and we may learn more by separating these in future research. Weinberg & Gould[19] and Biddle[47] give a review of recent research findings in much greater detail than is possible in this text. The following is a selection of findings that relate to motivation and participation in sport and exercise.

- Twelve-year-old British children have a strong interest in PE and sport.[48]

- Sport mastery motives are strong for young children (6–9 years), whereas social status is an important motive for youths (10–16 years).[49]
- Boys are more interested than girls in achieving success in competition.
- Fitness motives tend only to be important for those actively involved in exercise.
- Participation in sport in North America peaks around age 12.
- Drop-out rates from a particular activity do not necessarily imply discontinuation of all activity; young people often make positive choices.
- Most young people withdraw from a particular activity to join another. Other reasons given for drop-out are lack of fun, disliking the leader, not improving, pressure (to perform better/win), boredom.[50]

Some of the reasons for participation or drop-out given above are surface-level responses. For example, a youngster may say he/she does not like the coach, whereas the more important underlying factor is that the coach makes him/her feel inadequate. Gould &

Petlichkoff[51] suggest three underlying motives for participation or drop-out:

- perceived competence (self-perception of ability to learn/perform well)
- goal orientation (what the performer wants to achieve: personal mastery or competitive success)
- stress response (ability to cope with perceived pressure).

So far we have considered motivation as a 'unitary concept', but there are different types of motivation.

1. **Positive and negative motivation.** Positive motivation makes us want to continue an activity; negative motivation will decrease our enthusiasm for it. Reasons for drop-out given above will lead to negative motivation.
2. **Primary and secondary motivation.** Primary motivation comes from the activity itself; secondary motivation is provided by something or somebody else, i.e. encouragement from the coach.
3. **Extrinsic and intrinsic motivation.** Figure 12.23 identifies a continuum between two forms of motivation, intrinsic and extrinsic. **Intrinsic** motivation arises when an activity is pursued for its own sake, for the pride and satisfaction that is achieved, regardless of what anyone else thinks of one's efforts. The motivation derives directly from participating in the activity and is self-perpetuating. **Extrinsic** motivation stems from other people, through positive and negative reinforcement, and from tangible rewards such as trophies, badges and payment (see Figure 12.24). Behavioural psychologists have, for many years, recognised the power of extrinsic rewards to develop and modify behaviour. A very basic

Extrinsic rewards		Intrinsic sources
Tangible	**Intangible**	
Badges	**negative** **positive**	Satisfaction
Trophies	criticism praise	Achievement
Certificates	defeat fame	Feeling good
Money	winning	

Fig. 12.24 Extrinsic rewards and intrinsic sources.

principle of human behaviour is the **law of effect**, which states that rewarding a particular behaviour increases the probability that the behaviour will be repeated. Coaches and teachers recognise this and many of the governing bodies of sport have produced award schemes which encourage youngsters to work at skills in order to increase their proficiency and thus be awarded a badge or certificate.

Investigation 12.5 To identify a range of governing body award schemes

Method: Go to your local school or college library and look up the magazines and journals produced by the governing bodies of sport, e.g. *The Swimming Times*. Note details of any award schemes that are described. As a class group, write to several governing bodies, asking for details of their award schemes. Analyse these schemes in terms of:

1. age range for which the award is designed
2. level of difficulty of each stage of the award
3. nature of the award (certificate, badge, etc.)
4. general attractiveness of the presentation
5. potential interest which the award might generate in its target population.

Until recently, few would have questioned the appropriateness or effectiveness of such schemes. It was assumed that extrinsic rewards would encourage initial participation and that adding an extrinsic reward to a situation in which youngsters were already intrinsically motivated at best increased motivation and at worst did no harm.

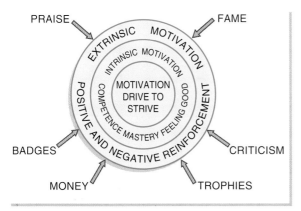

Fig. 12.23 Intrinsic and extrinsic motivation.

Recent research has led us to question this, however. Deci[52] and Lepper & Greene[53] showed that, in certain circumstances, adding external reward to a situation that is already intrinsically motivating actually decreases that intrinsic motivation and may eventually replace it, so that when the reward is no longer available, interest in the activity wanes.

Can you suggest some explanations for these findings? Can you think of any occasions when you have found the receipt of an extrinsic reward irrelevant or even demotivating?

Explanations that have been suggested are as follows.

- **Pace**. The reward acts as a distraction to the sportsperson's intrinsic desire to work at his/her own pace.
- **Play becomes work**. Individuals may feel that being given a reward turns what they thought of as play into work and thus changes the nature of (i) the relationship between themselves and the person giving the reward, (ii) the activity itself.
- **Control**. People like to determine their own behaviour; participating for the sake of a reward makes them feel that someone or something else is in control.
- **Competence**. If the reward is given in such a way that it increases the performer's confidence and perceived competence then it will act as a motivator. If, however, it does not do this, then it will not act as a motivator and may cause a temporary decrease in motivation. This sometimes happens in junior sport awards schemes when children receive a badge or certificate for something they found very easy.

Does this mean that we should scrap all award schemes, leagues, certificates, etc.? Certainly not – rewards do not automatically undermine intrinsic motivation. They may be used to attract youngsters to an activity they might not otherwise try or to revive flagging motivation or to help an athlete over a bad period in his/her training. The psychological borderline between intangible extrinsic rewards, such as praise and fame, and the intrinsic rewards of satisfaction and sense of achievement is by no means clear. Thus, if extrinsic rewards provide information about levels of achievement and competence, they enhance motivation. However, current thinking does suggest that as intrinsic motivation and participation for its own sake develop, so tangible rewards become

> **KEY POINTS**
>
> - Motivation to participate varies across age groups, gender groups and sport/exercise.
> - There are many different motives to participate in activity and people often participate for several reasons.
> - Intrinsic motivation derives from the activity itself and is a powerful motive.
> - Extrinsic motivation derives from tangible rewards and positive/negative social reinforcement.
> - Extrinsic rewards can have a positive or negative effect on motivation depending on how the performer perceives them in relation to pace, play, control and competence.

redundant and should be withdrawn or used very sparingly.

Measuring motivation

The predominant method for identifying and measuring motives is to use verbal or written inventories and ask respondents to list motives and attitudes which apply to them. An inventory may be 'closed' or 'open'. A **closed** inventory seeks responses to a given list of attitude statements. An **open** inventory would ask questions such as 'List three reasons why you are a member of this sports club. Put them in order of importance'. It is possible, of course, to combine the two forms. Such inventories are most effective when:

- they relate to specific activities and situations
- there is no perceived need to give socially acceptable answers.

Achievement motivation

So far we have considered motivation in terms of the sportsperson's interest in participating in physical activity. In taking this stance, we recognise that an important part of intrinsic motivation stems from perceived success in achieving competence and mastery. An individual's drive to achieve success for its own sake is known as **achievement motivation**. In sportspeople, this is closely related to competitiveness;

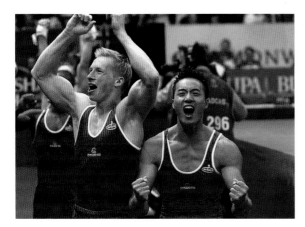

Fig. 12.25 Success contributes to motivation.

in other aspects of physical activity, this is (for example) the persistence of a climber in the face of difficulties or the striving for perfection of a dancer. Achievement motivation theory is about what happens when we are faced with a choice to seek out or to avoid situations where we might or might not be successful. For example, you might have a choice of routes to climb on a rock face or of opponents to make up your school or college fixture list. Which or who do you choose? Research shows that two factors contribute to the decision: personality and situation.

Personality factors

Atkinson[54] suggests that there are two personality factors that contribute to achievement motivation (Figure 12.26):

- the need to achieve (*Nach*)
- the need to avoid failure (*Naf*).

We all have both characteristics but those with a high need to achieve usually tend to have a low need to avoid failure (subject A) and those who have a high need to avoid failure generally have a low need to achieve (subject B). What is not so clear to sport psychologists are the characteristics of people who might appear in the other two quadrants of Figure 12.26.[32]

This aspect of personality explains why some people seek out success while others avoid situations where they might be seen to fail, but it does not give the full picture or account for behaviour in those situations where someone is committed to participate but can choose the level of task difficulty; for example, deciding on an easy or difficult rock route once a climber has arrived at the base of the cliff.

Situational factors

We judge the situation in terms of:

- the probability of success
- the incentive value of that success.

This is shown in Figure 12.27 and is derived from the work of Atkinson.[54]

The model shows that if the probability of success is low (for example, if you are playing squash against a world-class player), the incentive value of success is high (you would be very excited if you won). Similarly, if you play against weak opposition, winning doesn't mean so much to you. Research (e.g.[55]) shows that people with a low achievement orientation (high failure avoidance) tend to choose tasks which are either very easy or very difficult. Can you suggest why this is? High achievers, however, tend to select tasks where there is a 50/50 chance of success. Thus, high achievers tend to be risk takers.

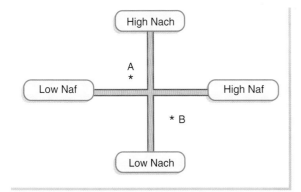

Fig. 12.26 The personality components of achievement motivation.

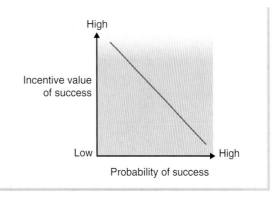

Fig. 12.27 Situational factors in achievement motivation.

Investigation 12.6 To investigate the hypothesis that high achievers are high risk takers

Method: Select a group of subjects who are not aware of the nature of the experiment.

1. Measure the achievement motivation of your subjects either by using the Lynn Survey of Achievement Motivation[56] or by means of the following scale (circle the score which most represents your feelings about each of the paired statements).

a.	Success in sport is very important to me	5 4 3 2 1	Winning doesn't matter; it's the game that counts
b.	I prefer to play opponents I know I can beat	1 2 3 4 5	I like playing opponents who are about my level
c.	I enjoy a challenge	5 4 3 2 1	I like doing things I know I will succeed in
d.	I don't enjoy close games	5 4 3 2 1	I enjoy a close game
e.	I don't worry about the result of a game	1 2 3 4 5	I don't like having to tell people I lost a game
f.	I tend to make errors when I'm under pressure	5 4 3 2 1	I play best when I'm under pressure

Scoring: Statements **a–c** are achievement orientation scores and statements **d–f** are failure avoidance scores.

6–11: Low achiever/avoider   12–22: Average achiever/avoider   23–30: High achiever/avoider

(Note that this is an informal scale and has not been tested for validity and reliability.)

2. Set up a basketball or netball shooting task. Each subject has 10 shots from a point of her/his choice on a line drawn at a radius of 4 m from the base of the post. Scores are noted.

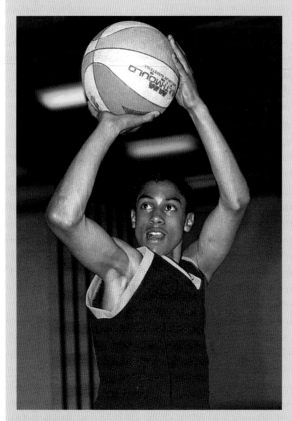

Fig. 12.28

The next 10 shots can be taken from anywhere. Subjects are told that successful shots will be added to their score, but they will be penalised for unsuccessful shots by the deduction of one point from their overall score. Record scores for feedback purposes but for the purposes of the research, note whether each of the second 10 shots was taken from nearer the post than the first 10 (1 point), from the same place (2 points) or from further away (3 points). Total the points (not the scores) for the 10 shots.

    10–15: Low risk taker

    16–24: Average risk taker

    25–30: High risk taker

Results: Draw two scattergrams that correlate:
(i) achievement and
(ii) failure avoidance

with risk taking.

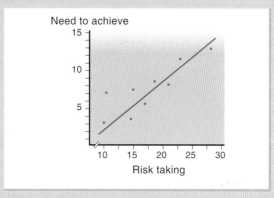

Fig. 12.29 The relationship between need to achieve and risk taking.

Atkinson's theory suggests that your achievement graph will look something like Figure 12.29. Does it? If it does not, can you suggest some reasons?

Discussion

1. Analyse your findings and discuss any discrepancies you note between your results and the hypothetical ones in Figure 12.29.
2. Debrief your subjects on what the experiment was about and what their shots scores were. Why is it important to do this? Bear in mind what you know about the ethics of psychological investigation.

Self-motivation

Self-motivation is an aspect of achievement motivation and represents the extent to which a person is able to persist in tasks or to generate action. It's seen in sport in situations where, for example, the competition gets tough or perhaps when training becomes hard or repetitive. It is closely related to intrinsic motivation, but refers to people who keep going on a task when the task itself is not immediately motivating.

Self-motivation approaches to theories of achievement motivation use achievement goal orientations.[57] The two main achievement goals are **mastery (task)** goals and **ego** goals. Sportspeople who adopt a mastery (task) orientation see success in terms of improving their personal performance. Those who have an ego orientation are concerned with winning or demonstrating ability that is superior to others.[47]

Research

Self-motivation has been studied in relation to fitness training. Biddle et al[58] used a children's self-motivation inventory (SMI-C) to compare children's self-motivation with their performances in an endurance run and found a significant correlation. An earlier, similar study[59] found that the highest levels of motivation in a 20 m progressive shuttle run were amongst children who were high in task orientation and low in ego orientation, regardless of how well they performed. For children who were less successful in the test and who were high in ego orientation and low in task orientation, fitness testing seems to be motivationally threatening. There are important lessons for coaches and teachers in this research and in many similar studies. Self-motivation appears to be highest when performers are concerned with mastery of skill and achieving personal best performances, rather than

comparing themselves with others. All children go through a phase of social comparison and this applies in sport as in other areas of life, but the mature performer will have learnt when such comparison is appropriate and when it is counterproductive. On the whole, coaches should aim to help performers set goals that relate to self-improvement. We shall return to this idea when considering goal setting in Chapter 13.

The attribution process

Investigation 12.7 To introduce the concept of attribution

Method: Play a small-number-a-side game, such as basketball, netball or five-a-side soccer. Play to a win/lose situation, i.e. avoid a draw. After the game, the players individually write down four reasons why they think their own team won or lost. In addition, each states whether or not he/she would like to play against the same team again, with the same teammates, in the near future.

Discussion: As a class group, pool these statements. Categorise them into groups of similar reasons, e.g. 'we played well as a team' with 'we had some good players'. These reasons are known as **attributions**.

1. How many categories did you construct?
2. Consider the relationship between wanting/not wanting to play again and winning/losing; does any pattern emerge?

Attribution is the process of ascribing reasons for, or causes to, events and behaviours. When something significant happens to us, such as winning or losing an important game, we ask ourselves 'why?'. The conclusions we come to tend to colour our approach to future similar events. Attribution theory thus suggests that motivation is due to cognitive processes. Sport psychologists have asked two important questions about this.

- What sorts of reasons do sportspersons give for success or failure?
- How does this affect their future participation and chances of success?

Weiner's[60] attribution theory of achievement behaviour has been widely applied to sport contexts. He suggests that one of the differences between high and low achievers is the way in which each group develops attributions about success and failure. He proposes a model with four types of attribution (though

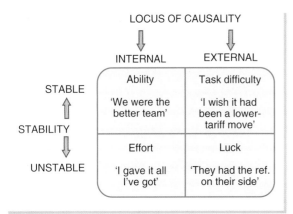

Fig. 12.30 Weiner's model of causal attribution.

recognises that these are not the only attributions), as shown in Figure 12.30.

- **Ability**. The extent of the performer's capacity to cope with the task.
- **Effort**. The amount of mental and physical effort the performer gives to the task.
- **Task difficulty**. The extent of the problems posed by the task, including the strength of the opposition.
- **Luck**. Factors attributable to chance, such as the weather or the state of the pitch.

To what extent did the categories you derived from Investigation 12.7 correspond to these? You may have found that with a little adaptation, your categories correspond to Weiner's. Or you may have used additional categories. Research by Duda & Nicholls[61] into students' beliefs about their success in sport, for example, replaced Weiner's 'task difficulty' category with 'deception' (unsportsmanlike behaviour). Weiner organised his categories into two dimensions (Figure 12.30), which he termed **locus of causality** and **stability**. The word 'locus' is derived from the Latin 'place'; thus the 'locus of causality' indicates where the individual perceives the cause of success or failure to lie. In this case, the two categories are **internal** (ability and effort) or **external** (task difficulty and luck). The stability dimension implies that two of the factors (ability and task difficulty) are relatively stable, i.e. not subject to change (in the short term at least), whereas the other two (effort and luck) can vary from competition to competition or even within an activity.

Weiner did not claim that these dimensions were exclusive. Also, although his original research was in achievement situations, it was concerned with students talking about examination success. When the model is applied to sport, the 'task difficulty' dimension does not always work as a stable attribute; if task difficulty means the strength of the opposition, this will vary as opponents change. In addition, although it is agreed that ability is a relatively stable attribute, 'form' (which is a crucial ingredient of sport success) is not necessarily so.[62] The model is still very useful, however, in understanding the implications of the dimensions for attribution analysis, as we shall see later. Further research[63] identified a third dimension, that of controllability. This is the extent to which the outcome of a situation is under our personal control or is uncontrollable. There are likely to be others.

ACTIVITY 12.7

To test out the usefulness of these ideas, video some TV sport broadcasts and discuss a selection of interviews with sportspeople immediately after an event. Try and place their statements about the competition into Weiner's categories and discuss the implications of what they are saying. Use Figure 12.30 to help you categorise.

The people whom you have recorded have successful careers in their sport, but they do not succeed all the time. It is particularly interesting to hear what they have to say when they do not win, for example when beaten by strong opposition in a soccer European Champions League game. 'We just didn't seem to "click" tonight, couldn't get our passing together': this is an internal attribution because it is about the team itself and they are taking responsibility for their own failure. It is also unstable because the player is implying that tonight's performance was unusual. They know it's something they can work on the training ground and get right next time. It's a question of effort. They may feel ashamed and that they have temporarily let down each other and their manager. 'We were always going to find it difficult to get through their defence': this player is recognising the difficulty of the task. The strength of the defence is an external attribution, the team can do nothing about it. It is also stable: they were expecting it and it is unlikely to change in the near future (stability). Thus although they do not like to lose, they do not feel any sense of shame in this defeat. They are probably not relishing the prospect of the return match, however, particularly if it is 'away'. 'It was a 50/50 decision and the ref decided to give the penalty against us: that's how your luck goes sometimes': here the player judges that the outcome of the game has been decided by an external factor (the referee's decision) but that in another situation, the decision might have been different (unstable attribution).

You are unlikely to hear successful players attributing failure to their own lack of ability. Ability is a stable attribute (i.e. it changes only slowly over time). Successful players know that they are able and have achieved success partly as a result of continuing reinforcement of their perceived competence and the confidence this gives. Listen to interviews with players from a winning team and they will almost certainly attribute success to their ability and good play. Only rarely will they concede that luck played a part. If they are forced to concede that they did not play well but that their opponents played even worse, then that will decrease feelings of satisfaction.

Attribution errors

Attribution is a cognitive process; it reflects the way we think about performance, but it is closely linked to personality factors such as self-confidence and self-esteem. Attribution is sometimes used to protect our self-esteem when it is threatened or to enhance it when we are given the opportunity. This is known as a **self-serving bias**. Thus we tend to attribute our successes to internal factors (our talent or our effort) and failure to external factors, e.g. the state of the pitch or the superiority of our opponents.

KEY POINTS

- Sportspeople analyse success and failure and attribute reasons. These reasons are called attributions.

- Confident, able performers tend to make internal attributions for success and external attributions for failure.

- Less confident performers tend to make external attributions for success and internal attributions for failure.

- Stable attributions lead performers to expect the same outcome next time; unstable attributions give hope for change.

- Stable attributions reinforce performers' perceived competence, whether it's low or high.

If this is an objective assessment of the situation, confirmed by the coach or significant spectators, then this is a natural process and provides useful feedback to us, particularly if we are self-confident. But less mature performers may use these particular attributions as a self-serving bias and may be wrong. For example, the pitch may have been uneven but it affected both teams in the same way and the coach knows that this was not the real reason for the defeat. If performers attribute wrongly on a regular basis, then they will not learn from errors and will not improve. This is particularly true if the attributions performers make are to do with the extent to which they are in control of the situation. Weiner calls this the **control dimension** and he differentiated personal control from external control. If things go wrong but performers feel that they can do something about it (i.e. they are in personal control), then they are motivated to work to put things right, but if they always believe that things are outside their control then they may develop a state known as **learned helplessness**.[64,65]

Learned helplessness is a psychological state that makes people give up very easily if a task seems difficult. If you ask some of your non-sporting friends why they don't join, for example, the badminton club, the initial response may well be 'I don't like sport'. However, if you persist you may get answers such as 'I'm no good at badminton', 'I never was any good and I never will be' or 'I'm useless at all sport'. Dweck[65] calls this learned helplessness and sees the cause as the individual attributing early difficulties to internal, stable, external control or global factors, usually a combination of these. The global-specific dimension relates to whether failure is seen to be specific to the particular activity or generalised to other areas of sport ('I'm useless at sport' is a global attribution). People who show learned helplessness in sport tend to attribute failure to causes which are internal, unchanging, outside their personal control and apply to most situations.

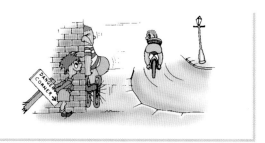

Fig. 12.31 The control dimension.

Outcome and task (mastery) orientations

Learned helplessness can be challenged by attribution retraining (see below). It also helps confidence if the teacher/coach emphasises task (mastery) goals and downplays outcome goals. Having an outcome goal orientation means that you focus your thoughts on comparing yourself with others. For example, an outcome goal plan for a race would be to win (or perhaps to be in the first three). The problem with this goal is that however well you run, if others are faster than you, you will not achieve your goal. A task (mastery) goal orientation means that you compare your performance with personal standards and improvement. Thus, a task goal plan for the same race would be to run a personal best or to improve your time on that of the previous race. In this case it is possible to achieve your goal regardless of how others perform.

KEY POINTS

Task (mastery) goal orientation leads to:

- Positive attitudes

- Increased effort

- Effective learning

- Self-confidence

Outcome goal orientation *may* lead to:

- Low persistence

- Low effort

- Fear of failure

- Low confidence

ACTIVITY 12.8 TASK VERSUS OUTCOME GOALS

- Which form of orientation, 'task' or 'outcome' do you think is best for long-term motivation? Why?

- For your own sport/activity, devise some task (mastery) and some outcome goals.

- Under what conditions might you use an outcome goal orientation?

The application of attribution theory: attribution retraining

Objective analysis by player and coach of attributions and the positive restructuring of these can help to increase motivation. Attribution training/retraining work can be an integral part of preparation for competition. This might be done by:

- recording, classifying and discussing attributions for success and defeat

- using video to analyse performance and adjust attribution

- devising a clear goal-setting programme which includes appropriate attribution strategies.

The application of attribution theory and research to coaching tells coaches that:

- performers are more likely to do well if they think they are going to do so, which in turn depends on how they attribute their success and failure in the past

- it is part of the coach's job to help the performer achieve initial success and then attribute this to stable, internal and controllable factors

- sportspeople do not always make logical attributions, based on the evidence of the competition. Even if attributions are logical, coaches need to help the athlete to ascribe success to internal, stable factors and failure to unstable factors.

An example of reattribution

Athletes with low self-esteem tend to ascribe internal and stable causes to failure and unstable causes to success and confident athletes the reverse. For example: 'I lost because my backhand is just not good enough at this level' or 'Well, I won that game, but only because she was serving so badly'. These are typical attributions of a player who has lost confidence; they are not helpful because they emphasise stable or external control factors, i.e. factors that cannot be changed easily. Because they cannot be changed, the player may feel it is not worth continuing and give up. They may or may not be an accurate reflection of the games but in any case, the coach should offer an alternative assessment (with evidence), so changing attributions from stable to unstable or emphasising internal control: 'No, your backhand's fine normally; you were just not getting into position quickly enough. Make that extra effort when you see it coming onto the backhand' (emphasising effort rather than technique). 'No, it wasn't weak serving; it was your good returns.

Keep returning the ball deep, as you are, and you've got him/her in real trouble' (emphasising ability and control).

Even if the player's attributions are an accurate reflection of what is happening, the coach should try to attribute failure to unstable causes, success to internal causes and engender a feeling of being in control: 'Yes, we need to work on your backhand, but I know what the problem is, and it's easily put right; work your strong forehand for now' (emphasising control). 'OK, she had some uncharacteristic double faults, but that shows you've got her worried. Keep the pressure on' (emphasising effort).

Feelings of pride and dissatisfaction (affective responses)

Figure 12.32 shows the results that were obtained when two teams of basketball players were asked to state the extent to which they felt satisfied with their performance after a game, in terms of the four categories of attribution. These results appear to be fairly typical[60] and suggest that if we attribute our success in an activity to internal factors, such as ability and effort, we are more likely to feel satisfaction with our performance than if we put our winning down to luck or the ease of the task. In the same way, we experience greater feelings of disappointment if we perceive our losing to be due to internal rather than external factors.

Expectancy

In addition to predicting the probability of a performer feeling satisfaction or disappointment with the outcome of an activity, attribution theory attempts to explain the way in which we come to **expect** certain

> **KEY POINTS**
>
> Attributions affect a sportsperson's view of his/her sport in three important ways:
>
> - feelings of pride and satisfaction
> - expectancy
> - confidence.
>
> These are expanded below.

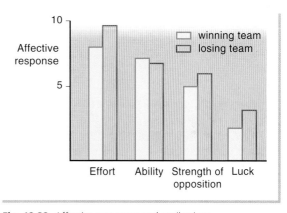

Fig. 12.32 Affective responses and attributions.

things to happen. If success or failure in a task is seen to be due to unstable (U) factors, then performers may be uncertain about how they will do in similar future tasks. If success or failure is seen to be due to stable (S) factors, then performers tend to expect similar results in their next outing (assuming conditions are generally similar).

Investigation 12.8 To investigate the effect of attribution on the expectation of subsequent success or failure

Method: Select a group of students who do not know the purpose of the task. Divide this group into four.

1. Devise four motor tasks, one for each group. The tasks should have a clear goal to be attained and should be as follows.
   a. Luck plays a major part in success or failure, e.g. throwing a dice for a specified number (code letter U).
   b. Effort plays a major part, e.g. improving previous performance on a simple strength task (code letter U).
   c. Ability is of importance – any novel motor task (code letter S).

   d. Task difficulty is central – this can be simulated by selecting a relatively simple task but distracting the performer during it (code letter S). The code letters refer to whether the task is likely to produce stable or unstable reasons for the result.

2. Measure the subjects' performance in their particular task by noting whether they succeed or fail.

3. Suggest to them that they are going to do the task again (in fact, they are not). Ask each subject whether they think they are going to succeed or fail at the second attempt. ▶

▶ **4.** Mark each subject in one of the boxes in Figure 12.33: for example, if they succeeded in their task but couldn't predict the outcome of the proposed second attempt, they would be marked in box 'C'. Mark the subject with the letter that corresponds to the attribution task they did, as in Figure 12.33.

Discussion: Theory suggests that you might obtain results as in Figure 12.33. If you did not, can you offer an explanation? Do you think the hypothesis is faulty or was there something different or special about your sample or your method? For example, do you think it is legitimate to assume that the subjects would attribute success or failure in the way suggested by the tasks? Figure 12.33 suggests that people who attribute success or failure in an activity to stable factors are more likely to expect the same outcome next time they perform than if unstable attributions are made.

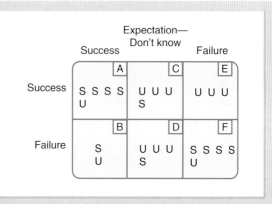

Fig. 12.33 Result of Investigation 12.8.

Self-confidence and self-efficacy

Self-confidence (a general personality trait) and self-efficacy (a situation-specific form of self-confidence) are essential for success in sport and physical activity generally. Coaches and teachers can increase self-confidence by careful planning of their teaching and by sensitive use of teaching or coaching style and interactions. We have earlier stressed the importance of the 'self concept wheel' (see Figure 12.16) in enhancing performance and ensuring success. In this section we study self-confidence and self-efficacy as aspects of self-esteem that are closely related to achievement motivation and that affect the way we make attributions in sport.

Self-confidence is probably one of the most important psychological prerequisites for success in sport. Self-confident athletes believe in their ability to develop the knowledge, skills and attitudes to succeed; athletes who lack self-confidence doubt their abilities or assume that opponents inevitably 'have the edge' over them. This represents what has been termed the **self-fulfilling prophecy**, i.e. that expecting something to happen tends to cause it to happen. We all recognise this phenomenon in others and ourselves, but how does it happen?

KEY POINTS

- **Self-confidence** is an aspect of self-esteem; it is an attitude, based on the belief that one can succeed.

- **Self-efficacy** is the perception of one's ability to perform a particular task successfully and is a situation-specific form of self-confidence.

- Weinberg & Gould[19] outline the psychology of self-confidence:

- Confidence arouses positive emotions, allowing the athlete to remain calm under pressure and assertive when required.

- Confidence facilitates concentration and a focus on the important aspects of the task. Lack of confidence causes stress under pressure and thus concentration on outside stressors, i.e. mistakes or spectators.

- Confidence affects goal setting. Confident athletes set challenging but realistic goals. Athletes lacking in confidence set goals for themselves that are either too easy or too difficult.

- Confidence increases effort.

- Confidence affects game strategies. A confident player plays to win, even if it means taking risks. A non-confident player tries to avoid mistakes.

- Confidence affects psychological momentum. Non-confident athletes find it difficult to reverse negative psychological momentum, i.e. once things start to go wrong they find it difficult to think positively, whereas confident athletes take each point or play at a time and never give up, even when defeat stares them in the face.

Of course, overconfidence or false confidence is dangerous because it leads to inadequate preparation and low motivation and/or arousal, both of which are difficult (though not impossible) to correct once the competition is under way.

There are a number of theoretical models of self-confidence (see[6]), of which the most widely reported is that of Bandura,[11] shown in Figure 12.34. This model brings together several ideas that have been discussed separately in this section. Bandura theorises that there are four factors that affect the expectations of future success that an athlete holds and thus determine self-efficacy. These are **performance accomplishments**, **modelling** (sometimes referred to as **vicarious experience**), **verbal persuasion** and **emotional arousal**. All are important and link to the attributions performers make for past success and failure.

Performance accomplishments: This refers to the previous success the performer has achieved. To build confidence the teacher/coach should focus the performer's attention on this success and attribute it to stable, internal factors.

Modelling: We discussed in Chapter 11 the coach's role in helping the athlete to model performance on someone who is already skilled and successful. Good demonstration by a successful model not only assists skill acquisition but helps the athlete to think, 'If I can perform like that, I'll be a good player too'. Vicarious experience means watching someone succeeding at something you are interested in achieving and imagining yourself doing the same thing.

Verbal persuasion: In Section 12.4 we discuss the role of persuasion in changing attitudes. In Bandura's model the coach establishes a positive attitude by convincing athletes that they are capable of performing well.

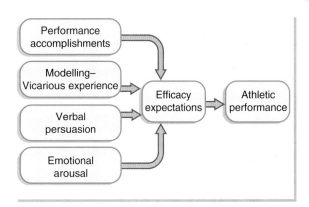

Fig. 12.34 Bandura's theory of self-efficacy.

Emotional arousal refers to the motivational component of all performance situations, how important it is to the performer to succeed. It relates to being appropriately 'psyched up', discussed in detail in Chapter 13.

Many sport psychologists claim that the most important of the four elements in developing self-efficacy is the 'performance accomplishments' element. This is because success (and failure) in sport is very obvious and clearcut. It gives the athlete very direct feedback and is an indication of current status and a signpost for the future. If you are successful in one competition, you will feel confident about the next; if you fail, you may worry about the next. This is why it is important for the teacher/coach to set realistic tasks and the appropriate level of competition.

Vealey[66] developed a model that specifically relates to sport confidence (Figure 12.35). This model differs from Bandura's in that it deals with how the performer's own beliefs and personality affect confidence and performance within a *sports* context.

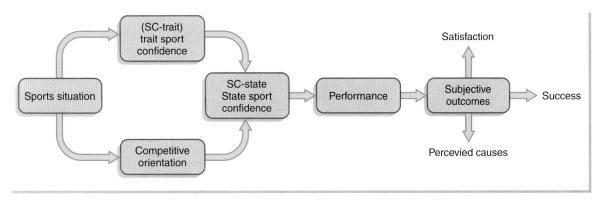

Fig. 12.35 Vealey's model of sport confidence.

Within the model:

- SC-trait is a personality trait, relating to confidence in sports contexts generally
- Competitive orientation is the extent to which the performer seeks and responds to competitive situations

- SC-state is the performer's confidence in a *particular* sport context and is determined by a combination of SC-trait and competitive orientation.

The model shows how the outcomes (satisfaction, success, attributions) feed back into competitiveness and SC-trait. It explains how confidence is affected by the experiences of the performer and thus how confidence can change over (for example) a season.

The attribution process is summarised in Figure 12.37.

> ### KEY POINTS
>
> The coach or teacher has a fundamental role to play in developing self-confidence and self-efficacy through successful achievement.
>
> - To ensure early and continued success during the learning process by the careful selection of goals, tasks and levels of competition.
>
> - The second Key Point is a fundamental one in all coaching and teaching and cannot be overstated. Success should be defined by how well athletes play or perform in relation to their ability and their 'personal best' and not by whether or not they win. Such an attitude was typified by the British men's 4 × 400 m track relay squad, interviewed after their run in the Atlanta Olympic Games. They had hoped to win gold and thought they could but in coming second, they took pride in having broken national and European records and were bubbling with confidence and optimism for future races. Weinberg & Gould's[19] 'recipe' for building confidence is shown in Figure 12.36.

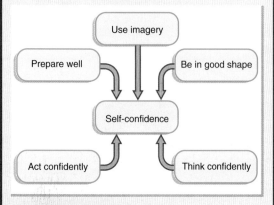

Fig. 12.36 Developing self-confidence.

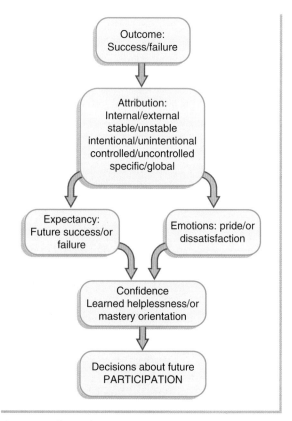

Fig. 12.37 The attribution process.

Review questions

1. Define the terms 'motivation' and 'motives' and distinguish between intrinsic and extrinsic rewards in sport, using examples.

2. List and explain Weiner's five components of motivation.[46]

3. Compare young people's motives for participating in sport/exercise with those of adults. Offer explanations for any differences.

4. Give three underlying motives for participation and drop-out in sport.

5. Why does intrinsic motivation plus extrinsic motivation not always lead to increased motivation?

6. Define achievement motivation. Show how personality and situational factors affect it.

7. Draw a diagram which contrasts high and low achievers in terms of (i) Nach/naf; (ii) attributions; (iii) goal orientation; (iv) task choice.

8. Sketch Weiner's[60] model of attributions and give sport-related examples of each component of the model. Explain 'locus of causality' and 'stability'.

9. Why should a performer seek to attribute lack of success to external and unstable factors?

10. What is meant by 'self-efficacy' in sport? Give at least five ways in which a coach can build an athlete's positive approach to competition

Exam-style questions

1. A number of PE students are attending trials at their chosen sport. Describe the Inverted U theory and explain how it might affect a student's performance at the trials. (5 marks)

2. a. Describe the characteristics of the positive motive: 'the need to achieve'. (4 marks)
   b. Describe an example from sport of someone who has a high motive to avoid failure. (1 mark)
   c. Identify factors which could affect the use of motives to achieve and to avoid failure in sporting situations. (3 marks)
   (Total 8 marks)

3. How would you promote the need to achieve motive, rather than the need to avoid failure motive? (8 marks)

4. a. Figure 12.38 partly illustrates Weiner's model of attribution. Explain the term attribution by using a sporting situation. (1 mark)
   b. Explain the terms locus of causality and stability when applied to attribution theory. (4 marks)
   c. Redraw the model and place on it relevant attributions for each of the four boxes. (4 marks)
   d. What attributions would you encourage if your team were playing well but often losing? (5 marks)
   (Total 14 marks)

5. a. Many young people claim to be 'hopeless' at gymnastics. Suggest three reasons why these youngsters might have a negative attitude to gymnastics. (3 marks)

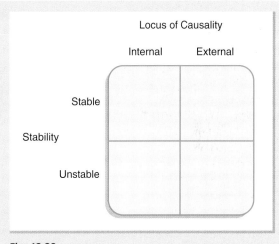

Fig. 12.38

   b. What is meant by learned helplessness (LH) and how is it caused? (3 marks)
   c. How would you attempt to attract beginners to a gymnastics class, and then change any negative attitudes? (4 marks)
   (Total 10 marks)

6. Those who achieve little in sport often attribute their failure to factors outside their control and **learned helplessness** can result. Using examples from sport, explain what is meant by learned helplessness and identify how self-motivational techniques may help to limit the effects of learned helplessness. (6 marks)

References

1. Kunath P 1995 *Future directions in exercise and sport psychology*. In: Biddle S H (ed) European perspectives on exercise and sport psychology. Human Kinetics, Champaign. Illinois
2. Triplett N 1898 *The dynamogenic factors in pacemaking and competition*. American Journal of Psychology 9:507–533
3. Beashel P, Taylor J eds 1996 *Advanced studies in physical education and sport*. Nelson, Walton-on-Thames
4. Tennenbaum G, Bar-Eli M 1995 *Contemporary issues in exercise and sport psychology research*. In: Biddle S H (ed) European perspectives on exercise and sport psychology. Human Kinetics, Champaign, Illinois
5. Eysenck H J 1969 *The biological basis of behaviour*. Thomas, London
6. Cox R 1998 *Sports psychology: concepts and applications*, 4th edn. WCB/McGraw-Hill, Boston
7. Apitzsch E 1995 *Psychodynamic theory of personality and sport performance*. In: Biddle S H (ed) European perspectives on exercise and sport psychology. Human Kinetics, Champaign, Illinois
8. Apitzsch E, Berggren B 1993 *The personality of the elite soccer player*. Lund, Sweden
9. Cattell R B 1965 *The scientific analysis of personality*. Penguin, Baltimore
10. Eysenck H J, Eysenck S B G 1968 *Eysenck personality inventory manual*. University of London Press, London
11. Bandura A 1977 *Self-efficacy: toward a unifying theory of behavioural change*. Psychological Review 84:191–215
12. McNair D M, Lorr M, Droppleman L F 1971 *Profile of mood states manual*. Educational and Industrial Testing Service, San Diego, California
13. Nideffer R 1976 *Test of attentional and interpersonal style*. Journal of Personality and Social Psychology 34:394–404
14. Spielberger C D, Gorsuch R L, Lushene R F 1970 *Manual for the state-trait anxiety inventory*. Consulting Psychologists Press, Palo Alto, California
15. Martens R 1977 *Sport competition anxiety test*. Human Kinetics, Champaign, Illinois
16. Martens R 1990 *Coaches' guide to sport psychology*. Human Kinetics, Champaign, Illinois
17. Van Schoyck S R, Grasha A F 1981 *Attentional style variations and athletic ability: the advantages of a sport-specific test*. Journal of Sport Psychology 3:149–165
18. Butt D S 1987 *Psychology of sport*. Van Nostrand Reinhold, New York
19. Weinberg W S, Gould D 1999 *Foundations of sport and exercise psychology*. Human Kinetics, Champaign, Illinois
20. Morgan W P 1980 *The trait psychology controversy*. Research Quarterly for Exercise and Sport 51:50–76
21. Terry P 1995 *The efficacy of mood state profiling with elite performers: a review and synthesis*. Sport Psychologist 9:309–324
22. Girdano D A, Everly G S, Dusek D E 1990 *Controlling stress and tension: a holistic approach*, 3rd edn. Prentice Hall, Englewood Cliffs, New Jersey
23. Sonstroem R J 1997 *Physical activity and self-esteem*. In: Morgan W P (ed) Physical activity and mental health. Hemisphere, Washington DC
24. Willis J D, Campbell L F 1992 *Exercise psychology*. Human Kinetics, Champaign, Illinois
25. Fox K R 1997 *The physical self: from motivation to well-being*. Human Kinetics, Champaign, Illinois
26. Triandis H C 1971 *Attitude and attitude change*. John Wiley, New York
27. Allport G W 1935 *Attitudes*. In: Fishbein M (ed) Readings in attitude theory and measurement. John Wiley, New York
28. Fishbein M, Ajzen I 1975 *Belief, attitude, intention and behavior*. Addison–Wesley, Reading, Massachussetts
29. Doganis G, Theodorakis Y 1995 *The influence of attitude on exercise participation*. In: Biddle S H (ed) European perspectives on exercise and sport psychology. Human Kinetics, Champaign, Illinois
30. Dishman R K, Ickes W, Morgan W P 1980 *Self-motivation and adherence to habitual physical activity*. Journal of Applied Psychology 10:115–132
31. Smith R A, Biddle S H 1991 *Exercise adherence in the commercial sector*. In: Proceedings of the 4th Annual Conference of the European Health Psychology Society, pp.154–155. British Psychological Society, Leicester
32. Gill D L 1986 *Psychological dynamics of sport*. Human Kinetics, Champaign, Illinois
33. Kenyon G S 1968 *Six scales for assessing attitudes towards physical education*. Research Quarterly 33:239–244
34. Sonstroem R J 1978 *Physical estimation and attraction scales: rationale and research*. Medicine and Science in Sports 10:97–102
35. Smoll F L, Schutz R W 1980 *Children's attitudes toward physical activity: a longitudinal analysis*. Journal of Sport Psychology 2:137–147
36. Hovland C I, Janis I L, Kelley H H et al 1953 *Communication and persuasion*. Yale University Press, New Haven, Connecticut
37. Festinger L A 1957 *A theory of cognitive dissonance*. Harper and Row, New York
38. Baron R A, Richardson D R 1994 *Human aggression*. Plenum, New York
39. Husman B F, Silva J M 1984 *Aggression in sport: definitions and theoretical considerations*. In: Silva J M, Weinberg R S (eds) Psychological foundations of sport. Human Kinetics, Champaign, Illinois
40. Lorenz K 1966 *On aggression*. Harcourt Brace, New York
41. Dollard J, Dobb J, Miller N, Mowrer O, Sears R 1939 *Frustration and aggression*. Yale University Press, New Haven, Connecticut
42. Bandura A 1973 *Aggression: a social learning analysis*. Prentice-Hall, Englewood Cliffs, New Jersey
43. Berkowitz L 1993 *Aggression: its causes, consequences and control*. Temple University Press, Philadelphia
44. Bredemeier B J 1985 *Moral reasoning and the perceived legitimacy of intentionally injurious sport acts*. Journal of Social Psychology 7:110–124
45. Tennenbaum G, Stewart E, Singer R N, Duda J 1997 *Aggression and violence in sport: an ISSP position stand*. ISSP Newsletter 1:14–17
46. Weiner B 1992 *Human motivation: metaphors, theories and research*. Sage, Newbury Park, California
47. Biddle S H (ed) 1995 *European perspectives on exercise and sport psychology*. Human Kinetics, Champaign, Illinois
48. Biddle S H, Brooke R 1992 *Intrinsic versus extrinsic motivational orientation in physical education and sport*. British Journal of Educational Psychology 62:247–256
49. Ashford B, Rickhuss J H 1992 *Life-span differences in motivation for participation in community sport and recreation (abstract)*. Journal of Sports Sciences 10(6):626
50. Gould D, Feltz D, Horn T, Weiss M 1982 *Reasons for attribution in competitive youth swimming*. Journal of Sport Behaviour 5:155–165
51. Gould D, Petlichkoff L 1988 *Participation motivation and attrition in young athletes*. In: Smoll F, Magill R, Ash M (eds) Children in sport, 3rd edn. Human Kinetics, Champaign, Illinois
52. Deci E 1971 *Effects of externally mediated rewards on*

intrinsic motivation. Journal of Personality and Social Psychology 18:105–115

53. Lepper M, Greene D 1975 *Turning play into work: the effects of adult surveillance and extrinsic rewards on children's intrinsic motivation*. Journal of Personality and Social Psychology 31:479–486

54. Atkinson J W 1974 *The mainsprings of achievement-oriented activity*. In: Atkinson J W, Raynor J O (eds) Motivation and achievement. Halstead, New York

55. Roberts G C 1974 *Effect of achievement motivation and social environment on performance of a motor task*. Journal of Motor Behaviour 4:37–46

56. Carron A V 1981 *Social psychology of sport: an experimental approach*. Mouvement Publications, Ithaca, New York

57. Roberts G C 1993 *Motivation in sport: understanding and enhancing the motivation and achievement of children*. In: Singer R N, Murphy M, Tenneant K L (eds) Handbook of research on sport psychology. Macmillan, New York

58. Biddle S H, Akande D, Armstrong N, Ashcroft M, Brooke R, Goudas M 1997 *The self-motivation inventory modified for children: evidence on psychometric properties and its use in physical exercise*. International Journal of Sport Psychology 14:237–250

59. Goudas M, Biddle S H, Fox K R 1994 *Achievement goal orientations and intrinsic motivation in physical fitness testing with children*. Pediatric Exercise Science 6:159–167

60. Weiner B 1986 *An attribution theory of motivation and emotion*. Springer-Verlag, New York

61. Duda J L, Nicholls J 1992 *Dimensions of achievement motivation in schoolwork and sport*. Journal of Educational Psychology 84:290–299

62. Biddle S H 1991 *Interpreting success and failure*. In: Bull S J (ed) Sport psychology: a self-help guide. Crowood, Marlborough

63. Weiner B 1979 *A theory of motivation for some classroom experiences*. Journal of Educational Psychology 71:3–25

64. Seligman M E P 1975 *Helplessness: on depression, development and death*. W H Freeman, San Francisco

65. Dweck C 1980 *Learned helplessness in sport*. In: Nedeau C et al (eds) Psychology of motor behavior and sport. Human Kinetics, Champaign, Illinois

66. Vealey R S 1986 *Conceptualisation of sport-confidence: preliminary investigation and instrument development*. Journal of Sport Psychology 8: 221-246

67. Hollander E 1971 *Principles and methods of social psychology*. Oxford University Press, New York

Psychology of sport: social influences on performance and mental preparation

13.1 Social learning

Learning objectives

On completion of this section, you will be able to:

1. Describe how young people may be socialised through and into sport and physical activity.

2. Define the role of significant others in this socialisation.

3. Use social learning theory to describe observational learning.

Keywords

- attention
- modelling
- motor reproduction
- norms
- observational learning
- reinforcement
- retention
- rules
- significant others
- social comparison
- socialisation
- social learning theory
- status

It is often claimed that physical education and sport have a variety of positive social effects: they build character, encourage teamwork and team spirit, develop the notion of fairness, teach adherence to rules and provide opportunity to let off extra energy and aggressive feelings in socially acceptable ways. While we do not have a great deal of research evidence for this, our common sense and experience suggest that sport and physical activity do have a **socialising effect**. In other words, we become socialised into some of the norms and values of our society *through* participation.

Sport itself has been, since the 19th century, a very important subculture of Western society; it is becoming a global subculture, as the modern Olympic Games demonstrate. A second socialising effect for youngsters entering sport is socialisation *into* sport culture, which is learning how to be a sportsperson. As in any culture, sport has **rules** that must be adhered to. We use demonstrations a great deal in physical education and Bandura[1] has suggested that we learn many of our behaviours through observation of others. As in any culture, sport has rules and values, which

must be learned and internalised. Some of these rules and values are formal, written down and public, such as the laws governing the playing of a particular game or the members' rules posted on the clubhouse noticeboard. Sanctions are likely to apply if these are not followed. Others are accepted by the sport community but are unwritten, such as applauding your opponents into the changing room in rugby union. Flouting these rules may be judged to be 'bad manners' but normally sanctions do not apply.

There are also the **norms and values**, certainly unwritten and often unexpressed, associated with being a member of a particular team or club: wearing the team kit in a particular way; always questioning the referee's decisions; playing 'hard but fair'. Some of these norms and values may be socially acceptable, others less so. A newcomer to the group must identify these characteristics of the group and decide (i) to accept them and become an integrated member of the group, (ii) to reject some but still stay a member or (iii) to leave the group. This sounds like a conscious decision process, but it is not necessarily so.

Through socialisation we also learn about our **status** within the sport group and we take on particular roles. There are formal roles such as captain or coach and informal roles such as humourist, peacemaker or motivator.

How do these socialisation processes work? There are a number of theories that explain socialisation. The one we use frequently in this text is Bandura's[1] **social learning theory**, also referred to as **observational learning theory**. We have used it to explain skill learning from demonstrations, the development of personality, aggressive behaviour and the development of self-efficacy.

Social learning theory has three component processes:

- **modelling** – observational learning: athletes learn behaviour (good and bad) and also skills and techniques by watching others
- **reinforcement** – this behaviour is reinforced or penalised
- **social comparison** – using other people as a 'yardstick' to evaluate our own skill, attitudes and behaviour.

These processes interact with each other whenever we are consciously or unconsciously aware of how others deal with situations. Such people are **models**. For us to learn from them, they have to be **significant**, i.e. we must want what they appear to have (skill, fame, power, etc.). People are significant to us because they are:

- influential or have high status, e.g. sport stars, heroes, coach, teacher, parent
- caring, e.g. friends, teammates, parents
- successful
- similar to ourselves, e.g. age, gender, physique, skill
- a combination of these.

We learn skills, attitudes, behaviour and language by observation. Bandura[1] claims that **observational learning** has four stages. These are shown in Figure 13.1.

- **Attention** – the learner consciously attends to what the model is doing. In the demonstration of a skill, a coach will identify a few important points and cues, which the learner should attend to.
- **Retention** – the model's behaviour will be committed to memory. For this to be most effective, what is being learnt must be interesting and relevant and the demonstration must be repeated.

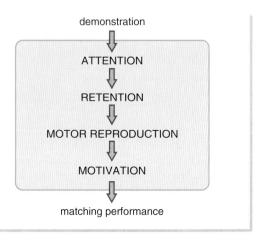

Fig. 13.1 Model of Bandura's observational learning.

- **Motor reproduction** – the learner must firstly be physically capable of performing the skill or copying the behaviour and secondly have opportunity to practise.
- **Motivation** – the learner must have reason or desire to acquire the modelled skill, behaviour or attitude.

You should note that the above process applies to:

1. **formal learning**, such as being coached in an athletic event (for example). In this case, research[2] suggests that it is not the expertise of the model that matters, but the quality of the feedback or commentary that accompanies the demonstration
2. **informal learning**, such as how to behave towards sport officials; in this case the model is usually either of high status or is a member of the peer group.

Review questions

1. Define social learning theory.[1]
2. Draw Bandura's model of observational learning.
3. Describe how observational learning theory explains how youngsters become socialised into a sport club.
4. Show how observational learning theory is used in skill acquisition.
5. Why is it important that professional players and/or athletes set good examples of behaviour in sport?

1. a. What is meant by the term socialisation and how can it be explained within the context of sport? (*3 marks*)

   b. Using Bandura's model of observational learning in Figure 13.1, show the importance of demonstration in motor skill learning. (*10 marks*)

   c. Videos are often used in the teaching and refining of motor skills as well as illustrating tactical strategies in sport. How would you use a video to encourage participation and to motivate performers in sport? (*6 marks*)
   (*Total 19 marks*)

2. a. When performing a demonstration, what are the key factors that influence observational learning? (*4 marks*)

   b. Social learning theory suggests that we learn through observation. How can this theory be applied to the teaching of sport to young people? (*4 marks*)
   (*Total 8 marks*)

13.2 Groups and teams

Learning objectives

On completion of this section, you will be able to:

1. Define the term 'group' and describe the formation and characteristics of sports groups.

2. Discuss the factors that lead to a cohesive sports team or group.

3. Describe and analyse models of group performance.

4. Discuss motivational factors within groups, including social loafing and the Ringelmann effect.

5. Describe coaching strategies that will ensure maximum effort from group or team members.

Keywords

➤ cohesion
➤ faulty processes
➤ formal role
➤ group processes
➤ informal role
➤ interaction
➤ interactive others
➤ norms
➤ passive others
➤ productivity
➤ Ringelmann effect
➤ social cohesion
➤ social interaction
➤ social loafing
➤ sociometry
➤ task cohesion
➤ task interaction

Most sports and activities take place within a social context. While there certainly are people who derive satisfaction from training and competing alone, dependent upon their own psychological and physical resources, most are drawn to activity because of the opportunity to join people who share their enthusiasm. Personal experience and research tell us that we tend to react differently when we are in a group from when we are alone and thus investigating these differences and considering their implications for teams and squads is important.

What is a group?

Shaw[3] defines it as 'two or more persons who are interacting with one another in such a manner that each person influences and is influenced by each other person'. McGrath[4] states that 'groups are those social aggregates that involve mutual awareness and potential interaction'.

Both definitions highlight the importance (whether actual or potential) of interaction. Shaw sees influence as an important component; McGrath prefers awareness of each other. There are many different forms of interaction within a group or team. **Social interaction** refers to the friendship groups that form. These can be very positive; they help integration and allow members to feel they are a real part of the group. But friendship groups can have negative effects if they become exclusive cliques. Verbal communication plays a large part in social interaction. **Task interaction** is the way in which participants cooperate with each other to win the competition. In some sports there is a high degree of task interaction; teams only succeed if players are very aware of and sensitive to the positioning and requirements of others, e.g. invasion games. Although verbal communication is often used (e.g. calling for the ball), non-verbal communication (signs, gestures) and the ability to 'read' movement cues are predominant.

Positive social interaction is important in all teams and groups, which is why good coaches will include social activities in their training programmes, to allow team members to get to know and like each other.

Investigation 13.1 Interaction within sports teams

Method: Make a list of sports included in the Olympic Games. Construct a continuum based on the extent to which the members of a particular team in each sport need to use task interaction during competition.

Results: You might have, for example, volleyball near one end (as a highly interactive sport) and archery near the other.

Discussion: Compare your list with those of others in your group and discuss any discrepancies.

ACTIVITY 13.1

1. Group discussion

   If you accept the definitions, would you consider a crowd at a football match, or a collection of people at a public swimming session, to be a group?

   Select some other examples of groups and non-groups in sports and activity contexts. Don't be concerned if you have some difficulty in deciding – the borderline between group and non-group is not clear-cut.

2. Make a list of as many different examples of sport and exercise groups as you can think of.

   Discuss the characteristics that these groups have in common (see the four components of the definition of a group, below).

   Discuss differences between these groups. For example, how does an athletics team differ from a hockey team, or a basketball team from a keep-fit class?

   All teams are groups but not all groups are teams. When is a sport/exercise group called a team? Part of your answer should include the importance of the interdependency of team members in working towards common goals.

For a collection of people to be defined as a group, the members must:

- interact with each other
- be socially aware of each other
- share goals or purposes
- have a shared identity, which distinguishes them from other groups. This may be represented by a uniform or by shared patterns of communication, behaviour and values.

Group/team structure

ACTIVITY 13.2

Consider a team or sports group of which you are a member.

1. Make two lists of the roles which people hold or play in the team. One list should be headed formal roles (e.g. captain) and the other informal roles (e.g. best player).

2. Discuss or list the norms of the group, i.e. the behaviour, dress style, beliefs and attitudes that are expected of group members.

These aspects, roles and norms, are two key factors in group structure. Teams and groups are strongest when these are recognised, understood and shared amongst members.

The **formal role** is the behaviour, rights and responsibilities expected of a person who has been given a particular job to do within a team. This may be a positional role (e.g. goalkeeper) or an organisational role (e.g. fixture secretary). The role player may have been appointed or elected and often needs to be trained in the role.

Informal roles are not part of the formal organisation of the team/group but nevertheless help (or occasionally hinder) its functioning. These roles usually evolve as the group members interact with and get to know each other and they arise from the personalities and strengths of the people who come to fill them. Examples of informal roles in sports groups are comedian, mediator (who solves disputes), motivator, mentor (who looks after newcomers).

Groups and teams can be made more effective by:

- ensuring that all members understand their own formal role and that of others (**role clarity**)

- making sure that members accept their formal role (and that of others) and understand the contribution of all roles to the overall objectives of the group (**role acceptance**)
- acknowledging informal roles where they are helpful to the group and dealing with unhelpful informal roles (e.g. troublemakers).

Team performance and productivity

A good team is more than the sum of its parts. Working together and interacting effectively is the key to good team performance. But this is not always easy to achieve and teams sometimes perform below expectations. Steiner[5] devised an equation to summarise this:

$$\frac{Actual}{productivity} = \frac{potential}{productivity} - \frac{losses\ due\ to}{faulty\ processes}$$

Put in sport team terms, this would be expressed as:

$$\frac{Team}{success} = \frac{potential}{for\ success} - \frac{effect\ of\ coordination\ and}{motivation\ problems}$$

This equation is explained below.

- **Potential for success** – in general, the most skilful individuals make up the best team. Jones[6] correlated the individual ability of members of a team against the overall success of the team and found high positive correlation in all his cases. The lowest correlation (0.6) was in basketball, a sport in which there is a great deal of interaction.
- High interaction presents **coordination problems** for players. If one player is being selfish or aggressive, or if a defence is not working together, overall team performance suffers.
- **Motivation problems** – people seem to work less hard in a group than they do on their own. For example, in the 1972 Olympics, the time of the winning double sculls was only 4% faster than that of the single sculls, and the eights only 6% faster than that of the fours. There might be a

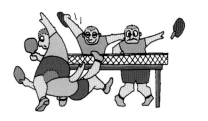

Fig. 13.2 Coordination and cooperation may be a problem.

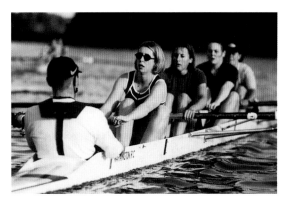

Fig. 13.3

technical reason for this in terms of the relative size and weights of the boats but experiments which control for this (e.g.[7]) suggest that it is motivational losses, rather than technical or coordination losses, which are the most significant.

Social loafing/the Ringelmann effect

Social loafing is the tendency for individuals to lessen their effort when they are part of a group. This loss of performance (**productivity**) is also known as the **Ringelmann effect** after an early experimenter who studied people's efforts in a tug-of-war competition. He found that as the number of people in the team increased, so the relative performance of each individual declined. Thus in a team of two each pulled at 93% of his potential; in teams of three this dropped to 85% and in eight-person teams, each only pulled 49% of his potential on average. More recent studies have tended to replicate these results in a range of activities and have shown that the overall reduction in performance is usually due to decrease in individual motivation and not to coordination problems.

Causes of social loafing in a sports team have been given as:

- individuals perceiving others to be working less hard than they themselves are, which gives an excuse to put in less effort
- individuals believing that their own efforts will have little effect on the outcome
- individuals disliking hard work and assuming that their lack of effort will not be noticed within the overall team performance
- individuals feeling 'off form' and believing that their teammates will cover for their lack of form or effort.

Social loafing can be minimised if players:

- believe that their contribution within the team is identifiable
- understand and accept their own particular responsibilities to the team
- know what it's like to play other roles in the team, e.g. another position in an invasion game or a different 'leg' in a track sprint relay.

Thus team coaches who are aware of this:

- identify situations where loafing might occur, recognising that fatigue is inevitable in lengthy competitions and that players sometimes need to coast temporarily
- publicly acknowledge individual performance in a game
- discuss loafing as a general issue with the team as a whole, but in private with individuals to determine possible reasons for loss of motivation or effort.

Cohesion

Earlier in the section we discussed the nature of interaction in groups and teams. Another way of looking at this is through the concept of **cohesion**. Cohesion is the extent to which members of a group exhibit a desire to achieve common goals and group identity. As with interaction, we identify **social cohesion**, the extent to which members of a group get on with each other, and **task cohesion**, the extent to which group members cooperate with each other in achieving the group's goals.

Carron[10] gives four factors which affect the development of cohesion.

- **Environmental**: factors which link a player with a particular team, e.g. nationality, location, friendship, contracts.
- **Personal**: motives and attitudes which the individual believes are fulfilled by membership of the team, e.g. status, success, friendship.
- **Leadership**: the style and behaviour of the manager, coach, captain.
- **Team**: identity, shared norms, targets.

Common sense suggests that the more cohesive a team is, the better they will perform. Cohesion is a popular subject for research studies[8,9] but the results of this research are equivocal. Some studies show that high group cohesion leads to better performances; others suggest that good performances lead to increased cohesion. Some results show a negative correlation between performance and cohesion, i.e. the less cohesive a team, the better they perform.

These differences may be explained by considering (i) how researchers measure cohesion and (ii) some of the factors that appear to be associated with cohesion.

ACTIVITY 13.3

In a small group take each of Carron's four factors affecting cohesion and discuss how the coach might demonstrate understanding of each in his/her work with a team. You might like to look at Section 13.3 (Leadership) before finalising your ideas. Share your examples with the whole class.

Measurement of cohesion

Cohesion is usually measured by questionnaire. Some examples from these are given in the Teacher's Guide that accompanies this book. The important thing is to differentiate between task and social cohesion (see above). When only social cohesion (interpersonal attraction/friendship) is measured, then often a negative relationship is found between team performance and cohesion, i.e. teams who are very friendly do not perform as well as teams who are not, when potential ability is taken into account. When task cohesion is measured, however, then results are mixed: in some instances a high degree of task cohesion leads to better performance but in others there is no strong relationship. This appears strange at first, for although common sense allows us to rationalise the negative relationship between social cohesion and performance, we would assume a positive relationship between performance and task cohesion, i.e. teams that are good at working together to achieve their goal should do better than teams that are not. To explain the fact that this is not always the case, we need to return to the concept of interaction.

Return to Investigation 13.1. At one end of your continuum you should have high interaction teams such as volleyball, basketball, hockey, soccer. At the other end you will have sports where, although the team will exist, its success will depend on completely independent performances, where there is no task interaction, e.g. skiing, archery. Between these two extremes are sports where there is some interaction during competition, e.g. tennis doubles, cricket, track and swimming relays.

Assume you are a researcher using a questionnaire to measure high, moderate and low degrees of task cohesion within teams. You have chosen a selection of consistently successful teams that represent the interaction continuum (high, moderate, low). Which teams do you hypothesise will show the highest task cohesion and why?

Research tends to support the idea that high-interaction teams need high task cohesion to be consistently successful, whereas for moderate- or low-interaction teams, cohesion of either form is less important to success.

Other factors associated with cohesion

A number of other factors have been found to relate to cohesion, but the ways in which this happens are not clear and patterns in the research findings are only just beginning to emerge. It is also not certain whether the factors listed below affect cohesion or whether cohesion leads to these characteristics.

Stability

The longer a group stays together, with the same members, the more likely it is to develop cohesiveness. The timing of dropping older players and the bringing in of new ones needs careful thought by team managers.

Similarity

The more similar group members are in terms of skill, age, attitudes, etc., the more cohesive the group is likely to be.

Size

Cohesion develops most quickly in small groups, unless there are any very disruptive members, who will have a much greater effect in a small group than in a larger one.

Support

Cohesive teams tend to have managers and captains who provide overt support to players and who encourage players to support each other. This support occurs before, during and after competition (task-related support) and at other times (personal and emotional support).

Satisfaction

Cohesion is associated with the extent to which team members are pleased with each others' performance, behaviour and conformity to the norms of the group.

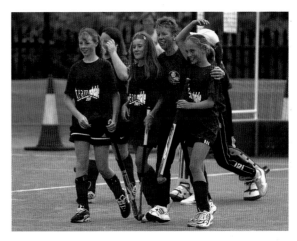

Fig. 13.4 Cohesion is made up of social and task elements.

For example, cohesion can be lessened if a player consistently lets the team down in some way. Conversely, it can be increased if a particular player is threatened from outside, for example a professional footballer that is 'picked on' by opposition fans or the media.

State of development of the group

Groups and teams take time to develop cohesion. Early in a group's formation, players will be getting to know their role and may be wary of each other. Later there will be some competition for roles and status and cohesion is likely to be threatened temporarily. Eventually, if the team is well managed, cooperation will replace competitiveness and cohesion will increase and maximise as stability is achieved and roles are clear and accepted.

Cohesion in a team can be measured by a technique known as **sociometry**. You will find more details of this in the Teacher's Guide that accompanies this textbook, but essentially it involves asking members of a group to nominate, in confidence, two or three other members who they would choose in the situation being investigated. The situation might be a friendship choice or it might be a task; the ways in which the technique can be used are very varied. These choices are then represented on a diagram, known as a sociogram.

Most coaches accept that members of a team interact more effectively in task-oriented situations if they like, or at least respect, one another. This does not apply in sport only. Consider the implications for a climbing team or a dance company if excessive rivalry develops between its members.

Investigation 13.2 To interpret a sociogram

Method: Look at the sociogram in Figure 13.5. The arrows represent choices; for example, 'N' has nominated 'K' as a friend.

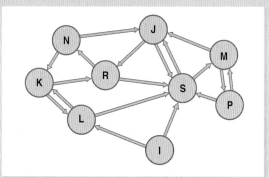

Fig. 13.5 A friendship sociogram within a sports team.

1. Organise a tournament in your class or college in a small-team sport, such as basketball or volleyball, so that the teams can be ranked at the end. Select the teams so that intrateam friendship groups are avoided as far as possible. Ask the individual members of the teams who were ranked highest and lowest to complete the following simple questionnaire to assess task cohesion (Q1) and social cohesion (Q2).

   • Q1. Did the members of your team play well together?

   | 9 | 8 | 7 | 6 | 5 | 4 | 3 | 2 | 1 |

   very much   not at all

   • Q2. Do the members of your team like one another?

   | 9 | 8 | 7 | 6 | 5 | 4 | 3 | 2 | 1 |

   very much   not at all

Results: Calculate a mean score on each question for each team. From your results, draw a bar chart similar to that given in Figure 13.6.

Discussion: What do your results tell you about the relationship between task cohesion, social cohesion and team success?

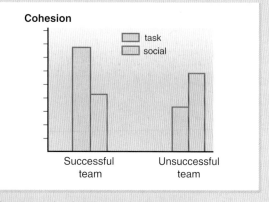

Fig. 13.6 Task cohesion, social and team success.

Coaching for maximum productivity

In order to perform to its potential, a team needs to ensure it makes the best use of the ability of its individual members (potential productivity), maximises team cooperation and minimises the negative effects of such factors as social loafing and lack of coordination (**faulty processes**).

Coaches, managers and leaders do this by:

• making the group distinct: a name, kit, slogans and songs
• having clear, group and individual goals that are shared and accepted (see later section)
• having clear formal roles, which as far as possible have equal status, and acknowledging useful informal roles
• encouraging shared decision making
• developing mutual respect

• ensuring that training is fun and interactive as well as individually demanding.

No doubt you can think of some more.

Review questions

1. Define a 'group'.
2. What are the factors that make a team or dance group 'cohesive'?
3. What is meant by the equation:

   actual team productivity = potential productivity – faulty processes?

4. **a.** What is meant by (i) the 'Ringelmann effect' and (ii) 'social loafing' in a sports context?

   b. How may these effects be overcome?

5. List at least five ways in which a coach might set about developing 'team spirit'.

Exam-style questions

1. a. (i) One definition of a group is that it consists of two or more people. Identify two other features of a sports group. (*2 marks*)

   (ii) The performance of a sports team can be explained using the following formula:

   actual productivity of team = potential productivity – faulty processes

   Using this formula, explain why a sports team might not always fulfil its potential. (*3 marks*)

   (iii) How could the coach of a sports team ensure that faulty processes are kept to a minimum? (*3 marks*)

   (*Total 8 marks*)

2. a. (i) What is meant by potential productivity? (*1 mark*)

   (ii) There may be motivational problems that contribute to the faulty processes. What is meant by the Ringelmann effect? (*2 marks*)

   (iii) Latane et al[7] identified one motivational problem as social loafing. Using your team as an example, briefly explain the concept of social loafing. What strategies could your coach use to stop social loafing occurring? (*6 marks*)

   b. (i) What two main personal qualities do you feel are important in a team captain? (*2 marks*)

   (ii) Using your knowledge of attribution theory, what reasons might you encourage your team members to give for losing a game? (*3 marks*)

   (*Total 14 marks*)

3. a. What is meant by cohesion in the context of teams? (*4 marks*)

   b. What factors stop a team ever performing to its true potential? (*6 marks*)

   (*Total 10 marks*)

4. Explain what is meant by social loafing by using examples from sport. (*3 marks*)

5. a. Explain what is meant by the term group cohesion. (4 marks)

   b. Briefly identify two methods of measuring the cohesiveness of a sports team. (*2 marks*)

   c. 'Two heads are better than one'; 'Too many cooks spoil the broth'. Discuss these apparently contradictory statements in relation to sports groups, with specific reference to group size and cohesion. (*8 marks*)

   d. Are cohesive groups in sport always more successful? Explain your answer. (*6 marks*)

   (*Total 20 marks*)

13.3 Leadership

Learning objectives

On completion of this section, you will be able to:

1. State reasons for the importance of effective leadership in sport.

2. Identify leadership roles in sport.

3. Use theoretical models to describe and analyse the characteristics of effective leaders.

4. Compare trait, social learning and interactionist theories of leadership and discuss these in sport contexts.

5. Explain Fiedler's contingency model and Chelladurai's multidimensional model of leadership.

6. Suggest practical guidelines for sport leaders within a sport or exercise activity with which you are familiar.

Keywords

➤ autocratic style
➤ Chelladurai's multidimensional model
➤ democratic style
➤ emergent (leader)
➤ Fiedler's contingency model
➤ laissez-faire style
➤ leader characteristics
➤ leadership
➤ members' characteristics
➤ person (relationship)-centred style
➤ prescribed (leader)
➤ task-centred style

In the previous chapter we considered the development of team cohesion. The development of team cohesion often depends on the **leadership** of the coach or team captain. Leadership is the process by which a particular individual fulfils the expectations of a group or team and develops an environment in which the group is motivated, rewarded and helped to achieve its goals. It should not be confused with management, which deals with routine organisation. Leadership is about vision.

Effective leadership is very important in sport. Sport and most exercise activities are social, organised and rule governed. Most take place within group or team contexts. The group tasks are complex and often tightly time constrained: the dance performance must start on time; a tournament will not be postponed because one player's preparation is not complete. Teams are complex social groups and the relationships within the group and between the members of the group and its leader will affect its success. Professional football provides some interesting examples of this. Team members look to the leadership for support, direction, organisation, motivation, strategy and discipline. A good sport leader provides the context in which the team can be successful and in which individual players feel supported and can thrive. Poor leadership leads to division, dissent, lack of motivation and frustration.

Theories of leadership

Early research into leadership, both in sport and generally, suggested that leaders are 'born, not made', i.e. they possess personality **traits** that suit them to a leadership role. Thus a leader must be (for example) courageous, tenacious, knowledgeable and a good communicator. People who have these attributes are likely to become leaders. This is sometimes referred to as the 'Great Man' theory of leadership. However, this has been largely superseded by the idea that there is not one particular set of personality traits that mark out a leader, but that certain combinations of traits might be useful in particular situations.

A more modern version of this theory takes an **interactionist** approach. Good leaders match their behaviour and approach to the situation. For example, a good team coach will treat players as individuals, being tough and demanding on some players and more encouraging with others, whilst maintaining a fair, supportive approach to all.

A third group of theories focus on the fact that these behaviours can be learned (**social learning theory**), so everyone has the potential to be an effective leader.

Leaders tend to come forward in one of two ways:[11] **emergent** leaders are those who come from the group itself, either informally because of their skills and abilities or formally through nomination and/or selection; **prescribed** leaders are those appointed by the organising body. What do you see to be the advantages and difficulties for leaders themselves of being in each of these two categories?

Characteristics of leaders

The characteristics of effective leadership are difficult to pin down, but it is generally recognised that there are three main factors that interact to affect a person's capacity to lead, as represented in Figure 13.7:

- **leader's characteristics**, in terms of the quality and style
- **the situation** in terms of the group's cohesion (individuality), the size and traditions of the group and the nature and difficulty of the tasks facing the group
- **members' characteristics**, in terms of their expectations and their preferred leadership style.

The theory is that the more the leader's actual behaviour matches the expectations and preferences of the members of the group and the specific demands of the situation, the greater the group's satisfaction, enjoyment and performance will be.

The problem is, however, that each group, and each activity context, is different, so defining just what these behaviours are is very difficult.

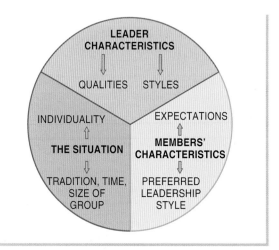

Fig. 13.7 Components of leadership.

Leadership style

Investigation 13.3 identifies leadership qualities or characteristics. An early categorisation of these identified three **leadership styles: autocratic, democratic** and **laissez-faire.** Autocratic leaders tend to want to control

Method: From your own experience, make a list of the qualities you would associate with a good team captain. Compare your list with those of others and derive a definitive list of about 12 qualities that you all agree on. Think of opposites for these. For example, if you choose 'self-confident', the opposite might be 'diffident'. Construct a questionnaire by separating your opposites on a five-point scale, for example:

| self-confident | 5 | 4 | 3 | 2 | 1 | diffident |
| unfriendly | 1 | 2 | 3 | 4 | 5 | friendly |

Try out your scale on yourself. To obtain an overall score you need to reverse the scoring on some items, e.g. unfriendly–friendly.

Discussion: How did you rate as a leader? Of course, you may have all these qualities and not be your team's captain – there are many other factors involved. Also, there may be times when a leader needs to be the opposite of what you have rated highly.

the group and they make most of the decisions. This style of leadership is useful in dangerous situations, when an immediate decision is needed, or with non-cohesive groups. Democratic leaders are interested in the opinions of the group as a whole and respect the views of the majority. It is a useful style for problem solving in a team, when time is not very important. A laissez-faire style is one in which the leader lets the group get on with the task without any guidance unless it is asked for or unless obvious problems arise. This style may be adopted consciously, because the leader wants the group to establish their own working patterns and strategies (it is sometimes used in counselling, therapy or education), or unknowingly, when the leader lacks confidence and skill. It works well if the group is achieving success, empowering group members and developing an internal locus of control (see Chapter 12) but can lead to frustration if success is not achieved quickly.

Fiedler[12] summarised leadership characteristics as a continuum between two styles:

1. **task-centred** leadership – the leader's focus is on what has to be done. The needs of individual group members are less important than the achievement of the group's goals. When this can be achieved through consensus, task-centred leaders will take the ideas of the group into account, but if not, they are autocratic

2. **person (or relationship)-centred** leadership – these leaders try to involve the group as much as possible in decision making and they may be willing to sacrifice success for good interpersonal relationships and the integrity of the group.

Can you see the link between the autocratic and task-centred styles and between the democratic and person-centred styles?

It is possible for a leader to adopt either style or a combination. A good coach, captain or manager does the latter, depending on the situation.

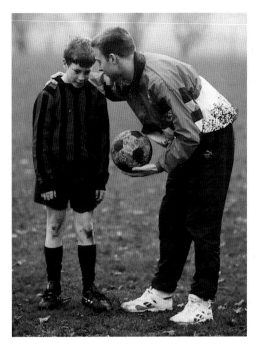

Fig. 13.8 A task-centred or a person-centred coach?

Situational factors

Fiedler's contingency model (Figure 13.9) relates effective leadership style to what he called 'situational favourableness'. If things are going well for the coach and the team or, alternatively, if the situation is un-favourable (e.g. poor facilities, little support, difficult opposition) then a sports leader needs to be very task centred. If the situation is moderately favourable then a person-centred approach is likely to work best. Thus, being an effective leader is about (contingent upon) adapting one's style to the situation.

There is a range of situational factors that a leader needs to be aware of in selecting an appropriate style. Research has shown that players in team sports look for a captain or coach who is directive and uses his/her

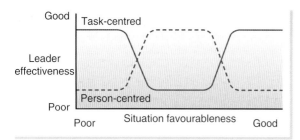

Fig. 13.9 Fiedler's contingency model.

ACTIVITY 13.4

Discuss a number of specific moments or situations in sport which demanded a leader's intervention and with which you are familiar either through participation or via the media.

Analyse them in the light of Fielder's contingency model. Do your examples fit the model or are there other factors that need to be taken into account?

---

authority to organise and structure the group in order to complete the task or achieve the group's ambitions (e.g. promotion to a higher league). Individuals, for example skaters and athletes, prefer a more person-oriented leader. This seems to relate to the size of the group – the more team members there are, the less easy it is to take each person's individual needs and preferences into account. Similarly, if decisions have to be made quickly, an autocratic style is usually adopted. Another interesting research finding, probably backed up by your own experience, is that groups tend to be traditional; once they have become used to a particular style, they resent change.

Members' characteristics

This leads us to the third section of the component model (see Figure 13.7). We tend to think of captains, coaches and leaders as influencing the behaviour of the group members, but of course it works the other way too. If, for example, a team captain senses that the team is hostile, he/she tends to develop a more autocratic style than if the team is friendly and cooperative. A team or group working towards a particular goal, an important competition, expedition or performance, looks towards the leader to help it succeed and has ideas about how this should be done, particularly if its members are experienced. Problems can arise if the strategies for training and preparation adopted by the leader do not match members' expectations. Good leaders are sensitive to the expectations, knowledge and experience of group members.

Figure 13.10 represents Chelladurai's interactional model of leadership.[13] He indicates that the athlete's **performance and satisfaction** are the required outcomes of the coaching process and that the extent to which these occur depends on the way in which three aspects of leader behaviour interact. 'Required leader behaviour' refers to the expectations that team management have of the coach or captain. 'Actual leader behaviour' refers to the way in which the coach/captain normally goes about his/her job, i.e. interaction with the team, coaching style, etc. 'Preferred leadership behaviour' is the way in which the players like their coach/captain to relate to them. The ideal team situation is when all three behaviours are congruent, i.e. when the coach/captain acts in ways that both management and the team like. If the coach behaves in a way that neither the management nor the players approve of, he/she is unlikely to last very long; an ambitious sport leader will ensure that either management or the players (and preferably both) are satisfied with how he/she deals with the team.

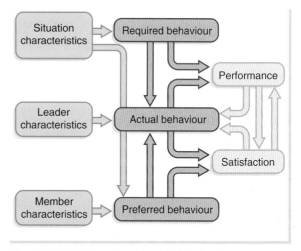

Fig. 13.10 Multidimensional model of leadership.

Chelladurai developed his multidimensional model to focus on preferred leadership behaviour and identified five types of coaching focus:

- training and instruction
- democratic approach
- autocratic approach
- social support
- rewards.

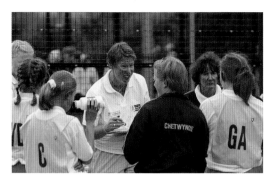

Fig. 13.11 Players prefer coaches who give plenty of feedback and reward.

Athletes seem to prefer a coaching focus that is strong on technical and tactical aspects (training and instruction) and in which the coach gives plentiful feedback and reward. Least preferred is an autocratic approach by a coach who only relies on authority and does not demonstrate an awareness of athletes' needs and preferences.

It is important to bear in mind, however, that different groups will have different preferences. For example, youngsters prefer and need a coach who provides plenty of social support; male athletes are more prepared to tolerate an authoritarian coach than are female athletes. This does not imply that other focuses are inappropriate; it is a question of emphasis.

Review questions

1. List at least three different leadership roles in a sport context. Indicate whether each is 'emergent' or 'prescribed'.

2. Discuss whether leaders are 'born' or 'made'.

3. Differentiate between a 'task-oriented' leadership style and a 'person- or relationship-oriented' leadership style.

4. When should a coach adopt a task-oriented style and when a person-oriented style?

Exam-style questions

1. **a.** What is meant by a leader and what sort of qualities would you expect to see in a leader within the context of sport? (*4 marks*)

   b. Using psychological theories, describe how an individual becomes a leader. (*4 marks*)

   (*Total 8 marks*)

2. **a.** Name three leadership styles. (*3 marks*)

   b. What factors should be taken into consideration when deciding upon which leadership style to adopt? (*6 marks*)

   (*Total 9 marks*)

3. **Look at Figure 13.10: Chelladurai's multidimensional model of leadership.**

   a. Explain each part of the model using examples from sport. (*3 marks*)

   b. Behaviour of the group associated with leadership can be viewed from three perspectives. Briefly name and explain each of these perspectives. (*3 marks*)

   c. Discuss the statement 'Good leaders are born not made' and explain whether you agree or disagree in the light of psychological theory. (*5 marks*)

   (*Total 11 marks*)

4. Fiedler's contingency model suggests that the effectiveness of a leader can change depending on the situation. Use sporting examples to explain this theory. (*4 marks*)

13.4 Competition effects on sport performance: social facilitation

Learning objectives

On completion of this section, you will be able to:

1. Describe and evaluate Zajonc's theory of social facilitation, Cottrell's evaluation apprehension theory and Baron's distraction-conflict theory.

2. Describe the positive and negative effects on sports performance of social facilitation and co-action, including the home advantage/disadvantage model.

Keywords

➤ audience (effects)
➤ co-action effects
➤ co-actors
➤ distraction-conflict theory
➤ dominant response
➤ evaluation apprehension
➤ home advantage
➤ social facilitation
➤ social inhibition

Most of us involved in sport or dance recognise the effect that the presence of spectators has on the way we play or perform. People watching us may tend to make us nervous and make mistakes (**social inhibition**), but their presence often means that we try a little bit harder (**social facilitation**). Investigating these effects experimentally has interested sports psychologists for a long time but there is still some difficulty in isolating the different variables that operate. Early research, which contrasted performance with an audience with performance without one, proved unexpectedly inconclusive until Zajonc[14] clarified the terms that were being used. He first defined different kinds of audience, as shown in Figure 13.12.

It is important for you to note that, in this model, the **audience** and co-actors are passive, i.e. not communicating in any significant way with the performer. **Co-actors** are involved in the same activity at the same time as the performer but are not competing directly. Competitors and supporters ('spectators' might be a more useful term) interact with the performer in a variety of ways.

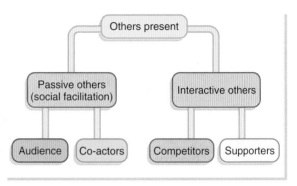

Fig. 13.12 Different types of audience.

Investigation 13.4 To interpret Figure 13.12

Method: Study Figure 13.12. Take each of the four categories, audience, co-actors, competitors and supporters, and give sport-related examples for each category. Remember that 'audience' and 'co-actors' do not interact or communicate with the performer. You may have to select particular periods in a game or event to illustrate these categories.

Discussion: Compare and discuss your ideas with others in the group.

Investigation 13.5 To investigate whether performance of a simple endurance task is improved by the presence of an audience or co-actors

Method: For the task, use a wall squat as illustrated in Figure 9.15. Make sure you have warmed up first. Divide the subjects available into three groups – A, B and C. Arrange your data collection so that all the subjects are timed on their ability to hold a wall squat under three different experimental conditions: **(i)** alone; **(ii)** in the presence of co-actors; **(iii)** in the presence of an audience. Measurements are taken in the following order:

• Group A: audience, alone, co-actors
• Group B: co-actors, audience, alone
• Group C: alone, audience, co-actors

Once you have got results from the three groups for the three conditions, treat all three groups as one.

Results: Obtain a mean score for the three conditions and plot these on a bar chart, as in Figure 13.13.

Discussion

1. To what extent do your results match those in Figure 13.13? Explain any discrepancies.

2. What is the reason for collecting the data in groups?

3. Does the presence of an experimenter pose a problem of validity?

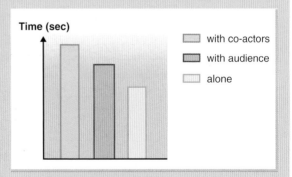

Fig. 13.13 The hypothetical relationships between scores on an endurance task, under three different experiment conditions.

Level of performance

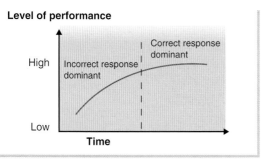

Fig. 13.14 A learning curve to show the development of a correct dominant response.

On the basis of work such as in Investigations 13.4 and 13.5, Zajonc[14] suggested that an audience affects a performer differentially, according to the part of the learning curve he/she is in (Figure 13.14).

Experiments show that learners perform better alone than with an audience, but that experienced performers do better with an audience. Zajonc explains this in terms of an increase in psychological arousal caused by the audience (Figure 13.15). For the inexperienced performer, still in the associative phase of learning, this increase causes interference with the production of the skill but for the expert, the increased level of arousal is motivating, as discussed in an earlier section.

Thus, according to Zajonc, the mere presence of others creates arousal (see Section 13.5) which then affects performance. Cottrell[15] disputes this model and suggests that it is not 'mere presence' which creates arousal but the fact that the audience may be

perceived as evaluating the performance, thus creating what Cottrell calls **evaluation apprehension**. If this is the case then what matters is *who* is in the audience; a 'scout' or selector in the crowd is likely to cause a young player more concern than a friend. The more expert and influential the observer, the more likely evaluation apprehension is to occur but remember that this can have either a positive or a negative effect, depending on the confidence of the player.

Baron's[16] **distraction-conflict theory** sought to explain the arousal engendered by spectators in a different way. He suggested that if a performer is able to concentrate solely on the activity, then arousal levels would be those generated by the activity itself. If, however, the performer is distracted by the audience, then this creates a conflict of attention since it is difficult to concentrate fully on both audience and performance. This conflict increases arousal level and leads to facilitation or inhibition. Football supporters try and use this effect when taunting individual members of the opposition team. Their chants are designed both to distract and make the player angry.

The home advantage/disadvantage phenomenon (performers do better on their home ground than they do away) is a theory which has 'common sense' value. We see it in the assignment of neutral grounds in the final stages of an important tournament. Research in the USA[17] gives overall support to the idea, though there are differences between sports and at different stages of a competition. There may be a familiarity/ unfamiliarity effect associated with the ground itself but home advantage is usually explained in terms of the balance of supporters and opposition in the crowd. For example, in sports where the spectators are near the field of play there is a greater advantage in playing at home than in sports where spectators are further away. Home advantage works most in the early stages of a competition. As the finals or the end of the season approaches, home games seem to put more pressure on teams and results are less certain. Can you suggest why this might be the case, using Cottrell's and Baron's theories? If you play in or follow a particular team, you could collect data on home and away results over a season and test out the theory.

Coaches recognise the negative effects of social inhibition and will work with performers to prevent these by incorporating strategies into training. Many of these strategies are to do with managing the negative effects of arousal (see Section 13.5). Others help performers to focus their attention on the task and avoid the distraction of spectators (see **attentional narrowing** in Section 13.5). A coach may use mental

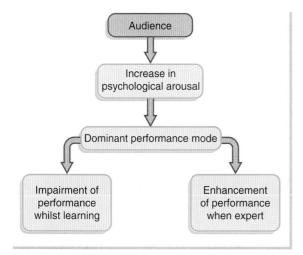

Fig. 13.15 The relationship between audience, arousal level and performance.

rehearsal (external imagery) to familiarise performers with the effects of spectators or to help them block them out of the mind. The coach can also manage the introduction of a young performer to spectators, by keeping them away during training and by (for example) bringing the youngster into a senior team when the outcome is not critical, thus minimising evaluation apprehension.

Review questions

1. a. Define the term 'social facilitation'.
   b. What different groups of 'others' in sport or dance does the theory define?

2. Draw a diagram of Zajonc's theory of audience effects. What are the implications of this model for competition in sport?

3. Explain Cottrell's evaluation apprehension theory and Baron's distraction-conflict theory.

4. How should a coach and/or performer prepare for audience effects in competition or performance?

5. Is there such a thing as 'home advantage'?

Exam-style questions

1. a. What is meant by social facilitation and what is its main effect? (*3 marks*)
   b. What effects can be experienced by an individual if there is an audience present? (*6 marks*)
   (*Total 9 marks*)

2. a. What is meant by evaluation apprehension? (*2 marks*)
   b. As a coach of an individual who is affected adversely by the presence of an audience, how would you help him or her to overcome the negative influences? (*4 marks*)
   (*Total 6 marks*)

3. Two groups of male sportspeople (of the same age) undertook an arm's length weight hold endurance test. Success at this exercise was measured by the length of time the weight was held. The table below shows the average times for group 1 (who did the exercise alone) and group 2 (who did the exercise in the presence of an audience).

	group 1 no audience	group 2 with audience
average time held in seconds	46.5	50.5

   a. What effect (if any) did the audience have on the performance of the exercise? (*1 mark*)

   b. How would you account for this effect (or lack of effect)? (*4 marks*)
   c. The audience in this exercise (for group 2) was not known to the participants. Explain any effect you think there would be if the audience was known to the group. (*6 marks*)
   (*Total 11 marks*)

4. a. Using examples from sport, explain what is meant by evaluation apprehension and outline the causes of it. (*3 marks*)

5. a. Social facilitation and social inhibition can be explained as the influence of the presence of others on performance.
   (i) Explain the factors that could affect performance when playing in front of a large crowd at an important local match. (*5 marks*)
   (ii) How could the coach of such a team help the players to cope with the effects of an audience? (*4 marks*)
   b. The main effect of an audience on a performer in sport is that the performer's arousal level is raised, which can have both positive and negative effects. Using drive theory, explain the relationship between arousal level and performance in a situation where an audience is present. (*4 marks*)
   (*Total 13 marks*)

13.5 Mental preparation for sports performance

Most sport and exercise participants can give a reasonably accurate account of how skilled they are in relation to a beginner or a top-class performer in their field. Leagues, times, distances, ladders, fitness norms, national and international ratings all help to provide a performer with competence information. Given a certain level of skill, experience and fitness, however, most performers recognise:

- that their own performance varies (sometimes they perform very well and sometimes badly in relation to their normal standard)
- that they may consistently perform better (or worse) than a colleague of apparently the same skill, fitness and experience.

These days these differences and fluctuations are attributed to the psychological state of the performer, when they cannot be accounted for by physical factors. Mental preparation for performance (sometimes referred to as psychological skills training) has become an important part of training. Mental training is a skilled task and any programme should be overseen by a qualified sport psychologist. Normally he/she would carry out an initial assessment of the performer. Extracts from some of the interview schedules and questionnaires that might be used are given on the CD-ROM that accompanies this book.

But many coaches have neither the luxury of a sport psychologist or psychological training; nevertheless, there are some key principles that can be followed. Sports coach UK (formerly the National Coaching Foundation: NCF) cites the 4 Cs of mental preparation for performance: **commitment, (self) confidence, concentration and (emotional) control.** We have considered self-confidence in Chapter 11 so to complete our study of sport psychology, we will concentrate here on the other three.

Commitment

Achieving success in sport and exercise takes time, persistence and hard work; in short, it demands **commitment**. Commitment stems from the performers themselves; it is a form of motivation. The coach or trainer can encourage it but cannot generate it. One of the factors which has been found to most enhance commitment is having clear, realistic goals.

Goal setting is important in sport and exercise because:

- learning is focused
- persistence and effort are increased
- uncertainty is reduced
- confidence is increased
- anxiety is reduced
- practice is planned and structured
- evaluation and feedback are specific.

If goals are structured so that they are relatively easily attained initially and then progressively become more difficult, the early success necessary for confidence building is more likely.

There are two important categories of goals: phased goals and objective goals. Knowledge of these is important in the goal-setting process.

Phased goals

Long-term goals are what the performer wants to achieve as the high point of the current stage of their involvement in the sport or activity. It might be the dream or a stage on the road to the dream. You might, for example, be aiming for a place in an Olympic team or for a particular competition score. This is then broken down into **intermediate** and **short-term** goals that lead to the long-term goal. For example, a skater might have the long-term goal of becoming the national junior champion in 12 months' time. One of the intermediate goals might then be to learn a routine that would catch the judge's eye and be awarded a high

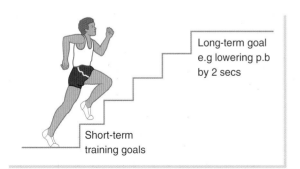

Fig. 13.16 Goal setting.

score; short-term goals would be mastering particular sections of this routine. Goals are often visualised as a series of steps on a stairway, each step taking the performer nearer to the top. This is a useful analogy because it reminds us that we can always pause on the staircase or even go back a few steps if one goal appears hard to achieve.

Objective goals

Outcome goals are to do with winning or performing better than someone else. To achieve an outcome goal, not only do you have to have done well but also your opponent(s) has to have done less well than you have. Thus, achieving your goal is partly dependent upon the opposition. Outcome goals are useful, particularly for confident, successful performers, but they should be balanced by the other two types of objective goals because maintaining confidence and motivation can be a problem if only outcome goals are used.

Performance goals specify a particular standard to be achieved. They can thus be realised independently of anyone else. You might set yourself a particular level of fitness to achieve or a specific sprint time or javelin distance or a particular percentage of returns in a game of tennis. Performance goals encourage the development of mastery and an internal locus of control; performers can feel satisfaction after a good performance, even if they did not win.

Process goals deal with the technique or strategy necessary to perform well. They are used particularly in training but can also be used in competition as long as they do not distract the performer from the broader requirements of the task. For example, a runner might have a goal of consciously relaxing in the back straight prior to the final bend or a defender might have been told to close mark a specific opponent at corners. Process goals help attention and focus and are very effective in helping to control anxiety.

Goals must be set according to the age, stage, confidence, ability and motivation of the performer. Beginners need very short-term, easily achievable goals to boost their confidence. The more experienced need challenge. There are two well-known acronyms to guide goal setting: SMARTER and SCCAMP.

SMARTER goals

- Specific: goals should indicate clearly what is to be achieved and the criteria for doing it well
- Measurable: goals should be quantifiable in terms of a time or a score, which can be recorded
- Action oriented: goals should indicate that something must be done

- Realistic: goals should be achievable by the person or group for whom they are set
- Timely: goals should be specified with a given time-frame, i.e. in 6 months' time we will have...[18]
- Effective: goals would be capable of delivering the results required
- Reviewed: goals should be reviewed regularly (with downward adjustment if necessary, e.g. in the case of injury). This implies that they should be written down.

SCCAMP goals

- Specific: as above
- Controllable: they are within the control of the performers themselves and do not depend on how others perform; this suggests that performance goals are preferable to outcome goals
- Challenging: goals that are too easily achieved can decrease motivation
- Attainable: motivation and commitment are enhanced by success in achieving a challenging goal but decreased by failure; this is equivalent to the 'realistic' goals above
- Measurable: as above
- Personal: goals should relate to the individual or the team and should always be either set by the performers themselves or negotiated. This ensures commitment.

ACTIVITY 13.5 SETTING GOALS

Select a sport or physical activity in which you participate regularly. Individually, plan a series of short-, intermediate- and long-term goals, to a specific time plan, under the following headings:

- individual skill
- fitness
- psychological skill.

Ensure that these goals meet the criteria indicated in the text. See if you can implement them and evaluate your progress.

1. What difficulties do you encounter in (a) goal setting and (b) implementing the goals?

How might you overcome these difficulties in the future?

Exam-style questions

1. a. What are the main positive effects of setting goals in sport? (*2 marks*)
   b. Show what is meant by short-term goals and long-term goals by using examples from sport. (*4 marks*)
   c. As a coach, how would you ensure that your goal setting was as effective as possible? (*4 marks*)

   (*Total 10 marks*)

Concentration

Concentration is the ability to focus and maintain attention on the important, relevant aspects of what is happening. It is one of the most important attributes of a sportsperson. Concentration in sport and exercise has three elements:

- focusing on the relevant cues in the environment (selective attention, see Chapter 10)
- maintaining that attentional focus over time (i.e. not allowing distraction)
- having full awareness of the situation.[19]

ACTIVITY 13.6 ATTENTIONAL FOCUS

Consider four activities: climbing, basketball, gymnastics and archery. All require concentration (**attentional focus**). What are the similarities and differences between the type of concentration needed to perform well in each of these?

Attentional focus and style

Nideffer[20] suggests that the kind of attentional focus required for different activities varies. His model is shown in Figure 13.17. Nideffer suggests that a person's attentional focus can be categorised on two continua:

- **internal** – focusing on thoughts and feelings; **external** – focusing on the environment, e.g. the positions of other players or the flight of the ball
- **broad** – focusing on the full range of what is happening, e.g. the changing positions of players in a game; **narrow** – focusing only on a few aspects of what is happening, e.g. concentrating on only your own lane and the tape in a 100 m track sprint.

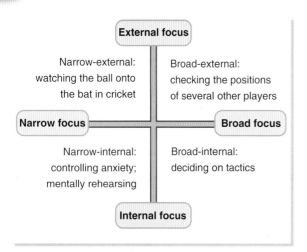

Fig. 13.17 Nideffer's model of attentional style.

The two continua are combined as in Figure 13.17 to produce four **attentional styles**.

Nideffer maintains that people have a preferred attentional style: broad-external, broad-internal, narrow-internal and narrow-external. This is not to say that we cannot change from one style to the other; clearly we can and do, but personal preference and other factors such as anxiety (see below) can affect how quickly and the extent to which we can change.

In general, closed skills require a narrow focus and open skills a broad focus. Most activities demand an external focus for performance but a switch to internal focusing will be required from time to time during planning, training and performance.

Concentration can be learned and practised and is an important part of mental training (see below). An effective attender:

- knows which cues and elements of the surroundings are important to attend to
- is able to 'shut out' unimportant or distracting stimuli, such as negative thoughts
- is good at broad focusing but can also switch quickly to narrow focusing when required, without losing any important information
- can cope with internal and external stimuli without becoming overloaded (see Chapter 10).

An ineffective attender has difficulty with the above skills and in addition may narrow attention so much that they miss important cues. For example, in concentrating too much on a difficult entry to a move

ACTIVITY 13.7 ATTENTIONAL STYLE

Using the Students' Attentional Style Questionnaire in the Teacher's Guide that accompanies this book, determine your own preferred style. Bear in mind that this is not a sport-specific measure.

The styles in column A below are wrongly matched to the actions in column B. Using the four attentional styles in Figure 13.17, correctly match the style with the action

Basketball	
A	B
Broad-internal	Player takes a free shot
Broad-external	Player prepares for a free shot by closing his eyes and trying to relax
Narrow-internal	Coach plans the next time-out
Narrow-external	Player moves up the court looking to make a pass

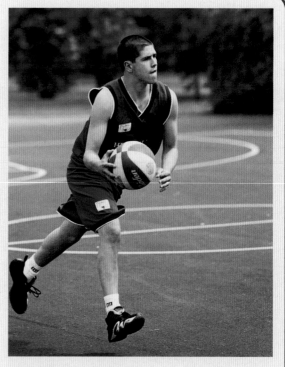

Fig. 13.18

in a sequence, a gymnast may lose the coordination of the move as a whole.

Attentional narrowing

Stress and anxiety alter the way in which performers attend and concentrate. At optimal levels of arousal for a soccer goalkeeper, for example, he/she can attend to all the significant players, including the defence (broad focus), whilst ignoring the off-putting chants of the crowd behind and can switch attention to a narrow focus as a shot is made. If he/she is unduly anxious, attention is automatically narrowed in several ways (in evolutionary terms, this allows undivided attention to sources of real danger to survival):

- peripheral vision is narrowed
- a narrow attentional focus is adopted (which may not be appropriate)
- an internal focus may be adopted ('worrying about worrying')
- switching attentional focus appropriately becomes difficult.

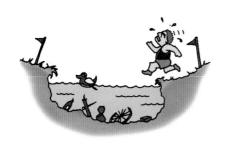

Fig. 13.19 Attentional narrowing.

Emotional control

In the above section we have considered the importance of being able to control our attentional focus. In sport and exercise, particularly in competition, we also need to be able to control our emotions, because these can have a very marked effect on levels of performance. We are all familiar with the feelings of nervousness before an important event. We do not want to let down our teammates, our coach, our family or ourselves. We do not want to appear to be incompetent or foolish. Yet we also want to be 'psyched up' to do our very best. The concept which psychologists use in this context is **arousal**. This section considers the theory of arousal before moving onto discussion about how it can be controlled.

Arousal is a state of mental and physical preparedness for action. It is closely associated with the concept of motivation (see Chapter 12). We know that as motivation increases so does a person's level of arousal. If you are tired and do not really feel like training one evening, then you will feel sluggish and perform indifferently; if you start to enjoy the session and forget your tiredness, arousal and performance will increase. The body gears itself up for action, both physically and psychologically. Your heart beats faster, your breathing quickens, you sweat more. Psychologically you focus on the task and concentrate. Arousal, then, has both physiological and cognitive components – the mind interacts with the body.

The purpose of arousal is to prepare the body for action. When we are just waking from sleep, arousal level is very low. As more demands are made on the body, so arousal level is raised to cope with these demands. Arousal is a function of the autonomic nervous system and is a response that was built into our central nervous system as we evolved. When danger threatened our primitive ancestors, they had to be immediately ready to fight or run and this response remains within our system.

Coaches and sport psychologists are very aware of arousal in sport and the effect it has on performers; they try to manipulate it, for example by 'psyching up' a team for an important event in the hope that a good performance will result or by calming down a nervous athlete. We need to be aware of it ourselves so that we can control our own level of arousal.

There are two forms of arousal:

- **physiological arousal** refers to physical readiness for action: heart and breathing rates, sweating, reaction times are all indicators of this. Warm-up activities are designed to increase physiological arousal in readiness for peak performance
- **psychological arousal** refers to the emotional and motivational state of the sportsperson and can range from indifference and boredom to alertness and then high excitement or tension.

There are a number of theories about how arousal relates to performance.

Drive theory

One influential approach is **drive theory**, which you also meet in other contexts (Figure 13.20). Drive theory proposes that as arousal increases to meet the perceived demands of the task, so the performance is more likely to reflect the most usual behaviour (dominant habit). If you have not learned a skill very well, the dominant performance habit is full of mistakes and, as arousal increases, so will the number

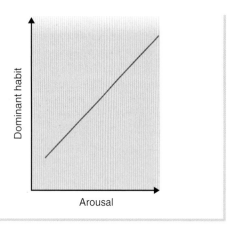

Fig. 13.20 Drive theory.

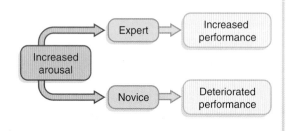

Fig. 13.21 The effect of arousal on experts and novices according to drive theory.

of mistakes you make. If you are an expert, the dominant habit is correct, with effective technique and judgement, so you may well play even better as your arousal level increases (Figure 13.21).

Inverted-U theory

The problem with drive theory is that it does not easily explain fluctuations in performance. A currently more accepted theory is the **inverted-U theory**. This suggests that, up to a certain point (A in Figure 13.22), arousal levels are too low for best performances. The sportsperson is just not 'psyched up' enough. But there comes a point (B in Figure 13.22) when arousal turns to anxiety and performance seems to deteriorate; the sportsperson is 'psyched out'. Between these two points is an area of optimal arousal, at which performers are able to give of their best. This has not been an easy theory to verify experimentally (see[21]) but most performers and coaches recognise the effects. Some critics[22] suggest that the inverted-U model is too

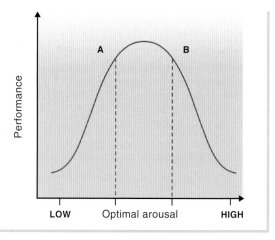

Fig. 13.22 The inverted-U theory.

simplistic to explain the complexity of the arousal–performance relationship and several alternatives (some derived from the inverted-U and some quite different) have been proposed. These are described when we consider anxiety later in this section.

The inverted-U curve shown in Figure 13.22 is very much a generalisation. Curves for particular individuals and tasks differ.

Individual differences

ACTIVITY 13.8 AROUSAL CURVES

In Figure 13.23, what do the arousal curves depicted tell you about the three athletes?

1. Who is capable of the best performance?
2. Who needs to be really psyched up before he performs at his best?

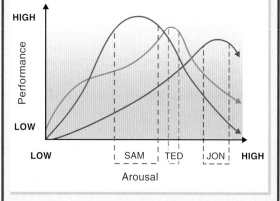

Fig. 13.23 Individual differences in the optimal arousal zone.

> 3. Whose level of arousal needs to be very carefully controlled for good performance?
>
> Your answers should be: 1. Sam; 2. Jon; 3. Ted. You should note, however, that these are stylised graphs. Actual arousal–performance curves are much more variable than these are.

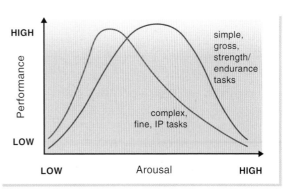

Fig. 13.24 Arousal–performance curves for gross/fine, simple/complex and strength/IP tasks.

Task differences

It is not possible to predict exactly what level of arousal is best for any one sport or activity – so much depends on circumstance and the personalities of the competitors, but there are some general rules that help competitors and coaches.

- **Simple and complex tasks.** We consider it to be easier to kick a penalty in rugby from in front of the posts than from the sideline. What we usually mean in saying that a task is easier is that there is a greater margin for deviation from the movement plan, while still staying within the boundaries of successful execution. Note that we are referring here to inherently simple and complex tasks. Obviously, a task becomes easier for an individual to perform as he/she becomes more practised at it. Thus, simple tasks have a broader optimal arousal zone than complex tasks, i.e. individuals can tolerate greater arousal levels before successful turns into unsuccessful performance.
- **Fine and gross tasks.** As with complex tasks, fine motor tasks have less margin for error than gross motor tasks; they require precision of movement. Compare putting in golf with weightlifting. If you watch these two sports on television you will notice that a golfer tries to relax and calm down before putting, while the weightlifter really tries to 'psych himself up'. Individuals tackling gross motor tasks can tolerate greater levels of arousal before errors appear than those dealing with fine motor tasks.
- **Strength or endurance and information processing tasks.** Another difference between golf putting and weightlifting is that the former has information processing as a key component. High arousal levels seem to interfere with information processing; thus skills in which this is important are more likely to be adversely affected than skills such as weightlifting in which the performer's concern is to summon as much of his/her strength and/or endurance as possible.

Figure 13.24 illustrates the optimal arousal levels for the six types of task discussed, but again you should note that these are largely hypothetical and that obtaining research data that confirms the relationships indicated is not easy. What seems to be clear from experience, however, is that:

- optimal arousal levels can be identified
- these vary across individuals and activities
- ability to control arousal is the key to successful performance.

Martens[23] put forward an interesting critique of arousal theory, suggesting that it is more useful to think in terms of positive and negative psychic energy. Such discussion is outside the scope of this book, but interested students might like to follow up his ideas by reading further.

Anxiety

You are now aware, from your work in Section 12.5, that a certain level of arousal is necessary for your best possible performance in sport. Arousal responses are generated by a variety of means – some are automatic, some are associated with emotion (you will recognise the physical symptoms of, for example, anger). Those associated with physical performance are generated by our perceptions of the demands of the situation. We know that in a practice or recreational game it is less important that we do not fail. In a championship game, however, it is very important that we live up to the demands of the situation, of our teammates and of our supporters; even the most confident of us has occasional doubts.

Arousal is a neutral concept. It can be triggered by both pleasant and unpleasant situations. If, however, arousal is associated with negative emotions such as worry, doubt or nervousness, we say someone is experiencing **anxiety**.

KEY POINTS

- **Anxiety** is a negative emotional state, similar to fear, associated with physiological (somatic) and psychological (cognitive) arousal and with feelings of nervousness and apprehension. Anxiety has four components: trait anxiety, state anxiety, cognitive anxiety and somatic anxiety.

- **Trait anxiety** is 'a *behavioural disposition*' which predisposes a person to perceive objectively non-dangerous circumstances as threatening and to respond to these with state anxiety levels disproportionate to the level of threat'.[24]

- **State anxiety** is an emotional response to particular situations, characterised by feelings of nervousness and apprehension.

Trait anxiety is a personality variable. If a person has high trait anxiety, he/she tends to be fearful of unfamiliar situations and to respond with obvious anxiety symptoms.

State anxiety is an emotional response, often temporary, which exists in relation to particular situations. For example, if you become nervous before a dance production but not a team game, you are showing state anxiety in relation to dance. People with high trait anxiety usually have higher state anxiety in competitive or evaluative situations than those with low trait anxiety.

Spielberger et al[25] developed a self-report inventory to measure levels of state and trait anxiety in general situations. It is known as the State Trait Anxiety Inventory (STAI). The full version is not easily obtained, but an excerpt from it can be found on the CD-ROM that accompanies this book. Martens[26] developed a sport-specific competitive trait anxiety measure, the Sport Competition Anxiety Test (SCAT). This has proved more helpful in investigating anxiety in sportspeople because it deals specifically with sport. You should note, however, that it is a test of competitive trait anxiety; that is, the tendency to be anxious in sport contexts in general. The state anxiety version of this test is the Competitive State Anxiety Inventory (CSAI) (Martens et al[27]).

Investigation 13.6 To investigate the relationship between competitive trait anxiety as measured by SCAT and state anxiety prior to an important sport event

Method: Select a group of people who are involved in competitive sport at a high level, for example your school or college first team or a local club team. Obtain their permission to administer two simple questionnaires, at a mutually convenient time. Use SCAT (Roberts et al[28]) to obtain a trait anxiety score and the following question (adapted from[28]) to obtain a crude state anxiety score for each player:

'Imagine that it is a few minutes before a very important league or championship game or event. You have been beaten only once this season, by today's opponent(s). How do you feel with a few minutes to go before the start of the game or event?'

Very anxious	9 8 7 6 5 4 3 2 1	Not at all anxious

Results: Follow the scoring system for SCAT in Roberts et al[28] or on the CD-ROM that accompanies this book. Using each respondent's SCAT and state anxiety (SA) scores, compute the Spearman's rank correlation coefficient.

Discussion: What does the correlation coefficient tell you about the relationship between SCAT and SA scores? Discuss the implications of this for the team's coach or for the sportspeople themselves.

Research along the lines of Investigation 13.6 suggests that:

- competitive trait anxiety and pre-game state anxiety are correlated
- high trait anxiety tends to cause high pre-game state anxiety
- winners tend to experience less post-game anxiety than do losers.

SCAT and STAI are self-report, psychometric approaches to anxiety measurement. In this sense they are equivalent to the personality tests (Eysenck and Cattell) discussed in Section 12.2. They are, however, generally available, but should only be used under the guidance of a qualified sport psychologist and with an awareness of the ethical principles of psychological testing. Simplified versions can be found in Webster[29] or Biddle.[30]

Zone of optimal functioning

Hanin[31] adapted the inverted-U curve to relate performance to state anxiety. His model is very similar to Figure 13.22, except that he is specifically concerned with state anxiety rather than the general concept of arousal. The points between the dotted lines are called individual zones of optimal functioning (IZOF) in Hanin's model. The implications of the model are that coaches and performers should work in training to identify and achieve the limits of their particular zone. Hanin claims that the model works for other emotions also, such as determination and relaxation, and that coaches should help performers generate the mixture of emotions that works best for them.

Multidimensional theory

The inverted-U model of the relationship between arousal and performance is useful in general terms but more recently, sport psychologists have suggested that (i) arousal is a neutral concept and (ii) anxiety is made up of three components which have differing effects on performance (McGrath[4]).

- **Cognitive state anxiety** is brought about by thoughts and perceptions and gives rise to the emotions of nervousness and apprehension which we normally associate with being anxious.
- **Somatic state anxiety** is the perception of, and concern about, high physiological arousal, i.e. the realisation that your mouth is dry, of the 'butterflies' in your stomach and that movement is not as well coordinated as usual.
- **Self-confidence**.

Multidimensional anxiety theory predicts that:

- cognitive state anxiety is directly negatively related to performance; that is, you will perform best when you are least worried and vice versa
- somatic state anxiety is related to performance as shown in the inverted-U curve; that is, low *and* high levels of somatic state anxiety lead to low levels of performance and the best performance is achieved with moderate levels of somatic state anxiety
- the levels of both forms of anxiety that can be tolerated by performers depend on their levels of self-confidence, i.e. if a team has a high level of confidence in each other and in their ability to win, they can cope with moments in the game when things seem to be going badly and when the outcome seems to be in doubt. They will still be worried, but this will not affect their game unduly.

ACTIVITY 13.9

Using multidimensional anxiety theory, draw a graph on the axes in Figure 13.25, illustrating bullet points one and two above. Label the lines 'cognitive state anxiety' and 'somatic state anxiety'. Check your graphs with a friend or tutor.

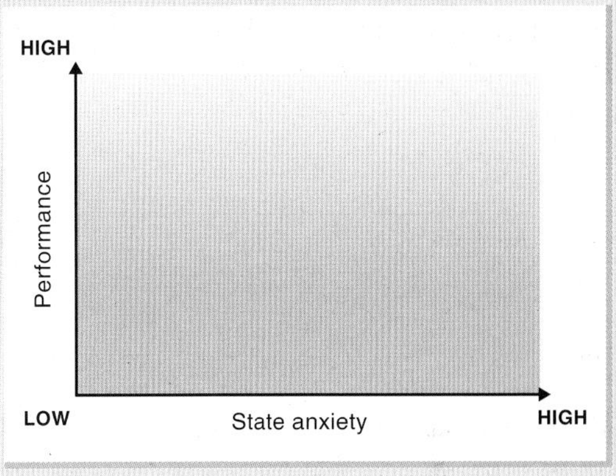

Fig. 13.25

Reversal theory

Kerr[32] is interested in the idea that arousal affects performance through the way in which it is perceived by the performer. Some people experience high levels of arousal as exciting and evidence that they are 'psyched up and ready to go'. Others find the physical and mental manifestations of arousal unpleasant and this leads to high levels of cognitive and somatic anxiety. We have discovered that these high levels are generally detrimental to performance, so coaches try and help performers to perceive arousal, even nervousness, as pleasant and evidence that they are in their optimal zone.

The catastrophe model

Hardy[33] takes the multidimensional view of arousal further by suggesting that performance depends on a complex interaction between arousal and cognitive state anxiety. His **catastrophe model** arose from the realisation that in some circumstances performance does not merely 'tail off' gradually as arousal increases, as shown on the inverted-U curve; it deteriorates rapidly and dramatically, i.e. catastrophically. He explained this by arguing that if a performer is not very worried (low level of cognitive state anxiety) then he/she performs best with a moderate level of

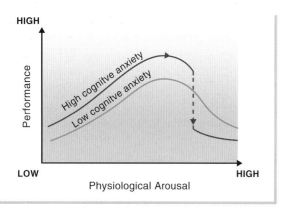

Fig. 13.26 The catastrophe model.

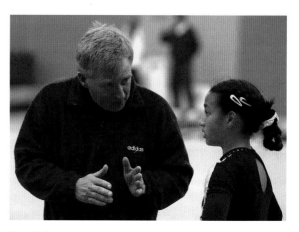

Fig. 13.27

physiological arousal, as predicted in the inverted-U model, and small increases in arousal will only cause minor problems with performance. If, however, the performer starts with a high level of cognitive anxiety, then even a small increase in physiological arousal can cause a 'catastrophic' deterioration in performance. This theory may explain, for example, uncharacteristic misses in football penalty shoot-outs. It is shown graphically in Figure 13.26.

ACTIVITY 13.10

Study Figure 13.26 and discuss what the model tells us about cognitive anxiety in sport. For example, do you think that it is a good or bad thing for a performer to be worried before an event? Does it depend on the type of activity?

In catastrophe theory, it is the *interaction* between cognitive state anxiety, somatic state anxiety and physiological arousal which seems to be causing the marked drop in the quality of performance. We can understand this better by briefly considering the concept of stress (see below).

KEY POINT

Stress is defined by Selye[34] as 'the non-specific response of the body to any demand made on it'. The sources of stress are referred to as **stressors**.

Some stressors are universal – everyone would be worried by a loud, unexplained noise in the night. But others, for example performing in front of an audience, may be stressful to one person but not to someone who is used to the experience and enjoys the challenge.

Stressors come in many forms:

- social
- chemical or biochemical
- bacterial
- physical
- climatic
- psychological.

Those involved in physical activity are very aware of the last three. The physical pain resulting from a sports injury, ill-fitting dancers' shoes or the final stages of a long-distance race or walk causes the participant considerable stress, as perhaps you know.

The weather can be a stressor. Heat stress is something that marathon runners have to be able to deal with and very cold, wet weather brings the danger of hypothermia for those involved in outdoor pursuits.

Psychological stress results from a mismatch between a person's perception of the demands of a situation and a self-assessment of his/her ability to cope, given that the outcome is important, as illustrated in Figure 13.28.

Selye's[34] theory of stress proposes that the body reacts to all these stressors in the same way. This is important for an understanding of catastrophe theory. He suggests that there is a General Adaptation Syndrome (GAS) which has three stages, as illustrated in Figure 13.29. In the alarm reaction stage, the body is alerted to deal with the stressor. This is when breathing and heart rate quicken and adrenaline is released.

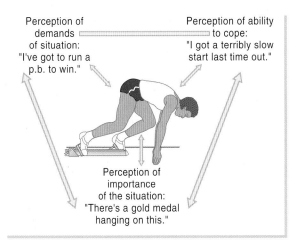

Fig. 13.28 Psychological stress.

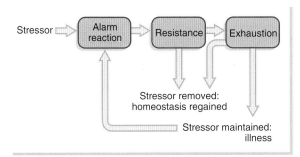

Fig. 13.29 The General Adaptation Syndrome.[34]

The stressor is there and the body is resisting but the individual enjoys, and may even seek out, the sensation. Mo Anthoine, a climber and mountaineer, has said:

> *The truth is, I like an unforgiving climate where if you make mistakes you suffer for it. That's what turns me on. I think it's because there is always a question mark about how you will perform.*[36]

In general, however, stress is something to be avoided in sport, for its effects, as with anxiety, may inhibit performance. Our awareness of being under stress may itself act as a stressor (Figure 13.30).

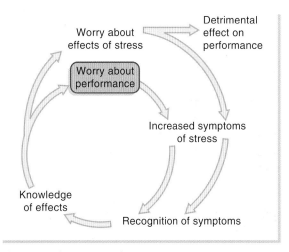

Fig. 13.30 The stress spiral.

During the resistance stage, a series of hormonal and chemical changes attempt to maintain homeostasis, that is, the delicate biochemical and fluid balance which allows our body to function effectively. A stressor is anything that disturbs this balance.

The final stage is that of exhaustion, when the product of the strength of the stressor and the length of time during which it acts is such that the body can no longer put up any resistance. Exhaustion is the body's last defence. If this stops the stressor (if, for example, you have been pushing yourself too hard in a 13 km run and you drop out), then the body recovers homeostasis. But if you drop exhausted in a blizzard on Ben Nevis without having gained shelter, then the stressor (the cold) persists in spite of your body having stopped and you may well not recover.

Psychological stressors do not have as powerful an effect on the body as the others, but over a long period of time will take their toll on general health.

You should note at this stage that several writers (e.g. Harris & Harris[35]) discuss **eustress**, or 'good' stress, associated with thrill and excitement. This should not be confused with optimal levels of arousal.

Returning to catastrophe theory, we can now see that cognitive state anxiety produces an 'alarm reaction' physiologically, thus preparing the body for action. Heart and breathing rates increase and adrenaline is produced. This reaction adds to existing levels of physiological arousal. So:

- if a performer is not properly warmed up at the start of a game, the anxiety of having a goal or point quickly scored against them is likely to increase both physiological arousal *and* performance
- if levels of physiological arousal are already high (either because the activity is well under way and challenging or because of high anxiety before the event), then something that causes more worry (e.g. a bad mistake) increases physiological arousal further. At some point this increase causes information processing and motor control systems to become dysfunctional and skill breaks down suddenly and catastrophically (arousal overload).

There are lessons here for the performer and coach:

- cognitive anxiety must be controlled because if it is too high, it can lead to catastrophe
- relaxation techniques and imagery can help to decrease physiological arousal (and thus avert catastrophe during an event) if there is 'time out', e.g. in self-paced situations such as penalty taking or end-changes in tennis
- if catastrophe occurs, arousal levels must be brought back to below that at which the catastrophe occurred before performance will recover. Usually this involves physical relaxation and cognitive techniques such as image refocusing and thought stopping. We deal with this in the next section.

Measurement of anxiety

Martens[23] suggests that there are three types of stress/anxiety symptoms: physiological, psychological and behavioural.

- **Physiological symptoms** – increased heart rate; increased blood pressure; increased sweating; increased respiration; decreased flow of blood to the skin; increased oxygen uptake; dry mouth.
- **Psychological symptoms** – worry; feeling overwhelmed; inability to make decisions; inability to concentrate; inability to direct attention appropriately; narrowing of attention; feeling out of control.
- **Behavioural symptoms** – rapid talking; nail biting; pacing; scowling; yawning; trembling; raised voice pitch; frequent urination.

These symptoms are used to identify and measure stress and anxiety. There are essentially three types of stress/anxiety measurement.

- **Self-report questionnaires** – two examples of these (CSAI and SCAT) are quoted above (see Investigation 13.6); there are many other similar inventories. As with all such measures, the full versions should only be used with the guidance of a qualified sport psychologist.
- **Observation techniques** – these are used extensively by coaches and consist of observing and monitoring the behavioural aspects of stress listed above in relation to particular aspects of competition and training; thus, over a period of time the coach learns what the athlete finds stressful and can work to avoid or overcome this.
- **Physiological responses** – many of the physiological responses listed above can be measured directly; for example, heart rate, temperature, oxygen uptake, sweating by a galvanic skin response apparatus. Under appropriate supervision, blood analysis can be carried out to measure hormonal responses. All these are useful to establish pre-game levels of stress, but it must be remembered that exercise itself produces similar responses and therefore measuring stress during or immediately after performance is very difficult.

The management of anxiety

It should now be clear to you that, in sport and other physical activities, the most damaging form of anxiety is that which is self-induced through worrying about the performance to come. Physical activity is inherently arousing, so in most cases becoming adequately 'psyched up' is no problem; the difficulty is in limiting anxiety to manageable levels. This means breaking the 'stress spiral' (see Figure 13.30). Since we know that the mind and body work in very close harmony in the production of skilled movement, it is no surprise that there are two places we can break the spiral; we can eliminate many of the harmful physiological responses to stress by persuading the body that the stressor does not exist (**somatic management**) and we can deal with the mind by replacing negative thoughts with positive ones (**cognitive management**).

Somatic techniques

For these we use relaxation. There are four forms of relaxation:

- imagery
- self-directed
- progressive relaxation training
- biofeedback.

Imagery relaxation involves picturing yourself in a place where you feel very comfortable and safe. You should try to see yourself there as vividly as you can, relaxed, warm, at ease; evoke the sounds, the smells, the whole 'feel' of the place. It helps if you are in a quiet and comfortable setting in reality, but eventually you learn to use the technique whenever you feel stressed. To make imagery relaxation work well, you need to:

- think of a place that has clear associations of warmth and relaxation
- possess good imagery skills
- practise the technique initially in non-stressful situations, before using it to control competitive stress.

Self-directed relaxation is a simplified form of progressive relaxation training (PRT), developed in the 1930s. PRT involves learning to tense and then deeply relax separate muscle groups. Tensing a muscle is not difficult, but thoroughly relaxing it is and takes several weeks of practice. Self-directed relaxation involves focusing on each of the major muscle groups in turn, simultaneously allowing the breathing to become slow and easy. As you focus on each muscle, visualise the tension flowing out of it until it is completely relaxed. Work through all the muscle groups in this way. Whereas initially you need to relax muscles separately to obtain the required relaxation effect, as you become more proficient you can combine groups and achieve total body relaxation very quickly. The Teacher's Guide contains a script which you can ask someone to read to you, or can tape, to help you start. Alternatively, there are many relaxation audiotapes on the market.

Benson[37] suggests a similar technique, but his focus is just on breathing and hence is closer to meditation than relaxation. You should find a quiet setting and concentrate totally on your breathing. As you breathe out, silently repeat a single syllable word that has no particular meaning for you. If you find your attention wandering, just bring your mind back to your breathing.

You may find that it is difficult to feel the difference between tension and relaxation in your muscles. In this case, biofeedback may be helpful, for it is a technique which gives you direct information about what is happening in your body. We have suggested that physiological responses to stress can be measured. Biofeedback does this and teaches you how to use your mind to change the reading. There are three main types of biofeedback.

- **Skin temperature**. When muscles are relaxed, more blood flows to the skin and skin temperature rises; this can be detected by sensitive electrothermometers taped to the skin. If you are stressed, blood is diverted from the skin to the tense muscles so the skin becomes cold. As you relax, using imagery relaxation techniques, the reading changes, which provides feedback and reinforces the relaxation.
- **Galvanic skin response**. A means of measuring the electrical conductivity of the skin, which increases when the skin is moist. When the muscles are tense, sweating occurs to remove the heat generated, thereby increasing the skin conductivity, which can be measured using a simple battery-operated device. This device provides immediate feedback on how successful you are at relaxing.
- **Electromyography (EMG)**. Electrodes are taped to the skin over specific muscles whose state of tension or relaxation can then be monitored. This is very helpful if you have a problem with tension in a specific muscle group during performance.

Relaxation techniques can be invaluable for reducing stress prior to an important sport event. They sound easy, but in fact it takes some time to learn to do them really effectively. The drawback is that whereas you do wish to remove stress, you do not want to remove all muscle tension before your game or event. Your aim, therefore, is to prepare the body to remove unhelpful tension, so that you can then effectively direct your thoughts and attention to the task in hand.

Cognitive techniques

Cognitive anxiety management involves controlling emotions and thought processes prior to, during and after competition or performance. Coaches and performers use it to:

- increase confidence
- control arousal
- focus on the positive and eliminate negative thoughts
- establish a feeling of 'flow'
- eliminate mental 'clutter' – unnecessary detail
- concentrate on key cues in technique and the surroundings.

Many techniques are used but there are two main methods: imagery (mental rehearsal) and self-talk, including thought stopping. An effectively planned and implemented goal-setting programme (see Chapter 12) also helps to boost confidence and ensures that performers are ready for the tasks demanded of them.

Imagery is the process of creating pictures in the mind. It is a form of simulation, i.e. running through an event or a feeling in your head without actually performing. It is increasingly being recognised as an important skill and many top-class sportspeople use it in some form, although it takes some time to learn how to use it. How effective it is depends on a combination of the nature of the task and the skill and imaging ability of the performer. Sally Gunnell (400 m hurdler) describes how she runs through the race in her head as she is waiting to get to the blocks: 'I've got to go hard out of the blocks, relax down the back straight, concentrate round that bend, and make sure I'm winning the whole time'.

There are several theories about how imagery works. These tend to focus on the interesting question of how mentally rehearsing a sequence of movements can actually help you to learn or improve them. In terms of anxiety management, the most useful idea is that using imagery consistently improves the psychological skills of concentration and attention management. In essence, it involves consciously imagining the performance, either by re-running a past experience, as if in 'action replay', or by pre-viewing a hoped-for success. There are two types of imagery:

- **internal**, i.e. visualising participating in the event; what it feels like to do. Coaches will often say something like 'Remember that time when you ran nearly a second faster than your PB – run it through again in your head and think about how it felt'
- **external**, i.e. visualising yourself from the outside, as if on video. You see yourself on the blocks, getting a fast start, running strongly and relaxed and winning, maybe even going up to get the medal.

Imagery can be used at any time, before and after competition and during breaks in the event and in spare time. It does take practice and some people find it easier to do than others.

Self-talk is, as you will guess, talking to oneself, either out loud or, more usually, by thinking. There are two types: positive and negative. Positive self-talk and thoughts are either:

- motivational, i.e. they keep performers focused and confident, or
- instructional, i.e. they remind a performer about a particular point of technique.

Negative self-talk or thinking is self-critical ('I'm useless on the backhand') or remembers past events ('I've missed the last two penalties I've taken') or is pessimistic about situations ('I'll never get rid of this injury'). It is important to change negative thoughts to positive thoughts because:

- negative thoughts may induce a self-fulfilling prophecy and
- negative thoughts are often irrational (just because you've missed the last two penalties does not

mean you are going to miss this one – you've been selected as a penalty taker for good reason).

Thought stopping is a particular technique for dealing with negative thoughts if they occur during practice or performance. It consists of recognising the thought briefly and then using a cue word or action to tell you to stop the thought and concentrate either on a positive thought or on a particular aspect of the performance. A young gymnast has begun to dread a particular tumble in her floor sequence. She knows she can do it most of the time but when it goes wrong, it goes badly wrong. Her coach has helped her to 'thought stop'. If she starts to worry as she prepares for the move, she says 'stop' under her breath and immediately visualises herself performing it perfectly.

Mental preparation for sport and exercise is a very important part of the training process. Whenever you are discussing or planning a training or fitness programme, remember the '4 Cs': commitment, confidence, concentration and control of emotion. When you talk to coaches, you will find that they say that confidence is the most valuable attribute a performer can possess. All their physical and psychological training techniques and strategies are designed, in the end, to produce performers who are confident that whatever happens, they will be able to do their best.

ACTIVITY 13.11 CHANGING NEGATIVE SELF-TALK TO POSITIVE SELF-TALK

In twos, each writes a list of negative statements that relate to specific sport or exercise situations (three examples are given above). Exchange lists and for each statement, write down a statement which reflects the reality of the situation but which reinterprets it in a positive way.

This is what a coach would do to help a performer who was expressing negative thoughts.

Review questions

1. What are the '4 Cs' of mental preparation for sport?
2. What are the main principles of goal setting for sport?
3. What are SMARTER goals? SCCAMP goals?
4. Why is it better to set performance goals?
5. Outline Nideffer's theory of attentional style.
6. What is the difference between 'arousal' and 'anxiety'?
7. Draw and explain the inverted-U model of the relationship between arousal and performance.
8. Briefly outline the following models of anxiety and performance: the catastrophe model, the multidimensional model, the zone of optimal functioning model and reversal theory.
9. Define 'stress'. What is the relationship between stress, motivation and anxiety?
10. What is the difference between 'state' and 'trait' anxiety and why is it important for coaches and athletes to recognise the difference?
11. List the techniques that can be used to manage stress in sport situations.

Exam-style questions

1. 'Stress can occur in a sportsperson when an imbalance is **perceived** between the performance demands of competition and the performer's ability to meet those demands successfully'.[26]
   a. What is the significance of the word **perceived**? Give **two** psychological symptoms of stress. (*3 marks*)
   b. High levels of **arousal** have often been linked with stress. Sketch a graph showing the relationship between performance of complex skill and low, moderate and high levels of arousal. Show how this relationship might change for the performance of **simple** skill by adding and labelling a second curve to your graph. (*3 marks*)
   c. Outline two methods of measuring stress in a sportsperson. (*2 marks*)
   d. What **strategies** might the coach employ to help a team member to cope with high levels of stress? (*3 marks*)

   (*Total 11 marks*)

2. a. i. Define **trait anxiety** and **state anxiety**.
      ii. Explain the implications of high **trait** and high **state** anxiety for performance in a competitive sport situation. (*5 marks*)
   b. Briefly describe Martens' Sport Competition Anxiety Test (SCAT) and Spielberger's State Trait Anxiety Inventory (STAI). (*5 marks*)
   c. A national squad gymnast, who has been performing very well, develops high state anxiety in the competitive situation.
      i. Sketch a graph to illustrate the kind of results you would expect and an appropriate schedule for use of Spielberger's STAI with this gymnast, over a 1-month period prior to a competition. (*3 marks*)

   ii. Suggest procedures the coach might use to help the gymnast reduce high levels of state anxiety. (*4 marks*)

   (*Total 17 marks*)

3. a. Define the terms **state anxiety** and **sport competition anxiety**. (*4 marks*)

   Figure 13.31 shows the levels of **state anxiety** reported by two wrestlers at intervals prior to a competition. One of the wrestlers is high, the other low in sport competition anxiety. Sketch the graph and extend each curve by suggesting **two** further points to show the levels of state anxiety experienced by each of the two wrestlers just after beginning a competition against:
      i. a tougher opponent
      ii. a weaker opponent. (*3 marks*)

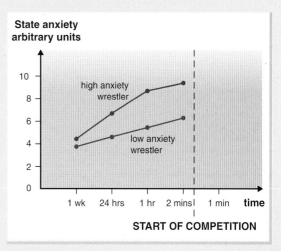

Fig. 13.31 After Gould et al.[38]

►   c. Give reasons to explain your extensions to the two curves. (*7 marks*)

     d. Describe procedures a coach might employ in an attempt to ensure that each of these wrestlers is mentally prepared to compete at his optimal level. (*6 marks*)

     (*Total 20 marks*)

4. Discuss the idea that a coach's half-time 'pep talk' significantly influences the performance of team members. Support your answer with reference to relevant theories and the use of appropriate examples from sport. (*20 marks*)

5. a. What is meant by the term stress? (*2 marks*)

     b. Explain two psychological symptoms of stress. (*2 marks*)

     c. Identify three main stressors in the context of sport. (*3 marks*)

     d. What is the difference between state and trait anxiety? (*2 marks*)

     e. What coping strategies should the anxious performer draw upon? (*5 marks*)

     (*Total 14 marks*)

6. a. Discuss the possible relationships between anxiety and performance in sporting activities. (*7 marks*)

     b. High levels of arousal have often been linked with stress. Sketch a graph showing the relationship between the performance of a complex skill and level of arousal. (*2 marks*)

     c. Add a second curve to your graph showing how the performance of a simple skill might be affected by arousal. (*2 marks*)

     (*Total 11 marks*)

7. With reference to sporting performance, explain how cognitive and somatic anxiety differ. (*5 marks*)

8. Many elite athletes identify an emotional response called the peak flow experience that is associated with success. Describe what is meant by peak flow experience and give reasons why it might occur. (*5 marks*)

References

1. Bandura A 1977 *Social learning theory*. Prentice Hall, New Jersey
2. McCullagh P, Meyer K N 1997 *Learning versus correct models: influence of model type on the learning of a free-weight squat lift*. Research Quarterly for Exercise and Sport 68:56–61
3. Shaw M E 1976 *Group dynamics*. McGraw Hill, New York
4. McGrath J E 1984 *Groups: interaction and performance*. Prentice Hall, New Jersey
5. Steiner I D 1972 *Group processes and productivity*. Academic Press, New York
6. Jones M B 1974 *Regressing group on individual effectiveness*. Organizational Behaviour and Human Performance 11:426–451
7. Latane B, Williams K D, Harkins S G 1979 *Many hands make light work: the causes and consequences of social loafing*. Journal of Personality and Social Psychology 37:823–832
8. Carron A V 1982 *Cohesiveness in sport groups: interpretations and considerations*. Journal of Sport Psychology 4:123–138
9. Widemeyer W N, Carron A V, Brawley L R 1993 *Group cohesion in sport and exercise*. In: Singer R, Murphy M, Tennant K (eds) Handbook of research in sport psychology. Macmillan, New York, pp 672–692
10. Carron A V, Spink K S, Prapavessis H 1997 *Team building and cohesiveness in the sport and exercise setting: use of indirect interventions*. Journal of Applied Sport Psychology 9:61–72
11. Carron A V 1981 *Social psychology of sport: an experimental approach*. Movement Publications, Ithaca, New York
12. Fiedler F E 1967 *A theory of leadership effectiveness*. McGraw Hill, New York
13. Chelladurai P 1984 *Leadership in sports*. In: Silva J M, Weinberg R S (eds) Psychological foundations of sport. Human Kinetics, Champaign, Illinois
14. Zajonc R B 1965 *Social facilitation*. Science 149: 269–274
15. Cottrell N B 1968 *Performance in the presence of other human beings: mere presence, audience and affiliation effects*. In: Simmell E C et al (eds) Social facilitation and imitative behavior. Allyn and Bacon, Boston
16. Baron R S 1986 *Distraction-conflict theory: progress and problems*. In: Berkowitz L (ed.) Advances in experimental social psychology, vol. 19. Academic Press, New York
17. Courneya K S, Carron A V 1992 *The home advantage in sport: a literature review*. Journal of Sport Psychology 14 (1): 13-27
18. Smith H W 1994 *The 10 natural laws of successful time and life management*. Warner, New York
19. Weinberg R S, Gould D 2004 *Foundations of sport and exercise psychology*, 3rd edn. Human Kinetics, Champaign, Illinois
20. Nideffer R 1976 *Test of attentional and interpersonal style*. Journal of Personality and Social Psychology 34:394–404
21. Landers D M, Boutcher S H (eds) 1998 *Arousal-performance relationships*. In: Williams J M (ed) 1998 Applied sport psychology: personal growth to peak performance. Mayfield, Palo Alto, California
22. Jones J G, Hardy L 1990 *Stress in sport: experiences of some elite performers*. In: Jones J G, Hardy L (eds) Stress and performance in sport. John Wiley, Chichester
23. Martens R 1989 *Coaches' guide to sport psychology*. Human Kinetics, Champaign, Illinois
24. Spielberger C D 1966 *Theory and research on anxiety*. In: Spielberger C D (ed) Anxiety and behavior. Academic Press, New York
25. Spielberger C D, Gorsuch R L, Lushene R F 1970 *Manual for the state-trait anxiety inventory*. Consulting Psychologists Press, Palo Alto, California
26. Martens R 1977 *Sport competition anxiety test*. Human Kinetics, Champaign, Illinois
27. Martens R, Vealey R S, Burton D 1990 *Competitive anxiety in sport*. Human Kinetics, Champaign, Illinois
28. Roberts G C, Spink K S, Pemberton C L 1986 *Learning experiences in sport psychology*. Human Kinetics, Champaign, Illinois

29. Webster S 2002 *AS/A2 sport psychology guide*. Jan Roscoe Publications, Widnes
30. Biddle S 1994 *Psychology of PE and sport – a practical guide for Teachers*. FIT Systems, Exeter
31. Hanin Y L 1997 *Emotions and athletic performance: individual zones of optimal functioning*. European Yearbook of Sport Psychology 1:29–72
32. Kerr J H 1997 *Motivation and emotion in sport: reversal theory*. Psychology Press, Brighton
33. Hardy L 1990 *A catastrophe model of performance in sport*. In: Jones J G, Hardy L (eds) Stress and performance in sport. John Wiley, Chichester, pp 81–106

34. Selye H 1976 *The stress of life*. McGraw Hill, New York
35. Harris D V, Harris B L 1984 *The athlete's guide to sports psychology: mental skills for physical people*. Leisure Press, New York
36. Alvarez A 1988 *Feeding the rat: profile of a climber*. Bloomsbury, London
37. Benson H, Proctor W 1984 *Beyond the relaxation response*. Berkley, New York
38. Gould D, Horn T, Spreeman J 1983 *Sources of stress in junior elite wrestlers*. Journal of Sport Psychology 5:159–171

Further reading (Chapters 12 and 13)

* = particularly recommended for students

Backley S 1996 *The winning mind*. Aurum Press, London
Biddle S 1994 *Psychology of PE and sport – a practical guide for Teachers*. FIT Systems, Exeter
Biddle S 1995 *European perspectives on exercise and sport psychology*. Human Kinetics, Champaign, Illinois
*Bull S J 1991 *Sport psychology: a self-help guide*. Crowood, Marlborough
*Butler R J 1998 *Sport psychology in action*. Butterworth-Heinemann, Oxford
Cashmore E 2002 *Sport psychology: the key concepts*. Routledge, London
*Clarkson M 1999 *Competitive fire*. Human Kinetics, Champaign, Illinois
Cockerill I (ed) 2002 *Solutions in sport psychology*. Thomson, London
Cox R 2003 *Sports psychology: concepts and* applications, 5th edn. WCB/McGraw Hill, Boston
Gill D 2000 *Psychological dynamics of sport and exercise*, 2nd edn. Human Kinetics, Champaign, Illinois
Hemery D 1991 *Sporting excellence: what makes a champion*, 2nd edn. John Wiley, Chichester
*Honeybourne J 2004 *Advanced PE and sport for A level*. Stanley Thornes, Cheltenham
Horn T S 1992 *Advances in sport psychology*. Human Kinetics, Champaign, Illinois
Ievleva 1997 *Inner sports: mental skills for peak performance* (audio edition). Human Kinetics, Champaign, Illinois
Jackson S A, Csikszentnihalyi M 1999 *Flow in sports*. Human Kinetics, Champaign, Illinois
*James R et al 2003 *Complete A–Z physical education handbook*, 2nd edn. Hodder and Stoughton, London
*National Coaching Foundation 1996 *Mental skills: an introduction for sports coaches*. NCF, Leeds
Nideffer R M 1992 *Psyched to win*. Human Kinetics, Champaign, Illinois
*Orlick T 1997 *Excel through mental training* (audio edition). Human Kinetics, Champaign, Illinois

Roberts G C 1992 *Motivation in sport and exercise*. Human Kinetics, Champaign, Illinois
*Roberts G C et al 1999 *Learning experiences in sport* psychology, 2nd edn. Human Kinetics, Champaign, Illinois
*Roscoe D A et al 2003 *PE and sport studies AS/A2 level revision guide*, 3rd edn. Jan Roscoe Publications, Widnes
Roscoe D A 2004 Teachers' guide to physical education and the study of sport, 5th edn. Part 2. The performer as a person, Psychology of Sport CD-Rom. Jan Roscoe Publications, Widnes
Schmidt R A, Wrisberg C A 2004 *motor learning and performance: a problem-based learning approach*. Human Kinetics, Champaign, Illinois
*Weinberg W S, Gould D 2004 *Foundations of sport and exercise psychology*. 3rd edn. Human Kinetics, Champaign, Illinois
*Webster S 2002 *AS/A2 sport psychology guide*. Jan Roscoe Publications, Widnes
Williams J M (ed) 1998 *Applied sport psychology: personal growth to peak performance*. Mayfield, Palo Alto, California
Willis J D, Campbell L F 1992 *Exercise psychology*. Human Kinetics, Champaign, Illinois
*Woods B 1998 *Applying psychology to sport*. Hodder and Stoughton, London
*Woods B 2001 *Psychology in practice*. Hodder and Stoughton, London

Multimedia/CD-Roms

Mace R 2002 *Switch on to Sport Psychology*. Sport in Mind, Droitwich Spa
Mace R 2002 *Mental Skills Training*. Sport in Mind, Droitwich Spa
Mace R 2003 *Sport Psychology in Action*. Sport in Mind, Droitwich Spa
Roscoe D A, Roscoe J V 2002 OCR/AQA/Edexcel Science and Sport Psychology Powerpoint Classroom Presentations. CD-Rom. Jan Roscoe Publications, Widnes
Roscoe D A, Roscoe J V, Honeybourne J, Davis R, Galligan F 2003 Physical Education and Sport Studies AS/A2 Level Student Revision Guide, 3rd edn. Jan Roscoe Publications, Widnes

Glossary of terms

Chapter 9–13

ability a stable, enduring, mainly genetically determined characteristic or trait that underlies skilled performance, e.g. reaction time.

achievement motivation the tendency to persist in difficult, challenging tasks or to avoid them.

aggression an action where the purpose is to cause harm, as distinct from assertive actions where no harm is intended.

aggressive cue hypothesis the theory that frustration leads to increased arousal but only to aggression if there are cues in the environment which draw out aggressive behaviour, e.g. playing a team which behaved aggressively in the previous match.

anxiety a subjective feeling of apprehension and worry.

arousal the state of readiness for action; arousal may be physiological (i.e. under control of the autonomic nervous system) or psychological (i.e. dependent on motivation and anxiety).

assertiveness unusual exertion or persistence in order to achieve; assertive play in an invasion game would be a safe, fair, strong tackle.

association theory a theory that suggests that learning happens when a stimulus and a response are connected in the mind of the performer: also known as S–R theory.

attention concentration on certain aspects of the environment, due to the limitations of the information processing system.

attentional focus a performer's ability to concentrate on relevant cues during action.

attentional narrowing narrowing of attentional focus due to increases in anxiety.

attentional style a performer's preferred way of concentrating. Nideffer identified four attentional styles: broad-internal, broad-external, narrow-internal and narrow-external.

attribution the process of giving reasons for events, such as believing that a game was lost because the team was unlucky with the refereeing decisions.

audition the process of hearing.

autocratic style a type of leadership in which the leader takes all the decisions.

biofeedback a relaxation programme in which performers learn to generate relaxation by using physiological (somatic) measures, e.g. heart rate, galvanic skin response.

body image the picture a person has of their own body; body image is composed mainly of physical characteristics such as height, weight and shape.

bracketed morality the idea that normal moral codes of behaviour do not necessarily apply in sport.

catastrophe theory a form of inverted-U theory in which it is predicated that beyond the optimal arousal zone, small increases in arousal may cause catastrophic decreases in performance.

catharsis the process whereby pent-up emotions and feelings of anger and frustration can be discharged through aggressive behaviour in sport.

central nervous system (CNS) the brain and the spinal cord.

choice reaction time the time it takes either to react to one stimulus selected from a number of stimuli or to match the right response to a particular stimulus.

chunking a memory process whereby items of information are grouped together in order to memorise more information, i.e. remembering a sequence of movement by making the end of one movement lead into the beginning of the next.

classical conditioning an explanation of learning in which one stimulus or event becomes associated with or predicts another.

closed loop control the execution of movements which are guided by feedback, i.e. there is a constant error detection mechanism operating.

closed skills skills performed in an environment which is stable and predictable, e.g. a shot in snooker.

co-active skills/sports activities in which competitors perform together but in which there is little interaction; for example, archery.

cognitive dissonance the tension which a person feels when two attitudes held are inconsistent.

cognitive anxiety management strategies which are planned to control anxiety and thus improve performance, e.g. imagery.

cognitive skills skills in which the main component is intellectual/mental, such as reading.

cognitive state anxiety the emotional feeling of worry or apprehension in a particular situation, i.e. just before an important game.

cohesion the extent to which a sports team or group get on with each other and work together to achieve their goals. There are two forms: social cohesion and task cohesion.

command style a style of teaching in which the teacher makes all the decisions about the learning situation and the learners follow instructions.

commitment one of the '4 Cs' of mental preparation for sport.

competence the ability to perform tasks effectively.

competence motivation the drive to become competent.

concentration one of the '4 Cs' of mental preparation for sport: associated with attention and focus.

concurrent feedback feedback that is given or occurs simultaneously with the action.

confidence one of the '4 Cs' of mental preparation for sport; associated with self-confidence and self-efficacy.

connectionist theory see *associationist theories*.

continuous skills skills which have no clear beginning or end, e.g. running.

controllability an attribution dimension which places events either within or outside a performer's control.

decision mechanism a theoretical component of the information processing model which uses incoming information and information stored in memory to select the most appropriate movement response.

decreasing errors graph a learning curve which plots a series of performances in terms of the number of errors in each performance and which demonstrates that errors are decreasing with each performance.

delayed feedback feedback which is only available after the performance is complete.

democratic leadership style a type of leadership in which the leader encourages discussion and joint decision making.

discovery style a style of teaching in which the learners are set structured tasks and questions in order to solve a movement problem without direct instruction from the teacher.

discrete skills skills which have a clear beginning and end, e.g. a tennis serve.

distributed practice a practice schedule or programme in which practice sessions are interspersed with rest periods which are longer than the practice sessions.

dominant response the response which is most likely to occur in a given situation, e.g. when a skill is well learned then a good performance is the dominant response.

drive theory a theory of motivation and arousal which predicts that as motivation and arousal increase, so the quality of performance increases and the relationship is linear.

effector mechanism a theoretical component of the information processing model which selects an appropriate motor programme and puts it into operation via the muscles.

ego orientation the tendency to see success in terms of winning or losing, i.e. in relation to the performance of others.

emergent leader a person who assumes the lead in a group because of their characteristics and competence and who is accepted as leader by the team.

EPI/Q Eysenck's Personality Inventory/ Questionnaire.

eustress pleasant stress whereby performers are excited by challenge.

evaluation apprehension a state of worry brought on by the presence of spectators (or co-actors) or significant others who are in a position to be critical of the performance.

executive programme the overall motor programme which governs the performance of a skill and which integrates the component subroutines.

external feedback feedback which is only available from a source outside the performer.

external focus of attention concentration on cues which are external to the performer, i.e. aspects of the environment.

externally paced skills skills whose timing is determined by someone or something other than the performer.

extrinsic motivation external factors which influence behaviour, such as rewards.

extroversion a personality dimension which is made up of a number of traits such as sociability, impulsiveness and willingness to take risks; the opposite end of the dimension is introversion. Extroverts are said to have lower levels of cortical activity and thus seek excitement and stimulation.

faulty processes social processes which prevent a group task being achieved efficiently and effectively, e.g. a new player who has not yet quite sorted out his position and tends to get in the way of other players.

feedback information about a movement which derives from the performance of the movement.

Fiedler's contingency model a theory of leadership which emphasises particular personality traits.

fine skills skills which require delicate muscular control, e.g. darts.

frustration–aggression theory a theory which suggests that aggressive behaviour is caused by the frustration of not being allowed to achieve one's goal, e.g. a defender is consistently being passed by a fast forward and eventually resorts to an aggressive tackle.

gestalt from the German meaning 'the whole picture'; it emphasises that the whole is more than the sum of its parts and that learning is most effective when the learner has a chance to see the whole picture.

goal setting the process of setting targets to increase motivation and aid performance. Goals may be long term, short term or intermediate.

gross skills skills which require large muscle and whole-body involvement, such as high jumping.

guidance processes by which a teacher or coach helps a learner to acquire a skill; these may be verbal (instruction), visual (demonstration) or manual (support or physically guiding the movement).

home advantage the idea that competing at home gives a team or individual an advantage because of spectator support.

hostile aggression behaviour which has the intention of harming another, with the specific intent to inflict pain or psychological suffering and which is accompanied by anger.

imagery the use of the imagination to visualise situations, in order to relax or to prepare for a forthcoming event.

individual skills skills in which the performer participates alone without the presence of either co-actors or interacting others.

information processing a theory that humans deal with information that passes into the central nervous system, rather than merely responding to it. Components of the process include perception, memory, decision making and action.

instinct theory the theory that aggression is innate and therefore cannot be eliminated but must be controlled.

instrumental aggression behaviour which has the intention of harming another in order to achieve a goal such as winning. Winning is the motivation, not causing suffering; there is no anger involved.

interactional theory a personality theory which stresses the importance of considering personality as interacting with the situation, i.e. a person might be shy amongst people they do not know well but show extrovert behaviour when with their teammates.

interactive skills/sports activities in which players must interact with each other during the game, e.g. volleyball.

internal/intrinsic feedback feedback which derives from the movement itself.

internal focus of attention concentration on one's own feelings, thoughts and emotions.

intrinsic motivation a drive to succeed which comes from within the performer and is inherent to the activity.

introversion one end of the extroversion–introversion personality dimension; introverts are not comfortable in new social situations and are more passive and controlled than extroverts; they are stimulus avoiders.

inverted-U theory a theory which takes its name from the graph which illustrates it; it predicts that performance will be at its highest at a medium level of arousal.

kinaesthesis feedback from muscles, tendons and joints; it gives the feelings and sensations associated with the movement.

knowledge of performance augmented feedback (i.e. from outside the performer) related to the quality of the performance.

knowledge of results augmented feedback related to the outcome of the action.

laissez-faire leadership style a style of leadership characterised by letting the group or team get on with the task without giving specific instructions; such leaders may interfere if things are going wrong.

law of effect behaviour which is rewarded tends to be repeated, whereas behaviour which is not rewarded gradually disappears.

law of exercise repeating an action makes it easier to perform and more accurate; this early theory of learning tended to ignore the effects of such things as motivation and rewards.

learned helplessness a tendency for a performer to give up or to avoid challenging situations because in the past they have been unsuccessful in similar situations; they feel that failure is inevitable.

learning a relatively permanent change in behaviour.

learning curve the diagrammatic representation of learning as a series of performances which become increasingly more refined, effective and error free.

linear graph a graph in which changes in one variable are directly related to changes in the other.

locus of causality/control the extent to which performers feel that they have control over what happens to them. An internal locus of control means people feel that they are in control: an external locus of control implies that control of events lies elsewhere.

long-term goals targets which are achieved over a relatively long period of time; short-term and intermediate goals contribute to long-term goals.

long-term memory the relatively permanent memory where information is stored for long periods and from which information is retrieved to be used. Information, including motor programmes, is stored in coded form.

manual guidance help given to a learner by a teacher or coach, by physical support or by physically guiding the learner through the movements, e.g. in the learning of a trampoline somersault.

massed practice a schedule or programme of practice interspersed with rest periods where the practice sessions are longer than the rest periods.

memory the process of storing information and motor programmes within the nervous system.

mental rehearsal practising a skill in the imagination without overt movements of the body.

modelling either the demonstration of a skill or task to show a good example of the technique or tactic or the copying of the demonstration or other behaviour by the learner.

motivation the internal state of a performer which drives them to behave or perform in a particular way.

motor programme a theoretical set of 'instructions' stored in the memory, which coordinates the muscles to produce the required action.

movement time the time from the start of the movement to its completion; reaction time plus movement time equals response time.

multidimensional anxiety theory a theory which suggests that arousal consists of both physiological and psychological elements and that these interact to affect performance.

multidimensional model of leadership Chelladurai's model predicts that performers' satisfaction and achievement are products of the interaction between three elements of leadership: prescribed leader behaviour, actual leader behaviour and preferred leader behaviour.

narrow attentional focus/style concentration which focuses on a narrow band of cues or events; these may be appropriate for the task or, if the performer is anxious, they may be inappropriate.

need to achieve the intrinsic motivation to be successful.

need to avoid failure a state of mind in which a performer avoids situations in which they think they might not be successful.

negative acceleration curve a learning curve which shows that in a series of performances, learning was effective early in the series but then the rate of learning slowed down.

negative reinforcement reinforcement of behaviour which inhibits that behaviour, i.e. it provides relief from something which is unpleasant.

negative transfer learning occurring in one situation which has a damaging effect on learning in another.

neuroticism one element of the personality dimension neuroticism–stability. Neurotics tend to be anxious and to worry, often unnecessarily.

noise in an information processing approach, noise is the operations of the nervous system which are not relevant to the task in hand.

observational learning learning which takes place by watching others; this can occur in a formal setting (e.g. a coaching session) or when a young player watches his sport hero in action.

open loop control a motor control system which operates without feedback or error detection, often because the movement is too fast for these to have an effect on the movement.

open skills skills which are performed in a constantly changing environment, e.g. an invasion game.

operant conditioning a method of teaching in which behaviours that approximate to the desired behaviour are rewarded to increase the likelihood of them occurring again.

optimal arousal the theory that for every skill and every person there is a 'best' level of arousal for maximum performance.

outcome goals targets that reflect winning or losing a competition; they depend on other performers doing less well and do not take account of the quality of the performance.

outcome orientation performers who judge their success in terms of winning or losing, rather than the quality of the performance.

pacing continuum skills which are categorised by the amount of control the performer has over the timing of the skill.

part–whole practice a programme of practice which breaks the skill down into its constituent parts for specific practice, then integrates the parts into the whole skill.

perceptual mechanism a component of the information processing model; the detection, comparison and recognition of cues from surroundings.

perceptual–motor skills skills which have both a perceptual and a movement component; most sport and exercise skills are of this type.

perceptual skills skills which are predominantly concerned with interpreting the environment.

performance a temporary occurrence of an action or skill, the level of which fluctuates because of influences such as motivation, fatigue and environment; trends in performance levels are used to indicate learning.

performance goals targets that are about the performer's own relative achievement, e.g. achieving a personal best. They do not depend on the performance of others.

performance orientation a tendency to judge performance on its quality in relation to what the performer is capable of, rather than on winning or losing.

peripheral nervous system the nerves leading to and from the spinal cord.

person (relationship)-centred leadership style in which the needs of the team or group are as important, if not more important, than achieving success.

plateau a period in learning when no appreciable gains in learning are taking place.

positive acceleration curve a learning curve which shows little increase in the quality of performance to start with and then there are rapid gains in learning towards the end of the period.

positive reinforcement rewards given to a learner to increase the likelihood of the desired learning taking place; praise and encouragement are often used as positive reinforcement in sport contexts.

positive transfer the process of getting better at one skill as a result of practice at another, e.g. practising passing with the left foot will also improve the ability to pass with the right.

practice style a teaching style in which the teacher sets the task but allows the class freedom to practise as they wish.

prescribed leader a leader who is appointed or elected.

process goals targets which focus on the quality of the performance and the means of achieving the target, rather than the outcome; they do not rely on the performance of others.

productivity the extent to which the members of a team 'pull their weight'.

progressive muscular relaxation a procedure for relaxing the body by systematically tensing and then gradually relaxing muscle groups in turn.

psychological refractory period the delay in the response to the second of two close stimuli.

psychometric methods methods of investigating people's behaviour and attitudes by measuring these using tests and inventories.

punishment an unpleasant response designed to prevent the occurrence of unwanted behaviour.

reaction time the time between the presentation of a stimulus (or stimuli) and the initiation of the response.

reciprocal style a teaching style in which the learners work with a partner and take it in turns to observe and comment upon each other's performance.

reinforcement the giving of a reward such that the rewarded behaviour will be repeated; praise for a well-timed pass in hockey would normally act as reinforcement.

response time the total period of time from the presentation of a stimulus to the completion of the response; reaction time plus movement time equals response time.

Ringelmann effect the observed phenomenon that the larger the sports group or team, the less each individual tends to contribute to the group effort.

SCCAMP goals targets which are specific, controllable, challenging, attainable, measurable and personal.

schema a rule or a concept or a relationship, which can relate to movement, and which is formed on the basis of experience.

selective attention the process whereby people concentrate on one cue or stimulus, to the exclusion of others.

self-concept the total view a person has of him/herself.

self-confidence a general belief in one's own competence.

self-efficacy belief in one's competence in a specific situation, e.g. a particular sport.

self-esteem the extent to which one values oneself.

self-talk a technique for changing negative attitudes to positive thoughts; literally, talking to oneself.

short-term goals targets that can be achieved in a short period of time.

short-term memory the part of the memory where information is held for a short time to determine its usefulness; if it is attended to and rehearsed, it will be passed to the long-term memory for permanent storage.

short-term sensory store a memory store which holds incoming literal information for less than a second to allow it to be selected for further processing.

simple reaction time the time taken to react to a single stimulus.

SMART goals targets which are specific, measurable, attainable and time bound.

social cohesion the degree to which members of a sport team or group like each other and relate socially to each other.

social facilitation support given to a performance by a non-interactive audience.

social inhibition the detrimental effect on performance of a non-interactive audience.

social learning theory a theory which suggests that we learn by being part of social groups and observing others.

social loafing the effect of performers believing that their lack of effort is masked by the performance of others.

sociometry the analysis of friendship and task groups, using a preferences questionnaire.

somatic management controlling anxiety by reducing the physiological symptoms of overarousal, e.g. heart and breathing rates, or by using imagery.

somatic state anxiety a physiological dimension of state anxiety, causing increases in heart and breathing rates, 'butterflies' and increased perspiration.

stability in attribution theory, the dimension that indicates whether an outcome or event will change or remain the same.

state anxiety worry and apprehension felt in relation to a particular event.

state measures measurements of state anxiety, such as Marten's Competitive State Anxiety Inventory (CSAI).

STEN score a standardised score out of 10 used in Cattell's 16 PF (personality factors) inventory.

stress: the response the body makes to any demand made on it; stress may result in cognitive or somatic anxiety or both.

subroutines motor programmes for specific parts of a skill which integrate to form the overall executive programme.

task cohesion the degree to which performers work together to achieve a team goal.

task orientation a tendency to view success in terms of personal performance rather than by comparison with the performance of others.

terminal feedback feedback available at the end of the performance.

thought stopping replacing negative thoughts by positive, achievement-orientated thoughts.

trait a general characteristic of a person which predisposes them to behave in a particular way.

trait anxiety a general tendency to be worried or apprehensive; a wide variety of situations are perceived as threatening and state anxiety is created.

transfer the process by which learning in one situation aids or hinders learning in another, often similar, situation.

translatory mechanism another term for the decision-making mechanism in the information processing model.

variable practice training which allows an open skill to be practised in a variety of situations to allow a strong schema to be established.

verbal guidance information about a task or skill, given to a learner in the form of instructions.

visual guidance images or demonstrations shown to a learner to help in the development of a skill.

whole method a method of teaching/learning whereby the whole skill is practised from the start, rather than breaking it down into parts.

whole–part–whole method a method of teaching/learning whereby the learner is introduced to the whole skill initially, or a modified version of it: the skill is then broken down into parts and these practised separately; they are integrated into the whole skill at the end.

zone of optimal functioning a modification (by Hanin) of the inverted-U theory; best performance levels of arousal are particular to individuals, to tasks and to situations.

Part 3

The performer in a social setting

Bob Davis

14. Important concepts in physical education and sport
15. Physical education and sport in the United Kingdom
16. Sociological considerations of physical education and sport
17. Some contemporary issues in physical education and sport

Glossary of terms

18. Physical education and sport on the continent of Europe with particular reference to France
19. Physical education and sport in Commonwealth countries with particular reference to Australia
20. Physical education and sport in North America with particular reference to the United States
21. Physical education and sport in Communist and post-Communist countries with particular reference to the Soviet Union (Russia)

Glossary of terms

22. Historical perspectives and popular recreation
23. Athleticism in 19th-century English public schools
24. The pattern of rational recreation in 19th-century Britain
25. Transitions in English elementary schools

Glossary of terms

It is very easy for us to turn to the sports pages and consider that information about players' performances is all there is to know. If we are to gain a useful knowledge and understanding of physical education and sport we must recognise that any group activity involves relationships between people and is influenced by the society to which it belongs.

There are three main dimensions to be examined under the title of The performer in a social setting. These consist of contemporary sociocultural aspects, comparative studies and historical perspectives of physical education and sport.

The increased significance of synoptic questioning means that links have to be made between contemporary, comparative and historical studies and so although each section is presented as a separate area of study, there is continual cross-reference to relationships with other sections.

The performer in a social setting starts with a critical analysis of concepts ranging from play to professional sport and involves the reader in the process of understanding words and notions. Having established what we mean by certain concepts, the second phase reviews the administration of these concepts in the United Kingdom, a rapidly changing picture, initiated by the publication *Raising the game* (1995) and influenced by the massive infusion of money through the National Lottery. The third phase involves an examination of physical education and sport using a number of sociological techniques as group interaction but also at a cultural level as it concerns different types of society. Finally, these components are integrated to examine a number of contemporary issues in physical education and sport.

Comparative studies takes us into the concepts, administrational frameworks and problems faced by a number of other countries but also synoptic comment on what the United Kingdom can learn from them in the context of physical education and sport. Particular reference is made to Australia, as a Commonwealth country with advanced policies in physical education and sport; France, as a fellow member of the European Union and a very successful sporting nation; the United States as a capitalist superpower, which dominates world sport at the moment; and Russia, as it goes through the transition from a communism regime to a socialist market economy. It also gives us a chance to look at Russia as an emergent country, with all the pressures on nation building, integration, health and defence, reflected in the commitment to physical culture and sport, following the political and economic U-turn of the 1991 reforms.

The historical perspective consists almost entirely of British sports history, on the grounds that this represents the nucleus from which most international sport has developed. It is presented in four phases: preindustrial popular recreation; athleticism in elite public schools; postindustrial rational recreation; and 20th-century developments in school physical education, as it changed from military drill and physical training. In addition to transitional links being established between these four phases, efforts are made to relate the recent past to the contemporary scene to facilitate synoptic analysis.

Bibliographies are presented at regular intervals to encourage additional reading and a large number of models and illustrative material are offered to involve the student in decision-making activities.

The main structural change in this fifth edition is to study each country separately but with the new focus on synoptic assessment, where there is a continual cross-reference from one section to another. This is reinforced through the availability of an associated CD-ROM, which looks at a number of synoptic themes.

Important concepts in physical education and sport

14.1 Introduction

Learning objectives

On completion of this section, you will be able to:

1. Develop a philosophical perspective of physical education as a field of study.
2. Understand the conceptual basis of leisure, recreation, physical recreation and sport in the United Kingdom.
3. Understand the role of physical education as a subject in schools and colleges.
4. Be aware of the outdoor and adventurous dimension as it concerns outdoor recreation and outdoor education.
5. Appreciate certain conceptual frameworks as they concern characteristics of sport and sporting competition.

You have read about the structure and function of our subject through the eyes of the scientist and the social scientist. It is now time to look at physical education and sport in a social setting. If we put this in the form of a model, it should look something like that shown in Figure 14.1.

Do you understand what each of the nine questions is trying to show? Can you give a brief answer to each of them? You need to know the meanings of the words and notions and be able to express them accurately. Get into the habit of asking two basic questions whenever you meet new words or situations: 'What do we mean by?' and 'How do we know?'.

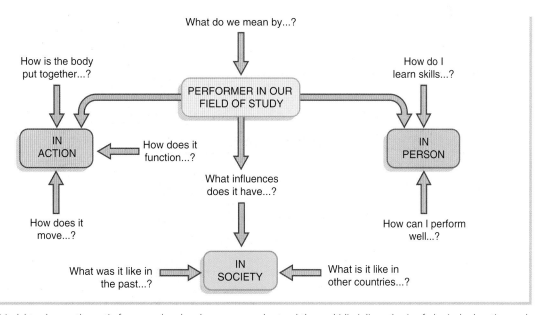

Fig. 14.1 Model to show a thematic framework, whereby we can understand the multidisciplinary basis of physical education and sport.

If you can answer this, you will be able to sort your definitions out, which will allow you to discuss things rationally.

How do we know?

If you go on to this second level of questioning and establish authoritative back-up to what you have said, you have changed a point of view into a worthwhile, public statement that will stand up to a certain amount of scrutiny.

So, what does this model tell us?

It would seem that most of what you have been reading has been centred on the **performer** and his or her involvement in a family of activities that we variously call **physical education**, **sport** or **physical recreation**.

You have looked at the **performer in action** through the eyes of the physiologist; at the **person involved in the activity** using the techniques of the psychologist; and you are about to examine the nature, structure and function of **physical performance in a social setting**.

This implies that you should know about physical education and sport in your own country; that it helps to know what it is like in other countries; and that it is important to know what influence the past has had.

Let's try to establish some **terms of reference**.

- We are concerned with a particular **field of study** that we have called **physical performance**.
- Our initial task, therefore, is to establish the boundaries of this term in this book.
- Our definition of physical performance is limited to activities that fall within the categories of **play, physical recreation, sport and physical education**.
- Other forms of physical performance exist and may have common features with those categories we have identified, but they are outside our present field of study.

All four categories can also be experienced in the natural environment, where alternative motives arise and different types of challenge have to be met, producing recreative and educative subcategories.

Having identified four categories, we now apply our questioning technique by asking, **what do we mean by them?** Figure 14.2 shows what they *might* mean.

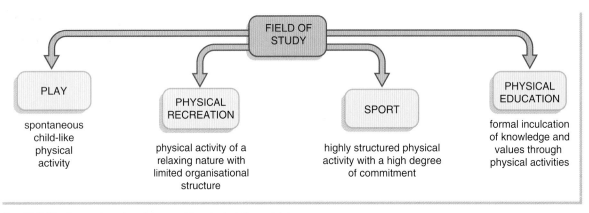

Fig. 14.2 The four categories of our model and what they might mean.

Review questions

To test the definitions

1. See if you can think of an experience you have had in each of the categories in Figure 14.2.

2. Put the following activities into these categories:
   a. two children playing hopscotch in the street
   b. Miami Dolphins playing the Redskins in the Superbowl
   c. a school gymnastics lesson
   d. a group of backpackers rambling in the English Lake District.

3. Make sure that you understand the words in each definition and try to find some exceptions.

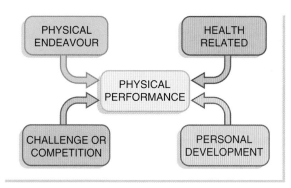

Fig. 14.3 Possible shared characteristics of the four categories.

If you have tackled the Review Questions in the right way, you will be starting to come up with some **characteristics** that all four categories share but you will also be aware that each has certain characteristics that make it **different** from the others. Do you agree with the **shared characteristics** shown in Figure 14.3?

Now let's look at a few other physical performances which we suggest are outside our terms of reference: acting in a play; playing chess; pulling a tooth out; and gardening. It is suggested that none of these fits into our notion of play, physical recreation, sport or physical education because they don't have a sufficient number of the shared characteristics we expect to find in our field of study.

See if you can establish why these four activities are outside our terms of reference. What you will find

is that there is a core of activities that can be applied to all four categories and others that may fit into only one. Motor racing, for example, is certainly a sport but it is hard to see it as play, physical recreation or physical education. Football, on the other hand, can consist of some children kicking a tin can down the road, being taught it at school, playing a game in the park with coats for goals or fulfilling a league fixture. It is all football but each of these examples fits into a different category of physical performance.

Most of the examples we are going to use will be like football; in other words, it depends on the players and the way they play as to whether they are involved in play, a formal educational experience, a sport or a recreation. Figure 14.4 identifies some of these core activities and 'dares' to classify them into five major groups.

We are suggesting that all these activities belong to the same family or field of study but that they have a number of unique features that make them rather like the fingers of one hand.

Try to identify some of these unique features. You will probably come up with words like game, combat and conquest; you might decide that some are objective while others have subjective elements; you might conclude that the key lies in the number of players and their relationship. It is always easier if you relate your definition to a specific activity and test it.

A combat, for example, involves you in beating an opponent in a stylised war game. Do you agree or is

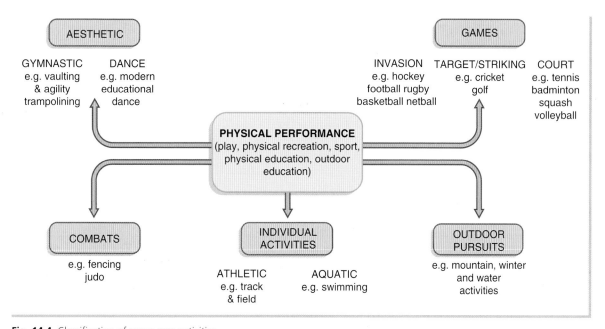

Fig. 14.4 Classification of some core activities.

there more to it than that? Test your definition by looking at judo or fencing. What do you think about archery being in this category?

Can you define a conquest activity? Does it involve competition or challenge? Is it against man or nature? Does it have to be the first time? What are its physical and psychological components? Is it basically an objective or a romantic experience? If you ask these questions and link them with an acknowledged conquest activity like mountaineering, you should come up with certain characteristics that will give you a clearer understanding of the term.

You are still left with the difficult notion of what a game is. For example, you might agree that basically it is a contrived competitive experience existing in its own time and space. That is quite a difficult statement. Can you simplify it and then pick a game to test it?

However, in Figure 14.4 the games are divided into partner and team. We also know that there are invasion games, such as hockey and football; court games, such as tennis and squash; and target games, such as cricket, baseball and golf. Can you set up some sets of characteristics to differentiate these types of game?

Unfortunately, this degree of analysis simply takes us into another round of what do you mean by and how do you know? For example, can you differentiate a contest from a game? Or what is the notion of combat? Is it a description of certain activities or a potential feature of all contests? Can you establish the difference between a competition and a challenge? We are probably raising more questions than answers by this point. Don't worry too much; the debate itself is valuable and the more we question, the more you will realise that there are very few absolutes.

Let's make a decisive statement and if it holds we are ready to make a start. Our field of study includes a number of specific activities that share a number of characteristics. There would seem to be four main categories within this field of study: play, physical recreation, sport and physical education. Most of the core activities can exist in each category, dependent on the attitude of the performer and the level of performance and organisation.

Test this statement by using different examples and different situations.

We now have one more basic step to take. Having just used the word 'situation', we need to recognise that we are concerned with a dynamic experience that is complete in itself, an intrinsic whole. Like a watch, once it is put together successfully, it works independently. Let's not forget, however, that we are not just a machine: our battery is an independent mind!

In model form, the components of this working dynamic can be arranged as in Figure 14.5. Can you make this model more meaningful by putting it into a real situation? For example, if you are performing, what are you performing? Where are you performing? Why are you performing? These are the most important components. Now, what about the influence of the coach, the spectators and the administrators? They all have a direct bearing on you as a performer and on the direct function of the activity.

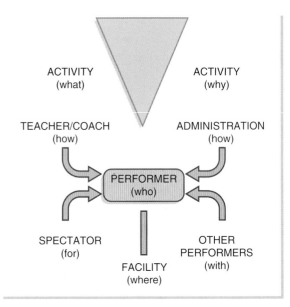

Fig. 14.5 Components for a model of the social setting of sport.

However, this activity does not exist in a vacuum. All the time, outside forces are acting on it. In the case of the watch, someone winds it up, wears it, looks after it, uses it, looks at it and values it. These outside influences are what we have called the social setting or they could be called **extrinsic factors**.

Terms like 'spheres of influence' and 'affective horizons' can help to explain the way in which society changes the performer and the performance. You probably belong to a sports club. What factors outside the club influence it? Are they human, financial, geographical or political or perhaps all four?

Figure 14.6 identifies the main extrinsic factors which have influenced the performance situation. It is often said that performance situations reflect the society and culture they exist in but there are occasions where such is the impact of sport on society or physical education on education that the opposite

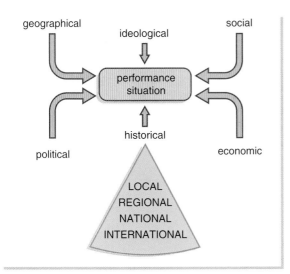

Fig. 14.6 Main extrinsic factors that influence the performance situation.

scale, you could assess the wave-like impact of the 2000 Olympic Games not only on Sydney itself but also on Australia, South East Asia and ultimately the whole world. These examples of interaction remind us that to understand the performance situation, we must be aware of its social setting. These relationships do not always reflect intrinsic values – for example, the selection of Atlanta instead of Athens for the Centenary Olympic Games in 1996 may well have hinged on the influence of the Coca Cola™ Company.

If these are the dimensions in which our field of study operates, we must appreciate the contemporary scene but we then need to unravel both traditional behaviour, through the **time** perspective of historical knowledge, and environmental influences, through the **spatial** perspective of comparative study, to understand parallel developments in other countries.

Clearly, for play, local influences are likely to predominate, whereas the impact of high-level sport can be worldwide. England being allowed to reenter European football is one example but the exclusion of South Africa from the Olympic Games had even wider implications.

In addition to dimensions, we need to be aware of perspectives if we are to obtain a coherent picture of the social setting. We will understand our own contemporary society more fully if we use historical perspective to establish what has **caused** the present and a comparative perspective to understand parallel developments in other countries.

occurs, so that our field of study changes aspects of society as well as some of its cultural patterns.

The extent to which this interaction takes place varies from a local influence to an international one, in waves of reaction which have been variously called 'spheres of influence' and 'affective horizons'. At a local level, you probably belong to a sports club and are aware of the influence of the local community on it. Conversely, you may be able to recognise the influence your club has on the town. Similarly, but on a wider

14.2 Towards a concept of leisure

The ordinary citizen has to work for a living. He or she then has certain obligatory activities that have to be performed, such as sleeping and eating. What is left is leisure time.

All the activities in our field of study either take place in leisure time, are themselves leisure activities or prepare us for active leisure and it is therefore essential that we understand what is meant by the term leisure. Let's start by making a list (Figure 14.7).

How clever are you at recognising differences between these activities? Well, there would seem to be two major variables.

1. Not all leisure involves physical performance; for example, watching TV sport.

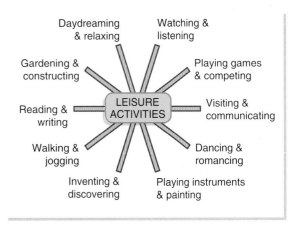

Fig. 14.7 Leisure activities.

2. Physical performance is not always a leisure-time experience; for example, professional sport has work connotations.

It looks as if it might not be as simple as we thought! Let's play safe and look at what other people think leisure is.

> *Leisure is time in which there is an opportunity for choice.*[1]

> *Leisure helps people to learn how to play their part in society; it helps them to achieve societal or collective aims; and it helps the society to keep together.*[2]

> *Leisure is a mental and spiritual attitude – a condition of the soul, not the inevitable result of spare time.*[3]

> *A necessary prerequisite for practising the more civilised virtues – the adoption of a critical attitude to life and developing a taste for excellence.*[4]

> *Leisure is the complex of self-fulfilling and self-enriching values achieved by the individual as he uses leisure time in self-chosen activities that recreate him.*[5]

> *Leisure is an activity – apart from the obligations of work, family and society – to which the individual turns at will.*[6]

Review questions

1. Remember, anyone can select quotations to make a biased case. Look for quotations by other authors and make an attempt at your own definition of leisure.
2. Before reading on, pick out the keywords in each quotation and assemble them in a model.

> *Leisure consists of relatively self-determining activity-experiences that fall into one's economically free-time roles.*[7]

These keywords should represent characteristics of leisure and you should try to fit them into a number of categories if you can. Compare your presentation (see Review Questions) of the concept of leisure with the analysis in Figure 14.8. Don't worry too much if your format differs from ours, as there are many ways of presenting characteristics of a complex experience like leisure. However, we tend to use the same order of presentation with all models: structure (what); function (how); interpretation (why); conclusion (key).

Well, we have produced a list of words in Figure 14.8, characteristics of leisure, maybe, but now you need to establish what each word means and explain it in a physical performance situation that you have experienced.

Investigation 14.1 The potential value of leisure

Read this short case study.

I'm John and I spend much of my leisure time gardening but my wife, Jane, prefers the theatre and my two children love swimming.

We all pursue our favoured activities when we have the free time to do so, but once in a while we share each other's hobbies. Both my wife and I work, but on summer evenings I am able to visit my allotment, while she settles down to a good play on the TV. We don't have to do either of these things, but we enjoy them and respect each other's right to choose. Similarly, the children swim whenever they have the chance, which amounts to two or three times a week. Mary is a little more serious than Bill and so she tends to train quite hard while he just plays around. Either way, they come home tired but happy.

Our hobbies certainly take us away from the boredom, conformity and stress of the working day and we find that we can relax within a few moments of tasting the atmosphere of our chosen activities. Funnily enough, although we often feel quite jaded when we start our various activities, the tiredness falls

away as we accept the responsibilities of our chosen activity. There are always new situations which are totally unpredictable and my wife tells me that her greatest joy is to experience a play unfolding for the first time. Nor is she limited to watching plays on the TV, as she belongs to a small amateur company, which puts on plays twice a year, and she also visits the West End in London occasionally, as a special treat.

It is as if we are genuinely part of the experience. I sometimes feel that I am actually growing with the plants and Jane says that she often loses herself in the story she's watching.

The children, of course, with their practical activity, are able to express themselves physically, as well as test their temperament in the hurly-burly of the swimming baths and they invariably come away from the pool exhausted but glowing inside.

Unfortunately, we find that our work is not very fulfilling. I work on a conveyor belt in a car factory and my wife is a typist in an office. We seem to spend each day doing the same thing, surrounded by the same noises and petty anxieties. Only our leisure ▶

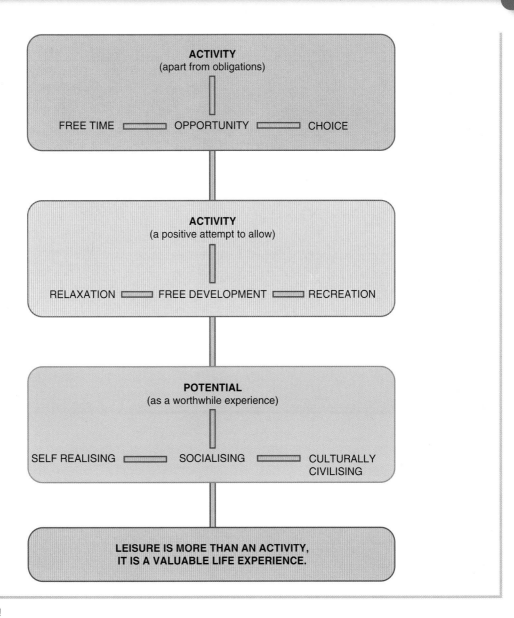

Fig. 14.8 Leisure!

activities seem to give us a chance to achieve something as individuals. I've learnt so much more about myself as a result of my leisure activity, sometimes reflecting on life's many foibles as I dig the ground each autumn; at other times realising, as I pick my own strawberries, that I am totally responsible for their existence; and, honestly, is there anything to equal the peace and quiet of a garden on a balmy summer evening?

Not that any of my family particularly want solitude – gosh, on the contrary, we seem to spend most of the time chatting to friends, sharing and caring, as they say, with a kind of sincerity that doesn't seem to occur very often at work.

I know I'm a better person as a result of the time I spend on the garden and the allotment; it's as if nature is slowing me down and actually giving me roots.

No one can tell me that gardening is just an activity. It is a diversion which is at once relaxing and invigorating; it broadens my experiences and has given me lasting friendships; it really is the free exercise of my creative capacity; and it's the only time in my life when I feel I actually taste excellence.

OK, so my family is involved in a pretty purposeful approach to leisure but if I can paraphrase John Ruskin:

True creative fulfilment comes from the exertion of body or mind to please ourselves.

1. Pick out the keywords that reflect the potential value of leisure. It is only a question of looking at Figure 14.8!
2. Establish your own role-play groups so that you can 'score points' in illustrating characteristics of leisure.

Always remember, however, that an **activity** is only the vehicle which allows a person to **experience** leisure.

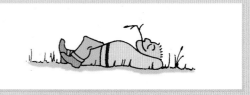

Fig. 14.9 Don't be a 'jock' all your life! Remember the reflective and the sportive should complement each other.

Leisure in a cultural setting

At first sight, it would seem that leisure is a universal concept. However, all activity-experiences are influenced by their cultural setting and so where there are societal differences between countries, there will also be variables in the structure and function of leisure. Kaplan produced a six-model analysis[7] but we will use the less sophisticated approach suggested by Jelfs.[8]

Leisure as spare time

The most common concept of leisure is the negative view that leisure is non-work. It presents work as the valued ethic in society and tends to devalue leisure, presenting it as a means of restoring individuals for work. This leaves leisure with little or no independent identity and minimal cultural status.

This view still exists in the United Kingdom as a result of the industrial revolution and the Protestant work ethic. To paraphrase Huizinga:[9] 'Work was first of all the IDEAL and then the IDOL of the age'.

This sums up 19th-century English industrial society and the ethic can still be seen today. Less evident in France and what was once the Soviet Union, it does have links with capitalist economics and so has found some favour in the United States.

Try to explain Figure 14.10, establishing what each term means and illustrating it wherever possible.

Leisure as an economic condition

This second concept of leisure is very closely identified with the first. An expression that describes it is that leisure is a reflection of cultural lifestyle – the point

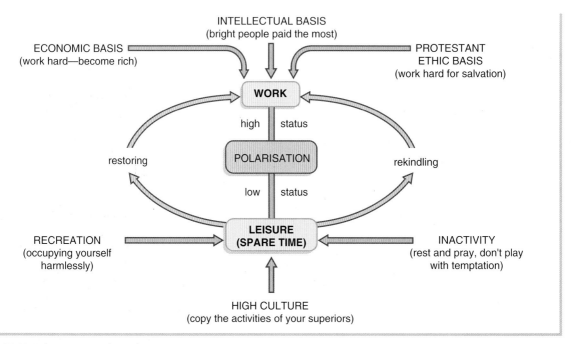

Fig. 14.10 Leisure as spare time – low status.

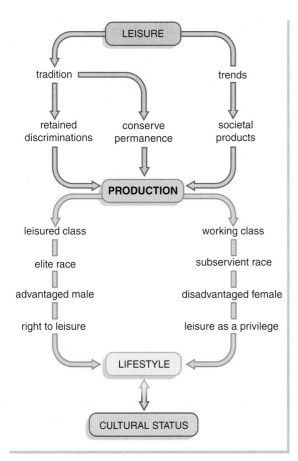

Fig. 14.11 Leisure as an economic condition – cultural lifestyle.

Leisure as a form of social control

This is identifiable in a society where social equality is very important but also where deviance from a culturally acceptable pattern of behaviour is not tolerated. The key phrase here is purposeful leisure.

So far, we have seen leisure as an optional extra and as a feature of privileged groups in society. In both cases the values have tended to be intrinsic, which means the activities are seen to have little value outside themselves. This view is common to most of the Western world and most strongly evident in Britain.

However, the former Soviet Union and other 'socialist' societies reflected this third concept much more strongly than America or the Common Market countries because the former Soviet Union tended to be, and still is, more authoritarian, even though committed to an egalitarian political system. Such statements as 'good socialist principles' and 'for the good of the state' were commonplace until the break-up of the Union. Leisure was given considerable social status, designed to reinforce sociopolitical values and based on the belief that leisure had extrinsic value – which meant that it could influence the social development of a society and also exist as a social process in its own right.

See if you can work your way through Figure 14.12 and try to grasp why leisure had such prominence in societies like the former Soviet Union.

being that any inherent form of social inequality will be evident in a society's pattern of leisure.

See if you can explain Figure 14.11 using illustrations from your experience.

If we look at the British and American leisure scene we find a high and a low culture, which are partly determined by status in society. This may reflect social class variables, racial discrimination or gender inequalities. In England it is evident in the group who play polo, as against those who play soccer. In the USA a comparison might be made between golf and baseball. Even in activities that involve a mixture of social groups, cultural demarcation is often evident, even if this is only a vestige of the past. The English Derby, for example, has the grandstand and enclosure for 'Society', and the Downs, where popular culture continues to thrive.

As egalitarian trends reduce these traditional boundaries, fewer leisure activities are completely exclusive but the traditional conservatism of many leisure activities gives them a permanence that resists change.

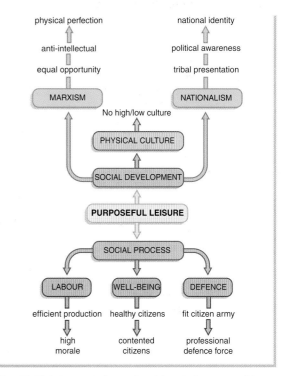

Fig. 14.12 Leisure as a form of social control – purposeful leisure.

Leisure as a basis of self-realisation

Finally, we have the most difficult concept to look at. We need to pick up the comments made by several of the authors we quoted earlier, where they wrote about humanistic values such as self-realisation and socialisation.

The potential of leisure as a medium for creative fulfilment is being increasingly recognised. It takes the social conditioning of the third model an extra step where, in addition to the extrinsic usefulness of leisure, it is felt that in the modern world of sedentary jobs, packaged goods and repetitious work, the only creative moments may arise in our leisure experiences; that only leisure can give us all a taste of excellence. Though you might think that all this is pretty revolutionary, the notion goes back to Aristotle, who argued that leisure is the most serious human occupation or activity. If you combine this with Ruskin's comment in the 19th century that leisure is the exertion of body or mind to please ourselves, we have an enlightened view of leisure as the key to personal development in a democratic society and as an art form in the context of cultural advancement. Select a leisure experience you have had and trace it through Figure 14.13.

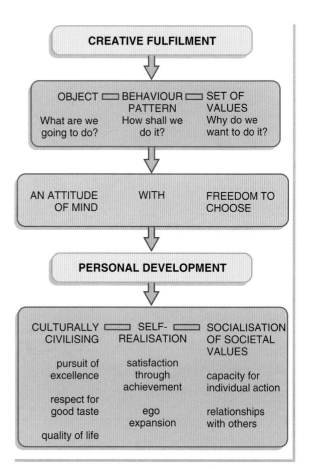

Fig. 14.13 Leisure as a basis of self-realisation – personal development.

Exam-style questions

1. Leisure is more than an activity; it is a valuable experience. Using examples:
   a. How can you recognise leisure? *(3 marks)*
   b. What is its function? *(3 marks)*
   c. What is its potential as an experience to improve the quality of our lives? *(3 marks)*
   (Total 9 marks)

2. The concept of leisure has a number of interpretations.

   a. What are the limits of a work–leisure analysis? *(4 marks)*
   b. How does the traditional view of leisure in Britain reflect its social class system? *(4 marks)*
   c. Explain ways in which leisure can be a form of social control, where a society presumes that leisure is purposeful. *(4 marks)*
   d. Explain leisure as an attitude of mind with freedom to choose. *(4 marks)*
   (Total 16 marks)

14.3 Towards a concept of play

It is very important to understand what we mean by the term 'play'. We use the word all the time and yet when we read about it in psychology books we find a highly complex area. Let's take it gradually.

Play is something we do. It involves ourselves and others in action. It tends to make us feel good but it has little or nothing to do with the real world; in fact, we often play to get away from the real world. Children play much more than adults and if it were not for the use of the word in the theatre and in sport, we would probably feel that it concerned children only. Play is not necessarily a physical experience but because it normally involves the whole person there is often a physical component.

When we are playing, we are behaving in such a way as to retain attitudes that have their origin in play and when we are playful we are having fun (Figure 14.14).

Let's compare war and a football match for a moment. War is real. You fight and the consequence may be death. The intention is to kill. Jokingly, you might suggest that you have seen football matches like that! Well, first of all, football is kicking a ball about, it is fun. A match is contrived to test the temperament and skill of one group against another, through football. It is played according to fixed rules with playing area and timing strictly controlled. When the whistle goes it is over.

These are all characteristics of play but occasionally rules are broken, violence breaks out and aggression goes on after the whistle. When this happens the game has left the world of play and become real; it can even become war!

Similarly, playing the game means you have made an undertaking to 'play the game'. If you cheat or commit fouls, you have stepped outside the play concept. We would argue that you have also stepped outside the moral concept of the game. The result of such behaviour will lead to the destruction of the

play element immediately and of the game situation eventually.

Can you identify any characteristics of play in Figures 14.15 and 14.16?

If you have an opportunity, do a critical review of the Pod Race in the 'Star Wars' film or the game of 'Quidditch' in Harry Potter to explain what has happened to the twin concepts of **play** and **game**.

Finally, you will find that theorists invariably look at a pure form of play, largely because it is much easier to categorise. However, when you see play operating, it is clear that you are looking not at a pure form of it but at elements of play mixed in with moments of

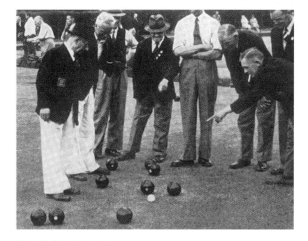

Fig. 14.15 It's mine!

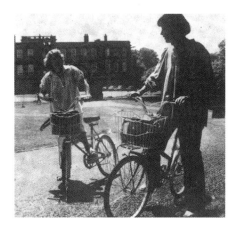

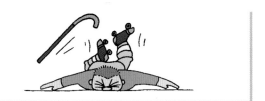

Fig. 14.14 Go on! Enjoy yourself!

Fig. 14.16 Let's go!

reality. This is almost always the case in our field of study.

Try to pick out the keywords that help to identify this thing called play from what has been written above. We have come up with the model in Figure 14.17. Compare it with your own.

Let us have a look at what other people think play is. Identify the keywords in the following definitions and use a play activity to explain what is being suggested.

Play consists of activities for immediate gratification.[10]

Play is play because the observer thinks it is.[11]

If it's fun it's play.[12]

Play requires an achievement of a social self.[12]

Play serves as adaptive problem solving for children.[13]

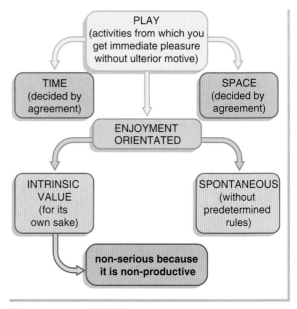

Fig. 14.17 A model of play.

Review questions

There has been a lot of theory written about play. What we need to do is to test some of these views against our own experiences.

1. Divide the following notions between members of the group, establishing the meaning of the different phrases and giving examples: civilisation preparation; role rehearsal; surplus energy; recreation; instinctive practice; recapitulation; transmission of culture; personality development; cathartic function; ego expansion.

   Alternatively, take a simple play activity like hide and seek and see how many of these interpretations can be linked with it.

   What we are discovering is that play has many sides to it and therefore can have a wide range of interpretations and uses.

2. Now explain Figure 14.18.

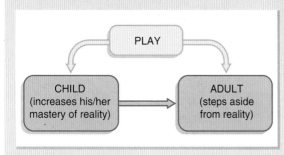

Fig. 14.18 Functions of play.

3. The final test as to whether we understand the term 'play' in the context of physical performance is to turn to Huizinga.[9] Select a physical performance activity that you have played. Test the extent to which you were really playing from the following criteria.

   a. Play is a voluntary activity, never a physical necessity or a moral duty. It is not a matter of leisure and free time, it is freedom.

   b. Play is not ordinary or real life, but this is not to say that play may not be intense or serious … an interlude in our daily lives, an end in itself.

   c. Play is a temporary world within and marked off from the ordinary world. It begins and is over in a specific moment and functions within limitations of time and space.

   d. Play creates order; in fact, it is order. Slight deviation from the rules spoils the game.

   e. The play community tends to become permanent, because in the course of playing you become part of an 'in-group', sharing a common existence.

If you have managed to understand these principles in the context of your chosen activity, you will realise that many of the components of play are immediately identifiable in physical recreation and sport. The more structured and commercially orientated sport is, the less play is evident and one might argue that the sheer joy of participation is often lost because of the work-orientated values that exist in high-level sport, resulting in an obsession with a 'win-at-all-costs' ethic.

And so we end with the Huizinga definition:[9]

Play is an activity which proceeds within certain limits of time and space, in a visible order according to rules freely accepted, and outside the sphere of necessity or material utility. The play mood is one of rapture and enthusiasm and is sacred or festive in accordance with the occasion. A feeling of exaltation and tension accompanies the action; mirth and relaxation follow.

You will no doubt recognise these characteristics from your own experiences of games, individual activities and outdoor pursuits and so there is every justification for us to continue to use the word 'play' freely in our field of study and to expect sport for all to live up to the qualities that are an inherent part of the play concept.

It may not be obvious but the application of play theory to playing games takes us away from the original emphasis by Huizinga[9] and Caillois[14] in that they stressed the temporary nature and spontaneity of play, largely discounting its developmental potential. The concept of play that we are adopting presumes that, given a retention of play attitudes, rules can facilitate rather than destroy a play situation. Secondly, that whether the game is won or lost, the experience can yet increase a person's ability to know themselves and others with greater emotional and social skill. The following list may help you to analyse potential learning experiences more accurately:

- Physical: effort and skilfulness
- Social: cooperative and competitive
- Cognitive: problem solving and strategy building
- Moral: accepting a moral code and able to made moral judgements
- Self-realising: knowing yourself and giving more of yourself
- Emotional: controlling your emotions and also expressing yourself
- Aesthetic: opportunities to taste excellence

This explanation is very much part of the **education** in physical education and the test of temperament that exists in most sporting situations. It is also a counter to the 'win-at-all-costs' ethic, which presumes that only winners gain from a sporting competition.

Exam-style questions

You will have seen play activities taking place in the playgrounds of schools. They may be recognisable by their intention, such as hide and seek, or by the equipment being used, such as a ball or skipping rope.

1. Play has been defined as 'activity from which you get immediate pleasure without ulterior motive'.
   a. Explain this definition, using a play activity to illustrate your answer. *(2 marks)*
   b. In what ways would you expect spontaneity to exist in your play activity? *(3 marks)*
   c. Explain how time and space constraints may operate in your play activity. *(3 marks)*
   (Total 8 marks)

2. It has also been said that 'play is a voluntary activity, never a physical necessity or moral duty'.
   a. How is this reflected in adult recreation? *(3 marks)*
   b. Explain the suggestion that in play a child increases mastery of reality, but an adult escapes from it. *(4 marks)*
   c. Figure 14.19 summarises the characteristics of play and physical recreation.
      i. How might a good physical education teacher make use of some of these characteristics of play? *(4 marks)*

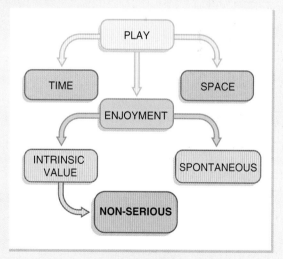

Fig. 14.19 Characteristics of play and recreation.

      ii. Use this diagram to identify why professional sport is different from physical recreation. *(6 marks)*
   (Total 17 marks)

14.4 Towards a concept of recreation

Recreation is a positive aspect of leisure and the word is widely used in the Western world to describe active leisure.

Two major problems with its universal acceptance concern its traditional association with the privileged classes and the built-in presumption that it has intrinsic value only. 'Socialist' societies have tended not to use the term on these grounds. Let's see how others define it.

> Activity voluntarily engaged in during leisure and motivated by the personal satisfactions which result from it ... a tool for mental and physical therapy.[7]

> Recreation embodies those experiences or activities that people take part in during their leisure for purposes of pleasure, satisfaction or education. Recreation is a human experience or activity, it is not necessarily instinctive, it may be considered purposeful.[15]

> Recreation carries away the individual from his usual concerns and problems. The attitudes derived from this are those involving feelings of relaxation. Contentment not complacency might best describe an attitude which is a product of a recreative experience.[16]

> Recreation is a concept closely related to play ... It means literally to re-create or to refresh oneself in body and/or engagement. Recreational activity is also limited in time and space by the actor and requires no preparation or training. Recreation is also non-utilitarian in product.[17]

If you go through the same exercise of selecting keywords, you will notice strong links with the analysis we have already done on leisure but also be aware of the conflict between those who label recreation non-utilitarian and others who acknowledge that it can be purposeful. Significantly, all the authors quoted are American and yet they cannot agree. Little wonder writers in the now disbanded Soviet Union find it an outmoded concept!

You will find that the four basic conceptual models we used to analyse leisure apply also to the slightly narrower field of recreation. We have taken characteristics mentioned in the quotations and built a model (Figure 14.20). Take a particular recreation and identify it in the context of each stage.

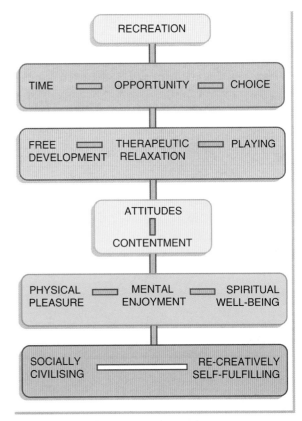

Fig. 14.20 Towards a concept of recreation.

14.5 What do we mean by physical recreation?

To date, you have been asked to identify the characteristics of leisure and recreation from a series of models and the occasional photograph. It is important that you should now get some practice in recognising the characteristics yourself, from a series of statements that we will call notional propositions. It is for you to think them through and decide whether you accept them or wish to question them. At the end of the exercise, however, you should have a list of the central characteristics of physical recreation.

Having made the progression from the general concept of leisure to the narrower experience of recreation, it should be a relatively straightforward step to reduce the field that much more to include only physical recreation. This notion of narrowing is an important one, because the conceptual elements identified in the leisure analysis still hold true but also because some of the cultural bias evident in recreation continues to operate in physical recreation.

The former Soviet Union, for example, tended to suspect that discrimination and non-functional values were still applied to the term 'physical recreation' in the West. They chose to use the term *massovost*, which avoided these limitations. In Britain and France, the slogan 'Sport for All' is extremely popular and tends to be replacing the term 'physical recreation' to describe physical performance opportunities for all members of the community, where emphasis is on participation rather than performance standards. In the United States, Loy[18] has used the phrase 'game occurrence' to describe physical activity that is playful, competitive and strategic, uses physical skill and prowess but is played at a relatively unsophisticated level.

Probably the main reason why the term 'physical recreation' is still used is simply tradition but it would also seem that none of the other expressions is able to replace it completely. It is a wider concept than 'game' and the recreative can be at odds with the sportive. Similarly, how can we still incorporate the concept of outdoor recreation, which is very much in vogue, when we are suggesting that the concept of physical recreation is outmoded?

Outdoor recreation

This term survives not only because of the traditional romanticism associated with the countryside but also because it invariably involves the challenge of self in the natural environment, which is more obviously recreative than the contrived competition of a game.

Outdoor recreation and the frontier spirit remain symbolic features of American ideology; also the former Soviet Union gave considerable political and national recognition to its outdoor policy, under the heading of tourism.

Participation for its own sake

This is the key to the identity of physical recreation and is also the reason why academics and politicians

have claimed that it is non-serious. The assumption here is that if there is no intellectual or commercial value, it is not functionally important in a society.

The fact that, in the 19th century, recreative opportunity was to some extent limited to wealthy people who had the 'right', the money and the time to participate is no more than an accident of history but may yet remain as a vestige of those times.

The privilege of a few has now become the right of the majority and so the social impact of physical recreation is that much broader. Now that almost everyone has the opportunity to recreate physically, we are increasingly motivated to gain from it – as a therapeutic experience; as a frontier experience, where we learn more about ourselves; and as a social experience, where we can make lasting friendships.

The key democratic factors are the right to choose; the opportunity to participate; and the provision to facilitate that freedom.

Little wonder that the Soviet Union was prepared to take these intrinsic elements and give them cultural status, on the grounds that here was an experience that would influence productivity and social well-being by improving health and increasing group morale.

American writers such as Slusher,[19] Vanderswaag[16] and Hellison[20] all argue that the self-realising potential of physical performance makes it a vital element in personal development. This would seem to be particularly true in a country where individual decision making is a cornerstone of the culture.

There may even be a case for using the term 'physical recreation' in a more general context, where sport is identified as one specialised aspect of it.

In societies where taking part is more highly valued than winning, the recreative component may be stronger than the competitive one (Figure 14.21). After all, there is not so much a conceptual difference between physical recreation and sport as a gradually increasing intensity of efficiency at the professionalised end of the continuum.

Hold on a minute: surely professional sport, as a means of livelihood, can hardly be identified as a physical recreation!

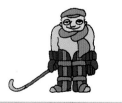

Fig. 14.21 This is my idea of heaven.

We have already made the point that physical activities can be recreational, sporting or educational, depending on the level of commitment. Furthermore, certain words specifically identify activities at a recreative level. For example, rambling, pony trekking, hill walking, paddling, cycle touring and boating reflect outdoor activities as pastimes rather than as sports; jogging, bathing and aerobics are recreative forms of individual activity; in addition, there are phrases like 'kick about at football', 'knock about at tennis' or 'a friendly game of golf' that imply that a game is being played at a low competitive key. These words and phrases tell us that the physical activity is recreative and being enjoyed with minimal organisation.

We have now gathered enough characteristics of physical recreation to produce our own conceptual model as a framework to test our understanding. It is most important that you should be able to operationalise this framework, so take a physical activity that you have experienced at a recreative level and use it to illustrate the keywords in Figure 14.22.

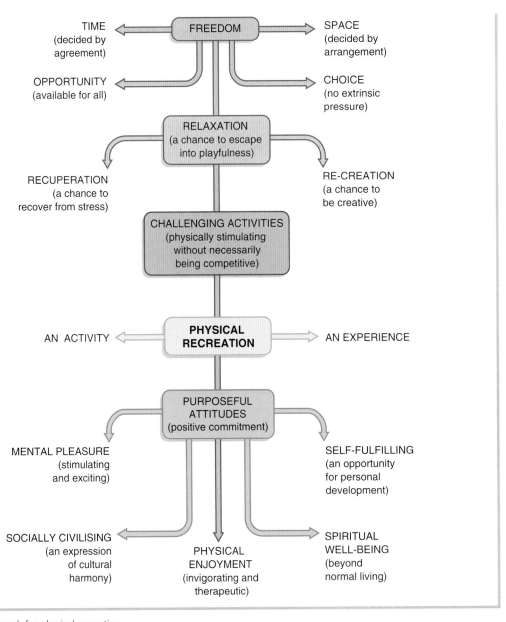

Fig. 14.22 Framework for physical recreation.

Review questions

You have your experience of recreating; you have made a systematic analysis of leisure characteristics earlier in this chapter; and you now have a range of notions outlining the qualities one would expect in physical recreation.

1. Using this knowledge, select one outdoor activity, one individual activity and one game from Figures 14.23–14.25 and describe the characteristics you would expect to find if you were playing these at a physical recreation level.

a. Outdoor activities. Study Figure 14.23 and identify what these outdoor pursuits have in common.

b. Individual activities. Why are the individual activities in Figure 14.24 'recreative' rather than 'sporting'?

c. Games. What clues are there in Figure 14.25 to suggest that the players have a recreative attitude? Could we be wrong?

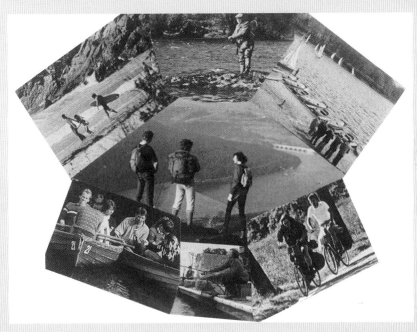

Fig. 14.23 Outdoor activities.

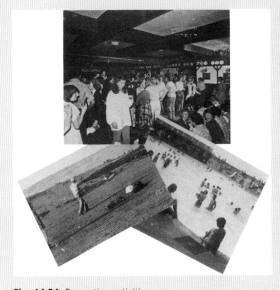

Fig. 14.24 Recreative activities.

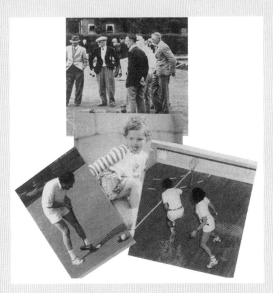

Fig. 14.25 Various games.

Exam-style questions

1. **a.** Outdoor recreation allows man and woman to re-create in ideal surroundings.

    i. What qualities are you likely to find in the natural environment that could lead to the use of the term 'romanticism'? *(4 marks)*

    ii. Use any one photograph in Figure 14.23 to explain the association of freedom and adventure. *(6 marks)*

    b. i. Explain how therapy appears to result from considerable effort in the outdoors. *(6 marks)*

    ii. Why do you think bonds of friendship are so strong after expeditions similar to those shown in Figure 14.23? *(9 marks)*

    (Total 25 marks)

2. **a.** Individual activities do not have to be based on competition.

    i. Explain the idea of being 'free to move'. *(3 marks)*

    ii. Select any one picture from Figure 14.24 and discuss the 'health-related' qualities depicted. *(3 marks)*

    iii. What can you learn about yourself if you become involved in an individual activity at a recreative level? *(4 marks)*

    b. The most important element in a game is the enjoyment that arises from taking part.

    i. Why do you think a game should always be 'friendly'? *(3 marks)*

    ii. Why is participation in a game so rewarding even when the standard of play is low? *(4 marks)*

    iii. We say that we 'play' a game. Explain the elements of play that can exist in any one of the games in Figure 14.25. *(8 marks)*

    (Total 25 marks)

14.6 Towards a concept of sport

Sport is commonplace and yet always controversial. It is universal in the sense that every country practises it and yet it does not always take the same form in each country. Everyone seems to know what it means but it doesn't always mean the same to everyone.

There are three levels at which we can attempt to explain these apparent contradictions.

1. Sports and pastimes are as old as civilisation and many features and values of modern sport are vestiges of the past.
2. Sport reflects the culture to which it belongs and therefore it also reflects cultural variables.
3. Sport is a sophisticated concept and, while it is relatively easy to identify its universal characteristics, the more we refine our definition, the more varied the cultural interpretation.

Let's first of all clarify the historical connotations. You must be well aware that sports and pastimes are as old as civilisation itself. There is ample archaeological evidence that ancient societies indulged in physical activities ranging from bull leaping in the Minoan culture of Crete to the football game of *tsu chu* played in China over 3000 years ago. You will be aware of the Ancient Greek Olympic Games but you may not realise that Olympian Games also took place in medieval England, as witnessed by the Dover Games, and re-emerged in Victorian England with the Much Wenlock Olympian Games, well before the 1896 modern Olympic Games were revived.

Review questions

1. Do you know a sport when you see one?

    a. Under the heading of games, football, hockey, baseball and tennis, for example, all seem to be acceptable – but what about poker, chess or table skittles?

    b. Individual activities, such as track and field, swimming and gymnastics, are unquestionably sports but what about sunbathing, skipping or body building?

    c. We have no doubts about outdoor pursuits such as canoeing and rock climbing but what about cycling, motor racing, hunting, angling and horse racing?

    Take some of these activities and discuss your reservations about them being part of sport. ▶

2. Look at Figures 14.26 and 14.27. What characteristics determine whether these are sports or not?

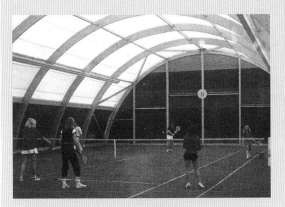

Fig. 14.26 How many for tennis?

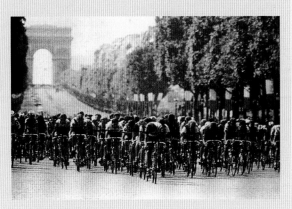

Fig. 14.27 And they're off!

In answering the Review Questions here, you have been determining what is necessary for an activity to be a sport. This is the first level of definition.

If, on the other hand, we look briefly at the cultural factors, there is ample evidence that different primitive cultures have evolved sports and pastimes that reflect their needs. The sports of the Canadian Eskimo may have little in common with those of the Australian aborigine. Even where cultures are geographically related, there are major differences. In Polynesia, for example, the war-like contests in Fiji are very different from the land-diving festival in the New Hebrides.

Controversially, a case has been made by Elias & Dunning[21] that these ancient and primitive sports are not sport in the modern definition of the term. They suggest that the genesis of sport is the product of the European industrial revolution in the 19th century and it is consequently a highly sophisticated institution matching the technology of such advanced societies as those in the United States and Western Europe.

Having made our own attempt to classify sport, let's find an authoritative view. The International Council for Sport and Physical Education (ICSPE)[22] has suggested that:

Any physical activity which has the character of play and which takes the form of a struggle with oneself or involves competition with others is a sport.

Did you pick out elements such as physical, play, struggle with self and competition when you were identifying those activities earlier?

Michener[23] has a similar definition of sport:

An athletic activity requiring physical prowess or skill and usually of a competitive nature.

Should we take the Kaplan[7] notion on board again and suggest that sports are more than activities in that they are also experiences? Certainly, we could argue that participation in a sport can be a most worthwhile experience.

The notion of sport as an experience is supported by Inglis[24] when he suggests that:

Sport is a scrapbook of memories which defines life. It involves a peculiar and intense awareness of yourself, a self-consciousness, in which the point of awareness is to get something right which is quite outside yourself.

Let's not forget our definition of physical recreation and the associated term, game occurrence. We have not defined anything which is exclusively sport as yet, have we? However, it is worth making the point that we are reinforcing the notion that sport is at one end of a physical recreation continuum.[25]

Don't worry if you are still unsure whether some activities are sports or not. Many others have also tried to define what are sports or not with only limited success.

Caillois,[14] in his analysis of *paida* to *ludus* (play to games), classified sports into four main categories:

- agon (competition)
- mimicry (pretence)

- alea (chance)
- ilinx (vertigo).

Huizinga[9] extended these to eight:

- pursuit (chase)
- enigma (mental)
- chance (gamble)
- vertigo (heady)
- strategy (planning)
- imitation (pretence)
- dexterity (skill)
- exultation (excitement).

McIntosh[26] suggested:

- competition
- aesthetic
- combat
- chance
- conquest.

There is considerable overlap between these three attempts at classification. It should also be clear that, whereas some activities or experiences fall within one criterion alone, other sports fall into two or more.

If you use the Huizinga[9] classification, it also seems reasonable to suggest that the more criteria that operate in any particular activity, the more secure its status as a sport.

Test these propositions by describing the sport criteria evident in:

1. horse racing
2. rowing.

We are now ready for a second level of analysis. Are there any set conditions as to how an activity should be performed before it can be accepted as a sport? The ICSPE[22] claimed that:

If this activity involves competition, then it should always be performed with a spirit of sportsmanship. There can be no true sport without the idea of fair play.

The assumption is that sport and sportsmanship are inseparable, definitive components of the sporting experience.

Noel-Baker[27] suggested that:

Fair play is the essence, the sine qua non, of any game or sport that is worthy of the name.

Similarly, the following words of Baron de Coubertin are displayed at all the modern Olympic Games:

The most important thing in the Olympic Games is not to win but to take part, just as the most important thing in life is not the triumph but the struggle.

This moral intention is further reinforced in the Olympic oath, where reference is made to:

...respecting and abiding by the rules that bind them, in the true spirit of sportsmanship, for the glory of sport and the honour of our teams.

Before you point to the cheating and corruption, the drug abuse and the political intrigue that are common-place in the modern Olympics, remember we are trying to establish what sport ought to be. Time enough later to recognise all the shortcomings.

An explanation of this moral requirement is best achieved at the three levels used earlier: historical, cultural and ideological.

Ancient and primitive societies have consistently used sport festivals as a ritual expression of their cultures. The ancient Olympic Games reflected the Man of Action concept held by citizen Greeks; the tournament reinforced the chivalric code in 12th-century Europe; the courtly mould was a cornerstone of Tudor England and Renaissance Europe; and the emergence of the gentleman amateur in 18th- and 19th-century England reflected the lifestyle of a leisured class.

In each case, the elite members of a civilisation used sport to reflect the ideals they held most dear. It is important to recognise that sport was the arena in which physical prowess and temperament were tested.

There were various times when these ethics were closely tied to religious beliefs: Greek gods were idealised humans; the chivalric code fuelled the Crusades; and muscular Christianity was inspired by gentlemen amateurs who were also social Christians. Nor must we forget that 19th-century athleticism in the English public schools was a duality of physical endeavour *and* moral integrity, not one or the other.

The bonding through tradition, therefore, is very clearly defined. However, we need to recognise that cultures differ and this means that, in addition to sport differing, the values associated with it vary from one country to another.

Gardner[28] examined the American 'win' ethic, linking it with the 'Lombardian' commitment of American professional sport and the pressures of capitalism and commercialism in American society. See if you can discover who Vince Lombardi was and why he is quoted so much by American sports commentators.

Little wonder that the European ethic of 'doing your best' has been regarded as an excuse for weakness.

Mind you, professional British sport is equally sceptical of this amateur ethic. Lombardism, on the other hand, defends the view that only winners matter in sport and society, turning the Olympic model on its head and emphasising the triumph rather than the struggle. If you want to continue this dialogue, it is probable that the humanist would reply that the struggle to do one's best is socially desirable and open to all, but that triumph is a reward for a few and a mark of failure for the rest.

There is a very interesting relationship here with rewards. The Greeks had a laurel wreath and 19th-century amateurs had medals – token reminders of the struggle. Today, an elite group of athletes receives great wealth, because commercialism idealises the champion in order to sell products to the envious. We find emergent cultures promoting their champions for such reasons as giving their citizens a sense of national pride or, more questionably, as an opium to forget hardship or revolution.

The Soviet culture, interestingly, needed winners to reinforce its political identity and yet could not justify the promotion of individualism in a so-called socialist society. Consequently, 'to do your best' was a very real Soviet concept, but it had to be for society rather than for self.

Fair play, therefore, is under attack from professional and commercial forces. Sport and sportsmanship have become political instruments and expedients. In both instances they represent a dominance of extrinsic factors that undermine the intrinsic values.

We must defend sport from these external excesses, if we believe that the essence of sport is sportsmanship.

As early as 1968 Lüschen[29] pointed out that sport had the potential to be functional or dysfunctional. It is an arena where 'man' is tested and may fail to cope with the situation. How many of you have fouled in a game in the heat of the moment, hopefully to regret it later?

If you want to achieve the highest moral experience from sport, you should be able to play to the rules regardless of having a referee present. Jimmy White, the professional snooker player, repeatedly acknowledges when he has committed a foul stroke, regardless of whether the referee has seen it. Here is the principle of 'walking' at cricket.

In life, there are those who would not steal on principle, while others do not steal because they are

high 3 (functional)	personal decision in the true spirit of the game	creative participation	inventive player/coach
2	personal decisions regarding the rules of play	active participation	playing the part: role-play
1	acceptance of the referee	emotional participation	observational appreciation
0	reluctant acceptance of the referee	entertainment amusement escape from monotony of killing time	antidote for boredom
−1	arguing with the referee	injury or detriment to self	excesses
−2 (dysfunctional)	retaliation	violence against other players	crime

Fig. 14.28 Application of Nash's model.

afraid of being caught. Similarly, some of us need the referee to be there to make decisions for us. Hopefully, we accept his decision even if we don't agree with it, but there are times when we argue with the referee or even retaliate against an offending player. When we do this the experience is detrimental to us as a person and detrimental to the game.

Nash[30] developed this concept in the context of recreation and leisure – Figure 14.28 is an adjustment of his model to match the sporting situation.

The third level of analysis is the one which allows us to distinguish between physical recreation (a game occurrence) and sport.

You will recall that Inglis[24] identified an 'intense awareness ... to get something right'. Similarly, McIntosh[26] wrote about 'striving for superiority against man and/or nature'. Weiss,[31] Loy[18] and Howell & Howell[32] all define sport as a highly organised game requiring physical prowess.

This is the identification of sport as an institution. To understand this we need to take it through three stages.

1. As an administrative feature. To paraphrase Elias & Dunning[21] – sport has a stringent organisation, fully standardised codification, a high level of permanence and regularity and technological sophistication.
2. It requires a performer to embark on a high level of physical preparation, involving fitness and skill ability.
3. It invariably demands an attitude of commitment, a struggle to focus the mind and body on attaining the goals of the competition or challenge situation.

We need only look at great athletes like Don Bradman (Australia), Daley Thompson (UK), Mark Spitz (USA), Jean-Claude Killy (France) and Ludmilla Turishcheva (former USSR) to identify the time and attitude commitment, the outstanding quality of performance and the administrative support system necessary for them to have achieved their optimum level of performance.

What we have, therefore, is a three-tier analysis: certain activities or experiences involving a spirit of fair play at the highest level of personal excellence.

What will have become obvious is that the more professionalised the sport, the less affinity there is with Huizinga's[9] play criteria. Edwards[17] goes so far as to say that sport has nothing in common with play, but this seems too categorical. Howell & Howell[32] seem nearer the mark when they write that:

An individual has to have satisfaction from playing the sport, otherwise it ceases to be a sport. A professional athlete whose only concern is money and who does not care for the activity itself would no longer be engaged in sport, but work.

It might seem that this combination necessarily excludes the Sport for All concept. However, though attention is automatically drawn to a professionalised elite, the term 'personal excellence' has been deliberately chosen because it describes any person with the commitment to strive for his or her own optimum level of achievement. The Sport for All campaign is designed to give everyone this opportunity; if they choose to retain a recreative attitude, so be it, but the provision, opportunity and esteem are all there to be grasped in the fullness and freedom of a leisure-time decision.

It is important that you should be able to illustrate Figure 14.29 from your own experience of a sport. You could trace a sport at which you have competed and then take the likely path of a successful professional performer. Comparing these two pathways is worthwhile but it is also important that you refer back to Figure 14.22 and compare it with Figure 14.29, explaining the extent to which the concepts of physical recreation and sport can differ.

Test your understanding of the concept of sport

Select a specific sport with which you are acquainted and use it to explain the following definition of sport.

Sport is an institutionalised competitive activity that involves vigorous physical exertion or the use of relatively complex physical skills by individuals whose participation is motivated by a combination of the intrinsic satisfaction associated with the activity itself and the external rewards earned through participation.[33]

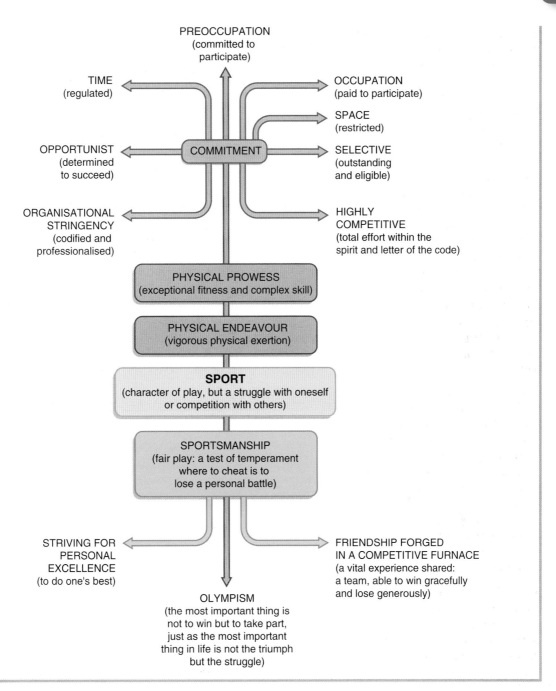

Fig. 14.29 Framework for sport.

Review questions

1. Test your understanding by identifying one of your own experiences in each of the labelled boxes in Figure 14.30, briefly explaining what is happening as you move from top left to bottom right.

2. This is a good time to reaffirm that no classification in our field of study is going to be perfect – and so have fun trying to point out the errors in this one. Then, if you are brave enough, produce your own format and defend it.

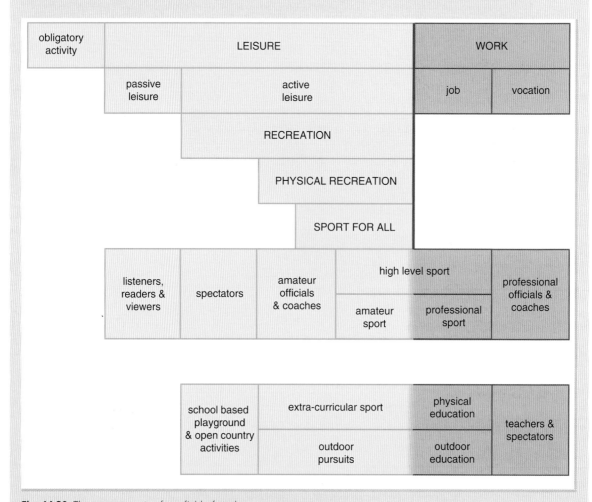

Fig. 14.30 The many aspects of our field of study.

Exam-style questions

Sport may be defined as a highly structured physical activity with a high degree of commitment. Use this definition and the model in Figure 14.31 to answer the following questions.

1. a. In terms of sporting commitment, what is the difference between preoccupation and occupation? *(4 marks)*

    b. How does the use of time and space differ between sport and children at play? *(4 marks)*

    c. Explain the differences between physical prowess and physical endeavour. *(4 marks)*

    (Total 12 marks)

2. Describe the main features of organisational stringency in sport. *(3 marks)*

3. Attitudes are a central factor in sport.

    a. What do we mean when we talk about the letter and the spirit of the game? *(2 marks)*

    b. Explain ideal relationships between competitors during and after a competition. *(4 marks)*

    c. Distinguish between sportsmanship and gamesmanship. *(4 marks)*

    (Total 10 marks)

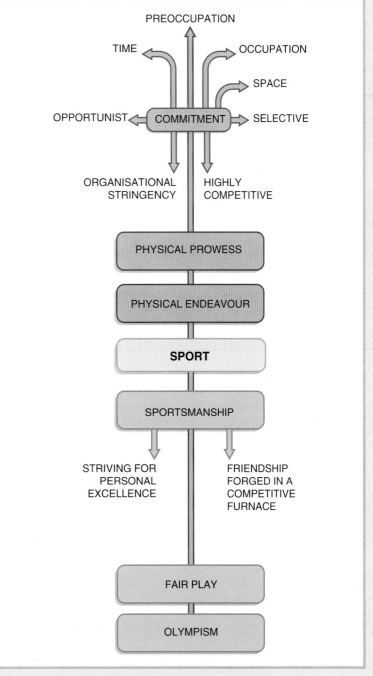

Fig. 14.31 Model for sport.

14.7 What is physical education?

It might help initially to establish where the term is used.

- Numerous universities award degrees in physical education (PE).
- It is a subject taught in all schools and is part of the core curriculum.
- The main administrative body is the Physical Education Association (PEA).
- The term is used to describe several GCSE and Advanced-level GCE syllabuses.

However, authors tend to write about physical education *and* sport and so presumably they are not one and the same thing. And although the term appears to have a similar currency in the United States, France and Britain, this is less the case in the diverse group of countries, federation of republics, etc. that once comprised the Soviet Union.

Let's look first at the situation in the former USSR. Though the term 'physical education' is used, physical 'culture' is a more common expression. Riordan[34] suggested that this more general concept could be defined as:

The sum total of social achievements connected with man's physical development and education.

If this is to be accepted, what was once the Soviet Union has a collective term for the whole of our field of study.

We intend to work from a very narrow definition of physical education, in which it is limited to:

The formal inculcation of knowledge and values through physical activity and/or experiences.

Review questions

1. **a.** Using your own school as an example, explain Figure 14.32 in terms of curriculum PE, extracurricular programmes and recreational activities.
   b. Why is a pyramid such a useful analogy?

2. **a.** Again using your own school as an example, explain Figure 14.33 in terms of relationships.
   b. Why are circles such a useful analogy in this context?

3. List the activities on your curriculum under two headings: core subjects and options.

4. Select one of your favourite physical education activities and use it to explain the three ways of knowing and understanding physical performance shown in Figures 14.32 and 14.33.

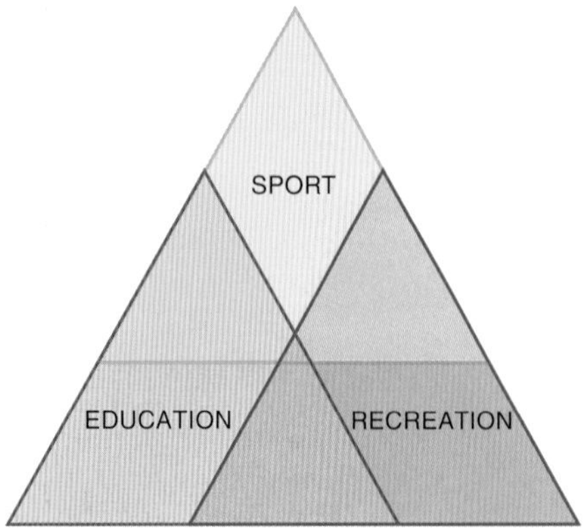

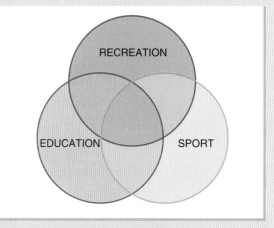

Fig. 14.32 Triangular model of physical performance opportunities in schools.

Fig. 14.33 Relationships within physical performance opportunities in schools.

As a direct result, physical education is most likely to be practised in educational institutions. The Leeds Study Group[35] defined physical education as:

A term used to describe an area of educational activity in which the main concern is with bodily movement.

(where the words 'educational activity' are presumed to mean the formal inculcation of socially desirable knowledge and values). The actual activities are often common to those already identified in play, physical recreation and sport and are those found in the school curriculum.

The core subjects will probably be common to most schools and include major games, gymnastics, track and field and swimming. These are normally compulsory activities but may vary according to gender and age group.

It is very important at this point to recognise that curriculum physical education is only one of a number of physical performance opportunities in the average school. Groves[36] produced two diagrams to illustrate this relationship between physical education, physical recreation and sport in schools (Figures 14.32 and 14.33).

The optional subjects will probably be less common because they have not been a traditional part of the curriculum, because they are less physical or because they are too expensive in terms of time, space or cost. Some of the activities we have recognised as sports may not be included in the school curriculum for these reasons but some sports may not be suitable for children; for example, they may be too dangerous to be pursued at school.

There are a number of traditional reasons why certain activities are included in the PE curriculum. For example, gymnastics has military and therapeutic roots; games owe much to the character-building ethic of the English public schools in the 19th century; and swimming has had links with cleanliness and safety.

There is also a very strong cultural association. Examples of high-prestige activities dominating the curriculum for economic and popularity reasons include American football and basketball in the United States; gymnastics and skiing in the one-time Soviet Union; and cricket and football in England.

However, the overriding reason for teaching a particular activity should be its potential as a medium for education. Lüschen,[29] for example, subdivided sports into functional and dysfunctional, meaning that the latter had a detrimental influence on society. In England today, the behaviour associated with professional soccer might lead educationists to the conclusion that the game should not be taught in schools.

Conversely, it can be argued that there is an even greater need to teach it, to reform its popular image.

It would seem that certain activities have more potential as a vehicle for the inculcation of desirable values. Currently, in England, gymnastics is regarded as an ideal medium by educationists, whereas table tennis is generally presumed to have only recreative value. These are dangerous presumptions as most sporting activities can become educational vehicles in the right hands.

A great deal also depends on the knowledge and values being promoted; for example, the choice of gymnastics in England is linked with heuristic, therapeutic and individualistic values, currently in vogue in educational circles. Alternatively, the importance of football in the American high school is tied to the significance of the sports ethic in the community and the socio-economic importance of competition and manliness.

We certainly need to tease out these societal variables before we can suggest what physical education ought to be in any one particular country. What we need to do, therefore, is to produce a series of models that can easily be adjusted to meet the needs of different societies.

First of all, we will look at knowledge. We teach physical education because we think it is a useful body of knowledge, the implication being that having this knowledge will make us better people and enhance our lifestyle.

We can assess its usefulness at three levels.

1. **Knowing about** physical activities should help us to understand them and enable us to talk about them.
2. **Knowing how** to perform allows us to express ourselves through physical skills and competitive performance.
3. **Knowing how it feels** to perform gives us an enriching experience that is possible only in a performance situation.

We teach physical education because we can promote desirable values both as an intrinsic experience and to achieve extrinsic ends. Let's look at these values under four main headings. Where you can, illustrate each one from your experience of a game, an individual activity, a contest and an outdoor pursuit.

1. **Instrumental values**: those directly linked with physical performance (Figure 14.34).
2. **Economic values**: those which are useful in everyday life and valuable to the community (Figure 14.35).

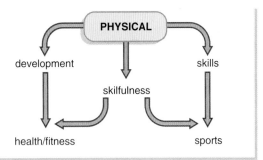

Fig. 14.34 Instrumental values.

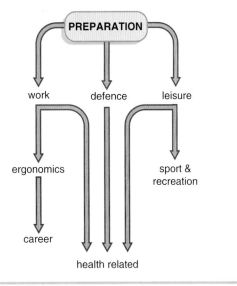

Fig. 14.35 Economic values.

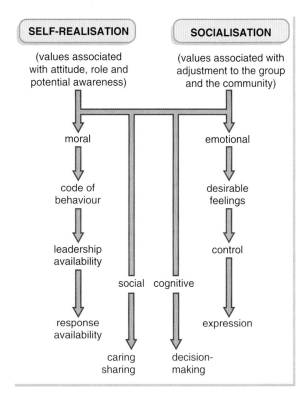

Fig. 14.36 Humanistic values.

3. **Humanistic values**: those which help in the development of a wholesome personality (Figure 14.36).
4. **Quality of life aspects**: those which carry experience beyond the ordinary in terms of awareness and commitment (Figure 14.37).

If you have explained each of these models in the context of a particular physical education activity, you should be aware of the potential range of intentions in the mind of a teacher. It is not enough to claim that this experience is physical education because the children are learning skills. Performance skills have obvious values in active leisure terms but a good teacher looks for an opportunity to educate the performer at each of the four levels identified.

    Remember, the first concern of a sports coach is performance but for the physical educationist, it is the person. The all-important factor is that if a comprehensive knowledge and a wide range of values are

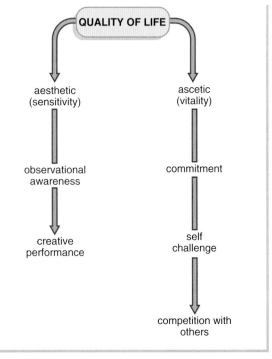

Fig. 14.37 Quality of life

inculcated through physical education during the formative years of childhood, it is more likely that physical recreation and sport will have a functional rather than a dysfunctional influence on adult lifestyle.

When looking at the concept of physical recreation, a special case was made for outdoor recreation. A similar situation arises between physical education and outdoor education. Conceptually, outdoor education is a part of physical education in that outdoor pursuits are sports that are included in the physical education curriculum and the use of the term 'education' implies that both involve the formal inculcation of knowledge and values.

However, we make special mention of outdoor education because, whereas games, contests and individual activities function in controlled surroundings, outdoor pursuits tend to be undertaken in a natural environment that is not entirely predictable. Also, in most physical activities, the environment simply regulates the activity but in outdoor education the natural environment stimulates the activity.

A series of definitions may be useful at this point.

Outdoor education is learning in and for the outdoors.[37]

Outdoor education contains within it a combination of outdoor pursuits and studies in the rural environment, but it is not necessary for them to be practised simultaneously or even in proportion to one another.[38]

Mortlock[39] advanced the understanding of outdoor education in his book *The adventure alternative*. His analysis of natural examination, the instinct for adventure and an awareness of risk suggests that outdoor education has an advantage over games and individual activities because it places the individual at the decision-making frontier.

Bonnington[40] examines this powerful element of adventure, an experience that is not always evident in other physical activities, and Mortlock[39] suggests that it requires an individual to differentiate between real and perceived risk and this helps a person to become a part of nature rather than a conqueror of it.

The word 'escape' is often used in sports history, where people have tried to find an alternative experience. In our urbanised society, the need for an escape to the simplicity of the natural environment has never been greater.

Review questions

1. Select an outdoor activity and use it to examine one of Mortlock's propositions (Figure 14.38).

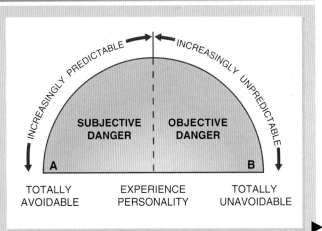

Fig. 14.38 Danger diagram. Subjective danger: that potentially under the control of the human being, e.g. correct choice and use of equipment. Objective danger: that over which the human being has no control, e.g. avalanches, blizzards, floods, storms. Beginners will be working at the left end of the baseline AB. Committed experts will be taking on challenges at the right end of the baseline.

2. We have now analysed the concepts of leisure, play, physical recreation, sport and physical education. As we have progressed from one to the other, relationships between them have been discussed. Test your understanding of these conceptual relationships by writing a critical evaluation of the model in Figure 14.39.

| PHYSICAL RECREATION | Latent values | SPORT | Manifest values | PHYSICAL EDUCATION |

a) Self-realisation in creative fulfilment — Self-realisation in action — Self-realisation

b) Socialisation in cohesion — Socialisation in conflict — Socialisation

c) Concept of play and mass participation — Concept of excellence — Concept of person

d) Joyful involvement — Artistic achievement — Aesthetic awareness

e) Preparation for work — Preparation for success — Preparation for leisure

f) Relaxation — Vigorous involvement — Balanced effort awareness

Re-creation — Commitment to challenge — Balanced lifestyle

Recuperation — Adventure & risk activity — Positive outlook

Fig. 14.39 Some conceptual relationships between physical recreation, sport and physical education.

Exam-style questions

1. Figures 14.32 and 14.33 are diagrams which show that curriculum physical education is only one of a number of physical performance opportunities in the average school.

   a. What does the outside perimeter to Figure 14.32 represent? (*3 marks*)

   b. What administrative units do the three main inner triangles represent? (*3 marks*)

   c. Explain the decision to overlap the triangles, using a PE curriculum activity as an example. (*5 marks*)

   d. Why would it be better to describe Figure 14.32 as a pyramid? (*3 marks*)

   e. Explain the additional relationships the set of circles shows in Figure 14.33, using your own school or college as an example. (*3 marks*)

   (*Total 17 marks*)

2. Figure 14.38 illustrates different types of danger in outdoor adventure activities.

   a. Using an outdoor adventure activity as an example, establish the difference between objective and subjective danger and explain how this varies according to the difficulty of the challenge. (*4 marks*)

   b. You are leading a group of young people on an extended walk or down a white-water river in canoes. Explain the difference between real and perceived risk in one of these situations. (*4 marks*).

   (*Total 8 marks*)

References

1. Arnold P J 1968 *Education, P. E. and personality development*. Heinemann, London
2. Parker S R 1971 *The future of work and leisure*. MacGibbon and Kee, London
3. Pieper J 1965 *Leisure and the basis of culture*. Fontana, London
4. Bell C 1947 *Civilisation*. Pelican, London
5. Miller N P, Robinson D H 1963 *The leisure age*. Wadsworth, Belmont, California
6. Dumazedier J 1967 *Towards a society of leisure*. Collier-Macmillan, New York
7. Kaplan M 1975 *Leisure, theory and policy*. John Wiley, New York
8. Jelfs B 1970 *Towards a concept of leisure*. ATCDE (PE) Conference Papers, London
9. Huizinga J 1964 *Homo ludens: a study of the play element in culture*. Beacon, Boston
10. Spencer H 1960 *The system of synthetic philosophy series*. London
11. Ellis M J 1973 *Why people play*. Prentice Hall, Englewood Cliffs, New Jersey
12. Beisty P 1986 *If it's fun, is it play?* In: Mergen B (ed) Cultural dimensions of play, games and sport. Human Kinetics, Champaign, Illinois
13. Johnson E P, Snyder K 1986 *The lighter side of play*. In: Mergen B (ed) Cultural dimensions of play, games and sport. Human Kinetics, Champaign, Illinois
14. Caillois R 1961 *Man, play and games*. Free Press, Dorsey
15. Zeigler E 1964 *Philosophical foundations of physical health and recreation*. Prentice Hall, Englewood, New Jersey
16. Vanderswaag H 1972 *Towards a philosophy of sport*. Addison Wesley, New York
17. Edwards H 1973 *Sociology of sport*. Homewood, Dorsey
18. Loy J W 1969 *The nature of sport*. In: Loy J, Kenyan G S (eds) Sport, culture and society. Macmillan, London
19. Slusher H 1967 *Man, sport and existence*. Kimpton, Philadelphia
20. Hellison D 1985 *Goals and strategies for teaching physical education*. Human Kinetics, Champaign, Illinois
21. Elias N, Dunning E 1970 *Sociology of sport*. Frank Cass, London
22. ICSPE 1964 *Definition of sport*. International Council of Sport and PE, Strasbourg
23. Michener J A 1977 *Sports in America*. Fawcett, New York
24. Inglis F 1977 *The name of the game*. Heinemann, London
25. Calhoun D W 1987 *Sport, culture and personality*. Human Kinetics, Champaign, Illinois
26. McIntosh P C 1987 *Sport in society*. West London Press, Twickenham, London
27. Noel-Baker P 1959 *Nobel Prize address*
28. Gardner P 1974 *Nice guys finish last*. Allen Lane, London
29. Lüschen G 1968 *Sociology of sport*. Mouton
30. Nash J B 1960 *Philosophy of recreation and leisure*. William Brown, Iowa
31. Weiss P 1969 *Sport: a philosophic inquiry*. South Illinois University Press, Illinois
32. Howell R, Howell M 1986 *Physical education foundations*. Brooks Waterloo, NSW, Australia
33. Coakley J J 1982 *Sport and society: issues and controversies*, 2nd edn. McGraw Hill, Boston, Massachusetts
34. Riordan J 1977 *Sport in Soviet society*. Cambridge University Press, Cambridge
35. Leeds Study Group 1970 *Statement of the concept of physical education*. PEA Conference Report
36. Groves R 1972 *PE, recreation and competitive sport*. PE Bulletin 9(3)
37. Patmore J 1972 *Land and leisure*. Penguin, Harmondsworth
38. Parker T H, Meldrum K I 1971 *An approach to outdoor activities*. National Association of Outdoor Education Publishers, London
39. Mortlock C 1984 *The adventure alternative*. Cicerone Press, Milnthorpe, Cumbria
40. Bonnington C 1981 *Quest for adventure*. Hodder and Stoughton, Sevenoaks, Kent

Further reading

Armstrong N (ed) 1990 *New directions in physical education*, vol 1. PEA, Human Kinetics, Champaign, Illinois
Armstrong N (ed) 1996 *New directions in physical education: change and innovation*. Cassell, London
Arnold P J 1978 *Notes on use and meaning of the term leisure*. Bulletin of PE 14(1)
Davis RJ 1997 *Understanding concepts*. Teachers' Guide. Pershore, Worcs.
Fine G A (ed) 1987 *Meaningful play, playful meaning*, TAASP, vol II. Human Kinetics, Champaign, Illinois
Haywood L et al 1990. *Understanding leisure*, 2nd edn. Stanley Thornes, Cheltenham
Hellison D 1975 *Humanistic PE*. Prentice Hall, Englewood Cliffs, New Jersey
Lumpkin A 1998 *Physical education and sport: a contemporary introduction*, 4th edn. McGraw Hill, Boston, Massachusetts
Kenyon G S, Loy J W Jr 1969 *Sociology of sport*. Athletic Institute, Chicago
Kretchmar R S 1994 *Practical philosophy of sport*. Human Kinetics, Champaign, Illinois
McIntosh P C 1979 *Fair play. Ethics in sport and education*. Heinemann, London

Morgan R E 1974 *Concerns and values in PE*. Bell, London
Roscoe D A, Roscoe J V, Honeybourne J, Davis R, Galligan F 2003 *Physical education and sports studies AS/A2 level student revision guides*. Jan Roscoe Publications, Widnes
Winnifrith T, Barrett C (eds) 1992 *Leisure in art and literature*. Macmillan, Basingstoke

Multimedia

Video

Sport in society. Video Education, Australia 1997. UK supplier Boulton and Hawker Films Ltd, Ipswich

CD-ROMs

Davis R J 2000 *Switch on to sport in society*. Sport in the Mind Publication, Droitwich Spa. Worcestershire
Davis R J, Mace R 2000 *Sport in society*. Sport in the Mind Publication, Droitwich Spa. Worcestershire.
Davis R J 2003 *Play & PE*. Pershore, Worcs.

Physical education and sport in the United Kingdom

15.1 The social setting

We need to have a knowledge of the **cultural background** before we can hope to understand how organised physical activity functions in the United Kingdom. We will call these influences **cultural determinants** and look at them under two main headings: **geographical** and **socio-economic**.

Geographical influences

Geography is a very broad field of study but is limited in the analysis here to comments on population, land area, topography, climate, urbanisation and communications in the context of sport and physical education.

Population

The population growth for the UK from 1851 to 2001 is shown in Table 15.1; the ethnic minority (Afro-Caribbean and Asian) has steadily increased from 2% in 1981, with the greater influx of asylum seekers since 2000. Over the past two decades the anticipated population increase did not occur but there were shifts in population from old industrial areas into rural districts, suburbs and new towns. There are also urban centres where there is a disproportionately high concentration of ethnic minorities.

Size

The area of the UK is 94 247 square miles.

Topography

England has mainly rolling country with the Pennines and the Cotswolds as its major hill features. The hills and meadows are ideal for rambling and field sports. The East Anglian Fens are very flat and popular for boating, angling and ice skating.

High mountains in the UK are limited to the Lake District, the Scottish Highlands and Wales and are attractive for climbing, game fishing and shooting, with skiing in Scotland. There are extensive coastal waters which are ideal for sailing and other water sports and, traditionally, the British have an annual holiday by the sea. Numerous rivers make angling the most popular individual sport in the country but

Table 15.1 UK population growth								
Year	*1851*	*1881*	*1921*	*1951*	*1961*	*1981*	*1991*	*2001*
Population (millions)	20	29	42	49	51	54.1	53.9	60

there are also a large number of canoe and inland sailing clubs.

Climate

The weather is temperate – Western maritime, with a moderating influence from the Gulf Stream drift. Generally, there is less rainfall on the east coast, which also has colder winters as a result of the continental influence.

The four clearly identifiable seasons have shaped the pattern of sport but the weather is so changeable and unpredictable that it may account for the durable British temperament, particularly in the context of sport. Though the area is small, the climate and terrain are so variable that the diversity of sporting opportunity is considerable, with the possible exception of winter sports.

Urbanisation

The population density is very high, 596 per square mile, with many urban industrial conurbations, surrounded by green belts.

Communications

There are six international ports. The railways were reduced after 1945 but there is a fast inter-city service, which includes a cross-channel link with France. Roads include major motorways, with A-roads radiating from London. There are airports serving each of the major cities. All areas in Britain can be reached in the same day for sporting fixtures and tourism.

Socio-economic factors

Nationalism

The UK consists of four major racial groups: the English, Scots, Welsh and Irish. In nationalist terms, an active minority in Northern Ireland, Scotland and Wales would prefer independence from a Union dominated by England. However, the recent devolution of political powers to individual elected assemblies has partly overcome this.

Sports fixtures between the four countries have been held annually for over a century and remain highly emotive but the sporting ethic normally prevails and so they may be seen to act as a safety valve in the long term. In these traditional international confrontations, England is invariably the 'old enemy' and constantly finds itself involved in the defence of ancient transgressions, well in excess of normal rivalry. Rugby against Wales, soccer against Scotland and cricket against Australia are all ritual battlefields.

In the Irish context, the Republican cause has been identified with Gaelic football; a divisive rivalry continues to exist in soccer, where Northern Ireland and Eire have separate administrations, but in rugby football there is the bridge-building situation of players from both sides of the border playing for the Irish Rugby Union.

Large numbers of Afro-Caribbean and Asian immigrants have settled in Britain since the Second World War and although they are full British citizens, they justifiably retain links with their mother countries. This is never more evident than during cricket tours by the West Indies, India and Pakistan. This can be seen to be separatist but at the same time it allows cultural identity to be retained and expressed.

Despite justifiable accusations of 'institutionalised discrimination', the Afro-Caribbean contribution to British athletics and both codes of football is considerable, as is the Pakistani and Indian influence on cricket, hockey and squash. Significantly, Afro-Caribbean women have successfully broken into British sport but cultural barriers still prevent widespread participation by Moslem girls. The film 'Bend it like Beckham' illustrates this issue.

There is also a tradition of regional loyalty being expressed through sport. The county championships in cricket and rugby are highly competitive and charged with territorial pride. Similarly, the sense of belonging to an urban community is achieved through loyalty to a professional soccer club, although the football fan may also be attracted for a variety of other reasons.

Internationalism

Ireland retains special links with the UK, particularly at a sporting level. Cheltenham races is probably the best example of this, where an English race meeting has become an occasion for the Irish in England and Ireland to unite annually.

The United Kingdom contribution to world sport has been significant, not least because of its colonial history and the development of international schools in those colonies. This influence is retained through Commonwealth links and particularly the Commonwealth Games, significantly known as the 'Friendly Games'. The contests between the northern and southern hemispheres and the Test matches regularly make us aware that we now have much to learn from them.

Political factors and the United Kingdom

The monarchy, with wealth and romantic influence but little political power, has a strong impact at

Commonwealth level. Sporting members of the royal family including Prince Philip, Prince Charles and the Princess Royal, have a considerable impact on national and world sport. The Queen Mother (deceased) and the Queen have maintained a lifelong love of horse racing.

With two elected Houses of Parliament, the Lords and the Commons, opposition parties function at local and national level. There is a UK Sports Minister with limited executive powers and a Sports Council that remains politically autonomous. In line with the policy of devolved government in the four home countries, there is now a sports council in each country under the guidance of the UK Sports Council, for example, the English Sports Council is known as Sport England.

Conservative governments over an extended period in power dramatically changed many features of the welfare state, moving it towards a market economy, but a 'New' Labour government favours devolution and closer ties with Europe. In terms of sport this new policy is not only reflected in national sports councils but the expansion of regional centres of excellence on the Australian model.

The Modernisation Programme launched by the Government in 2001 is administered by UK Sport. The English Institute of Sport (EIS), with Steve Cram as chairman in 2004, is responsible for a set of regional High Performance (Training) Centres (HPCs) which are currently situated in Bath, Loughborough, Birmingham, Manchester and Sheffield and linked with the universities in these towns. An additional centre is planned for Gateshead, with the eventual allocation of eight HPCs throughout England. We are some 20 years behind Australia and France with this provision, but the older centres of excellence, such as Bisham Abbey and Holme Pierrepont, will probably become HPCs when their facilities are upgraded, and there are also centres of excellence for specific sports run by individual governing bodies. With planned HPCs in the other home countries, the gap between Britain and other advanced countries in sport should be markedly reduced over the next decade.

Finance and resources in the United Kingdom

The UK owes its status to industrialisation, to the raw products of coal and iron ore, but most of all to its skilled workforce and business expertise. The 1980s saw a decline in heavy industry and now it is technological advance that holds the key to the future.

Depression and resultant unemployment are major social problems but this may yet promote a more

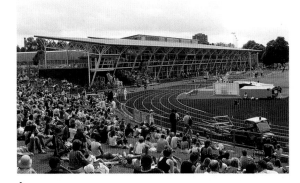

A

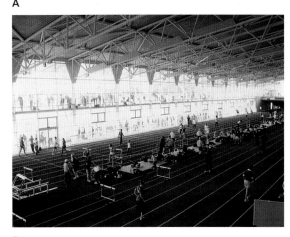

B

Fig. 15.1 Loughborough University High Performance Centre (HPC) **A.** Outside **B.** Inside. Photographer: Helen Roscoe

enlightened view of leisure in the future. The increasing importance of tourism is also highly relevant as package holidays increase and the tourist trade is increasingly recognised as a major factor in economic terms.

The 1988 Sports Council publication *Into the 90s* gave detailed figures of grant aid from central government and local government on expenditure on sports excellence in 1985–86, as shown in Table 15.2. It was anticipated at this time that there would be a rise in revenue from tourism and from the commercial and voluntary sections, but not on the scale achieved with the arrival of the National Lottery.

For a long period it has been felt that revenue from the football pools should go directly to sports aid, as in France, rather than to the general Exchequer but this and other tax measures have not been adopted as yet. In 1990 overall central government expenditure on sport was £533 million compared with a government

Table 15.2

1985–86	£m
Sports Council	7.1
Local authorities	4.0
Governing bodies (net of Sports Council grants)	16.0
Sponsorship	109.5
Sports Aid Foundation	0.5
British Olympic Appeal	2.0
TOTAL	£139.1 million

income of some £3556 million, predominantly from the taxation of sport-related activities.

The National Lottery was introduced in 1994 and has averaged first prizes of over £8 million each week, with an additional mid-week draw, which commenced in January 1997. Although it is argued that the Exchequer benefits most and many charities lose from it, sport's estimated share is some £320 million a year. This sum dwarfs the reducing central government grant to the Sports Council of £47.4 m in 1996–97.

Initially, Lottery money was only made available for capital projects, where the applicant had to find 30%. However, the initiative was expanded in 1996 to what is called the 'four-pack', where money is allocated for capital projects; governing body awards; coach education; and subsistence awards for promising athletes. The latter is controlled under the World Class Performance Plan with means-tested grants of up to £30 000 a year on a rolling four-year basis and this is supported by the World Class Potential Plan which involves partial funding for promising performers. This is supported by government action such as the £125 million scheme to 'bring back our playing fields' in 1999.

There is a general fear that the National Lottery will produce less money in the future. If this occurs problems could exist for the HPCs. Sheffield alone costs £1 million a year to keep open. The 2000 elite athletes from all sports who use these new EIS centres are not sufficient to allow the centres to flourish and so increased numbers of elite and club performers are needed to attend regularly with additional coaching support.

Review question

1. Discuss the likely advantages to UK sport of the National Lottery.

Discrimination

Cultural variables have inevitably led to certain groups being discriminated against in a specific community and in a society. Normally, whatever form this takes, it is reflected in a country's sport.

In order to compare one community or society with another, it is useful to have a structural framework that helps us to tease out the variables. Three basic questions need to be asked.

- What **opportunities** do you have to participate in sport and physical recreation?

  CHOICE OF ACTIVITY, TIME TO PLAY, MONEY TO PAY, SUITABLE STANDARD, ACCEPTABLE COMPANY.

- What **provision** is there for you to participate in sport and physical recreation?

  VARIED TYPES, ACCESSIBLE, REASONABLE COST, SUFFICIENT SPACE, EQUIPMENT FOR USE, SOCIAL AMENITIES, DEGREES OF PRIVACY, SOCIALLY ACCEPTABLE.

- Do you have sufficient **esteem** to play a full part in sport and physical recreation?

  SELF (how do you see yourself?), OTHERS (how do others see you?), STATUS, EXPECTATIONS, RESPECT, SELF-FULFILLING, SOCIALLY STRATIFIED.

Regional

In the UK, regional differences have always existed between England, Scotland, Wales and Ireland and between the industrial Midlands and the North, the rural South West and South, and suburbanised London and the Home Counties.

This has influenced the pattern of sport, largely on a class and/or occupation basis, but with the decline in the industrial economy there is now a North–South divide in wealth terms, which directly influences the pattern of leisure.

Class

Clearly identifiable cultural patterns, particularly in tourism, become a major problem when associated with racial and gender discrimination. Traditional divisions are:

- upper-class: exclusivity, land ownership and schooling; dominance of field sports

- middle-class: salaried, urban influence; dominates many sports with strong club control
- working-class: wage earning, traditional sports; soccer spectator dominance.

There is a gradual breakdown of elitist divisions, evident in such sports as rowing and sailing.

Gender

The pattern is linked with the class variable. Upper-class women are fully emancipated but Victorian values have delayed equal opportunity for other women. Some problem areas remain in sport, e.g. girls and soccer; femininity and aggressive sports; and payment of professionals.

Religion

Divisions still exist in Northern Ireland and Scotland with the separatism between Catholics and Protestants. This influences community recreation and determines sporting loyalty. However, sport does have a bridge-building potential; for example, the 1988 Irish Olympic boxing team was drawn from Northern Ireland and Eire and included boxers from both religious groups. The rivalry between Glasgow Rangers and Celtic is a classic example of religious allegiance being expressed on the terraces.

There is still some conflict over sport on Sundays (sabbatarianism) in Britain, but the 'continental Sunday' is very much a day for sport. The limited sporting opportunities for Moslem females is an area for concern.

Race

Until 1948, there was only a very small non-white community in the UK and sports like professional boxing helped Jewish and black boxers to improve their social status.

This picture has changed dramatically since 1948, with the influx of Afro-Caribbean and Asian immigrants into Britain, Algerians into France and Turkish workers into what was then West Germany. Legally, there is no discrimination but colour, language and cultural variables result in social discrimination still being practised. The baiting of professional black soccer players and cricketers still occurs in England (even though it is the country of their birth). Generally it is not simply colour but rather the combination of race and class in traditional activities that has prevented black performers from having full access to certain sports.

Age

All age groups should be catered for equally. Schools are of a high standard nationally but the United Kingdom has failed to retain the strong links between youth and sport established by public schools a century ago (Figure 15.2). In sporting terms, the post-school

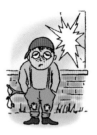

Fig. 15.2 'If only I'd been given a chance to participate in organised sport!'

'gap' highlighted by the Wolfenden Report[1] is still evident in the UK.

Disability

There is an increasing awareness that physical education, sport and physical recreation concern the whole of society, not just the able-bodied. If we start from our own interest and ability, it should be possible for all of us to express ourselves through a physical experience. To exclude those with special needs is unfair and fails to recognise the potential of our field of study to make life more worthwhile. Most of us have special needs in some way or other and it is for society to help us through these problems. Regrettably, in Western Europe, societies tend to separate, forget and even deny the disabled.

The Sports Council publications *The next ten years*,[2] *Which way forward*[3] and *Into the 90s*[4] identified 'target groups' that did not make full use of Britain's sports provision. These groups are invariably the ones that are still discriminated against socially.

Investigation 15.1 Discrimination

1. One of the most necessary tasks for you to undertake is to establish the extent to which our society handicaps the disabled.

2. This involves all problems of discrimination. You must attempt to assess the suitability of separation, pluralism and/or assimilation in any discriminatory situation.

15.2 Administration of physical education

Traditionally, the British educational system has been divided into a private sector for a social elite and a state sector for other children. At the end of the Second World War, a major building programme was necessary following the widespread destruction due to bombing. The victory resulted in a general feeling of well-being and a need for an extension of recreational opportunity and a tripartite system of education allowed some children to receive a free grammar or technical education. In the 1960s, the tripartite system was largely replaced by comprehensive schools but the old-style grammar schools persisted in some authorities and the private schools continued as a separate system, functioning as private institutions or as charitable trusts (Figure 15.3). Then, in the 1980s, central government encouraged schools to consider becoming independent from local authority control as grant-maintained schools.

Throughout these changes, the British educational system has remained **decentralised**. This means that the basis of decision making is in the hands of the teacher responsible for physical education in the individual school. That person can select from a variety of objectives, activities and teaching styles. There are a number of common features that operate, however. Teachers appear to retain habits and interests from their own school experiences; they often select colleges which reflect these interests but they are also influenced by innovations experienced at college; they are very much at the mercy of local attitudes and provision in the school; and, although they are 'responsible', the Head of the school always has the final word (Figure 15.4).

The considerable increase in the quality of physical and human resources in physical education has had a marked effect on the PE curriculum. On the physical resources side, the new sports halls and swimming pools have broadened PE beyond gymnastics and field games and the introduction of an all-graduate profession has increased the general quality of input and the status of the subject. The latest innovation is the state sports college system. The Youth Sports Trust has been responsible for the validation of this special category of 11–16 school. These colleges have a large additional funding package above that of normal schools for extra facilities and specialist staff.

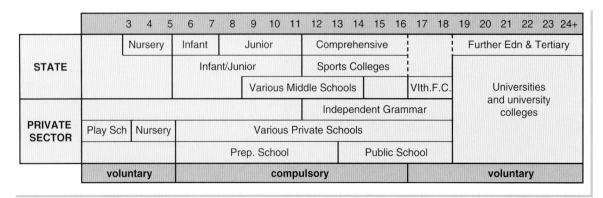

Fig. 15.3 English and Welsh school system.

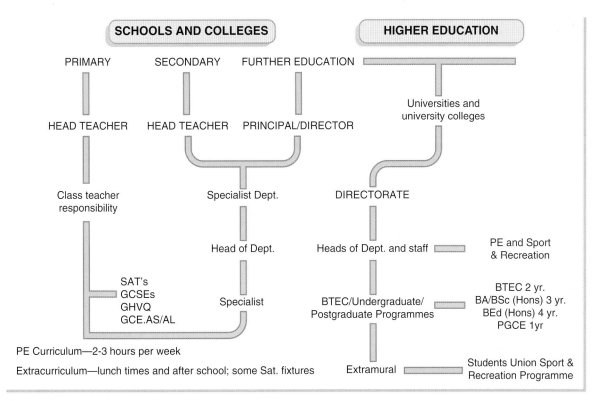

Fig. 15.4 Institutions.

With 16 operating in 1998, there were 46 by the end of 1999 and a prediction of 400 by 2005.

Another major area of change arises from the cluster of ethnic minorities. In certain schools, the proportional dominance of Asian and Afro-Caribbean children is such that the traditional PE programme is being questioned. The overall trend of increased coeducational PE is being criticised by Asian parents; many also prefer their boys to play hockey rather than traditional soccer and rugby and swimming for Moslem girls is a particular problem.

The local authorities, which represent shire counties and urban conurbations, are the pivot on which decentralised administration functions. They have the communicative role of relaying government policy and maintaining local standards. The personnel involved are professionally qualified and highly experienced and, despite the recent move to give them inspectorate status, their traditional role has always been as advisers – helping teachers with their problems, initiating in-service programmes, recommending and supplying equipment and stimulating innovation.

Finally, central government is responsible for general educational legislation and has maintained a decentralised policy. However, the 1988 Educational Reform Act resulted in a number of major changes being directed by the government which, apparently, reduce the level of decentralised autonomy. The 1988 Act introduced a National Curriculum; increased the extent to which schools are open to public scrutiny, through the increased powers of school governors; increased the influence of parents; and increased the extent to which market forces can determine the success of schools. While on the one hand this would appear to increase governmental control, it significantly reduces the powers of local government, particularly where schools decide to 'opt out' of local government control (Figure 15.5).

There was an initial adverse affect on physical education as the local management of schools (LMS) made policy decisions on the basis of costs rather than benefits, such as reducing the priority of swimming, closing school facilities to the public and selling off part of their playing fields.

This policy has now been checked as a result of pressure from the Sports Council, PE associations and parents and most recently by the government policy document *Green space initiative* (1999). It has become obvious that sports facilities can generate a steady income for a school; that a successful record by

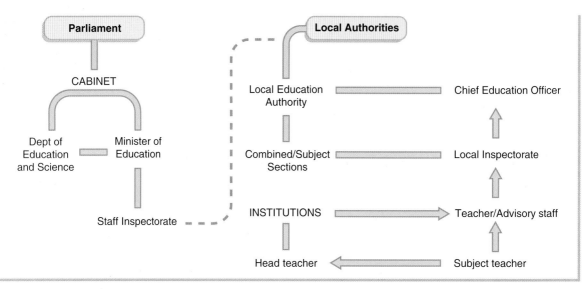

Fig. 15.5 Government and local government authorities.

sports teams and PE examinations can increase status and improve admissions; and that, as a subject on the core curriculum, PE remains a vital part of education.

This last has become increasingly apparent as attainment targets and programmes of study have been written for PE (The Education Order 1992), where the purpose of the attainment target for PE is to 'demonstrate the knowledge, skills and understanding involved in areas of activity encompassing athletic activities, dance, games, gymnastic activities, outdoor and adventurous activities and swimming'. There are four Key Stage tests (SATs): Stages 1–3 came into effect in August 1992 and Stage 4 in August 1995. Stages will take place in years 1, 3, 7 and 10 of schooling, respectively, and be followed by the national examinations of General Certificate of School Education (GCSE) and Advanced GCE (AS/A2-level) at an optional level. Several of the key stage tests are under attack on the grounds that they reduce positive teaching time and may be phased out.

Courses for young people in the 16–18 age group have been rationalised under the general title of General National Vocational Qualifications (GNVQs), which are vocationally orientated programmes for those not taking AS/A2-level courses.

Key Stage 1 programmes meet the needs of children aged 5–7 years and include five areas of activity: athletic activities, dance, games, gymnastic activities, and outdoor and adventurous activities, but if the school wishes, swimming can also be included. Stage 2 is for children aged 8–11 years, where the six

activities include swimming. Stage 3 is for 12–14 year olds and requires children to cover four areas, one of which must be games, with choices from the other areas. Stage 4 is for 14–16 year olds and is for children not doing GCSE in PE and they will select two activities for practical assessment.

GCSE PE has been under some government criticism because of the variations in content and standard but these were rationalised by the School Curriculum and Assessment Authority (SCAA) in 1996. The two A-Level programmes, Physical Education and Sport Studies, which had been administered by the Association of Examining Boards (AEB) since 1986, were merged into one syllabus and the Oxford and Cambridge Board (OCEAC) introduced a new Physical Education syllabus in 1996. In 1996 more than 1000 centres were teaching A-Level in Physical Education and Sport Studies, which amounts to more than 10 000 candidates a year. September 2000 marked the introduction of new syllabuses by QCA (replacing SCAA) from four boards, AQA (AEB), OCR (OCEAC), Edexcel and the Welsh Board, where alternative AS and A2 level programmes are available.

With the worst abuses of LMS now in the past, the value of accountability in raising standards in schools and departments could make the National Curriculum a positive step, provided testing does not reduce learning and as long as the ambitious schools and teachers are free to do more than the national requirement. It would seem, however, that the ambitious content of the PE attainment tests will require either the provision of specialist PE teachers in the primary sector or increased professional training in PE for prospective general teachers.

Finally, with much of the government policy driven by a desire to improve the standard of sport, several new initiatives have been introduced by different agencies to improve the standard of sport at school level. The first scheme was Champion Coaching set up by the National Coaching Foundation in 1991; the English Sports Council established the National Junior Sport Programme (NJSP) in 1995; and more recently the Youth Sports Trust has promoted Sportsmark, Sportsmark Gold and Top Sport.

Investigation 15.2 The administrative levels

Trace the following three administrative processes from ministerial level to the child in the school.

1. A school is in need of a new swimming pool.

2. A parent asks a teacher about safety regulations in the gymnasium.

3. A pupil wants to study an A-Level PE programme.

Local administrative framework

Having produced a structural framework for the administration of physical education in the United Kingdom, we now want you to examine the level at which it operates in your own school. Four research models are presented in Investigations 15.4–15.7. The suggestion is that the class should be separated into four sets, with each set researching one investigation.

These exercises should help us to obtain a balanced picture of what is actually happening in our own institutions but will also be useful when we try to look across at physical education in other societies.

If we visit a school we see a curriculum in action; if we read articles on curriculum theory, we begin to appreciate what the curriculum ought to consist of; but most important, we should be able to use our theoretical knowledge to draw the most out of the limited provision in any given situation. This can be simplified into a model called the **credibility gap** (Figure 15.6).

We can't always achieve what **ought** to happen, because of limitations in staff ability, provision, finance, children's attitudes, etc., but with effort we could probably improve upon what we are doing at the moment (Investigation 15.3).

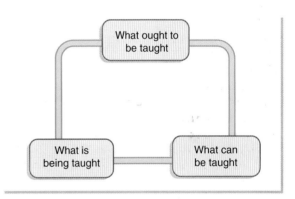

Fig. 15.6 The credibility gap.

Investigation 15.3 Session organisation

You will have all played either basketball or hockey. You know quite a bit about how an ideal session should be organised. You go to another school and you see 30 children being given a 1-hour lesson in basketball or hockey. Throughout the period they use only one ball in a game situation, with those not selected in the teams acting as spectators.

Suggest what limitations may have brought this situation about and then describe how you would use your knowledge of what *ought* to be happening to produce the best experience for the children that the limitations will allow.

If we are going to understand the British PE curriculum, it should be possible to produce a model which will act as a series of 'coat-pegs' for us to analyse what is happening or what **might** happen in any given school (Investigation 15.4).

Investigation 15.4 Curriculum theory analysis

Select an individual pursuit (athletics, swimming or gymnastics) and show how each of the conditions in Figure 15.6 can be met in a half-hour practical session.

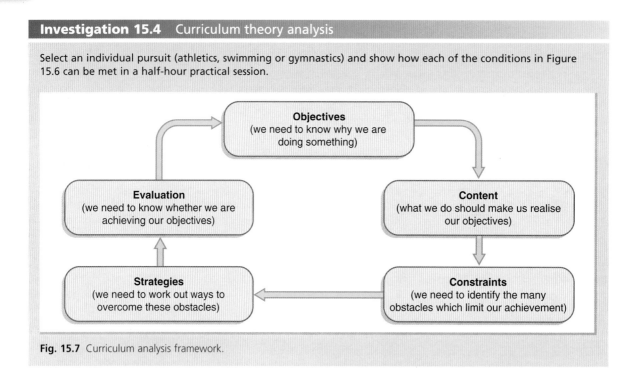

Fig. 15.7 Curriculum analysis framework.

In the early 1970s, the Schools Council researched the PE objectives favoured by teachers of secondary-school boys and girls. They asked the teachers to rank in order nine objectives – the results are listed in Table 15.3.

We are going back some 35 years for this information. Very few PE teachers were graduates in those days and most of the teacher-training programmes were practical in content. In addition, general attitudes have changed as regards the role of women in society and there has been an extensive campaign by the Sports Council in the shape of Sport for All (Investigation 15.5).

Investigation 15.5 Rank order of PE objectives

1. Ask all the members of your PE staff to make their own rank order.
2. Ask the group to rank order these objectives.
3. See if you can account for the changes that have occurred over the last 35 years as well as for the differences you might find between the views of staff and students on the rank order of these objectives.

Finally, let's put all this together with the framework in Figure 15.8 (Investigation 15.6).

Table 15.3 Teachers' rank order of PE objectives	
Boys	*Girls*
1. Motor skills	1. Emotional stability
2. Self-realisation	2. Self-realisation
3. Preparation for leisure	3. Preparation for leisure
4. Emotional stability	4. Social competence
5. Moral development	5. Moral development
6. Social competence	6. Organic development
7. Organic development	7. Motor skills
8. Cognitive development	8. Aesthetic appreciation
9. Aesthetic appreciation	9. Cognitive development

Investigation 15.6 Objectives and outcomes of physical education

With the help of the staff, see if you can gather the information to explain the relationships between objectives, programme and outcomes in the teaching of physical education in your school or one PE class in your school.

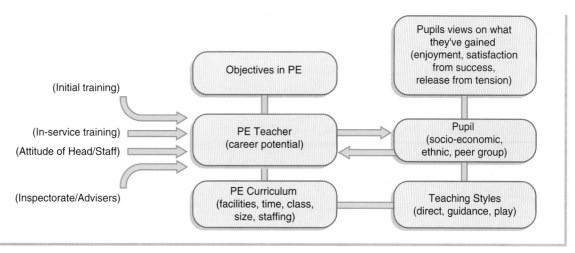

Fig. 15.8 Objectives and outcomes of the British PE system.

Things you ought to know about British physical education

Local authority

With senior advisers increasingly involved in the inspection of standards arising from the central directive on accountability, a number of advisory teachers have been appointed to retain the close liaison between the local authority and individual schools. Finance for courses and in-service training was distributed by local authorities but is becoming the responsibility of individual schools. Increasingly funding for TOPS courses and teacher/coaching courses is being put in the hands of local authorities and their recreational officers (Refer to Figure 15.9).

Teachers

In-service is now a compulsory part of the teacher's contract. There is concern at the degree of wastage, as a large proportion of PE teachers leave the profession.

There have been problems over a reduction in the birth rate which has led to a cut-back in the number of teachers being trained and also a number of redundancies and job reallocation. New contractual regulations for teachers are having a detrimental effect on extracurricular activities.

Examinations

The introduction of GCSE and AS/A2 level examinations in PE has led to more graduate knowledge being brought into play. Increasingly, examination boards, local authorities, colleges and schools are structuring in-service programmes at a local level.

Teacher training

Although physical education is a graduate profession, there are still a number of older teachers who are only certificated.

Undergraduate programmes have changed dramatically over the past 15 years in terms of the increased proportion of theoretical study and also in the delay of professional studies until the third or fourth year. It is felt in some quarters that this has had an adverse effect on teaching standards.

Extracurricular

City schools have established league fixture programmes in most sports, whereas their rural counterparts tend to retain friendly fixtures with schools in the locality. The **English Schools Sports Associations** are very well organised and there is a creaming system in most games and sports from area level through to national representation in each of the four home countries.

Figure 15.9 shows the diversity of award schemes occurring in sport education; however, it is difficult to separate policy from implementation at the moment. The NCF, as part of a ministerial strategy, initiated **Champion Coaching** in 1991 (as part of the TOP programme offering coaching for 11–16-year-old students after school). All the major administrative sports bodies were involved, including the British **Council for Physical Education** and the **National Council for Schools' Sport**. This was a major breakthrough, reducing the rivalry between sports coaching and physical educators. Twenty schemes went into operation, two in each of the 10 regional Sports Council areas in England. Each scheme provided 6 weeks of top-quality coaching in a number of target sports and involved around 3500 children. Progress was published in 1992 as *Champion coaching*[5] and the success of the project brought more funding and a second phase, which was in turn evaluated in 1993 in the publication *More recipes for action*.[6] Meanwhile, the other three National Sports Councils are following suit; Northern Ireland, for example, has already produced a **Corporate Plan, 1993–97** to raise standards in sport for children aged 11–14 years.

It is in the context of these projects that the political initiative, known as the John Major Initiative, July 1995, must be viewed. John Major, as Prime Minister, endorsed the publication *Raising the game*[7] by saying that his ambition was to 'put sport back at the heart of weekly life in every school, to re-establish sport as one of the great pillars of education alongside the academic, the vocational and the moral. It should not be relegated to be just one part of one subject in the curriculum' (Figure 15.10). These words need to be backed up with a detailed, fully sponsored programme. The Lottery is a potential source of money to pay for this and a strategic plan being operated in Victoria, Australia, **Physical and Sport Education**, may be the blueprint to work from. There are strategies to sponsor coaching courses for teachers and capital grants for schools hoping to specialise as sports colleges.

Schools

The schools in the private sector still tend to give more credibility to PE and have PE lessons and games afternoons.

There has been a tradition of so-called 'sports schools' in the UK. These include public schools such as Kelly College, Llandovery, Millfield and Gordonstoun, where scholarships or special arrangements are made for talented performers. Alternatively, governing bodies are setting up 'schools' in conjunction with local education authorities. The Football Association (FA) soccer school at Lilleshall is an example of a governing body establishing a selective school. It was opened in 1984 and 16 boys per year have been selected to spend 2 years at this boarding institution, where they have special coaching facilities and complete their normal schooling in Telford.

To date, this experiment has had only limited success and it may be that community ventures like the Manchester United Soccer School and the Aston Villa Community Project will more closely meet the

'More People, More Places, More Medals'

National Junior Sport Programme				
Lead Agency	**Foundation**	**Participation**	**Performance**	**Excellence**
Governing bodies of sport (including sports clubs)		Development plans for young people including facility development		
	Sport specific mini games			
			Competitive opportunities	
		TOP Club		
		Junior Club Development		
Community (local authority lead)	ACTIVE Programme	Local authority young people schemes		
		Sports Fair		
		Champion Coaching		
Schools	TOP Play 4 - 9	TOP Sport 7 - 11		
		Health related exercise 14-18		
	Curriculum resources and in-service training			
	Teaching children to play games	*Teaching students to play games*		

Fig. 15.9 New sports award schemes.

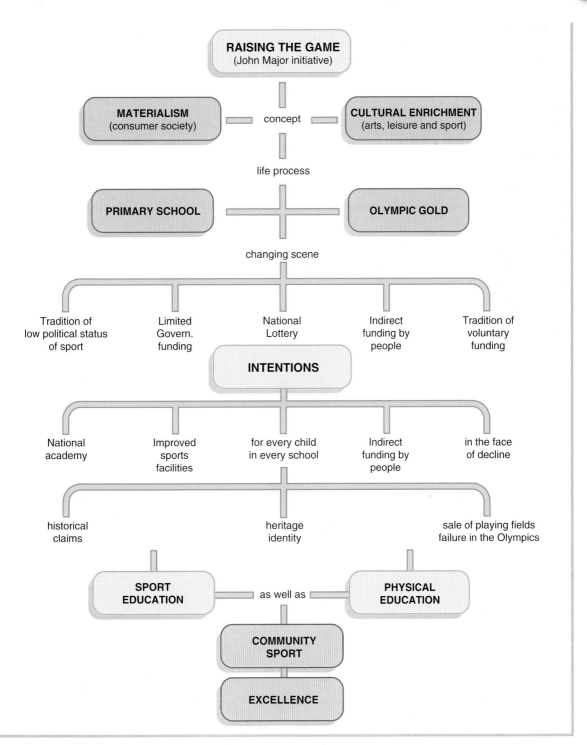

Fig. 15.10 Raising the Game framework.

needs of aspiring young footballers. Since 1998, soccer academies associated with premiership and league clubs have mushroomed around the country.

Dual use and joint provision of major facilities are being encouraged to increase participant use and to share costs.

However, the most significant advance was in 1997 when the Department of Education and Employment announced that specialist colleges in technology, language, sport and art were to be set up to act as 'beacon' schools in a locality and link the specialism with all local schools and the community. No limit has been set on the number of sports colleges to be established in the country and with some 46 in 1999, there was a projected target of 400 by 2005. With the focus on 11–16 year olds, these colleges with exceptional facilities and specialist staff can eventually act as 'beacons' for youth sport throughout the country (Figure 15.11).

Parents

Parents are being encouraged to play a more active part in school management. There is a long history of support from parent–teacher associations (PTAs), and parent governors will increase parental influence.

Curriculum

PE is one of 10 core subjects on the National Curriculum. It recommends a minimum of 10% of the timetable for PE and some LMS committees have opted for this minimum. Market forces, particularly examinations, may lead to many schools offering more than the statutory minimum.

Gymnastics tends to be taught in most primary schools as 'movement' rather than formal skill gymnastics; games teaching is following this proactive teaching style through 'games making' and 'games for understanding' approaches.

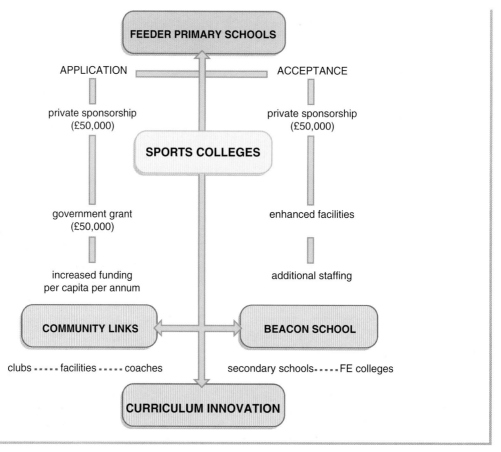

Fig. 15.11 Sports colleges.

15.3 Administration of sport

The **Department of the Environment**, now DEFRA used to be the government department primarily responsible for government policy regarding provision and public expenditure in the development of sport. Since 1962 there has been a **Minister for Sport**, with each of the home countries having their own minister with respon-sibility for sport. It is important to note that they are not Ministers of Sport and have only an advisory role in Britain's decentralised organisation of sport. In 1990 the Ministry was moved to the Department of Education and Science, but in 1992 it achieved Cabinet status as part of the responsibility of the **Secretary of State for the National Heritage** (Figure 15.12B). The devolution of the UK Sports Council to include Sports Councils for each of the home coun-tries in 1997 also led to sport becoming accountable to Parliament through the **Secretary of State for Culture, Media and Sport (DCMS)**. Kate Hoey was appointed as the Sports Minister in 1999, setting the scene for a dynamic but balanced future for sport in the United Kingdom. Richard Caborn held the office at the end of 2003.

The **Countryside Commission** is an independent statutory body, which reviews matters relating to the conservation and enhancement of the landscape and the provision and improvement of facilities of the countryside for enjoyment, including the need to secure access for open-air recreation.

The **Sports Council** was established in 1965 and received its charter in 1972. It is an independent statu-tory body with overall responsibility for British sport, but in effect a devolved policy is now in the hands of the separate Councils for England, Scotland, Wales and Northern Ireland. The Council(s) have four main aims:

- to increase participation in sport and physical recreation
- to increase the quality and quantity of sports facilities
- to raise standards of performance
- to provide information for and about sport.

They have been given the responsibility of distributing Lottery money for capital projects for sport and recrea-tion provision. A Modernisation Programme was launched in 2001 and is administered by UK Sport.

The **English Sports Council**, now working under the title **Sport England**, has nine regional offices which work closely with regional and governing bodies, local sports councils and many other agencies to develop and implement regional strategies for sport. The most recent development has been the formation of the English Institute of Sport (EIS) with High Performance Centres (HPCs) at Bath, Loughborough, Birmingham, Manchester and Sheffield in operation in 2004, and another in Gateshead in the near future. Money has already been allocated for eight HPCs in England together with examples in the other home countries. Governing bodies have access to these HPCs with more popular sports, such as athletics, having so-called 'hubs' in the UK, with most of these in the HPCs with professional coaches for each sport represented (Figure 15.12A) Photographer Helen Roscoe.

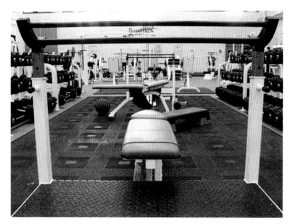

Fig. 15.12A Loughborough University HPC Power Base where Power matters!

The **National Coaching Foundation** has changed its name to **sports coach UK** and is the education service for coaches in the UK. Based in Leeds, the network comprises 16 **national coaching centres** in different higher education institutions in England (11), Scotland (2), Wales (2) and Northern Ireland (1). Its function is to improve the quality of coaching in this country by providing introductory packs, a programme of key courses for practising coaches, advanced workshops and a diploma for experienced coaches, and a documentary resource. Sports coach UK has been given many additional responsibilities as a result of the latest government initiatives, including direct access to the HPCs. These include sponsored courses for teachers and the negotiation of funds for elite performers and coaches.

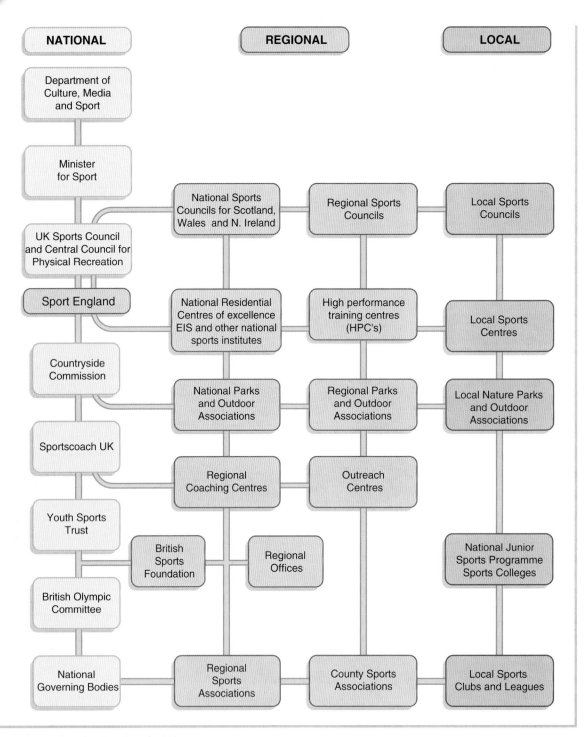

Fig. 15.12B The administration of British sport.

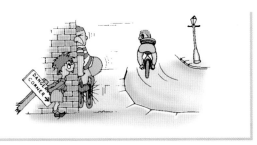

Fig. 15.13 Sport is all about getting it right on the day with a little help from others.

The **Youth Sports Trust**, sometimes entitled the United Kingdom Sports Trust (UKST), is the most recently established sports agency and has the responsibility for the development of sport for younger people, but also has the resources from government and the National Lottery to facilitate programmes like TOPSPORT and sports colleges.

The **Sport Aid Foundation** (SAF), renamed the British Sports Foundation (BSF), is an autonomous fund-raising body. It grants aid to individual established sportspersons for their financial needs in relation to training, preparations and medical treatment. It raises funds from commercial and industrial backing and distributes its grants through the governing bodies of sport. It aims to place Britain's talented performers on the same footing in relation to training and preparation as those in the USA and Eastern Europe (Figure 15.13). The BSF has national offices in Scotland, Wales and Northern Ireland and regional offices in England to encourage local fund raising and to help local competitors reach national standards. In 1997, the central role of sponsoring promising athletes and coaches was taken over by the Sports Council(s), sports coach UK, governing bodies and LEAs with the BSF supporting a second tier of performers.

The **Central Council of Physical Recreation (CCPR)** is an independent national voluntary organisation representing over 240 governing and representative bodies of sport and physical recreative activities. It is the 'collective voice' of British sport, a representative body which formulates and promotes measures to improve and develop sport and physical recreation in the UK and a consultative body to UK Sport. The CCPR receives financial support from UK Sport by contract, in addition to its members' donations. The Council has introduced a Community Sports Leaders Award scheme to encourage young people to assist in coaching sports groups.

The **British Olympic Committee** (BOC) enters competitors in the Olympic Games. It is autonomous and must resist all political, religious and commercial pressures. It is also responsible for fund raising in conjunction with the governing bodies of sport.

The **governing bodies of British sport** are completely autonomous. They are responsible for the organisation and codification of their individual sport and for financial solvency.

National sports centres

There are five national residential sports centres managed and financed wholly or partly by the Sports Council. Priority of use is given to national team training, competition and the training of leaders and officials. When these needs have been met, however, the centres are available for general courses to improve personal performance and to introduce beginners to new activities.

- **Crystal Palace**: Established in 1964 in Norwood, London, it was Britain's first multisports centre, built by the Greater London Council and managed by UK Sport.
- **Lilleshall Hall**: Established in 1951, near Newport, Shropshire, it is set in secluded grounds. In 1977 the Sports Council and the FA launched their development scheme to make Lilleshall the country's premier soccer school. There is also a sports injuries clinic.
- **Bisham Abbey**: Established in 1946, near Marlow, Bucks, it is a 12th-century abbey foundation adapted to the needs of 20th-century sport. There is now an established tennis school for promising young players, which parallels the football and gymnastics at Lilleshall.
- **Holme Pierrepont**: Established in 1973 in Nottingham, this is a national water sports centre developed on derelict land as a joint project with Nottinghamshire County Council.
- **Plas y Brenin National Centre for Mountain Activities:** Established in 1955 at Capel Curig, North Wales, it provides an outlet for adventure through the mountains and outdoor activities.

The UK Sports Institute (UKSI) was established, with each of the home countries having their own Institute of Sport. After some reshuffling, the English Institute of Sport (EIS) became London based and an initial five high performance centres (HPCs) were established, closely associated with local universities, with a further three envisaged in the future. These are very high-quality, multisport facilities, with major sports science units, and though intended for elite performers, the plans are to give access to local clubs and sports associations. It is likely that several of the national centres of excellence will eventually be upgraded to the HPC status.

Future developments

Subject to the resources being made available, the policy of UK Sport is to seek the development of more HPCs and high-quality facilities for various sports. These projections have included a national indoor velodrome for cycling, a national ice skating training centre, a national centre and arena for movement and dance, a national indoor athletics training centre, a national outdoor competition centre for bowls and elite training facilities for judo, boxing, modern pentathlon, sailing, alpine skiing and hockey.

Many of these projections have now been completed as government initiatives to promote sport using National Lottery money. The so-called 'four-pack' consists of capital schemes for sports provision; expansion of coaching; increased sponsorship for elite performers; and regional capital schemes for the provision of high performance centres and sports colleges.

Review questions

The Sports Council has published details on all governing bodies of sport and the Palmer Report[8] on **eligibility** is available from the CCPR.
See if you can use these publications to:

1. build up an organisational structure for your own sport
2. list the main regulations for amateur performers in your sport.

Exam-style questions

1. **a.** To achieve excellence in sport, a high level of commitment, resources and expertise is necessary.
   i. Explain these three conditions, using illustrations from your own experience in a sport. (*3 marks*)
   ii. Suggest three ways that a games club might be elitist. (*3 marks*)
   b. There are only a limited number of sports schools in England and Wales compared with certain continental countries. Give three advantages and three disadvantages likely to be experienced at an existing residential school of excellence in association football or gymnastics. (*6 marks*)

   c. The National Coaching Foundation (now sports coach UK) was set up by the Sports Council in 1983.
   i. Briefly describe the work of sports coach UK. (*3 marks*)
   ii. Explain the TOP sport project in the context of the Major Initiative. (*4 marks*)
   d. The UK has been largely responsible for the development of racket games throughout the world. Why is Britain still not producing many performers of an international standard in tennis? (*6 marks*)

   (*Total 25 marks*)

15.4 Organisation of outdoor recreation and outdoor education

Outdoor recreation is taken to mean recreational activities in the natural environment. While it is fundamentally concerned with enjoying and appreciating natural scenery, there is an element of escape in that many outdoor recreationists are 'getting away from' the urban environment. There is also a concern for conservation, with environmentalists reminding us that abuse and excessive use of the countryside can lead to pollution and erosion.

When different ways of exploring the natural environment are considered, we are studying the area of **outdoor pursuits**. At the most recreational level, this can simply be the use of skills like canoeing or climbing to travel and reach places or it can mean engaging in the challenge of nature and the elements, through canoeing on wild water or attempting classified rock climbs. Finally, there is the sporting dimension, evident in sailing and canoeing, where contests are held on fixed courses.

The use of the term **outdoor education** implies the inculcation of educational values in the natural environment and may involve physical, personal and social development, as well as learning more about the natural environment.

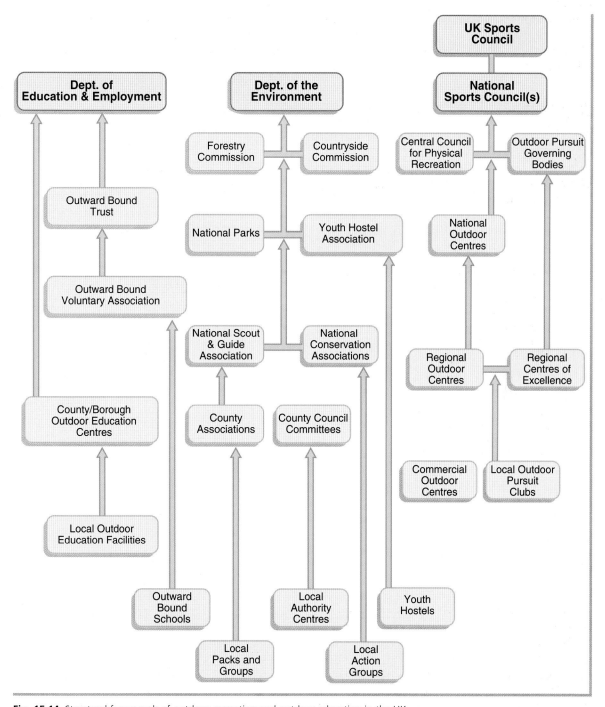

Fig. 15.14 Structural framework of outdoor recreation and outdoor education in the UK.

The **Department of the Environment** (DoE) was established in 1970 and took over three existing ministries. It has recently been changed to DEFRA. It is led by the Secretary of State for the Environment and one area of responsibility is conservation of the countryside and the provision and upkeep of amenities (Figure 15.14).

National parks

The 10 national parks cover a total of 13 600 square kilometres or more than 9% of the land area of England and Wales, much of it open countryside in the mountains or on the high moors. This is land considered to be of such great scenic importance that it has been given a special legal status to protect it against inappropriate development, but the fact that an area has been designated a 'national park' does not mean it is in public ownership. As in the rest of the country, all land in the national parks is owned, much of it privately, and farmed, forested or used in some other way, even on the moors. In the past there was no general right of public access simply because the land was within a national park and the normal rules about access to open land applied,[9] but a Government Act has now extended the legality of rights of way.

Open country

'Open country' is just what the term suggests. It is any area consisting wholly or mainly of mountain, moor, heath, down, cliff, sea foreshore, beach or sand dunes. The term also includes woodland, as well as rivers and canals and their banks.

Although this is usually private land, local authorities are able to make access agreements or orders giving the public a legal right of access to it. Generally, access will be only on foot subject to certain restrictions. You may not be able to camp, for example, and you may have to keep a dog on a lead and even where public access is guaranteed through an agreement or order, it may be suspended temporarily – for example, to reduce the risk of fire during very dry weather, especially in woodlands, or to prevent the spread of a livestock disease.

Picnic sites and country parks

Throughout England and Wales there are hundreds of picnic sites, some opened with the support and collaboration of the Countryside Commission, others

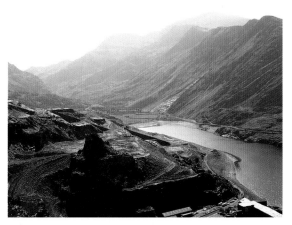

Fig. 15.15 A view of Snowdon from the Padarn Country Park. Photographer Helen Roscoe

provided by the Forestry Commission or bodies such as the National Trust. Each occupies a few acres, with seats and tables for picnics and car parking nearby, and is chosen for the beauty of its surroundings.

There are about 170 country parks supported by the Countryside Commission, ranging in size from a few to several hundred acres. They cover a wide range of scenery, from open parkland and woodland to parks where abandoned industrial land or a worked-out quarry or gravel pit or even a disused reservoir has been transformed to create an attractive landscape. Depending on the site, it will have woods, streams and pools, good habitat for a variety of wildlife, and it may also include a golf course, enough open water for sailing and space for horse riding. The Countryside Commission advises on the planning of country parks and awards grants to help pay for them. A few are owned and managed privately, some by the National Trust for example, but most belong to local authorities or other public bodies. Country parks exist for the enjoyment of the public and within them you may go where you choose, although occasionally small areas may be reserved for wildlife.[9]

Administration

Although there are a number of very influential national bodies, like the **National Trust**, the **Youth Hostel Association** and various outdoor pursuit **governing bodies**, the emphasis is on a decentralised organisation, which is controlled at local authority level and exercised with a great deal of freedom for individuals, families and organised parties. County councils and urban councils have **town and country** planning committees, responsible for matters to do with public access to the countryside. As with all British leisure administration, there is a mixture of state and private provision for community and school use.

The **Countryside Commission** is an advisory and promotional body which aims to conserve the landscape beauty of the countryside; to develop and improve facilities for recreation and access in the countryside (Table 15.4); and to advise government on countryside interests. There is a separate commission for each of the home countries.

The **National Trust** owns and protects more than 603 000 acres of Britain's finest countryside, 575 miles of unspoilt coastline and 276 houses which are open to the public. The Trust now has up to 3 million members who are entitled to free entry to its properties. Parks and areas open for rambling purposes may be privately owned (where access permission is needed), commercially based or belong to the local authority.

The **Duke of Edinburgh's Award Scheme** is an attempt to help young people to make the best use of leisure time. Established in 1956, it involves boys and girls aged 14–20 years in a series of challenging alternatives designed to help them with their personal development and their social awareness. There are bronze, silver and gold awards, which are valued by both participants and employers.

A wide range of **outdoor education centres** is owned by local education authorities (LEAs). The centres are a fully subsidised part of the education system and the majority have residential facilities. The warden and staff receive children from the authority and the majority of state school children have an opportunity to attend at least one field week during their school career. Young children have programmes in environmental studies mixed with simple open country activities; older children have programmes in outdoor education involving outdoor activities; and youth groups have leadership courses involving outdoor pursuits.

In addition, college students and others attend award courses for proficiency and coaching, such as the **Mountain Leadership Certificate** and awards organised by the British Canoe Union (BCU) and Royal Yacht Association (RYA).

The **Outward Bound Trust** is a registered charity whose patron is the Duke of Edinburgh. It was formed in 1946 to promote personal development training for young people and today administers five Outward Bound centres in the UK and has inspired some 35 centres of a similar type overseas. The Trust is supported by 35 Outward Bound Associations which consist of groups of people who voluntarily promote the Trust and raise funds to assist deserving cases financially.

A wide range of courses include Outward Bound, Expedition and Outdoor Skill Courses; the Duke of Edinburgh Award; City Challenge courses, an urban equivalent to Outward Bound; the Gateway and Senior Gateway courses, which are associated with business management skills; and Contract courses, which can be arranged by individual companies and organisations.

All the programmes are 'intensive experiences involving personal development experience, designed for young people to develop skills, judgement and confidence to meet the future with its problems, uncertainties and new responsibilities' (Outward Bound brochure, 1991).

Table 15.4 Long-distance routes in England and Wales

Long-distance routes designated by the Countryside Commission	Length (km)	(miles)
Pennine Way	402	250
Cleveland Way	150	93
Pembrokeshire Coast Path	290	180
Offa's Dyke Path	270	168
South Downs Way	129	80
South-West Peninsula Coast Path:		
Somerset and North Devon	132	82
Cornwall	431	268
South Devon	150	93
Dorset	116	72
Ridgeway Path	137	85
North Downs Way	227	141
Wolds Way	127	79
Peddars Way and Norfolk Coast Path (opened 1986)	150	93
Total	2711	1684

The South Downs Way and parts of the Ridgeway and the North Downs Way are open to horse riders and cyclists as well as walkers.

References

1. Wolfenden Committee 1970 *Sport and the community*. CCPR, London
2. Sports Council 1982 *The next ten years*. Sports Council, London
3. Sports Council 1987 *Which way forward*. Sports Council, London
4. Sports Council 1988 *Into the 90s*. Sports Council, London
5. NCF 1991 *Champion coaching*. NCF, Leeds
6. NCF 1993 *More recipes for action*. NCF, Leeds
7. DfNH 1995 *Raising the game*. DfNH, London
8. CCPR 1988 *The Palmer Report: amateur status*. CCPR, London
9. Countryside Commission 1987 Countryside Commission, London

Further reading

Anthony D 1980 *A strategy for British sport*. Hurst, London
Armstrong N (ed) 1990 *New directions in PE*. Human Kinetics, Champaign, Illinois
Bailey S, Vamplew W 1999 *100 years of physical education 1899–1999*. Physical Education Association, London
Bale J 1982 *Sport and place*. Hurst, London
Cashmore E 2000 *Making sense of sport*, 3rd edn. Routledge, London
CCPR 1983 *The Howell Report: sports sponsorship*. CCPR, London
CCPR 1991 *Organization of sport and recreation in Britain*. CCPR, London
Coe S et al 1992 *More than a game*. BBC Books, London
Coghlan J F 1990 *Sport and British politics*. Falmer, Basingstoke
DES 1992 *Physical education in the curriculum*. HMSO, London
Hendry L B 1978 *Sport, school and leisure*. Lepus, London
Houlihan B 1992 *The government and politics of sport*. Routledge, London
Houlihan B 1997 *Sport, policy and politics: a comparative analysis*. Routledge, London
Macfarlane N 1986 *Sport and politics*. Collins and Willow, London

McIntosh P C 1987 *Sport and society*. West London Press, Twickenham, London
OPCS Census 1991 *Preliminary report for England and Wales*. HMSO, London
Polley M 1998 *Moving the goalposts*. Routledge, London
Roscoe D A, Roscoe J V, Honeybourne J, Davis R, Galligan F 2003 Physical education and sports studies AS/A2 level student revision guides. 3rd edn. Jan Roscoe Publications, Widnes
Sports Council 1994 *New horizons*. Sports Council, London
Sports Council 1997 *England, the sporting nation*. English Sports Council, London

Multimedia

Internet

www.dcms.gov.uk
www.eis.2win.gov.uk
www.info@uksport.gov.uk
www.olympics.org.uk

Sociological considerations of physical education and sport

16.1 Towards an understanding of sports sociology

It is not intended to go into any detailed analysis of sociology as a discipline. The feeling is that in your reading you may need to be able to interpret certain sociological articles and it will help you to understand some of the contemporary issues in our society if you can use sociology as an analytical tool. Unfortunately, the lay person is sometimes frustrated by the technical language and meanings used by some sociologists and so it is hoped to make you conversant with the main terms and concepts as they concern physical education, sport and outdoor recreation.

Two sociologists were asked to define their discipline.

1. **Sociology deals with the way individuals interact with one another to make up a social structure.** (Given that there is a great deal of group action in physical education and sport, there should be plenty to interest a sociologist!)

2. **Sociology is the scientific discipline that describes and explains human social organisation.** The size of the human group under study can range from two people wrestling, to a sports club, a governing body, the leisure pattern of a community or the place of sport in a society. The sociologist is interested in the patterns that emerge whenever people interact over periods of time. Although groups may differ in size and purpose, there are similarities in structure and in the processes that create, sustain and transform the structure. In other words, although one group may be involved in aerobics while another is striving to win a football match, they will share many features. For example, they will have **a division of labour; a ranking structure; rules of procedure; punishments for rule breaking; special language and gestures; and cooperation to achieve group objectives.**

It is probable that most of you will want to adopt the first definition and if you think the longer definition is rather repetitive and verbose, then you are probably right. However, if you take the second one step by step you will have a better working framework.

A sociologist makes an objective evaluation of what exists. Developmental treatment of what is established is left to 'professional' groups to interpret. Much of what follows includes both stages insofar as we are using sociology only to help us recognise how to achieve desirable social objectives.

Some basic sociological theories

1. **Relationships** (Figure 16.1) are what happens in a group or between groups. The study of **intrapersonal relationships** is a part of social psychology. It means looking at the interaction within a group and the resultant influence on individual members. The study of **interpersonal relationships** tends to focus on the influence of one group on another.

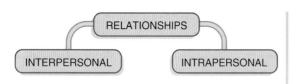

Fig. 16.1 Relationships.

2. **Structure** (Figure 16.2) is the organisation of a group – *what* it is. **Function** is the behaviour of the group – *how* it operates. **Deviance** is what occurs when members, or the group as a whole, break with the accepted structure and function of a group to achieve alternative objectives. In an **authoritarian** situation, deviance is automatically presumed to be **destructive**. In an **open** situation, it might be termed 'divergent thinking' and result in **creative possibilities**.

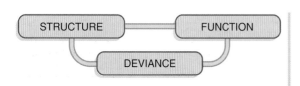

Fig. 16.2 Structure, function and deviance.

The **structure–function** model (Figure 16.3) is useful when we classify the largest groups in a society down to the smallest.

3. **Role theory** (Figure 16.4) suggests that people react to certain stimuli and adopt the role that circumstance dictates. **Action theory** suggests that though the stimuli are received by a person, he or she has the capacity to make an individual interpretation.

4. **Conflict theory** (Figure 16.5) suggests that change and/or progress are made by one group at the expense of another. **Balanced tension** theory suggests that a degree of stress can be productive if it is controlled and channelled.

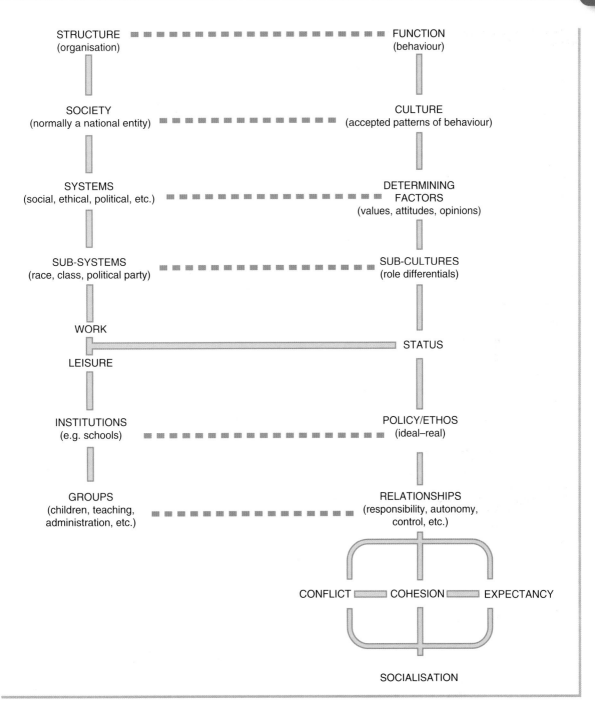

Fig. 16.3 Structure–function model.

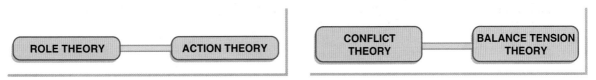

Fig. 16.4 Role and action.

Fig. 16.5 Conflict and balance.

1. Can you describe the action of a hockey umpire who sees an offside? Is it predictable?

2. A climber has an injured friend several miles from civilisation. What does the climber do? If you decide that he or she has several alternatives, identify them and justify one.

16.2 Society, culture and sport

You have been introduced to a number of sociological theories and each one has been examined in a sporting situation. We are now ready to look at a few of these in more detail.

We have decided that **society** is the structural composition of a community of people. We will be considering society as a national identity, in which a large group of people has an organisation that is unique.

Secondly, we have decided that **culture** explains the way this society functions. It describes the unique patterns of a society, summarised in the term **lifestyle**. It reflects the customs, attitudes and values of the people and can be analysed at ethical, socio-economic and artistic levels.

Societies have **institutions** as organisations within their structure and these normally have a degree of autonomy with their own unique cultural interpretation.

Sport is one such institution. It has its own traditions and values but these normally reflect the patterns in society at large. The same applies to physical education but in this case we are concerned with a subject within a school institution and so PE may be influenced by educational factors which do not directly apply to sport.

The intention is to look at different types of culture and to see how they affect organised physical activity. We haven't used the term 'sport' at this point because we might find that it is too sophisticated a notion to exist in some simple communal groups. Figure 16.6 attempts to frame the different levels at which sport exists in a society and show variables determined by culture. These societies are identified as ancient, tribal, emergent and advanced, with the cultural dimension of high and low behavioural patterns.

There are two additional dimensions which cut across time and scope which need to be appreciated to get the whole picture of sport, society and culture. **Ethnic sport** cannot be completely explained as a set of tribal sports and pastimes as they still exist in a semi-reformed format in advanced societies. They have survived the passage of time and social change and yet in terms of scope remain essentially localised. Alternatively, the **Olympic Movement**, originating in Ancient Greece, re-emerged with the European Renaissance and was re-established through the 1896 Modern Olympics to become a global sporting festival today, changing as societies and communications changed but retaining a basic code which attempts to maintain sport as a model of high culture.

See if you can work your way through Figure 16.6 from left to right. Look at the social scientific section first.

1. To what extent was the sport of the ancient Romans functional, ideological and concerned with ritual?

2. How was physical activity in the life of the Native American (American Red Indian) ritualised, natural and concerned with survival?

3. Look at an emergent country such as Kenya and see if sport is linked with cultural survival and whether it is selective and nationalistic.

4. Take a Western democracy, Britain if you like, and decide whether sport is based on recreation and excellence and explain how this is linked with commercialism.

5. Test your knowledge of Soviet sport by assessing the importance of excellence in the context of political ideology and purposeful intention.

6. Why does it appear that most ethnic festivals in Britain are in isolated areas of the country?

7. Why is it generally accepted that the Sydney 2000 Olympic Games were such a success?

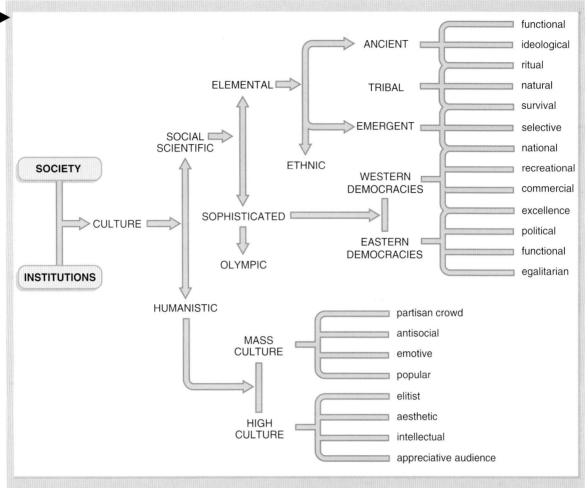

Fig. 16.6 A descriptive framework for societies, institutions and culture.

In Investigation 16.5 you should have thought about five different cultures, using the keywords to trigger your response. You may have agreed with the suitability of these words or questioned them. Most of your suggestions will have been **value judgements** but you may have had some genuine evidence or obtained some information from a published article.

The important point to be made is that your own ideas are useful but they do not represent social scientific evidence. A sociologist, archaeologist or anthropologist has systematically to collect and collate data and present them for public scrutiny. We need, therefore, to take this extra step and read what researchers have found. If we do this we are attempting to comment accurately on what is or was the situation in these cultures.

Ancient cultures, physical activity and archaeology

Minoan Crete

We have frescoes and vases which were retrieved from ruins. They show acrobats in the activity of bull leaping, a ritual to please the Minoan god Minos who was half bull, half man. This type of bull fighting combined piety and courage and reflected an affluent society, which used captives to fight the bulls while the citizens enjoyed the festival.

Ancient Egypt

There is considerable evidence in stone carvings on tombs. The best example is Beni Hasan's tomb (2000–1500 BC), which shows the technical development of wrestling and also boxing, fencing, swimming, rowing, running, archery and horse riding. These contests seem to have advanced beyond the level of religious ceremony to a sporting experience. Perhaps more directly linked with ritual, there are frescoes which show women engaged in various partner activities, like juggling.

Ancient Greece

The earliest evidence concerns the funeral games, contained in Homer's *Iliad* and *Odyssey*, books which were written around 800 BC. They are legendary and so not an accurate record but athletic feats, violent contests and chariot racing were part of a need to maintain fighting fitness, appease the gods and express the Greek ideology of 'Man of Action'. It is from these ancient myths and stories that the ancient Olympic Games derived as religious ceremonies connected with Zeus and lesser gods. Formal contests were held between city states despite the fact that they were constantly at war. Evidence of the diversity of activities and the athletic form which was idolised is to be seen on a wide range of frescoes, painted objects and sculptures.

Ancient Rome

Recorded in written form, sculpture and as monuments like the Colosseum, evidence suggests that the *ludi* or Roman Games were spectacles of extreme brutality, serving to illustrate the status of the patricians (ruling class) and the attempts to **appease** the plebeians (subject races). Affluence led the Romans away from vigorous participation to the spectator situation of the Games and the recreational pastimes of the *thermae* (baths).

It is unlikely that direct questions will be asked on this ancient sports history but basic values do re-emerge and so general concepts like ritual, militarism, Olympism and appeasement will have synoptic relevance in modern history and contemporary studies of sport.

Tribal societies, physical activity and the social anthropologist

General

The suggestion that tribal societies had functional physical activities is supported by the popularity of competitive foot racing among the Sioux tribe in North America, where the ability to cover large distances on the Plains was economically necessary. Log racing

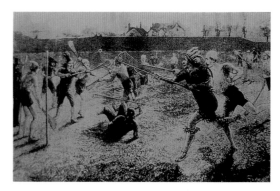

Fig. 16.7 Native Americans playing baggataway.

by the Timbira tribe in South America was not competitive but assessed on team success in getting logs down the river, another economic strategy. In terms of **ritual**, the ball symbolised the supernatural in the case of the Aztecs, the Arizona Indians and in the old Celtic game of hurling. An extension of ritual into **victory ceremony** is demonstrated in the Native American game of baggataway, later refined into lacrosse (Figure 16.7). Similarly, Peruvian Indians played with a feathered object like a shuttlecock, in a simple version of badminton.

Aborigines

Salter[2] studied the Australian aborigines. He suggested that group pastimes, such as tribal dancing, were most popular, followed by group games, which included hide and seek, mock battles, throwing the boomerang and plunging from a height. He felt that cooperational activities were much more common than competitions, because the aborigines were few in number and needed one another to survive. Weapons were also necessary for survival and the various ritual dances were intended to please the gods.

Polynesia

Jones[3] looked at 10 Polynesian cultures, including Hawaii, New Zealand, Fiji and Tonga. He observed their games, which consisted of canoeing, hide and seek, spear throwing, dart games, bandy (primitive hockey) and sham fights. They played string games and hand clapping, kites and surfboard riding were all in evidence. He found that the social and psychological need for group interaction was the major influence on the choice of activities; there were strong self-preservation and government control factors very few family activities, because of the Polynesian group culture, and a great deal of ritual significance.

Samoa

Dunlap[1] suggested that games were a central part of Samoan culture. In terms of the fulfilment of **social needs**, she identified social mixing, outlets for rivalry, opportunities for leadership, opportunities for prestige and honour to be won and an outlet for excessive emotions connected with birth, marriage and death. As a fulfilment of religious **ritual needs**, she suggested that erotic dancing was intended to stimulate the gods; fertility festivals were linked with nature and the tribe; and the flow of blood served to demonstrate devotion to the gods. Finally, at the third level, she identified fulfilment of **militaristic needs** partly through skill with weapons and partly through the physical strength essential for military preparedness.

The significance of **outside influence** was also considered. Missionaries prevented the association of vigorous amusements with the old religion; certain sports like bonito fishing were denied their ritual and tribal status; and erotic dances and tumbling were banned. The **colonial** influences changed the method of warfare by introducing guns, reduced the freedom of travel between the islands and introduced colonial games, some of which were eventually modified to meet local methods of play. The success of the Fijians and Western Samoans in rugby union, particularly at seven-a-side, is an interesting phenomenon. **They have adopted the colonial game but incorporated the aggression and flair of their culture to produce a unique variation of that game.** The Haka is a typical re-emergence of ritual from a precolonial culture (Figure 16.8).

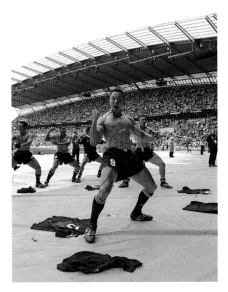

Fig. 16.8 The New Zealand Team performs the Haka after winning the Cup Competition 2002 Manchester Commonwealth Games. Photographer Glyn Kirk/Action Plus.

Pueblo baseball

Fox[4] noted that ancient Indian witchcraft was being mixed with a superimposed Catholicism to produce a non-competitive culture. With the importation of baseball, the competitive game conflicted with the culture and there was an emergence of witchcraft strategies within the game.

There is a considerable overlap of this tribal culture with the Comparative Studies programme as these minority ethnic groups are not only part of North American and Australasian studies but tribalism is still evident in the ethnic sports and pastimes of the United Kingdom, France and Russia.

Emergent countries and sport as a national identity

Riordan[5] suggested that all developing countries are in the process of **nation building**, which normally entails the authoritarian integration of a variety of tribal groups to establish stability. In turn, this can be achieved only if the nation is healthy and strong, which leads to emphasis on the **health** of the people and their **military preparedness**. One outcome in the modern world is the recognition that **sport** is a competitive frontier which draws a nation together without bloodshed. However, technological and financial limitations mean that an **elitist** route is necessary, where focus has to be on a specific activity that is straightforward to establish. Funding and effort are then **disproportionately** allocated to achieve **excellence** in this one area. The reward for international success is the production of a **role model**, which at once inspires and appeases less fortunate members of the society under one banner and gives the developing country international **exposure** and **recognition** (Figure 16.9).

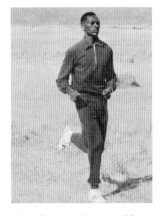

Fig. 16.9 Kip Keino, the great Kenyan athlete, training at altitude.

Africa

The world prominence of middle-distance and long-distance runners in East Africa and boxers in West Africa is out of all proportion to the sporting population of these countries. Tribal traditions and altitude have made athletics a natural choice in the East and the heavier build of Ghanaians and Nigerians has made boxing a natural choice for them. There is no need for sophisticated coaching methods or technological infrastructure and both athletics and boxing have the world stage, resulting in a few elite athletes stimulating tremendous national pride as well as international respect.

Kenya

This country is a particularly good example to use because it shows a tribal sporting development focusing on the development of one national sport and the emergence of sport as a more general vehicle for the development of sport. The initial identification of middle-distance running was the result of the impact of an Olympic gold medal and the political recognition that this could have internal and global value. One unsophisticated activity, in one sport, by one male, from one advantaged tribe, with a suited body type and the advantage of living at altitude, led to disproportional funding being made available. This initial trend, clearly elitist, led to world recognition of Kenyan dominance in this event and subsequently to a gradual expansion of involvement and political recognition of sport in Kenya so that today a wide range of track and field events are attempted by Kenyans. Women are also strongly represented in this sport and cricket and football are now played at an international standard, which opens sport to wider tribal participation and so sport as a whole is now viewed not only as an vehicle for internal appeasement but also for global recognition, gaining considerable economic and political support in that country.

Far East

The colonial impact on the old British colonies has had a widespread influence on the development and choice of sports. Success in these activities reflects the success of the family as a relic of colonial superiority. Cricket, hockey, badminton, table tennis and squash are games which have considerable cultural importance. Holding the Olympic Games in South Korea allowed it to express its particular form of nationalism; the use of the sports arena to demonstrate a political identity and the opportunity of showing the world the richness of Korean culture through a variety of artistic displays gave a small country the world stage.

South America

Here, the sport and culture link lies in the pre-eminence of football. Each of the South American countries uses the game to express its national identity, to allow its volatile emotions to be expressed, to appease the underprivileged and to provide an escape route for a few of them to earn lasting fame and fortune. This is particularly true of Brazil but Argentina is worthy of particular mention because there are major ethnic European minorities dominating certain regions of Argentina and their strength of identity has produced polo and, more recently, rugby union as national games.

West Indies

The popularity and success of cricket in the West Indies is an excellent example of the association between the natural lifestyle of tropical island communities and the pursuit of a colonial game, which was initially elitist but has now become an expression of the people, played in a style which is uniquely their own. The proximity and commercial influence of the United States, however, have made basketball an alternative to cricket, weakening the disproportionate focus and consequently the standard of play of the older game.

Advanced democracies and sport as a commercial and political vehicle

You will be realising that the roots of many of our games and individual activities lie in the inventiveness of ancient and primitive cultures and, more importantly, that changes which have occurred to these events are the result of changes in society in general. Three revolutions have been at the heart of this change: agrarian, industrial and urban, leading to the present structure of a sophisticated technological administration, based on a large, affluent population.

A sociologist looking at sport in such a country would be likely to say that sport is a solution to the problem of increased leisure time; a release of physical energy and aggression in a harmless way; a challenge which is artificially created to give an ensuing sense of achievement; and a part of institutionalised education through physical exercise. The more complex social structure leads to a more sophisticated sporting system but, as Loy & Kenyon[6] have pointed out, sport exists as **a social institution**, thereby having a considerable influence on society; and also as a **social situation**, so helping in the socialisation process in a group, community or society (Figure 16.10).

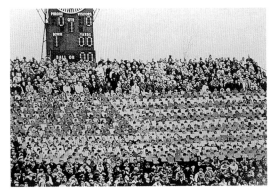

Fig. 16.10 USA: a case of the game giving the crowd a sense of identity.

The complexity of an industrialised society results in a number of **primary** determinants, such as the mode of production, relationships between rural and urban society, the division of labour and the distribution of power, in economic and political terms. It is also possible to produce a number of **consequential** determinants, such as the centralisation of authority, the provision of communications, social class and racial divisions and the provision of specialised facilities, which are a necessary part of maintaining an advanced society (Figure 16.11).

The tribal chief, elders and family could cope with all these social issues in a tribal community,

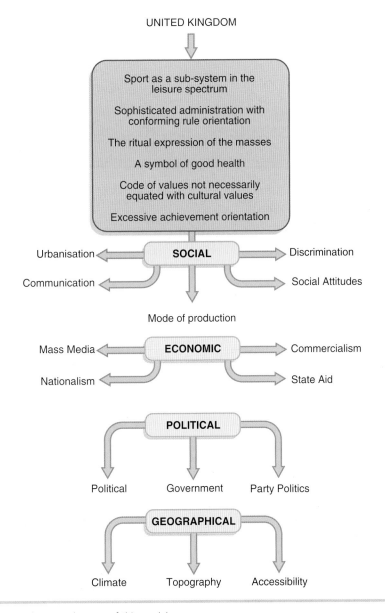

Fig. 16.11 Try to put examples to each stage of this model.

but this level of administration would not work in the UK, France or the USA. Some sociologists might argue, however, that at a local level these simple, self-nurturing groups continue to operate even in an advanced society. It is important to recognise the hypothesis by Luschen[7] and others that, in a sophisticated society, sport has a codification of rules which may not be the same as the cultural values outside sport. Things are done legitimately on the football field which would be common assault on the streets. Critics of sport also say that it is excessively achievement orientated, a situation which is already too strongly identified in our materialistic society. Finally, this **dysfunctional** possibility is carried to an extreme in the behaviour of some sports crowds, where it is suggested that antisocial behaviour is promoted in the sports situation and overflows into society at large.

The reforms in the Soviet Union do not mean an end to communist or socialist influence in the world. China and Cuba still have communist political systems, even though they are increasingly adopting free market economies. Russia and other old Soviet republics may yet retain socialism as a moderate version of stressing the community rather than the individual. It is also important that it might be single-party authoritarianism as against democracy which is critical. Similarly, some advanced countries, like France, are prepared to give their sport considerable state funding, partially because they see it as a political vehicle to empower feelings of nationalism.

Today, we can see so much in common between the West and the East, but it is important to realise that the political principle of putting the individual or the community first can give rise to a different interpretation of the function of sport (Figure 16.12). The focus in America is certainly on the commercial value of sport and as such sport itself is controlled by advertising and the media rather than sport for its own sake. This can be advantageous in terms of wealth becoming available to sports development and top performers, but there is a price to pay where business factors sometimes conflict with sporting values. This process is associated with the democratic rights of an individual and claimed to be a central part of the **American Dream**. There is truth in this in terms of opportunity for some and role impact on others, but the win ethic in much of American sport means that only a few winners make the top in a society which remains unequal in terms of the rights of race and gender. It is because of this that the humanistic view is presented as a counter-culture, where many Americans and Europeans support the notion of sport as a valuable experience in its own right for all

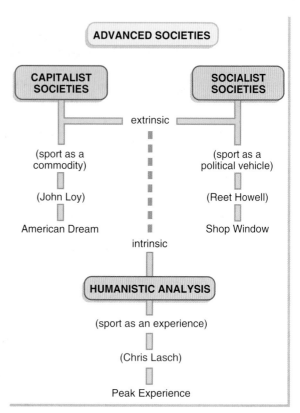

Fig. 16.12 A framework for Western and Marxist ideologies.

participants, not just winners and not as a commercial product.

Conversely, the phrase '**shop window**' reflects the view that if politics controls sport, the drive to produce winners can lead to the exploitation of individuals to the extent of risking lives and can also lead to the funding of a minority at the expense of the majority. In this case the propagandic process satisfies the citizens who are deprived and impresses the world with the presumption that excellence in sport is a product of excellent government.

This brief analysis of capitalist as against socialist, expressed by the phrases **American Dream** and **shop window**, is a simple way of reviewing two extremes in advanced societies. In synoptic terms, this material links directly with more detailed comparative study of the USA, Australia and France, where the impact of sport as a commercial product and sport as a political vehicle become significant, particularly as it explains the phenoneon of **stacking** in sport.

Ethnic sport in the UK and the emergence of local sports festivals

There are a number of sports festivals in the UK and other parts of the world which have ancient origins, but still play a major part in the fabric of sport. Many of them still retain traditional characteristics and have yet changed to satisfy the values in contemporary society.

They encourage us to become aware of traditional sports in our locality, as well as nationally, and increase a sense of local identity and pride. The twin notions of ritual and festival are dominant, where ancient beliefs are often symbolically re-enacted in an atmosphere of celebration and community well-being (Figure 16.13).

As a definition, therefore, ethnic sports are normally traditional, annual events, with merriment as a feature and with unique, local characteristics. These festival occasions can be usefully divided into four main groups.

Olympian rural games

Although these were relatively widespread in 16th-century Britain, there are now only three which have this long history, the Highland Games, the Lakeland Games and the Cotswold Games. The first two are regional games held annually in townships in that area of Britain, whereas in the case of the Cotswold Games, they were developed by Robert Dover in the town of Chipping Campden during the Restoration. In each case they are annual, multi-sports festivals, each with their own unique characteristics, many of which reflect traditional local pastimes. A fourth rural games which is sometimes included with these three is the Penny Brookes Sports at Much Wenlock in Shropshire. These originated as a local wake, but their development as an Olympic festival was due to the singular efforts of Dr. Penny Brookes in the late 19th century as an attempt to revive the Olympic Movement well before de Coubertin. However, though the Wenlock Games still exist today, they now have all the characteristics of a modern athletic sports meeting.

Holy Day festivals

In preindustrial Britain, holy days tended to be the major holidays and as there was no employment on these days, they became days with a traditional dual involvement of the **sacred**, with a church service, followed by the **profane**, as a major festival of merriment. In many cases this format was the case of a new Christian institution trying to fit in with old pagan customs. The most notable festival days of this type were Boxing Day, Shrove Tuesday, Eastertide and Whitsuntide, with May Day Spring festivals also in this group. Into this category of ethnic sports there are most of the traditional mob football events, such as those at Ashbourne, Alnwick and Atherstone, but also regionally unique occasions like Hurling in Cornwall, the Haxey Hood Game, Gloucestershire Cheese Rolling and the Hallaton Bottle Game. In each of these festivals, there remains a strong community involvement, often with violent elements.

Local wakes

In the villages and small towns of rural Britain, each church had a veneration (foundation) day. This became a local holiday which involved a visit to church followed by festivities. By the late 19th century many of these were becoming more and more debased in terms of behaviour, not least because people from the industrial cities used the railways to take advantage of the festivity and the alcohol. As a result many wakes were stopped or redefined as garden fetes, with an emphasis on respectability. Many of these local, annual occasions still exist, each in their own format, where the old fashioned 'smock races' have become family athletic events, just as the old maypole events have changed from courting rituals to children's entertainment.

Fairs and mops

The market towns in rural Britain, whilst influenced by church wakes, also had a strong commercial focus. The markets meant that agricultural work took second place on market days and, in addition to commerce, there became a tradition of associated merriment or fair. From medieval times, each market town also had its own Grand Fair which grew out of a statute for an annual market. The rights of this fair was and still is very much out of the hands of local councils and remains a period of festival entertainment. In addition to commercial markets and fairs, there was also annual statute or mop days, when agricultural and domestic workers were annually employed. Traditionally, this day included festivities after the employment transactions had been completed and many towns still have these mop fairs, even though the unacceptable old custom of public employment has long since gone.

It is important not to lose sight of the impact of these ethnic sports on a local community today and particularly in our case, the synoptic links between our reformed ethnic sports and their format in the past, as well as numerous examples of similar occasions in other countries.

The global impact of the Modern Olympic Games

The study of the Olympic Movement, though reflecting ancient and recent history, remains the ultimate

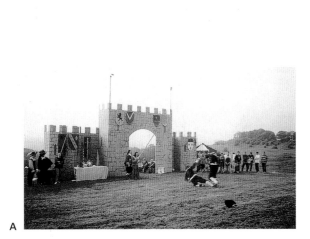

A

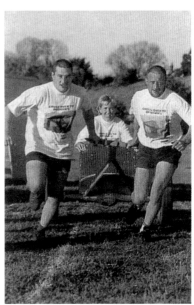

B

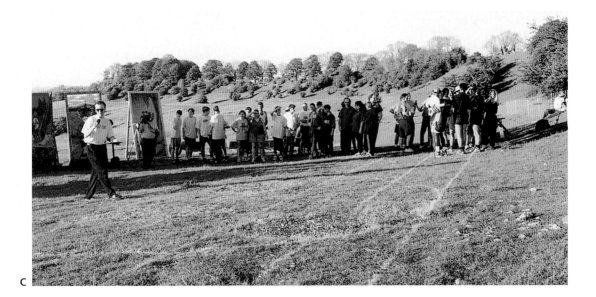

C

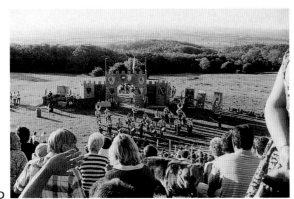

D

Fig. 16.13 How do the pictures reflect the characteristics of ethnic sport?

athletic challenge of today. To ignore the history is to reduce our understanding of developmental features and causational factors linked with social changes, but the central focus needs to be with our latest experience of a most successful Sydney 2000, the potential of Athens 2004 and the need to recognise the changes which might be necessary to maintain the place of the Olympic Games as the premier athletic occasion in the future.

The popular view is that the Modern Olympics reflect the Ancient Greek Olympics. However, though we have inherited a few of the ideals of classical Greek society, it had little in common with the sophisticated global society of today. Equally, the philosophy of de Coubertin was more attuned to aristocratic French society and the athleticism propounded by the English public school system than any ancient religious festival. It is important to remember that the Greek games had involved a small number of male athletes in a small variety of war-like contests between a few city states, with a common language and culture. These games were a religious ritual dedicated to Zeus, having little in common with our muscular Christianity and dedication to athleticism, the pursuit of happiness in a technological age or our obligations to commercialism and politics. What we can say is that we share certain values of physical endeavour and moral integrity and we have followed a similar pathway from amateurism to professionalism, even if there is little similarity in our interpretation of the two codes. However, there might be a warning for us in that affluence and corruption destroyed the ancient games and we may not be doing enough to prevent the same thing happening again.

In terms of recent history, that is the developments which have occurred since 1896, we only need to be aware of significant events over the last century to explain the critical moments when positive and negative situations have had a major impact. These would include the early aristocratic involvement; the effects of increased scope; the interpretation of amateurism, as identified in *Chariots of Fire*; the blatant nationalism of the 1936 Berlin Games; and the effects of the Games being used as a political arena, such as hostage taking, boycotts and possible terrorist activity. With these events being important in developmental terms, the real focus needs to be on current factors, such as excessive commercialism, drug abuse, the emergence of professionalism and the need for a professional administration.

It is important to be aware of the underlying values which the Modern Olympic Movement has promoted

at different times. The original aims in 1896 were **'the promotion and development of those fine physical and moral qualities which were the basis of amateur sport and to bring together the athletes of the world in a great quadrennial festival of sports thereby creating international respect and goodwill and thus helping to construct a better and more peaceful world'**. These words still ring true, but it is important to remember that at the time only aristocrats from a few wealthy nations were able to compete, women were deliberately excluded and later Games faced nationalist, terrorist and political intrigue.

By 1921, the Olympic motto emerged as '**Citius, Altius, Fortius**' (faster, higher, stronger) and so athletic excellence rather than participation was becoming centre stage.

Today, we have the Olympic Oath which requires athletes to 'swear that we will take part in these Olympic Games in the true spirit of sportsmanship and that we will abide by the rules that govern them, for the glory of sport and the honour of our country'. One wonders what the East Europeans had in mind during the years of drug-induced performances and the notion that the initial motive was one of individual effort rather than flag waving. The saving grace, however, is that the Olympic Code still retains the original concept despite drugs, death and boycotts. 'The most important thing in the Olympic Games is not to win but to take part, just as the most important thing in life is not the triumph but the struggle.' There are those who feel that after years of a downward spiral of the win-at-all-costs ethic and the failure of the IOC to face the sickness of drugs in modern sport, the Sydney 2000 Games had at last turned the corner (Figure 16.14).

It is important for us to recognise the progress the Olympic Games has made in terms of the steady expansion of the number of countries, activities and participants involved. The increased standards of performance, rational organisation and provision over the last century. The involvement of a greater social diversity in terms of age, wealth, race, gender and disability.

We also need to be able to explain these developments in terms of social and cultural changes. To be aware of the performance and resilience of the fine thread of athleticism, particularly in the face of increased affluence and obesity in wealthy nations. Thankful that the rise in democracy has enabled sport to advance from the gentleman amateur to an increasingly open competition for all countries. Aware that the steady emancipation of the female is leading to an increased opportunity for the sportswoman. However, we need to recognise how, inevitably, the

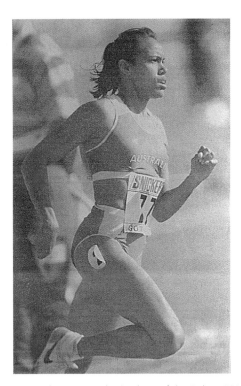

Fig. 16.14 Kathy Freeman, lasting hero of the Sydney 2000 Games.

media make the Games a target for dissenting groups and also a target for commercial exploitation.

If Sydney 2000 is thought to have 'turned the corner' as a result of its efficient organisation, its focus on the needs of athletes and the overall friendliness of the whole occasion, there still remain weaknesses which need to be rectified. Has the Olympics grown too big? Surely, the number of athletes, activities and events needs to be questioned given the logistics of housing athletes, building facilities and running the event over a shorter period at a reasonable cost. Such a reform will not be easy to achieve, given that world governing bodies will be unwilling to reduce their representation.

Without doubt a strong IOC is needed and yet we have officials who are appointed rather than elected and surely athletes and coaches should be represented. The IOC principle of a president for life with the power to select members is surely outmoded.[9]

The cost of the Games seems totally out of hand. There is the massive building programme every 4 years. One must ask if such excessive celebrations are necessary, with so much spent on the opening and closing ceremonies and the expenses claimed by IOC members as they inspect each bidding nation. The only way for this bill to be paid is putting the Games in the hands of commercial businesses and television companies. They inevitably want to sell their products, control the presentation of the Games and even the selection of venues.

The Ancient Games were destroyed by corruption and the loss of ideals. We are close to that in the context of performance-enhancing drugs. The small number of athletes found guilty of taking drugs during the Olympics, given recent East German revelations, suggests that the cheats are winning and that the IOC has not been vigilant enough for fear of damaging themselves. This is not a problem which can be solved by an amateur organisation which meets every 4 years. The Olympic Oath demands action but global involvement and commitment are also necessary.

Finally, there is the recurring question as to whether it is time to have one permanent Olympic venue. We have Athens 2004, the home of the original Olympic Games. Is it not time to put international money into a permanent symbolic site, with an object programme of activities, where commercialism and politics take a second place to athletes and a global festival of sport?

Investigation 16.6 Social influence on sport

Attempt to link Western sport with a social influence, e.g. how does commercialism influence high-level sport in the USA?

Review question

Explain why East European countries have used sporting success as a political agency.

Sport and low (mass) culture

An alternative way of studying sport and culture is to look at the behaviour of groups of people from a humanist viewpoint. Our basic model identifies two polarised patterns of behaviour: mass culture and high culture.

Mass culture is normally associated with modern industrialised societies with large population groups (Figure 16.15). It suggests that these groups can have common unifying values which may not match those held by other groups in the community. They are bound by a code of behaviour and emotional sharing, where a sport might bring them together as a group and stimulate them to act collectively. The behaviour

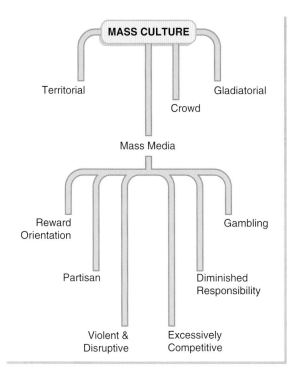

Fig. 16.15 Elements of mass culture.

of such a group represents the standard of the lowest member of the group, in a gravitation of standards permitted by the diminished responsibility of an individual in a crowd. It is generally felt that membership leads to a coarsening of human expression.

A mass culture sporting situation might be a fight between players in a rugby league game, a tag-wrestling contest or the football crowd at a local derby game.

1. Select one of these and use Figure 16.14 to establish any mass culture elements.

2. Link your popular sport with the four basic interpretations and then continue the analysis of sport as a mass medium.

In attempting to identify examples of mass culture operating in sport, you should be looking for situations with limited intellectual expression but considerable immediate excitement. Certainly, the most common example of mass culture in British sport at the present time is hooligan behaviour by members of a soccer crowd.

A great deal has been written on this topic, where almost everyone points to a different set of causes. Some blame society; others criticise the way the game is played and the attitude of players; some suggest that the facilities are at fault; others blame media hype and commercialism while probably most point the finger at the excessive use of alcohol. The Harrington, Popplewell and Taylor Reports made many recommendations but the problem is still with us.

You could visit a ground and assemble some data. Then, armed with some facts, we might have more than points of view to offer.

1. a. Does my ground fit a **mass culture** classification?
   b. Does a faction in my club bring violence to the ground?
   c. Does the game trigger violence or is it a combination of the two?

2. a. Is there a domination of certain **subcultures** in the hooligan element?
   b. Can you identify a **youth cult; a class cult; a regional cult;** or/and a **religious cult**?

3. Can you see the crowd being driven towards antisocial behaviour by the **code of the game**; by the **attitude of the players**; by the **condition of the facilities**; or by some other factor?

4. What are the **group dynamics** operating in the crowd? Can you pinpoint aggression, conflicting aspiration, collective bravado and protective reaction?

5. Is there evidence as to what incidents cause excessive stimulation or frustration and to what extent is this loss of control carried into the streets?

6. Can you point to similar examples of group misbehaviour in the community at large and, if so, what evidence have you that this is a law-and-order problem in your town?

7. Is this a **territorial** issue, resulting from away fans invading and home fans protecting their territory?

Sport and high culture

High culture is the training, development and refinement of the mind, taste and manners in society. It identifies with the highest moral, social, intellectual and physical qualities of a culture (Figure 16.16).

In a society where there are differentials of class, gender or race, the underprivileged are unlikely to be included in the activities which make up this quality of life. It might be argued that such people have their own ethnic or communal qualities which offset this. Arguably, in a 'socialist' state, such as the old Soviet Union, social discrimination should not exist and so these activities must be available and sought after by the whole of society. However, high culture tends to be based on affluence and intellect and it may be that the Soviet Union did not have sufficient resources to fulfil high culture right across society; it may be that intellectualism and the stain of Tsarist culture stood in the way of its full expression. It now seems likely that there was so much corruption taking place that major inequalities continued to exist in the Soviet Union, which may have been one of the causes for its decline. Similarly, if we look at the commercialism and the

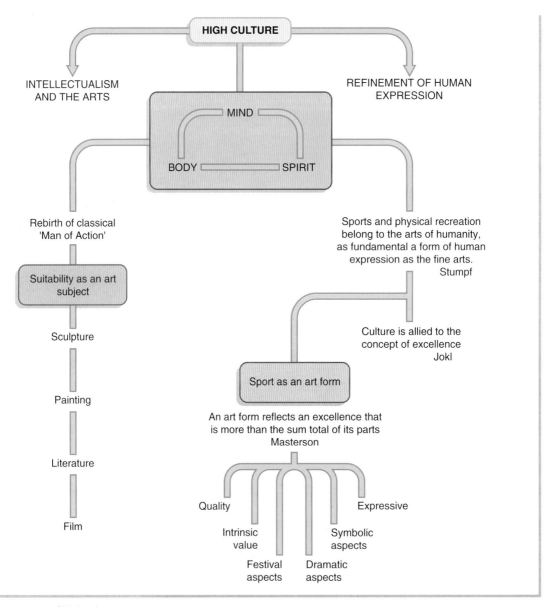

Fig. 16.16 Aspects of high culture.

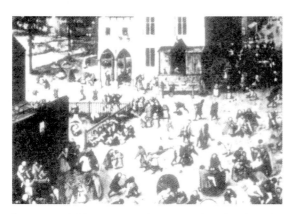

Fig. 16.17 'Children's Games', by P. Bruegel. Explain how the artist justified sport as an art subject.

competitiveness of American culture and particularly sport, there is a brashness which makes high culture activities part of the counter-culture. It is in the older cultures of Britain and France that high culture is at its strongest and where sport has had difficulty in achieving acceptance as a subject for aesthetic expression or as an art form in its own right.

The biggest problem with sport being accepted as an art form has been the inability to capture it for public appraisal. In sport, the moment of beauty is transitory (Figure 16.17). Today, we have film and video to capture the moment and to relay it in slow motion, providing time for its moments of artistry to be appreciated and stand up to critical reflection.

The analysis of culture from this behavioural perspective links directly with historical studies in that existing patterns are the result of causational factors in the 19th and early 20th century. In addition, the comparative study of certain other countries will establish that there are similarities and differences in behaviour patterns in different societies. Both these dimensions will be assessed as part of any synoptic questioning.

Review questions

1. Play is universal and yet each culture is responsible for the form and function it has. Suggest explanations why Aboriginal and Eskimo versions of hide and seek involve sending one person off to hide while the others seek but in the British Isles we expect one person to find everyone else in the game.

2. Western Samoa and Fiji play a particularly committed game of rugby football. Attempt an explanation of this in the context of ethnic culture, colonialism and postcolonialism.

3. Many emergent and/or developing countries justify elitism in the name of stability, integration and aspiration. Explain this using at least one such country as an example and explain why this elitism may be only a temporary necessity.

4. Discuss the theory that the 'win-at-all-costs ethic' in sport is strongly applied in both capitalist and Communist societies but that many of the motives differ.

5. Association football in this country can claim to be an art form on the one hand and a vehicle for the expression of mass culture on the other. Explain the duality of the English game, identifying the good and bad of both cultural forms.

6. Select an ethnic festival, like the Highland Games or Ashbourne Shrovetide football, and explain the significance of tradition and reasons for its uniqueness.

7. How do you think the Olympic Oath is jeopardised by the pressure to win at all costs?

Exam-style questions

1. All societies have engaged in physical activities and these tend to reflect the level of cultural sophistication of the society. Figure 16.18 shows one model of this relationship.
   a. How did the ancient Roman *ludi* (gladiatorial games) meet the three characteristics of functional, ideological and ritual? *(3 marks)*
   b. Explain why wrestling appears to have been very popular in many primitive cultures. *(4 marks)*
   c. Using the information in the diagram to help you, explain why Kenya has outstanding middle-distance runners. *(5 marks)*
   d. Explain why Western democracies seem to have a commercial basis to their sport, while Communist democracies have tended to stress political ideology. *(5 marks)*

   (Total 17 marks)

2. Figure 16.19 represents an alternative model of the relationships between Western democratic culture and physical activity. Explain the implied behavioural variables, using a soccer crowd and a gymnastics audience as examples. *(8 marks)*

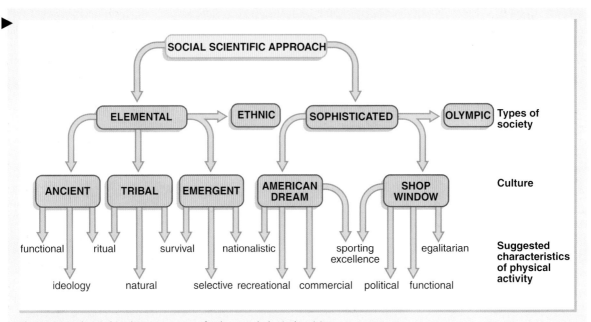

Fig. 16.18 Relationships between types of culture and physical activity.

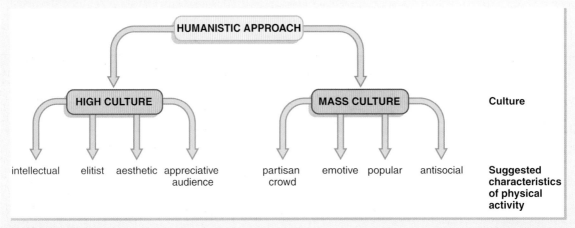

Fig. 16.19 Physical activity in the context of high and low culture.

16.3 Group dynamics in sporting situations

Now that we have examined the interaction between sporting groups and the social setting in which they exist, we need to look inside a sports group to see how it works. This may enable us to overcome problems which might arise from something going wrong at the **intrapersonal** level. You've probably all played in a team which has 'cracked up'.

The term '**group dynamics**' suggests simply that within a group there are constantly changing relationships which influence the outcome of what the group is trying to achieve (Figure 16.20).

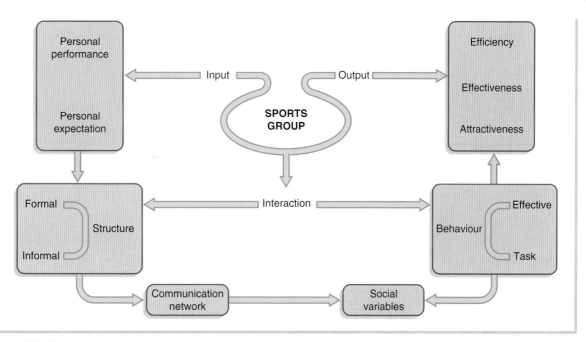

Fig. 16.20 The dynamics of a sports group.

Investigation 16.9 Group dynamics

Get into sets of 4–5 people, decide on a sporting activity and play for a time. Don't just choose a game; include a contest and an individual activity too. Then decide:

1. What did we have to do to make this a group?

2. What are the main objectives of the group?

3. What strategies should we employ to achieve these objectives within the spirit and rules of the activity?

Let's see if you reached similar conclusions to leading theorists in this area. Cratty[10] suggested that a group (sports group) is a *collection of people mutually*

interacting to solve a common problem or general type of problem.

4. Were you mutually interactive? (That is, everyone contributing!)

5. Did your objectives tease out the problem(s)? Or didn't you even consider what you were playing for?

6. Will your strategies solve the problem(s) by helping you to work together to achieve your objectives, albeit as a group involved in basketball, fencing or a cross-country race?

You'll quickly become aware that a group in sport has a **structure**, which allows it to work successfully.[10] This could involve fixture arrangements, playing positions, conventions or rules. Similarly, a group involves many **relationships**, which determine how well it works. Here we mean the sort of roles you might adopt in playing the activity. These may make you a successful group or perhaps merely a contented one. In sport we have this very meaningful word 'team', which describes group structure, and the expression 'team spirit', which describes desirable group relationships.

The **input** of a group is all about **personal performance** and **personal expectation**. Here we have a

mixture of ability and enthusiasm which will make you a worthwhile member. While the group is operating there is always **interaction** going on (Figure 16.21).

Investigation 16.10 What makes a good team?

1. List what you consider to be the characteristics of a good team and the qualities identifiable with team spirit.

2. Compare your ideas with those of other members of your work group.

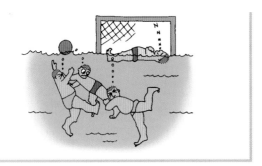

Fig. 16.21 Things aren't always what they appear on the surface.

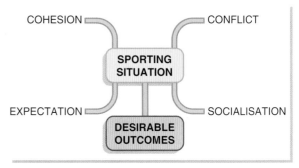

Fig. 16.22 Group motives.

When you play a game of football or hockey, for example:

1. is the structure **formal** or **informal**? (Are you playing in fixed positions or not?)
2. what is the **communication network** like? (Are you using an agreed code?)
3. are you committed to **effective** or **task** behaviour? (Are you letting the run of the game decide or have you been given a fixed job to do?)
4. What **social variables** are operating on the group? (What are the pressures on winning? What are the rewards? What attitudes are acceptable within the group? Do you have restrictions on membership?)

If we watched an interschool match, we would soon be able to answer these questions and it would be interesting to compare this interaction with the operation of a professional team. If we are going to understand the **output** of a group we need to look at its **efficiency** (how much does it achieve?); its **effectiveness** (how valuable is it to the group?); and its **attractiveness** (how valuable has it been to each individual?). It should be easy enough to sit down and do this after a match.

A physical performance group is almost invariably held together by the challenges it sets itself. This may be the competitive element in games, the contest of combat, the perfection seeking of many individual activities or the adventure of outdoor recreation. Let's call this the **sporting situation**.

It is important to reassert that these challenges are self- or group inspired and are couched in the experiential medium of play and self-realisation. The deliberate infliction of injury, on oneself or others, is not compatible with the desired values of a sporting situation.

The survival of the group is very much dependent on the balanced satisfaction of the four group motives shown in Figure 16.22.

Sporting challenge and competition are contrived situations where cohesion, conflict and expectation are channelled to give a desirable outcome.

Cohesion

Cohesiveness of a group is the result of all the members wanting to remain in the group. It embodies an underlying sense of cooperation (Figure 16.23).

- It can be identified as the essence of team spirit, where there is an **attraction** in belonging to a group with high **morale** and **shared responsibility**.
- It almost always involves the development of friendships, many of which may be long-lasting through mutual interest, e.g. Dr Roger Bannister's famous phrase 'friendships forged in the fire of competition'.
- An individual member tends to follow the collective will of the group in a form of mutual mimicry.

The basic cohesive ingredient of a match is the **contract** between two teams to engage in a fixture.

Given that the match always involves **opposition**, the team is drawn together by this outside threat. However, the opposition is required to **conform** to the same rules and this in itself is a cohesive element.

For the winning team there is the **shared reward** of victory and, in a well-orientated losing side, there is a tendency to **close ranks** and work for future success.

When the game ends with the final whistle, opposing sides should be **drawn together**, having put each other to the test. Similarly, the completed expedition, where risk and adventure are shared, results in the cementing of **life-long relationships**.

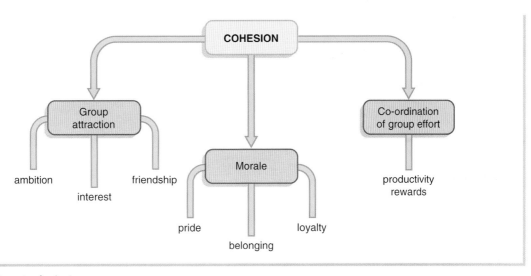

Fig. 16.23 Aspects of cohesion.

1. What are the cohesive elements evident in Figure 16.24?

2. Engage in a game of basketball, making a mental note of the cohesive elements and stopping at intervals for discussion; or play a game of volleyball with exaggerated elements of group reinforcement and cooperation, subsequently discussing the advantages of such an approach.

3. Select a sporting activity and explain the cohesive elements within it.

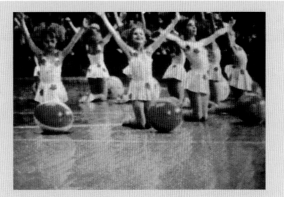

Fig. 16.24 A cohesive sport.

Conflict

Testing your mettle, temperamentally and physically, is the essence of physical performance. It is invariably a question of competing **against** self, others and/or nature.

The level of conflict varies in different types of activity and in different specific situations. In games conflict can arise playing against another team, winning a place in your own team or confronting match conditions. Individual activities such as swimming and athletics also include rivalry and conditions but are concerned mainly with pitting yourself against a previous best performance. In gymnastics, performance also includes subjective assessment and so

the contest involves impressing the judges. Finally, the outdoor pursuit situation may involve competition against others and self but the emphasis is normally on the challenge of the environment.

This is a good point at which to compare functional conflict with instances of outright aggression which lie outside the rules of play. Sport can claim to be culturally valuable only if it can be seen to give individuals and teams an opportunity to discipline themselves in the face of provocation.

This takes us into the conflict which occurs as a result of frustration. Here is a possible cause of instances of outright aggression. Fighting on the field and among spectators may reflect tensions which the game itself has promoted. Some educationists are concerned that sport stimulates aggression in a society which some claim is already excessively competitive.

Man is aggressive; the sporting activity requires commitment and effort; the heat of the moment and the desire to win test temperament control to the maximum. The key, therefore, is **channelled aggression** or **balanced tension**. The coach and athlete work to produce a top performance and this involves lawful strategies to make the most of that particular sporting situation.

If we learn to control aggression through sporting competition, if we satisfy the human need to be aggressive without overstimulation, then educationists may begin to recognise the socialisation potential of the sports group.

Review questions

1. Discuss the specific conflict elements in an athletics squad, a hockey team, a judo squad and an expedition party.

2. Look at Figure 16.25 and decide what the headings mean before allocating your different conflict elements to them.

3. Try to relate the following statements to Figure 16.25.
   a. The level of aggression should always be within the spirit and letter of the rules of play but should also satisfy the needs of the occasion.

   b. The required aggression of a combat sport would be much greater than that needed for an afternoon sail on a lake.

   c. Winning a ball in hockey with the need for commitment against opposition is very different from the personal discipline of refining a gymnastic routine.

   d. Surviving a difficult rapid in a canoe is real and unpredictable, as compared with the tension which exists in the controlled environment of target archery.

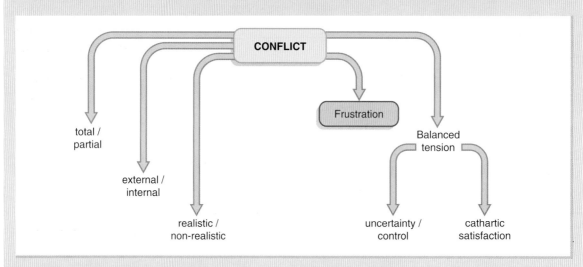

Fig. 16.25 Aspects of conflict.

Investigation 16.12   Effects of conflict

Set up some practical conflict role-play situations and monitor the effects, e.g.:

1. an example of gamesmanship
2. weak refereeing
3. excluding a player from receiving passes
4. verbal criticism of team mates.

Expectation or aspiration

The desire to succeed is fundamental to all sporting groups and to individuals within each group. Problems arise when the aspirations of an individual are not shared by the group.

We can be aware of how good we are and consequently what is feasible; alternatively, we can believe in our potential and speculate on our hopes. In both cases the significant factor is that the expectations

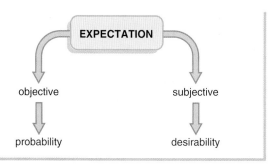

Fig. 16.26 Aspects of expectation.

should be realisable. Given the challenging motives underlying sport, however, it is important that these expectations should be at the limit of potential achievement in order to challenge the individual and the group (Figure 16.26).

It has been suggested that an individual's aspiration level is related to his perceived standing in the group. If this is not the case, there is likely to be dissension. Frustration exists at an individual and group level when expectations are too high.

It is also important to recognise that an individual who lacks ambition is as counterproductive in a group as someone with unreasonable expectations. Expectation is conditioned by the degree of role freedom in the group. For example, in American football, with the exception perhaps of the quarterback, players have a very **closed** role.

It is necessary for the player to fulfil his or her role to the satisfaction of the coach, other players, supporters and him or herself. Try to tease out expectations **in** this game and then expectations **from** this game.

Netball is another example of individuals accepting specific roles, which may require them to condition their own ambitions.

Saunders & White,[11] in looking at rugby football, suggested that it has a closed structure in terms of rules but an open system of relationships. In British mini-rugby a wide range of alternatives are open to the young person. He or she is free to explore various alternatives and other members of the group are likely to be extremely permissive.

Remember, a good team player subsumes personal aspirations for the advancement of the team and a sound coach invariably promotes a variety of objectives along an achievement continuum to stimulate the squad with a succession of small victories on the way to a major challenge.

Socialisation

At a societal level, socialisation (Figure 16.27) is **man's adjustment to his culture**. At a more specific level, it follows that it is also the **sportsman's adjustment to sport as a subculture**. In relationship terms it would seem that **social adjustments in sport may influence behaviour in society at large**.

It is worth remembering that Lüschen[7] points out that this might be a **functional** or **dysfunctional** process. We have the potential to produce heroes or villains!

In the field of physical education the teacher uses the sporting experience to inculcate socially desirable skills, norms and values, whereas sport tends to leave the ethics and rules to promote these indirectly.

The degree to which a group is **open** or **closed** decides the extent to which an individual can hope to

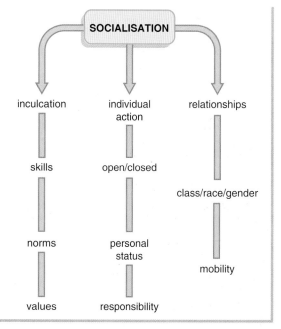

Fig. 16.27 Aspects of socialisation.

inculcate social changes. The status of the individual is also significant, e.g. a captain would probably be able to influence the group, a talented player might be able to but a newcomer would probably not.

At what levels might we presume socialisation can take place in a sporting situation? Simply being accepted into a sports group is a social experience. The ethics and rules of the group, team or club require the individual to make a social adjustment.

In the competitive or challenging situation, the individual and the group are required to meet the requirements of the sport in skill and behaviour terms. In playing together with others, the individual learns to submerge his or her own interests in favour of the group. Similarly, he or she has to accept the outcomes regardless of personal disappointments (Figure 16.28).

A sports group may include members from different racial or social class minorities where sport can help in the removal of discriminatory barriers. The sports group which is based on physical performance is a vehicle for social mobility where social constraints still operate in society at large.

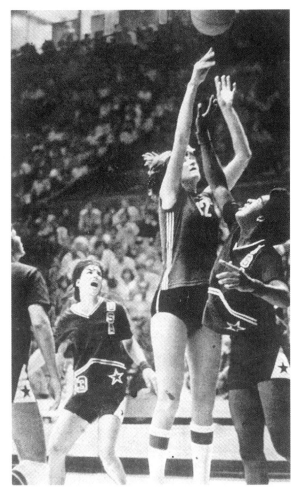

Fig. 16.28 Why was it so important for the Soviets to beat the Americans at women's basketball?

Exam-style questions

1. You will have all played in a games team and will realise that this involves not only the players themselves and what they bring to the team but also the interaction between team members. A flow chart of this experience is shown in Figure 16.19.

   a. Selecting a game of your choice, explain what you would expect to offer the team on becoming a member. *(2 marks)*

   b. During a game you would need to communicate effectively with your team. Identify two ways in which this might be done and the advantages of each. *(3 marks)*

   c. Describe the social relationships which might exist in a team selected solely on ability. *(3 marks)*

   d. Give a number of reasons for wanting to play for the same team the following season. *(3 marks)*
   (Total 11 marks)

2. It has been presumed that your team has been selected and run with an emphasis on participation values.

   a. What pressures would be applied to your games dynamic if the person in control promoted a 'win-at-all-costs' ethic? *(6 marks)*

   b. Explain the change of focus from cohesion to conflict if a win ethic was adopted. *(4 marks)*

   c. How would the adoption of a win ethic change the structure, formal and informal, and behaviour, task and effective, in a game? *(4 marks)*
   (Total 14 marks)

It should be clear from the text and illustrations that this sociological analysis of intrapersonal relationships involves considerable international material, establishing the probability of synoptic linking with Comparative Studies.

16.4 Roles in sport and physical education

When people find themselves in a social situation they behave in a specific way: in other words, an individual has one or more roles to play in every sports group. There are a number of variables operating which decide what that role is and how it is determined.

Your **status** in the group is probably the most significant single factor; to quote Linton,[12] 'Role represents the dynamic aspect of status'. This means simply that your standing in the group decides how you behave. You might be leader of an expedition, playing your first game in a hockey team or coaching an Olympic athlete. How you act depends on your status in the relationship.

The second variable in role concerns your own **make-up** and, therefore, the way you like to behave with others. How you act depends very much on your personality and while you can be 'someone else' for a time, this is difficult to maintain and there is usually a 'reversion to type'.

In addition to personal traits, there is the **impact** of the group on the individual or group make-up. How rigidly is your behaviour controlled by others in the group, by the dynamic of the game or by the rules imposed by an authoritative body?

If you want to know more about these dimensions, then you can look into **autonomous** (self-directed) roles and **authoritarian** (imposed) roles.[13]

If we stay within the spheres of play and games, then you will recall that children's play is very much a set of make-believe experiences, which may involve self-development as well as social development. If you look at games, you will recognise that we artificially restrict our actions to the needs of the team and the game's code: that, as with play, our experiences might lead to personal and social development.

The complexity of the game situation, according to Mead,[14] is that instead of just taking over the role of someone else, for example the striker in a soccer team, you also take on the role of the whole team: that is, you have to maintain your place in the fluid interaction of players and situations for the good of the team. If this is the case, then the value of group role play in a 'serious' sporting situation involves continual judgements and these experiences may overflow into a more effective lifestyle.

An extension of this hypothesis takes you into the 'reality' of a role: the view that for roles to be effective, they must be internalised. If we only 'play' a role, our commitment lacks the intensity required to fulfil it adequately. An American school for actors uses the technique of 'method acting'. They attempt to internalise the character totally – they 'become' the character. In sport we talk about 'intensity of focus'; the performer closes the world down to the immediate objectives of the contest. Incidentally, some opponents use gamesmanship tactics to break down that concentration. When we think of great tennis players like Laver, Ashe and Borg, we realise that when their focus was complete the 'strategies' of Nastase and Connors, who were also great players, did not succeed.

Because so much of a person's role is visual, the easiest way to establish it is by observation or by attempting to recreate situations. This is also the best way to understand what can appear to be complicated hypotheses.

Investigation 16.13 Role play in sport

Case Study 1
A PE teacher is teaching a group of children soccer. He is very keen to establish the spirit of the game as well as the rules, recognising that the game, if played with a high moral content, might help to reinforce desirable values. The teacher knows that the game itself tests the self-control of the player; that in games against other schools there is the temptation to retaliate in reaction to fouls and gamesmanship; that the players have the professional game as their model and so may see their heroes practising gamesmanship (Figure 16.29).

▶

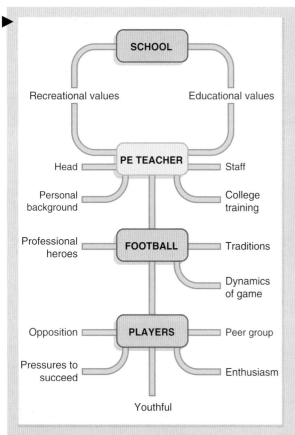

Fig. 16.29 A sociogram for Case Study 1, Investigation 16.13.

1. Set up a role-play situation where there is a teacher and a team of young players. The teacher explains why he intends to punish the players severely for any acts of gamesmanship or retaliation during a forthcoming game. Try to establish all the reasons why gamesmanship is counterproductive and antisocial but encourage the players to voice their reasons for allowing it to take place.

2. Having done this, what would you say if one of the players claimed to have seen you, the PE teacher, playing in a club game on a Saturday afternoon, where you were sent off for a deliberate foul?

Case Study 2

A party of four are high on an isolated mountain in extreme winter conditions. The group has made camp in a snow hole to decide whether to make a final assault on the summit. The leader is very experienced but willing to listen to the views of the others. The next most experienced person is a member of the opposite sex, suffering a little from mountain sickness. The third member of the party is young and aggressively headstrong. Throughout the climb he has

been difficult, unwilling to accept group decisions or the authority of the leader. There is a particularly dangerous rivalry between this young person and the second-in-command. The fourth person is the least experienced and it is her first time ever in such difficult conditions. The leader has had a lot of problems with this person, who is completely lacking in confidence and desperately afraid (Figure 16.30).

1. Set up the four roles and engage the team in a discussion on whether to go for the summit. Before you start, try to establish the individual status of each member; establish their personal feelings and the levels of group responsibility felt by each one.

2. Let's presume the decision was to go for the top. Unfortunately, the experienced climber falls, breaks a leg and has internal bleeding. They manage to get back to the snow hole but face a 12-hour journey, in white-out conditions, to make it down. With only a day's emergency rations they have to decide what to do. The leader listens to the arguments and decides. The alternatives would

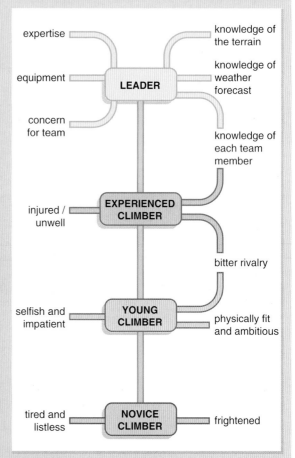

Fig. 16.30 A sociogram for Case Study 2, Investigation 16.13.

▶ seem to be: all stay; one or two go for help (but who?); three go, presumably leaving the injured one; or all struggle down with the injured person. Discuss these alternatives and the possible consequences of your decision.

Case Study 3

The coach of a mixed hockey squad is preparing her team for a major championship game. Together with two selectors, the coach watches a practice game and decides that the captain is so out of form that she will have to be dropped for the all-important game. The captain is recovering from injury but has also suffered the anguish of a relative involved in a car crash. The members of the team have loyalties to their captain and their coach but also a desire to win this championship game.

1. Set up a role-play situation (see Figure 16.31).

2. When you have decided whether the captain should play or not, discuss the degree to which the coach's authority has been compromised if:

   a. the game is won, either without the captain or with the captain

   b. the game is lost, either with the captain or without the captain.

   Select one of these and act it out.

3. As a result of this study of the coach, are you aware how many different roles she has to play in a situation like this? Each member of the group should take one of the roles shown in Figure 16.32 and explain how he or she would act given this problem with the captain.

The result of the two role-play situations will be markedly different, depending on the role(s) the coach decides are most important for each occasion. The lesson to be learnt is that you may have many choices in the way you behave but, by internalising and thinking through the consequences, your judgement can completely change the process and the product of any given sporting situation.

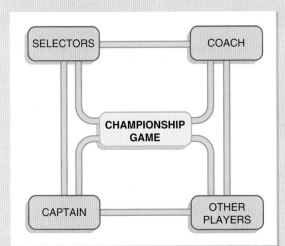

Fig. 16.31 The role-play situation for Case Study 3, Investigation 16.13.

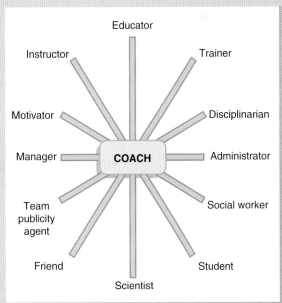

Fig. 16.32 Roles of a coach.

The role of the coach

Armstrong[15] produced a series of role-play situations which might serve to broaden the understanding of what might be expected of a coach in sport.

Coach and chairperson of selectors

The coach feels that she or he has too little say in selection, discussions and decisions and that selectors do not really know what they are doing. There is a history of poor communication between them.

The chairperson feels the coach is too autocratic and not sufficiently dispassionate. The chairperson has years of experience.

Coach and captain

The coach is worried that the strong personality of the captain is undermining his or her authority – the captain is talking of alternative strategies to the players without acknowledging the coach.

The captain feels that the coach's knowledge is inadequate in certain respects and that the players know best because they are the ones facing the challenges.

Coach and physiotherapist

The coach is concerned that a performer is becoming psychologically dependent on the physiotherapist and treatment and that his or her selection decisions are undermined by this.

The physiotherapist sticks to the point of view that medical assessment comes first to safeguard the future health of the athlete.

Coach and player

The coach wants a full squad to attend a residential training weekend to help develop team cohesion, even though it is expensive.

The player lives locally and can accommodate a couple of others, all on student grants, and therefore does not see why they need to be resident.

Coach and referee

The coach has been asked by the squad to broach the subject of bias with one of the competition officials.

The official or referee defends his or her position as the objective arbiter of performance.

Review questions

1. How does the role of the PE teacher compare with the role of the sports coach?
2. With the professionalisation of rugby union, how will the role of the amateur player differ from that of the professional player?
3. Compare the role of a teacher with an outdoor education group with the leader of an outdoor pursuit expedition.

Exam-style questions

1. The coach plays an important part in sport at all levels.
   a. Use a swimming, athletics or gymnastics situation to explain the need for a coach to adopt the role of an instructor, a trainer and an educator. *(6 marks)*
   b. There are always things to learn in coaching. Explain the roles of scientist and student which the coach might need to adopt in swimming, athletics or gymnastics to achieve effectiveness. *(4 marks)*
   c. When you are coaching children, how would you balance discipline and motivation? *(4 marks)*
   (Total 14 marks)

2. Sometimes the coach has to make difficult decisions to achieve short-term objectives. How would you explain that your captain should stand down for an important match? *(4 marks)*

3. You are a PE teacher who expects a high standard of behaviour from the players in your school team.
   a. On what grounds would you justify never condoning gamesmanship? *(3 marks)*
   b. How would you explain being sent off in a weekend club game, when confronted with this by the school team on the following Monday? *(4 marks)*
   (Total 7 marks)

References

1. Dunlap H 1969 *Games, sports, dancing and other activities and their function in Samoan culture.* In: Loy J, Kenyon G (eds) Sports, culture and society. Macmillan, London
2. Jones K 1967 *Polynesian games.* Unpublished MA thesis, University of Alberta, Canada
3. Salter M 1967 *Games of the Australian Aborigines.* Unpublished MA thesis, University of Alberta, Canada
4. Fox J R 1969 *Pueblo baseball: a new use for old witchcraft.* In: Loy J, Kenyon G (eds) Sport, culture and society. Macmillan, London
5. Riordan J 1988 *Comparative PE and sport*, vol 5. ISCPES, Human Kinetics, Champaign, Illinois
6. Loy J, Kenyon G 1969 *Sport, culture and society.* Macmillan, London
7. Lüschen G 1968 *Sociology of sport.* Mouton, Paris
8. Wohl A 1966 *Conception and range of sport sociology.* International Review of Sport Sociology 1:5–17
9. Clark R 1999 *Fixing the Olympics.* Information Australia, Melbourne
10. Cratty B J 1967 *Social dimensions of physical activity.* Prentice Hall, Englewood Cliffs, New Jersey
11. Saunders E, White G 1977 *Social investigations in PE and sport.* Lepus, London
12. Linton R M 1936 *The study of man.* Appleton Century Crofts, New York

13. Calhoun D W 1987 *Sport, culture and personality*. Human Kinetics, Champaign, Illinois
14. Mead G H 1967 *Mind, self and society*. University of Chicago Press, Chicago
15. Armstrong M 1984 *Effective coaching*, pack 13. NCF, Leeds

Further reading

Baker W J 1982 *Sports in the Western world*. University of Illinois, Chicago

Burns F 2000 *Heigh for Cotswold!* Robert Dover's Games Society, Chipping Campden

Coakley J J 2003 *Sports and society: issues and controversies,* 7th edn. McGraw Hill, Boston, Massachusetts

Davis R J 1998 *Sociological consideration*. Teachers' Guide. Privately published. Pershore, Worcs WR10 1EA

Dunning E (ed) 1970 *Sociology of sport*. Frank Cass, London

Edwards H 1973 *Sociology of sport*. Dorsey, Homewood, Illinois

Gardiner E N 1970 *Greek athletic sports and festivals*. Brown, Dubuque, Indiana

Gleeson G 1986 *The growing child in competitive sport*. Hodder and Stoughton, Sevenoaks

Greendorfer S L, Hasbrook C A 1991 *Learning experiences in the sociology of sport*. Human Kinetics, Champaign, Illinois

Guttmann A 1994 *The Olympics*. University of Illinois, Chicago

Hargreaves J 1986 *Sport, power and culture*. Polity Press, Cambridge

Hendry L B 1975 *The role of the PE teacher*. Education Review 17(2)

Hendry L B 1978 *School, sport and leisure*. Lepus, London

Horn J et al 1999 *Understanding sport*. E & FN Spon, London

Houlihan B 1997 *Sport, policy and politics*. Routledge, London

Maguire J 1999 *Global sport*. Polity Press, Oxford

Mills T M 1967 *The sociology of small groups*. Prentice Hall, Englewood Cliffs, New Jersey

Rees C R, Miracle A W (eds) 1986 *Sports and social theory*. Human Kinetics, Champaign, Illinois

Roscoe D A, Roscoe J V, Honeybourne J, Davis R, Galligan F 2003 *Physical education and sports studies AS/A2 level student revision guide*, 3rd edn. Jan Roscoe Publications, Widnes

Multimedia

Video

Sport in society. Video Education, Australia 1997. UK supplier Boulton and Hawker Films Ltd, Ipswich

CD-ROMs

Davis R J 2003 *Sport and culture*. Privately published. Pershore, Worcs WR10 1EA

Roscoe D A, Roscoe J V, Honeybourne J, Davis R, Galligan F 2003 *Physical education and sports studies AS/A2 level student revision guide*, 3rd edn. Jan Roscoe Publications, Widnes

Some contemporary issues in physical education and sport

Learning objectives

On completion of this section, you will be able to:

1. Develop a problem-solving perspective in physical education as a field of study.

2. Understand the issues of sporting excellence and mass participation in sport as cultural problems in the United Kingdom.

3. Be aware of specific issues arising in these two areas such as equal opportunity, performance-enhancing drugs and media impact.

4. Understand issues arising at an institutional level with particular reference to physical education variables.

5. Understand problems arising at subcultural levels, particularly as they concern such minority groups as race, gender, age and disability.

6. Be aware of the need for constructive policies and strategies to act as a reformative process in solving existing problems.

The issues approach to the study of physical education and sport allows the student to use a range of disciplines to establish the root of a particular contested area. Having completed a contemporary analysis of any issue in our country, it is valuable to study it from the **historical** perspective, where focus would be on causation, or from the **comparative** perspective, where we might learn from studying other countries.

The suggested order of study is as follows.

- **The issue** – the group needs to make a serious attempt to identify the different parameters of the problem.
- **Definitive** – analysis should start by establishing the meaning of the main words being used to describe the problem. In each of the three examples in this chapter, this definitive aspect is

covered in some detail but each group should discuss the accuracy of the definitions being offered.

- **Structural framework** – you need a series of headings to work under, which outline the structural basis of the study area. Only the framework is offered here and so it is necessary for each group to collect and collate data specific to the particular problem area. Some of the information has been included in earlier parts of this text but additional specialised articles and books need to be studied. For this reason a specialised reading list is given with each topic. Students should be encouraged to build files of contemporary articles and the school should make use of the National Documentation Centre at Birmingham University and the Web.
- **Functional** – the data you have collected should also help you to explain how the issue operates in this country and you may also wish to consider how it functions in a number of other countries to give you a global perspective.
- **Cultural analysis** – regardless of whether you embark on this comparative analysis, it is essential that you put the problem in a social setting. The 'cultural determinant' framework is offered to help you to explain how certain cultural factors might influence the problem.
- **Reformative** – finally, it is important that you should be able to suggest a series of reform procedures. This may be reorganising your own country's policy, provision and administration or may involve the introduction of certain ideas used abroad. The important point here is to recognise the problems which might be associated with the recommended changes.

Issues seem to exist at three main levels: **social**, **institutional** and **subcultural**. A sample issue in each of these has been selected for examination together with a list of alternative topics.

17.1 Societal: excellence in sport

The issue

There is a debate on the social ethics of elitism in sport: whether emphasis should be placed on the success of a few or participation by the majority. At an administrative level, the issue is whether a particular society has the right balance or whether we can learn from the policies and procedures of other countries.

A structural dynamic of sport is shown in Figure 17.1.

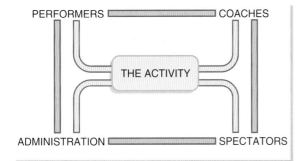

Fig. 17.1 Structural dynamic of sport.

Definitive

For **excellence** to be achieved a high level of **commitment**, **resources** and **expertise** is necessary from each group involved.

Excellence
This is the objective assessment of **quality**. Though in sport the end-product is the level of performance in competition, it should not be separated from the support role played by coaches, supporters and administrators.

This can be **elitist** in the sense that certain privileged individuals are given opportunities not available to the majority. If the reward is sufficient, societies may accept this social inequality. If everyone has the opportunity in terms of selection, where the talented are given every opportunity to attain their optimum level of achievement, this is a form of meritocracy which is widely accepted. This justifies rewards given to a few as a result of open selection.

There is an alternative, personalised notion that any enthusiast who achieves his or her optimum level of performance is on an excellence continuum. Where this view is individualised, we have a Western cultural

analysis; where it is collectivised, as in communist cultures, the society is presumed to reap the reward.

Status
A great deal depends on the status of sport in a society. Where there is recognition of the cultural importance of sport at national, political and commercial levels, the ideological and financial support will be greater.

The status of the performer is also important. In a country where professionalism exists with high financial rewards and where the professionals are drawn from the middle class, there is high status. Where there is a strong amateur tradition involving the middle classes, the same may apply but, in financial terms, the performers may be left to their own resources and prestige may exist only at a personal level (Figure 17.2). However, where amateurism is strongly reinforced by state aid and political significance, the status of the performer will be high.

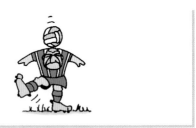

Fig. 17.2 Commitment and pain may be the price of success.

Structure

This is outlined in Figure 17.3.

Function

Policy and practice for children
1. Preparation for excellence in curriculum PE.
2. Extracurricular programmes for excellence.
3. The sports school/colleges in operation.

Youth opportunities and the Olympic Reserve
1. Club and/or community facilities for youth excellence.
2. Industrial provision for youth excellence.
3. Higher education and sporting excellence.

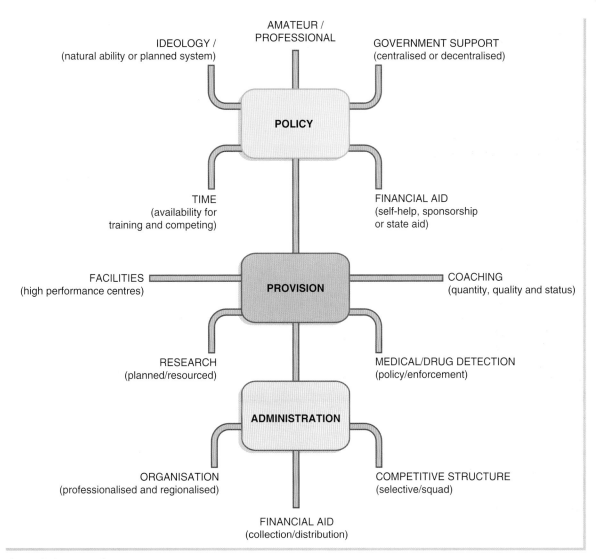

Fig. 17.3 Structure of sport.

Organisation and sporting excellence
1. Efficiency of the administrative framework for selection.
2. Distribution of financial aid.
3. Equality and use of the UK Sports Councils, English Institute of Sport, centres of excellence and high performance centres.

Status and human factors
1. Effects of status on development.
2. Level of opportunity and esteem for performers. The temptations of drug abuse.
3. Preparation and proliferation of coaches.

Investigation 17.1 Centres of excellence

Figures 17.4–17.7 reflect excellence: the organisation and performance standard of the Tour de France; the Australian Institute of Sport as a centre of excellence; the Astrodome as an outstanding facility; and a Soviet sports school. What is there in the UK to compare with these?

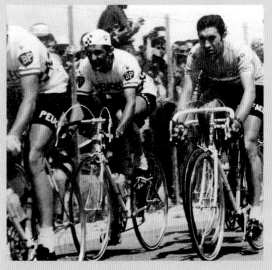

Fig. 17.4 The Tour de France cycle race.

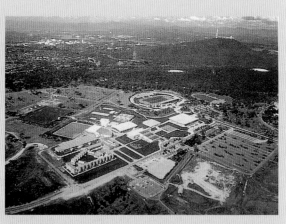

Fig. 17.5 The Australian Institute of Sport.

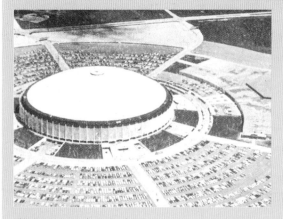

Fig. 17.6 Astrodome in the USA.

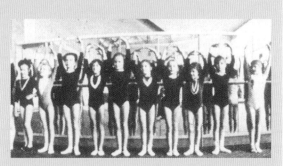

Fig. 17.7 A sports school in the former Soviet Union.

Cultural determinants

Some major determinants are shown in Figure 17.8.

If one of these sub-systems is analysed, such as **ranking structure**, it will become clear how much additional knowledge is required to understand links between a problem in sport and the society in which it exists.

Ranking structure

This refers to the status of specific groups of people in a society. Arguably, in the egalitarian Soviet society efforts were made to live up to a socialist philosophy by giving everyone equal opportunity but history has shown us that the political ideal is not always achieved. In European countries like France and Britain there is a very powerful democratic ideal but tradition tends

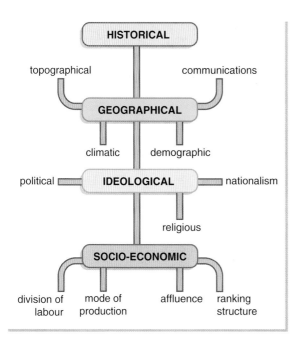

Fig. 17.8 Cultural determinants.

to give certain groups an advantage which they try to retain. Thirdly, it is important to recognise that in addition to some people starting off with an advantage, abilities and attitudes vary and so, in a 'free' society, able people 'get on' better than those who are less able. In economic terms, a capitalist market economy encourages this and so status is fluid, reflecting the material success of an individual, which brings them cultural as well as material advantages. American society does have strong 'ranking', explained in the initials WASP (white Anglo-Saxon Protestant), and can be defined as 'hegemony' but allows more opportunities for 'excellence' to be achieved through the ideological support given to opportunism – as they would say, 'rags to riches'.

Social ranking, therefore, is one of the major factors that determines the opportunity to participate in sport – adequate access to provisions for sport and sufficient self-esteem and social acceptability to enter fully into a high-level sports programme.

The suggestion is that, in an unequal society, certain groups find it difficult to play a full part in sport: that society is **ranked** according to **status**. This may be the consequence of restrictions put on these groups by the dominant groups or may reflect a lack of confidence or affluence among the members of that minority group.

In Britain, there is the traditional influence of **social class** which lies at the root of most discrimination but **gender** bias is also the result of values cemented in Victorian tradition.

Many Afro-Caribbean and Asian people have settled in Britain in the past 50 years and have tended to move into an industrial working-class social stratum, which combines the existing class discrimination with the additional problems of occupational rivalry and racism. These negatives are made worse for females, because ethnic minorities tend to retain their own cultural taboos in an adopted social system that already discriminates against females. This is a particularly powerful factor when **religion** also plays a part in gender roles.

Sport, particularly high-level sport, has always been dominated by the dynamic **young** male adult and consequently **age**, particularly in the case of the very young and the elderly, has also been a target for discrimination. Young people are often exploited to achieve excellence or are excluded because adults find their presence disruptive. Older people suffer from the accusation of 'being over the hill' and there are still only a few sports where 'veteran' events are actively encouraged. 'Lifetime sport' is a concept which has still to be fully realised in Britain.

Finally, elite sport is normally focused on **physical ability**, so that anyone who is not able-bodied is discriminated against. The notion of 'a disabled person being handicapped by society' suggests that discrimination is not limited to sport; in fact, sport offers a solution to the problem of people being handicapped by a disability through contests where individuals are able to test themselves against their peers.

Class, gender, race, age and disability: these are the factors by which our social system classifies and stratifies, ranking individuals and, in so doing, influencing their likelihood of achieving excellence in sport. It is equally important to recognise that the Sports Council's target groups also reflect this social ranking and, as a result, highlight the constraints operating against the successful implementation of a Sport for All policy.

Reformative

Development potential

1. What might we usefully consider at school level?
2. What youth policies abroad could help in Britain?
3. What organisational and financial improvements might the British adopt?
4. How might we change things at personal and status levels?

Constraints which might operate

1. Cultural resistance to the imposition of foreign methods.
2. Unacceptable influence on the status quo.

Final comments

The model used for this analysis should be adaptable for any national policy or campaign (Figure 17.9).

In addition, the framework allows other societal issues to be analysed, such as Sport for All, recreation and the countryside, and health and exercise.

As a thematic component, it is essential that other parts of this textbook are used to increase understanding and to give supportive information. For example, the issue cannot be comprehended without clear conceptual understanding; determinants may include physiological variables and so there must be an accurate input from the biological sciences; and it may be advantageous to use your knowledge of other countries to clarify the issue.

Finally, the exposure of a societal issue is bound to take you into more specific areas. These may be institutional or subcultural frameworks and an outline

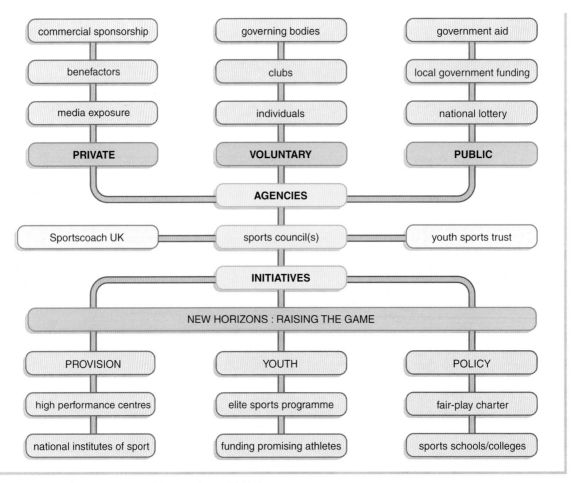

Fig. 17.9 Raising the Game: sponsorship, agencies and initiatives.

of these follows on from this section but they can also be specific problems that require special analysis. The National Lottery and its distribution; professionalism and elite performance; media and sport; advertising and the star performer; and drugs and sport, for example, warrant more than a passing mention and require understanding of the more general issue of **excellence**. In order to open some of these doors, a relatively simple outline can frame the issue and enable knowledge to be added as required (Figures 17.10–17.14).

These frameworks can only act as a starting point and it is necessary to produce a more detailed analysis even before supportive information can be added. An example of this second phase is reflected in Figure 17.15, a conceptual map for **drugs and sport**, produced by Glen Cummins in 1993, which includes four suggested levels of analysis.

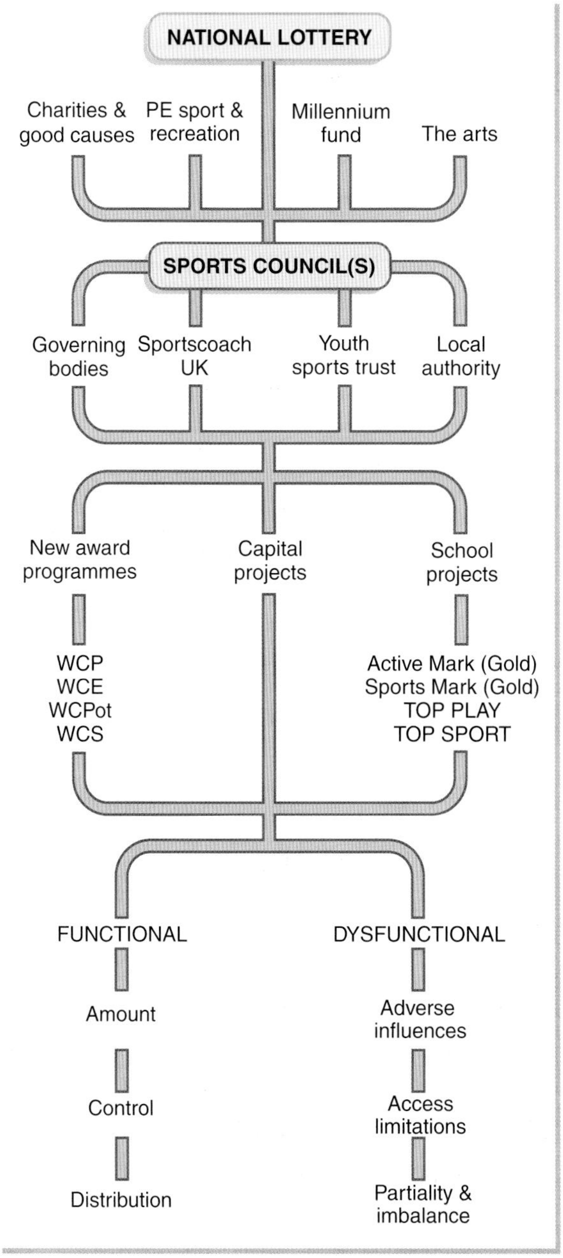

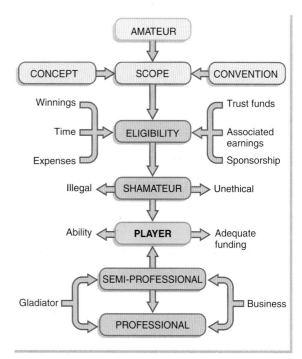

Fig. 17.10 National Lottery and its distribution.

Fig. 17.11 Professionalism and elite performance.

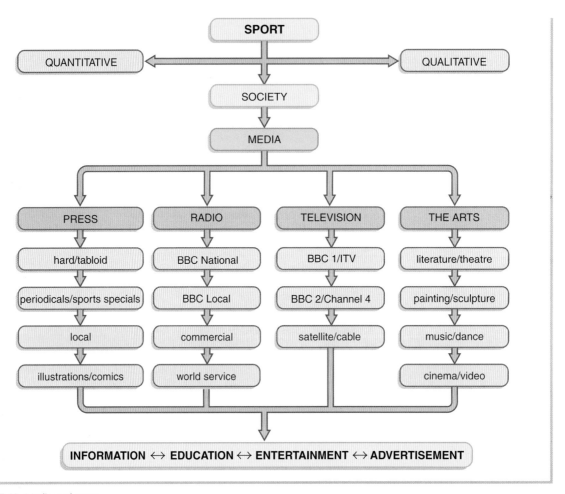

Fig. 17.12 Media and sport.

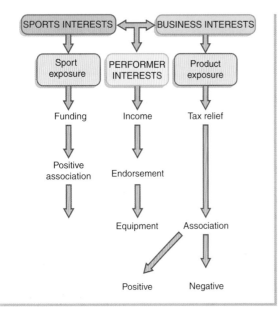

Fig. 17.13A Advertising and the star performer.

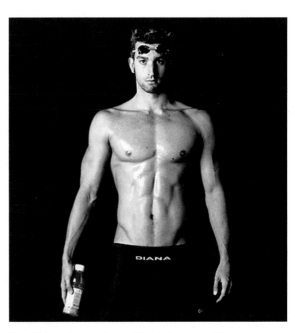

Fig. 17.13B James Gibson. World Champion 50m breaststroke.

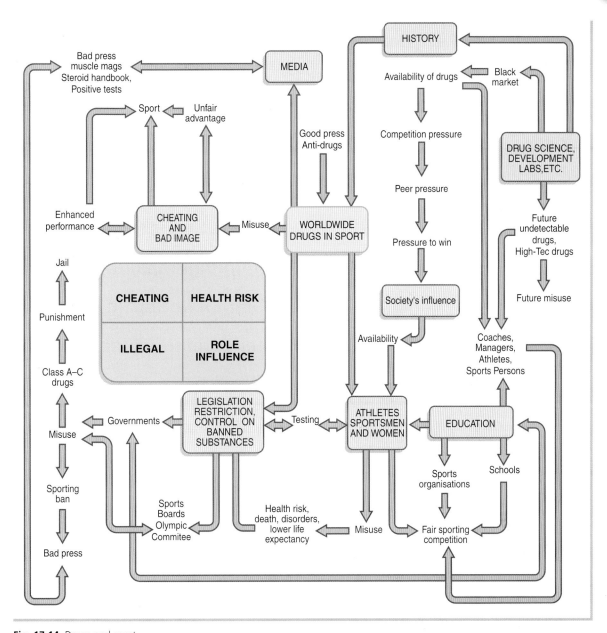

Fig. 17.14 Drugs and sport.

Review questions

1. Use a particular sport to show the extent to which excellence is being achieved as a result of elitist ideology, administrative structure and coaching expertise in the UK.

2. Examine the extent to which Sport for All remains a myth in this country given limits in opportunity, provision and esteem.

3. Discuss the use of drugs as a sport issue, which involves the notion of cheating and the risk to health and identity.

4. Advertising can make a star athlete little more than a billboard, where product association can undermine the performer and the sport. Discuss.

5. The media serves its audience but not always the interests of the sport. Discuss.

6. Rugby Union is going down a new path to professionalism. Explain the opportunities and pitfalls.

7. Analyse the proposed recent initiatives to improve the standard of sport in the UK.

1. To achieve excellence in sport, a high level of commitment, resources and expertise is necessary.

a. Explain these three conditions, using illustrations from your own experience in sport. *(6 marks)*

b. What is meant when a sport organisation is said to be elitist? Explain this in the context of a games club. *(4 marks)*

(Total 10 marks)

2. Sportscoach UK and the Youth Sports Trust are agencies designed to improve standards in British sport. Explain how they attempt to achieve this and the constraints they face. *(8 marks)*

3. Even in the UK not all games have the same opportunity to achieve excellence. Why is it that badminton appears to attract far less money than tennis in Britain but neither seems able to produce world champions? *(7 marks)*

17.2 Institutional: outdoor education

The issue

There is an accountability argument as to whether the expense and time needed for outdoor education are justified by the experience it offers. It might be suggested that the objectives would be better served through a recreational programme. At an administrative level, the issue is whether a particular society's outdoor education programme can be improved by looking at other systems.

Definitive

Formal education

This is an **institutional** focus. Concern is with what happens in a school or college. It may be part of the curriculum or part of the intramural or extracurricular activity of the institution.

Informal education

A broader concept of education acknowledges that there is a form of social education operating when recreational **institutions** exist to promote a particular lifestyle, where the outcome may be a transmission of desirable cultural values.

Outdoor education

This is a means of approaching educational or cultural objectives through direct experiences in the natural environment, using its resources as learning materials.

In all recent school curriculum documents, the term **outdoor and adventurous education** has been used. This may be to avoid some outdoor activity being

wrongly assigned but it also identifies the focus of the activities. There are occasions when very young children may go no farther than the playground to taste adventurous activity and in these cases the natural hazardous environment is replaced by contrived challenging situations.

Outdoor pursuits

These are physical activities in the natural environment which place the individual in decision-making adventure situations and as such are a central part of outdoor education.

Vacation camps

Though recreational, these offer adventure situations in the natural environment and indirectly promote the same values as outdoor education centres.

Escape

There is a strong feeling of escape: from work, from urban existence, as a holiday; as a return to rural simplicity and basic survival; as a return to one's cultural roots; but also as romantic and/or religious awareness of natural beauty, which is an escape to enlightenment.

Desired values

These are outlined in Figure 17.15.

Structure

This is outlined in Figure 17.17.

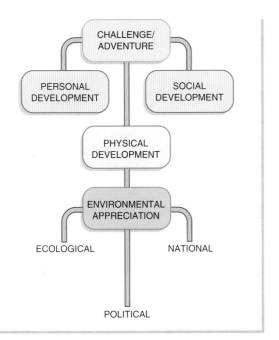

Fig. 17.15 Desired values of outdoor education.

Fig. 17.16 Decision making in adventure situations. Photographer Helen Roscoe.

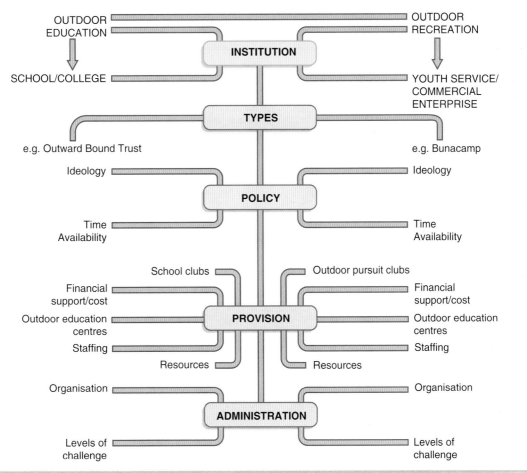

Fig. 17.17 Structure of outdoor education.

Function

Policy and practice in schools

1. Outdoor activity curriculum programmes in primary, secondary and higher education departments.
2. Extracurricular and/or intramural clubs in outdoor activities.
3. Schools and/or colleges with special interests in outdoor activities, e.g. Gordonstoun and Charlotte Mason College (St Martin's College, Ambleside, Lancaster University).

Policy and practice in outdoor education centres

1. Outdoor centres belonging to specific schools.
2. Local government outdoor education centres.
3. National outdoor education centres, e.g. Plas y Brenin and Holme Pierrepont.
4. Outward Bound Trust and other adventure schools, e.g. Aberdovey.

Policy and practice of specific associations and schemes

1. Youth associations and their facilities, e.g. Scouts, Pioneers, etc.
2. Adventure youth schemes, e.g. Duke of Edinburgh Award.

Organisation of outdoor recreation holiday schemes

1. State-sponsored outdoor facilities, e.g. Pioneer camps, former USSR, and Colonie de Vacance, France.
2. Commercially sponsored facilities, e.g. Manor Adventure, UK, and Bunacamp, USA.

Organisation of natural areas of beauty

1. Administration of national and local parks.
2. Promotion of conservation.

Cultural determinants

These are outlined in Figure 17.18.

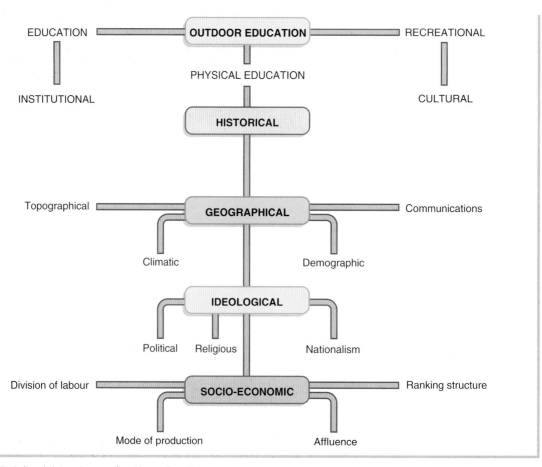

Fig. 17.18 Cultural determinants of outdoor education.

Reformative

Development potential

1. Can we improve the relationship between physical education and outdoor education?
2. How might we usefully improve outdoor education in and around the school?
3. How might the function of outdoor education centres be improved?
4. How might we extend special schools?
5. How might we broaden opportunities for summer camps and winter holidays for children?
6. How might we communicate the message of conservation more effectively?

Investigation 17.2   Outdoor education institutions

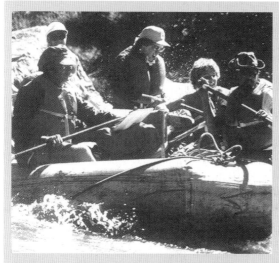

What are the fundamental differences between a camp school and an Outward Bound school in the USA and how did these compare with a Soviet Pioneer camp (Figures 17.19 and 17.20)?

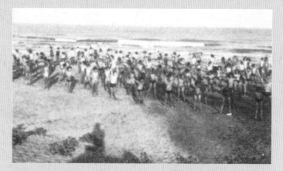

Fig. 17.19 An adventure situation on the Colorado.

Fig. 17.20 Orlyonok camp on the Black Sea.

Constraints which might operate

1. Limits imposed by our educational and physical educational philosophies and administrations.
2. Cultural resistance to the introduction of foreign methods.
3. Limits imposed by the geographical determinants.

Final comments

There appears to be a serious attempt to educate young people to respect and conserve the natural environment. This education is particularly necessary in a world that is becoming increasingly materialistic and where population expansion puts the natural environment at risk. In a world which is becoming increasingly urbanised and technological, there is a need for a renaissance of rusticity on the one hand and the opportunity for adventure on the other.

The model used for this analysis should be adaptable to any major institutional issue. It need not be limited to education but could focus on industry or the armed forces, where one facet of an institution may have to operate alongside others.

There are a number of **educational issues** that are worthy of analysis. Most of these are linked with **sport education**, a term used regularly in Australia and reflecting the place of sport on the school curriculum. TOP sport and other YST programmes, sports colleges and Raising the Game are UK policies and programmes which are now being implemented. Alternatively, there are major areas of education which can be looked at, such as undergraduate programmes, teacher training, play and nursery education and coach education. Finally, there are other institutions which involve physical education and sports issues, such as sport and the Army, sport and industry, sports injuries and physiotherapy.

Review questions

1. Justify the inclusion of outdoor and adventurous education on the national physical education curriculum in the UK.

2. What progressions would you expect to see in programmes in outdoor and adventurous education from key stage 1 to A-Level Physical Education (OCR)?

3. Explain the qualities of the Sports Mark and Top Sport as the first steps towards an integrated programme of **sport education**.

4. Describe the organisation of English sports colleges.

5. Discuss the potential and constraints of the John Major Initiative as identified in *Sport: raising the game*.[1]

6. Discuss the modularisation and study of **sport** and **physical education** in higher education.

Exam-style questions

1. Many people have classified different sports by identifying certain characteristics which they feel are central components. P C McIntosh suggested that there were five key characteristics: competition, combat, conquest, aesthetic and chance.

   a. Explain a canoeing or climbing **outdoor pursuit** in the context of conquest. *(4 marks)*

   b. In the context of this outdoor pursuit, explain the potential existence of the other four characteristics. *(5 marks)*

   (Total 9 marks)

2. According to the Leeds Study Group,[2] **physical education** is an area of educational activity in which the main concern is with bodily movement.

   a. Given that this suggests both physical development and the development of temperament, explain the particular contribution outdoor education can make within the physical education programme. *(4 marks)*

   b. You are leading a group of young people on a canoeing or climbing expedition. Explain the difference between real and perceived risk. *(4 marks)*

   (Total 8 marks)

3. The high population density of the UK results in a conflict between different agencies in the countryside. Identify the problems and suggest strategies for:

   a. Problems arising in outdoor adventurous activities which have to share limited provision *(3 marks)*

   b. The potential conflicts between **recreation** and **conservation**. *(5 marks)*

   (Total 8 marks)

17.3 Subcultural: women in sport

The issue

In many societies women do not have an equal opportunity to participate in sport. It is necessary to tease out the differences in role from culturally induced discrimination and to look at other countries to see if we can learn from them.

Definitive

It is important to recognise that this is not fundamentally a sport issue but a case of social inequality which also manifests itself in sport.

The physiological differences between males and females are the source of sexual stereotyping but cultural traditions and trends distort and exaggerate the male and female roles in society to the extent that basic freedoms are denied.

Where social inequality exists, the forces of a democratic society can press for reform. However, an additional problem exists when social inequality is justified on biological grounds and a policy is enacted which presumes women's predisposition for certain sports.

In Britain, for example, the resistance to women's soccer is based on traditional stereotyping and the conservatism of the Football Association (FA). This does not appear to be the case in the USA, where the game is played by both sexes largely because it is a recent innovation and does not rival the prestigious male preserve of grid iron football. In the former Soviet Union, the 'official' view was that women's soccer was physiologically harmful and morally degrading and every effort was made to discourage it. The view that certain sports undermine femininity is the most difficult to overcome, because it often has the support of many women.

The differentiation of sex roles in society stems from the traditional notion of family life. This tradition recognises the role of the woman as a wife and mother, where her leisure time is committed to home and family. Though it was originally very much a middle-class concept, it became a feature of the respectable working-class family, replacing the survival role of the wife as a bread-winner. The development of this stereotype coincided with the emergence of modern sport and this resulted in a dominance by men. However, career women now render the stereotype outmoded.

It is easy to see this as a female problem but when sex discrimination operates it can result in constraints on males as well as females, as certain sports are considered feminine and so unsuitable for men.

It is this feminine stereotype in sport and society at large which prevents freedom of the individual to operate and so 'women in sport' will remain an issue until every person is free to participate in a full range of sports with equal support from the community.

There are a number of routes which may be taken to increase female opportunity in sport. The right to participate could include the right to remain separate from mixed sport but the choice must be available to the individual. The American Title IX legislation (1972) presumed that for children to have an equal opportunity in an unequal culture, physical education had to be co-educational. The problem with a categorical decision like this is that it stimulates a counteraction from male teachers, who see sports standards slipping. The fact that Title IX applies only to federally aided institutions also presents another anomaly but there are few educational institutions which do not receive some federal support financially.

There are a large number of myths about the capacity of women to cope in sport. Many of these are being refuted, as illustrated by the successful inclusion of a women's marathon in the 1988 Olympic Games, but it is a slow process of eroding traditional attitudes. In Britain, the Equal Pay Act (1970) and the Sex Discrimination Act (1975) now allow women in sport to go to court if their rights are abused but it is important to recognise that sex discrimination in itself is not unlawful, only instances where discrimination creates financial consequences. In addition, Section 44 makes concessions in cases:

> where the physical strength, stamina or physique of the average woman puts her at a disadvantage to the average man ... as a competitor...

This clause may have been designed to protect the female but can be used to exclude her (Figure 17.21). Similarly, Rule 29 of the Olympic Charter (1983) states that female competitors must be registered female. These so-called sex tests may have been designed to protect genuine female competitors but feminists might want to know why males should not also be tested.

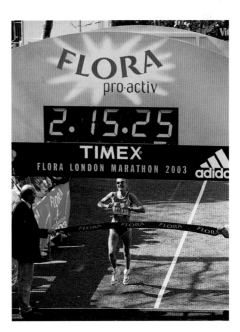

Fig. 17.21 Paula Radcliffe long distance superstar wins the 2003 Flora London Marathon in a world record time. Photographer Chris Brown/Action Plus

Structure

This is outlined in Figure 17.22.

Function

It is worthwhile to consider function in terms of the UK, France, the USA, Australia and the former Soviet Union.

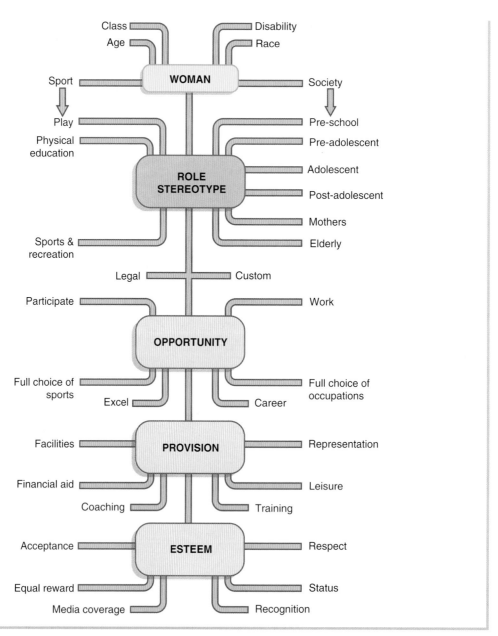

Fig. 17.22 Structure to illustrate the place of women in sport and society.

Policy and practice in school PE programmes

1. Inequalities in the PE curriculum.
2. Inequalities in extracurricular sport.
3. Inequalities in outdoor education.

Policy and practice in Sport for All programmes

1. Differences in proportional involvement.
2. Differences in the availability of facilities.
3. Differences in the variety of activities.

Policy and practice in sports excellence programmes

1. Variations in selection and coaching.
2. Variations in the distribution of financial aid and income.
3. Variations in career possibilities in sport.

Organisational inequalities

1. Sporting activities not open to females.
2. Sporting activities where sexes are not mixed.
3. Sporting activities where female involvement is taboo.

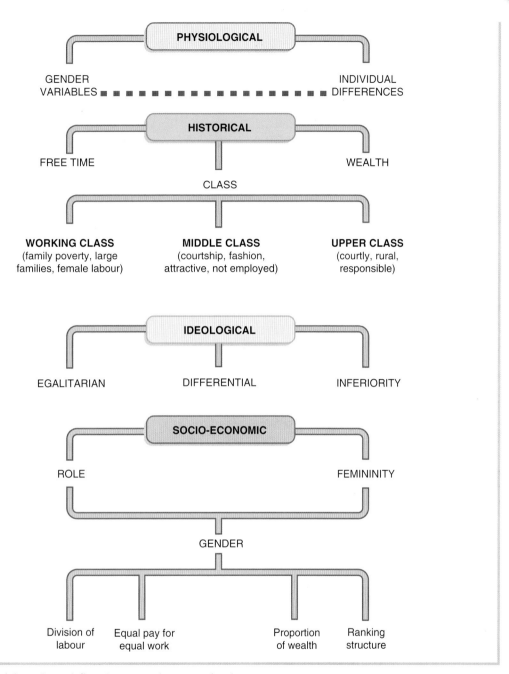

Fig. 17.23 Cultural determinants influencing women in sport and society.

Cultural determinants

These are outlined in Figure 17.23.

Reformative

Development potential
1. What might we usefully change at school level?
2. What organisational and financial improvements might we adopt?

> **REFORMATIVE?**
>
> It takes a great deal of courage and independence to decide to design your own image instead of the one that society rewards, but it gets easier as you go along.
>
> Germaine Greer, *The female eunuch*, 1971

3. How might we change things at a personal and status level?

Constraints which might operate
1. Cultural resistance to the imposition of foreign methods.
2. Unacceptable influence on the status quo.

Final comments

The right of the individual to a free choice of legitimate activities or lifestyles is a cornerstone of a free society. As yet, these rights are not being observed in the context of women in sport. Even if social attitudes are slow to change, there can be no excuse for administrational and financial discrimination to operate. The different contribution that men and women bring to sport enriches the total experience. What is at fault is the singular stereotype of what it is to be a sportsperson.

The model used for this analysis should be adaptable to any major area of discrimination in physical education, sport or outdoor recreation. Other recommended issues for study in this category are ethnic minorities, people with special needs, opportunities for the unemployed, social class discrimination, opportunities for the elderly, potential abuse of young people and regional discrimination. It is essential to acknowledge, however, that these exist on an opportunity ladder, sometimes called cultural stacking, whereby multiples of problems arise; for example, an elderly woman with special needs meets problems from three sources at least (see Further Reading).

Finally, although these are contemporary problems in our society, the source of the issue lies in the past and the solution may lie in other countries, so you must use knowledge from historical and comparative sources to help produce reformative strategies.

There are a number of theoretical principles which need to be explored in the context of subcultures and subsystems in the context of inequality.

1. No **culture** is homogeneous and even within egalitarian societies, inequalities are either caused by unfair **systems** or by advantaged attitudes of certain individuals and subcultures; this is normally reflected in **sport**. This social phenomenon is called **hegemony**.
2. The British upper class is traditionally so privileged that they do not enter the public arena in society or sport.
3. The **advantaged** public group in society and sport is the 23–30-year-old **white, able-bodied, middle-class male**.
4. This gives us a number of disadvantaged subcultures: young and elderly, women, the disabled, a variety of ethnic minorities and individuals and families caught in a poverty trap as members of the so-called working classes and/or unemployed.
5. The three main dimensions in the investigation of these disadvantaged subcultures are constraints on **opportunity**, **provision** and **esteem**.
6. Recognise the two-way process of society imposing sanctions on certain people but also certain people acquiescing in an acceptance of inferiority **or** claiming to be different **or** claiming disinterest.
7. The **radical** group within a disadvantaged subculture is often quite small because of the risk of ridicule and isolation.
8. There will always be resistance from a **conservative** elite who will lose advantage by accepting equality. Radicals suggest that this may arise from feelings of inferiority if the traditional advantages are removed.
9. Though not mentioned, **cultural tradition** and **religion** can also play a major part as illustrated by the limited number of **Moslem women** who participate in sport in this country.
10. Recognise that discrimination seldom comes singly: **women** in **sport** are disadvantaged but don't forget the **young girl** or **elderly woman**, the woman from a poor family, the **black woman** or the **disabled woman** and, perhaps worst of all, the **battered woman**. Each constraining feature reduces opportunity and self-esteem.

Review questions

These have been directed towards physical education but could be adjusted to review subcultural influences on sport and recreation in society.

1. **Girls and physical education in schools.**

a. What are the links between self-esteem and girls' reluctance to participate in school sport?
b. What is the place of rugby football for girls in the PE curriculum?

▶

► c. Can girls throw or not?

d. Is there a possibility that girls are threatening the notion that sport makes boys into men in school PE?

e. Is separatism the answer for girls' PE?

2. **Ethnic minorities and physical education in schools**.

a. What do you say to the young Afro-Caribbean child during the swimming lesson?

b. How do you rationalise the problem of teaching Moslem girls to swim?

c. Can you separate society from culture and explain the case of a Pakistani child supporting the Pakistan cricket team when they are on tour in this country?

d. What effect does Linford Christie continue to have on the aspirations of black schoolboys?

e. How is physical education countering the resistance to the production of male Asian footballers and female Asian hockey players?

3. **Young children and sporting excellence**.

a. What are the problems of early specialisation in tennis and why do we do it?

b. What are the dangers of training methods used by some gymnastic coaches and some PE teachers?

c. Can we be physical educators and teach gamesmanship in our extracurricular sessions?

d. What risks are we taking when we treat children like little adults?

e. What are the advantages of integrating recreative notions of play with educative notions of personal development?

4. **Disability and adaptive physical education**.

a. Integration or separation in physical education: what are the pros and cons?

b. Explain the reasons for allowing an able-bodied tennis player to play a wheelchair player.

c. What are your experiences of limitations of **access** for an impaired person in a PE, school or sport situation?

d. What are your views on the encouragement of wheelchair basketball for the able-bodied in any club you run?

e. To what extent does a child with impairments suffer from 'a cycle of oppression' in his or her experience of sport in school?

Some problems occur because disadvantaged subcultures do not easily adjust into society, so some groups are not directly involved in formal schooling and thus some additional questions arise.

5. **The elderly and sport**.

a. Should we attempt to integrate or separate elderly people who wish to be physically active?

b. How can we separate the elderly from the stereotype often held in sport?

c. How might the notion of **veteran** in sport enhance the club scene?

d. Examine the presumption that to be elderly is to be senile.

e. What strategies can we adopt to establish a lifetime sport concept for all citizens?

6. **Some mixed 'smart' questions in sport**.

a. Young at heart is not a question of chronological age in sport. Discuss.

b. 'Let's not patronise people by watering down able-bodied sports, but allow an alternative focus to evolve.' Discuss.

c. What are the genuine links between the athletic and the cosmetic in female sport?

d. 'Let's escape from the constraints of centrality and stacking and allow people to follow their inclinations and talents in sport.' Discuss.

Some of the answers may lie in looking at the privileged group in our society, i.e. wealthy young white males and their masculine identity in sport.

7. a. To what extent is sport a social construction of **masculinity**?

b. Can it be true that sport turns boys into men?

c. Muscles and morality: does the achievement of manhood involve physical prowess combined with moral integrity?

d. **Masculine or effeminate**? Does sport empower young men to demonstrate force and physical skill (manliness from experiencing their bodies in action) as against sensitivity and appearance which dictates femininity (leading to the demeaning and objectifying of women)?

e. Is it really a question of male vulnerability and is there a basic case of women threatening men's traditional roles in our society in the name of sporting equality.

Exam-style questions

1. In 1982, the Sports Council released figures which suggested that the relative popularity of sport varied within different socio-economic groups. Suggest reasons why the middle-class professional group has participated in sport more than members of the unskilled group. *(4 marks)*

2. The Sports Council uses the term **target group** in encouraging Sport for All.

a. What is the meaning of the term **target group**? Identify sections of the community who fit into it. *(4 marks)*

▶ **b.** What are the strategies recommended by the Sports Council? *(4 marks)*

(Total 8 marks)

3. The concept of excellence in sport is often accused of being elitist – it can mean that certain groups of people are disadvantaged.

   a. Select one such group and explain how their access is limited in terms of reaching the top in sport. *(4 marks)*

b. Explain the part played by self-esteem and role modelling in influencing participation at the top level by your chosen group. Use a sporting example to illustrate your answer. *(4 marks)*

(Total 8 marks)

4. Discuss the cultural factors which are responsible for such inequalities still existing in sport in the UK. Refer to any disadvantaged group in your answer. *(5 marks)*

References

1. DNH 1995 *Sport: raising the game*. Department of National Heritage, London
2. Leeds Study Group 1970 Conference paper

Further reading

Societal: excellence in sport

Anthony D 1980 *A strategy for British sport*. Hurst, London
Calhoun D W 1987 *Sport, culture and personality*. Human Kinetics, Champaign, Illinois
Cashmore E 1996 *Making sense of sport*. Routledge, London
Coakley J J 1998 *Sport in society: issues and controversies*, 6th edn. McGraw Hill, Boston, Massachusetts
Coe S et al. 1992 *More than a game*. BBC, London
Cummins G 1993 *Drugs in sport project*. Manchester Metropolitan University, Manchester
Dunning E G et al (eds) 1993 *The sports process*. Human Kinetics, Champaign, Illinois
Elias N, Dunning E 1986 *Quest for excitement*. Blackwell, Oxford
French Information 1985 *125 sports in France*. French Embassy, London
Hargreaves J 1986 *Sport, power and culture*. Polity Press, Cambridge
Hemery D 1986 *Sporting excellence*. Willow, London
Hoolihan B 1991 *The government and politics of sport*. Routledge, London
Hoolihan B 1994 *Sport and international politics*. Harvester Wheatsheaf, London
Lapchick R E 1996 *Sport in society*. Sage, Thousand Oaks, California
Lawton J 1984 *The American war game*. Basil Blackwell, Oxford
Macfarlane N 1986 *Sport and politics*. Willow, London
McPherson B D et al 1989 *The social significance of sport*. Human Kinetics, Champaign, Illinois
Nixon H L 1984 *Sport and the American dream*. Leisure Press, New York
Riordan J 1977 *Sport in Soviet society*. Cambridge University Press, Cambridge
Roscoe D A, Roscoe J V, Honeybourne J, Davis R, Galligan F 2003 *Physical education and sport studies AS/A2 level student revision guide*. 3rd edn. Jan Roscoe Publications, Widnes
Sage G H 1998 *Power and ideology in American sport*, 2nd edn. Human Kinetics, Champaign, Illinois
Sports Council 1995 *New horizons*. Sports Council, London
Sports Council 1997 *England, the sporting nation*. English Sports Council, London
Walton G M 1992 *Beyond winning*. Leisure Press, Champaign, Illinois

Youth Sports Trust 1998 *You can be part of our sporting future*. Youth Sports Trust, Loughborough
Youth Sports Trust 1998 *Bringing sports to life*. Youth Sports Trust, Loughborough

Institutional: outdoor education

Almond L et al 1994 *An introduction to implementing the physical education curriculum: a practical guide*. Loughborough, 17878/159
Bank J 1983 *Outdoor development*. Leadership and Organisation Development Journal 4(3):
Department of Education and Science 1983 *Learning out of doors*. HMSO, London
DSE 1993 *Physical and sport education for Victorian schools*. Directorate of School Education, Melbourne
Gray D 1977 *Access to open country*. Sport and Recreation 18(3):
Johnson A 1979 *School it isn't: education it is*. School Sport 4(4):
Journal of Health, Physical Education and Recreation (editorials) *Intramurals*, February 1983; *Leisure and tourism*, April 1983; *Family recreation*, October 1984; *Leisure today*, October 1988
Manor Adventure (brochure). The Manor, Craven Arms, Shropshire
Mason T 1993 *Only a game*. Cambridge University Press, Cambridge
Mortlock C 1984 *The adventure alternative*. Cicerone, Milnthorpe, Cumbria
Mottram D R 2003 *Drugs in sport*, 3rd edn. E & F N Spon, London
Rhudy E 1979 *An alternative to outward bound programmes*. Journal of Health, Physical Education and Recreation, January
Voy R 1991 *Drugs, sport and politics*. Human Kinetics, Champaign, Illinois
Youth Sports Trust 1998 *You can be part of our sporting future*. Youth Sports Trust, Loughborough
Youth Sports Trust 1998 *Bringing sport to life*. Youth Sports Trust, Loughborough

Recommended periodicals

Jeunesse au Plein Air
Journal of Health, Physical Education and Recreation
Outdoors (PEA)

Age

Gleeson G 1986 *The growing child in competitive sport*. Hodder and Stoughton, Sevenoaks

Grisogono V 1991 *Children and sport*. John Murray, London

Sports Council 1994 *Young people and sport in England*. Sports Council, London

Sports Council 1994 *All to play for 50+*. Sports Council, London

Disability

Butterfield S A 1991 *PE and sport for the deaf*. Adapted Physical Activity Quarterly 8:

Department of the Environment 1989 *Sport for people with disabilities*. HMSO, London

National Coaching Foundation 1990 *Coaching people with a disability*. NCF, Leeds

Race

Allison L (ed) 1986 *The politics of sport*. Manchester University Press, Manchester

Cashmore E 1982 *Black sportsmen*. Routledge and Kegan Paul, London

Sports Council 1991 *Sport and racial equality*. Sports Council, London

Sports Council 1993 *Black and ethnic minorities in sport*. Sports Council, London

Women

Birrell S, Cole C L 1994 *Women, sport and culture*. Human Kinetics, Champaign, Illinois

Blue A 1987 *Grace under pressure*. Sidgwick and Jackson, London

Editorial 1986 *The role of women in sports*. Journal of Health, Physical Education and Recreation, March:

Fletcher S 1983 *Women first: the female tradition in English physical education, 1890–1990*. Athlone Press, London

Lenskiyj H 1986 *Out of bounds. Women, sport and sexuality*. The Women's Press. Toronto

Mangan J A, Park R J 1987 *From 'fair sex' to feminism*. Frank Cass, London

Riordan J 1977 *Sport in Soviet society*. Cambridge University Press, Cambridge

Sports Council 1994 *Women in sport, people with disabilities, young people and sport (policy and frameworks for action)*. Sport and Leisure supplement. Sports Council, London

Talbot M 1982 *Women and leisure*. Sports Council, London

Women's Sports Foundation 1980–1996 *Women in sport booklets*. Women's Sports Foundation, London

General

Cashmore E 2000 *Making sense of sport*, 3rd edn. Routledge, London

Kew F 1997 *Sport, social problems and issues*. Butterworth Heinemann, Oxford

McPherson B D et al 1989 *Social significance of sport*. Human Kinetics, Champaign, Illinois

Polley M 1998 *Moving the goalposts*. Routledge, London

Sage G 1998 *Power and ideology in American sport*, 2nd edn. Human Kinetics, Champaign, Illinois

Multimedia

CD-roms

Davis R J 1999 *Contemporary issues*. Teachers' Guide. Private Pershaw, Worcs.

Roscoe D A, Roscoe J V, Honeybourne J, Davis R, Galligan F 2003 *Physical education and sports studies AS/A2 level student revision guide*, 3rd edn. Jan Roscoe Publications, Widnes

Glossary of terms

academies though this term is used to describe centres of sporting excellence, particularly in Australia, the normal use in the UK is to describe football schools being run by Premiership and League soccer clubs to improve local standards in boys' football.

adventure the challenge of entering the unknown to test oneself, existing at the upper level of competence, where to go beyond this is to risk misadventure.

ageism discrimination over age; in sport this tends to be at the two extremes of young people and the elderly, where both are target groups for Sport England.

agencies bodies working under the Sports Council(s) and individual governing bodies to facilitate sport in the UK. The main three are the National Coaching Foundation, the Sports Youth Trust and the Sports Aid Foundation.

amateurism the participation in sport for the love of it rather than for extrinsic gain

assimilation the absorption of different cultural groups into a single society. It can be an ideal form of equality or it can be conditioned by an authoritarian government.

challenge a primary element of competition in sport, where targets are set and enthusiastically achieved to test oneself physically and temperamentally.

chance an essential element of all sport in that the result is not predetermined. Huizinga characteristic.

civilisation the development and stabilising of a society to reflect a set of higher values.

combat in sport, the level of experience where the performer is at risk from physical and mental danger.

combats a profile of specific activities where physical contact occurs as part of the codification, with a view to testing character through sport.

competition in sport, it is a contract to compete with and against time, distance, height, other competitors, the environment and self for intrinsic and possibly extrinsic reasons.

conquest a challenging contest where you achieve a new level of experience.

contest a challenging experience where you can win or lose to a chosen opponent.

crowd behaviour a large congested group of people, where individual identity is lost in an excess of emotion and is often driven by a specific motive where behaviour reflects that of the lowest member of that crowd.

culture represents the accepted behaviour patterns of a stable society. In all cultures there are subcultures or minority groups which retain a level of separate identity and may be on a social, racial or gender basis.

disability on an ability–disability continuum, we all have special needs. Our disabilities should be recognised in facilitating access to sport but unfortunately, society still handicaps the less able.

drugs in sport taking drugs to enhance performance is unethical, a health risk, illegal and a dangerous role model.

education can be the drawing out of knowledge and understanding or the inculcation of knowledge and values, depending on the liberal or authoritarian bias of the society.

elitism the policy to give unfair advantage to privileged members of society. In our case it is a focus on excellence in sport, where disproportionate funding is limited to an exclusive group of sports or performers.

emergent a complex society which has moved out of the tribal stage of development and is focused on nation building, the integration of its tribal groups, concern over public health and a strong desire to defend its cultural and political status.

enigma the mystery or puzzle that sport can sometimes hold for you. Huizinga characteristic.

exultation a feeling of great joy after a wonderful experience. Huizinga characteristic.

ethnic sports are traditional sports festivals which are localised and have unique features. They range from grand rural sports like the Highland Games to mob games and specific pastimes like the 'obby oss' in Padstow.

fair play a moral contract to play within the letter and spirit of the rules.

fundamental motor skills is a programme for primary school physical education adopted in progressive schools as a copy of an Australian programme and recognising the need for young children to learn a series of basic skills such as throwing, catching, kicking, cartwheels, etc.

game a contrived competitive activity based on fixed rules and with a beginning and end.

games there are three main profiles offered: invasion games, where territory is gained to score goals, e.g. soccer; target/striking games, where these two roles are played alternately, e.g. cricket; and court games, where a net/wall separates players in alternate play, e.g. tennis.

hegemony an unusual term used to describe a society where there is an ascendent power group, e.g. the WASP dominance in the USA.

high culture a subculture which reflects the highest values in a society and associated with privilege, intellect and art.

high performance centres are new centres with the highest quality of facilities, designed to satisfy the needs of elite performers in the UK. It is intended to have at least 8 in England for squad training and scientific research programmes, but some provision is made for use by local performers.

institutes of sport is the new title for the administration of elite sport in the UK. There is to be one in each of the home countries with the resonsibility of programming the high performance centres and developing sport research.

institution an organisation which functions within a society, but has some focus and values which do not necessarily match that society, e.g. educational institutions.

leisure more than an activity, it is an experience in free time where there is the opportunity to choose.

minorities normally, we identify social class, race, gender, age and disability as the main minority groups but some societies would involve regional and religious. In each case the focus is one of discrimination.

Olympic Games is the quadrennial global games, which represents the biggest multi-sport competition and functions within an acknowledged Olympic code.

outdoor education a controlled, adventurous, educational experience of the outdoors, normally involving the natural environment.

outdoor pursuits experiences which normally involve specific activities in the natural environment at an adventurous level.

outdoor recreation an experience in the natural environment which is adventurous, but based on the notions of freedom and fun.

outward bound a challenging and adventurous approach to the outdoors as a character-building experience which is supported by a specific organisation/trust.

personal development an experience involving self-realisation and socialisation, where there may be physical, cognitive, moral, emotional and aesthetic elements involved in the learning process.

physical education (1) a field of study which includes play, physical recreation, sport and institutionalised physical education.

physical education (2) formal inculcation of knowledge and values in, about and through physical activities in an educational institution.

physical endeavour the desire to do one's best in any physically challenging sporting situation by virtue of being physically prepared in terms of fitness and positive attitudes.

physical prowess the ability to utilise general skilfulness and specific skills in a challenging sporting situation and the ability to use strategies to facilitate these skills.

physical recreation physical activity of a relaxing nature with limited organisational structure and in an atmosphere of freedom and fun.

pluralism established in a society where individual subcultures are encouraged to retain their ethnicity. Particularly common in the USA where you not only have New Yorkers but Irish-American New Yorkers.

professionalism earning one's living from sport, where intrinsic values tend to be dwarfed by the full-time commitment in sport with all the commercial connotations this brings with it.

quest the ultimate target of people engaged in sporting activity where memorable moments of high personal and/or team achievement are experienced.

racism the discrimination against certain ethnic minorities to the extent that in sport and society, these people do not have equal access in terms of opportunity, provision and esteem.

recreation a positive activity in a leisure context, where the freedom and fun make it a worthwhile experience.

risk part of all sporting activity, it is part of the dynamic of self-testing in an adventurous situation and while on occasions these risks are real, they are often only perceived.

separatism the separation of subcultures to allow coexistence of each one. The example of apartheid in South Africa demonstrated that if one group is advantaged others become more disadvantaged in this system. This can go beyond economic discrimination into the racial hatred reflected in ethnic cleansing.

society the structural basis of a country, reflecting its traditions, administration and policy.

sport best described through a triple analysis of certain activities which are highly structured and which involve attitudes of considerable commitment. Within this context there is normally the duality of sport and sportsmanship, given that the organisation and associated attitudes are morally based.

Sport for All a campaign organised to increase mass participation in sport.

sporting excellence exists at two levels: the identification of an elite few who aspire to be champions and the notion of personal achievement where each individual can strive to reach their optimal level of performance.

sports colleges these are the latest developments in special schools (DfEE) where each community is being encouraged to apply for special provision as beacon schools in a locality, where they stimulate feeder primary schools, support other secondary schools and develop major community links.

sportsmanship the belief that rational sport can only usefully exist in an atmosphere of fair play, where the spirit of play is more important than winning at all costs.

systems the means by which a society functions: normally political, economic, social systems, but can include institutions, e.g. educational systems.

tribal the most elemental division of a community or country, where the society and its cultural development is at a specific (primitive) level, e.g. Samoan culture and its commitment to rugby football.

vertigo a feeling of giddiness which accompanies an unusual experience, e.g. exposure in a high rock climb. Huizinga characteristic.

Physical education and sport on the continent of Europe with particular reference to France

18

Learning objectives

On completion of this section, you will be able to:

1. Develop a global perspective, particularly as it concerns the European Community.

2. Appreciate the shared and specific cultural variables which exist in France and Britain.

3. Be aware of the structure and function of physical education in France and links between school sport and the community.

4. Understand the basis of French sport and the reasons for their recent successes.

5. Appreciate the concept of *le plein air* as an expression of French love of rural France.

The increasing significance of global studies in the context of physical education and sport, with the academic links through international studies programmes, makes it essential that we have a general grasp of similarities and differences, traditions and trends and cultural development from tribal through emergent to advanced societies.

The tribal and emergent countries have already been reviewed in Chapter 16 and the following four chapters will focus on four advanced societies as part of a synoptic analysis reflecting developments in the United Kingdom. At the same time, with world focus so much on reforming programmes and getting the best for each national community, nations are continually looking at other countries to help them to re-evaluate their own policies and practices. There are dangers in this procedure which we must be aware of, not least because each country has built up its own cultural characteristics which directly influence development and where conflicting cultural features in different countries can make the borrowing of policies unproductive and undesirable.

It is also important not to work within a structure of separate countries but recognise the historical, geographical and sociocultural ties which exist between some groups of nations.

18.1 The social setting of physical education and sport in France

We need to have a knowledge of the **cultural background** before we can hope to understand how organised physical activity functions in different societies. We will call these influences **cultural determinants** and look at them under three main headings: **geographical**, **historical** and **socio-economic**.

In all these three determinants European countries have considerable common elements, ranging from topographical and communicational environmental links to a history of tribal movement eventually leading to nation building. There has been constant rivalry and outright aggression and the development of sport festivals on a European scale and the recent emergence of an economic community had been temporarily limited by the divide caused by the Cold War.

Geographical influences on physical education and sport in France

Geography is a very broad field of study, but is limited in the analysis here to comments on population, land area, topography, climate, urbanisation and communications in the context of sport and physical education.

Population

The population growth for France from 1931 to 2001 is shown in Table 18.1. The ethnic minority (so-called foreign residents) was approximately 2% in 1982, mainly North African Arabs and Portuguese. The population of 60 million in 2001 is misleading in the sports context because France claims access to elite performers from Greater France. These overseas departments have a population of 58 million

Size

The area of France is 210 000 square miles. In comparative terms, France and the UK have populations of approximately the same size but France is twice as large, with the result that provincial France retains its rural nature.

Topography

A wide plain covers half the country, with the Massif Central, a mountainous plateau, in the centre. The Alps are famous for winter sports and climbing and there are numerous canoeing rivers in the Massif Central. An extensive coastline makes sailing and other water sports as popular in France as in Britain.

Climate

This is much more varied than in Britain, with *Western maritime* in Normandy and Brittany, *Continental* inland from Paris, *Alpine* in the mountainous areas and *Mediterranean* along the South coast. The French follow a clear pattern of winter skiing holidays in the Alps and seaside summer holidays on the Landes (Atlantic) and Mediterranean coasts.

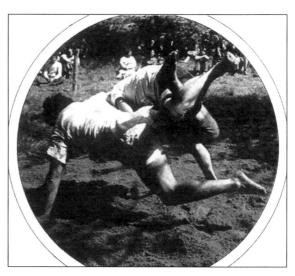

Fig. 18.1 Breton wrestling (125 Sports in France, 1985).

Urbanisation

The population density is 108 per square km (less than half that of Britain). France is dominated by Paris but there is an industrialised North East, where soccer has been popular, and extensive vineyards in the South West, where the main game is rugby football. Ethnic activities include Breton wrestling (Figure 18.1), kick boxing or 'savate', boule or petanque (a form of street bowls) and pelota and bull fighting in Basque districts.

Communications

These are totally dominated by Paris, with roads and railways radiating from it. Marseilles, Le Havre, Nantes, Bordeaux and Rouen are the main ports, with numerous ferry ports along the English Channel. The country is geared for tourism but the French themselves tend to have fixed holidays at Eastertide and in July and/or August.

Historical influences on sport and physical education in France

The first comment about sport in France must belong to the high culture of Louis XIV and with it the extension of the 'courtly mould' and the art of fencing,

Table 18.1 French population growth[1]							
Year	*1931*	*1954*	*1962*	*1982*	*1989*	*1994*	*2001*
Population (millions)	42	43	47	54	56.2	58.3	60

Review questions

1. What are the significant features of rural France?

2. Explain the suggestion that communications in France are like the spokes of a wheel.

associated with the sophistication of real tennis in the 17th century.

This elite culture finally collapsed as a result of the French Revolution, which in turn led to the Napoleonic period. From this time, militarism and nationalism have dominated French physical activity, reflecting the phrase 'every Frenchman is born a soldier'.

As early as 1817, Amoros was invited to Paris to open a gymnasium to match the German and Scandinavian developments. It was built at Joinville and destined to be the centre of French military and sporting endeavour for well over a century.

By 1845 Clias was at Joinville, training school PT instructors as well as military personnel. Drill was central, particularly after France had lost a war with Prussia, but in 1887 Demeny identified therapeutic exercises and in 1906 Hebert introduced his 'Natural Method', a lasting influence partly because it so closely reflected the philosophy of Rousseau.

Teacher training, as we know it today, began at Joinville in 1920 and, in 1934, despite Hebert's condemnation of sport, attempts were made to quantify PE with a series of *brevets sportives* (tests). Throughout these years sport had been excluded from PE and even today PE is often known as 'la Gym'. Sports development consisted of popular recreations, as in England, but very clearly provincially orientated.

Conversely, rational recreations radiated from Paris and, stimulated by such aristocrats as Baron de Coubertin, amateur sport spread among the middle classes in the last quarter of the 19th century, based very much on the Olympic ideals.

Although professionalism did not occur in games, there were semi-professional cycling races between Rouen and Paris as early as 1869, which eventually developed into the Tour de France.

Sporting links with schools were established with the formation of the Association du Sport Scolaire et Universitaire (ASSU – School and University Sports Association), where university sports clubs helped in the coaching of school children, changing to the Union National du Sport Scolaire (UNSS – National Union of School Sport) in 1978.

The collapse of France in the Second World War, followed by failure in the 1952 Olympics, led to an upsurge of nationalism, which was encouraged by President de Gaulle.

M Herzog, alpinist, led a High Commission for Youth and Sport in 1958 to improve the organisation and finance of sport and this was followed in 1961 by a 4-year plan and £46.5 million to improve sports facilities nationwide.

Review question

1. Explain the dominance of gymnastics in French physical education.

Socio-economic factors influencing sport and physical education in France

Nationalism

France has a very strong sense of national identity, largely because of the constant threat from outside. In sporting terms this is more closely associated with amateur representation, as in rugby union, than with professional soccer and cycling, which are seen to be commercially based. Even in the case of rugby, however, appearances are deceptive. The French cockerel is displayed with great pride against England but a closer scrutiny shows that the players are largely drawn from provincial clubs in the South of the country, suggesting that the game has national appeal only when representing the 'tricolor'. There are similarities here with rugby league in the North of England. The recent professionalisation of rugby union has not reduced the nationalist appeal and the success at World Cup level of the French soccer team has made the game a focal part of French identity.

The extreme centralist administration was initially revised in 1982 with their devolutionary policy and in 1984 with their legislation which established regional and departmental bodies to coordinate the financial contributions from central and local government as well as private sources. This has had a dramatic recent effect on the devolution of education including physical education and the provision of sport for local and regional communities.

In France, as in Britain, there are powerful ethnic minorities, like the Basques and the Bretons, who are trying to maintain a cultural and a political identity. In addition to retaining their own language, there is a major attempt to revive many of their old ethnic sports.

A second comparative point is that sport and nationalism have never had political ties in England but President de Gaulle made French sport a rallying point for the revival of national pride.

Unlike the British, the French have always regarded their colonies as part of Greater France. Consequently, there is a substantial North African minority resident in the country with little evidence of discrimination in terms of sport participation. Significantly, middle-distance runner Said Aouita, the Moroccan Olympic

Review question

1. Compare the ways used by France and the United Kingdom to establish nationalism through sport.

gold medallist, received a great deal of his coaching in France. The make-up of the French soccer squad also demonstrates the number of Africans qualified to play for them.

Internationalism

Undoubtedly, the European Union has drawn Western Europe together in sporting and tourist links. More recently, commercial interests have broadened with several European soccer competitions and the European Athletics Grand Prix.

France also has the Tour de France cycle race, which is probably the biggest annual international event in Europe and which has included a UK stage – emphasising, with the Channel Tunnel, the ever-growing European unity. This is reflected in the number of European leagues and championships.

As a continental country, France has close sporting and recreative ties with various European countries: for example, the special relationship with Britain and Ireland in rugby union and horse racing; the shared winter sports and tourist amenity of the Alps and the business of attracting tourists to its Mediterranean resorts and casinos.

Political

A republic with an elected president, France tends to be identified as a bureaucracy. It is a Western democracy but has a larger number of minority parties than in the UK and a much wider political spectrum. There is a disturbingly influential right-wing Nationalist Party and an equally large Communist Party. This results in moderate parties having to establish coalitions with extremists to gain a majority. It is very much a mixed economy.

Finance and resources

Much less urban than the UK, France depends a great deal more on agriculture and the tourist industry.

The significance of sport in France can be measured in the increases in the size of the sports budget since 1958 (Figure 18.2), when President de Gaulle recognised the need to disproportionately fund sport. Additionally, in 1985 a sports lottery was introduced with an expected 3 billion francs available for sports federations and clubs each year. This political and economic support is reflected today in France's world status in cycling, fencing, judo, rugby union, soccer and tennis but also in the quality of urban sports facilities.

Discrimination

Cultural variables have inevitably led to certain groups being discriminated against in a specific community and in all European societies. Normally, whatever form this takes, it is reflected in a country's sport. There is a level of 'institutionalised discrimination' in France as in Britain. The traditional minority cultures of the Basques, Bretons and Normans continue to seek their own identity, much as the Welsh and Scots have done in the UK, and whereas immigration into Britain has been largely Caribbean and Asian, North Africans, particularly Algerians, are the dominant immigrant minority in France and there is a perceivable level of discrimination against them. However, there is a much broader racial spread in France than in the United Kingdom as a result of their colonial policy, which gave all members of 'colonial' France the right to French citizenship and allowed the home country to 'adopt' promising footballers and athletes from around the world.

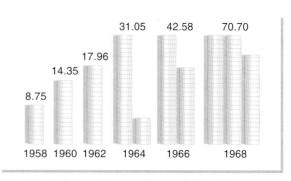

Fig. 18.2 Evolution of the French sports budget (francs).

Review question

1. Discuss the role of different football codes in international relations in France.

Review question

1. Discuss the influence of government aid on sport in France.

18.2 The administration of physical education in France

The traditional structure of the French educational system is similar to that in the UK in that it has a private and state sector, where private schools have tended to attract a wealthier clientele. However, French private schools and colleges are largely Roman Catholic institutions whereas in Britain, though many private schools have church associations, only a minority are directly managed by church bodies. A second similarity has been the gradual change in the state sector from a tripartite system, where the *lycée* (grammar school) had considerable status, to a predominantly comprehensive system (Table 18.2). As in Britain, the private sector has been left relatively unchanged by successive governments and has retained the attraction of *lycées* in a society which values intellectualism.

The French educational system remains **centralised** and as such it has a uniform, authoritarian basis which makes it totally different from the British model in decision-making terms (Figure 18.3). Any structural analysis, therefore, must start from the government and involves government-administered official instruction. The communication of these directives is carried out by regional authorities but, unlike the British equivalent, policy is implemented and not initiated at this level. The 1984 Regional and Departmental Administration Acts changed this to some extent in that although most of the funding continued to come from central government, regional and departmental (county) administrations were given the right to coordinate and distribute administrative and financial contributions. As a result of this devolution, a much more effective level of local administration and funding was achieved and with it the provision of staffing and facilities to meet local needs.

The present organisation of physical education dates from the 1967 Official Instructions and in 1969 new provisions in respect of PE and sport in schools were made in a weekly timetable in primary and secondary schools. This is called the **programme** and is a syllabus equivalent. The credibility gap mentioned in the British situation certainly operates in the presentation of this programme. Schools are required to teach it but human resources, such as the quality of teaching, and physical resources, such as equipment, do not always allow this to happen.

Central authority structure

Unlike the British system of virtual head teacher autonomy, administration is directed through bureaucratic channels (see Figure 18.3). Similarly, unlike the British local inspectorate and advisers, the French regional director and his inspectors had little autonomy until 1984.

The most obvious example of centralist policy was in the '*tiers-temps pedagogique*' – primary instructions that 6 hours per week should be devoted to PE and sport (Table 18.3). A practising French teacher from Brive suggested in 1987 that this was a 'beautiful dream'. However, he did say that the problem over physical resources was much less than in the 1970s. He claimed that 'infant school children' in the area had about 6 hours of PE a week and primary school children between 1 and 3 hours. He suggested that the most interesting developments were occurring in extracurricular sport in the primary schools. Formerly, about 25% of the pupils took part in sport on a Wednesday afternoon and about 30% within the *tiers-temps* programme. By 1987, this had increased to 50%

Age	Education	Establishment	Curriculum
2 to 5	Pre-school (non-compulsory)	Nursery school	All-round development, physical, motor skills, co-ordination of movement, spatial awareness
6 to 10	Primary	Primary school	
11 to 16	Secondary – 1st stage	Collège	Wide range of developmental possibilities (in theory) – many schools still concerned with social control through physical situation
16 to 18	Secondary – 2nd stage	Lycée	
18+	Higher	University *Grandes écoles*	

Table 18.2 The French school system

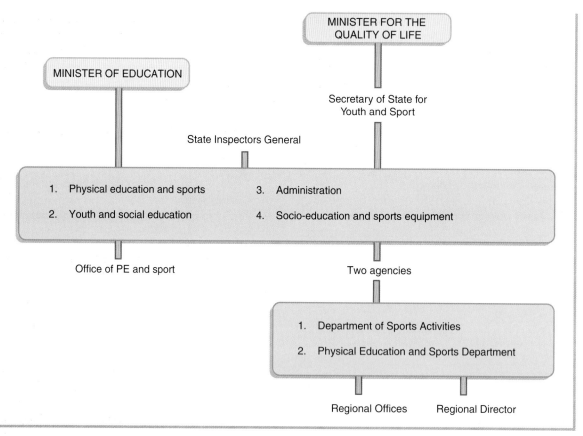

Fig. 18.3 Central authority structure.

Notes:

1. Unlike the British system of virtual head teacher autonomy, French authority is directed through central bureaucratic channels, down to regional and departmental committees.
2. Similarly, the British local inspectorate and advisory teachers have more autonomy than the French regional directors, but the gap is closing.
3. The greater the distance from Paris, the less notice is taken of government directives while the regularity of OFSTED inspections has maintained a tight control over schools throughout England and Wales.
4. The key stage tests are much more formal and ambitious than the 'brevets' in French PE.
5. The secondary PE curriculum retains a focus on 'la gym' as part of a long tradition but from 1990 a much broader curriculum was developed involving individual activities and games.

Table 18.3 Weekly hours of PE and sport

	Primary	*Secondary*	
		Stage 1	*Stage 2*
PE & sport (compulsory)	1/3 teaching time 6 hours	PE & sport 3 hours **SPORT** (CAS) 2 hours	PE & sport 2 hours **SPORT** (CAS) 3 hours
SPORT (optional)	USEP 1/2 day	1/2 day UNSS (formerly ASSU)	

during *tiers-temps* with only 7% on Wednesdays. It is important to note that primary school teachers assist programmes on a voluntary basis and so there is a great range from one school to another. The *tiers-*temps programme is part of the teachers' paid commitment.

All these sporting activities are administered by an independent association (Union Sportive de l'Enseignement Primaire, USEP – Primary Schools Sports Union), acknowledged by the Ministry of Education and reflecting the centralisation policy. In addition, agreements are being reached by which staff and coaches from individual sports federations go into schools to initiate interest in specific sports. In the Brive school this has so far involved rugby, riding, climbing and athletics federations.

The comment from Brive reflected the influence of devolution and the late 1990s has produced not only a dramatic improvement in local community facilities but the introduction of primary sports schools, where most '*departments*' have their own specialist school for children with sporting promise. Note this is a primary school development, unlike the British sports college equivalent which is in the 11–16 age group.

France is even more 'examination conscious' than the UK and physical education is assessed formally at three levels: Brevet des Collèges – 15 year olds; Brevet d'Enseignement Professionel – 17 year olds; and Baccalauréat (Higher Education Entrance) – 18 year olds or older. In the Baccalauréat, besides the compulsory PE section, candidates who are specially gifted can take an optional complementary exam in a definite sport or activity, thus scoring extra marks which are added to their overall mark. This also occurs in music, art, handicraft and languages. In each of the three PE examinations, there is a system of continuous assessment throughout the final year, which mainly concerns practical performance but also includes marks for general attitude and behaviour, goodwill shown and effort made.

The unfortunate consequence of these tests is that they can dominate the PE curriculum and act as a focus of interest for the candidates to the extent that attempts to extend the physical education experience are frustrated. It is hoped that the GCSE and AS/A2 level programmes in Britain will have the opposite effect because they are given additional time and also include extensive theoretical components.

If the overall impression is that the French PE curriculum is stilted compared with the British equivalent, then the opposite would seem to be the case in the context of **extracurricular** sporting activities.

Britain has a tradition of games afternoons and school fixtures from a public school and grammar school system, but over recent years political and financial constraints have reduced these activities in many state schools. The opposite is the case in France. All French schools have had Saturday morning school and a games afternoon in the week as a long tradition. However, these sports afternoons, now normally a Wednesday, were optional and therefore extracurricular, but instead of being administered by the individual schools they were controlled by a national sporting body, the Association du Sport Scolaire et Universitaire (ASSU, 1962–1978). More recently, the organisation of school sport has been taken over by the Union National du Sport Scolaire (UNSS, Figure 18.4). Once again this is part of a centralised policy which takes the organisational responsibility away from individual schools. Nevertheless, it gives the children in poorly organised schools a better chance to participate and ensures a pyramid structure for the promotion of talented performers. This system has also facilitated the policy of licensing sports competitors in France.

One of the inherent problems of PE in schools was the lack of status of the PE teacher. Other teachers were answerable to the Ministry of Education but PE teachers came under the Department for Youth and Sport. This was changed in 1982 and the status of the staff and the subject has increased since then.

There had always been a very restricted allocation of places for specialist teachers of PE at a specialist college (Ecoles Normales Supérieures d'Education Physique et Sportive, ENSEPS – Training Colleges for Sports and Physical Education), but in 1982 the ENSEPS stopped teacher training and became the National Institute of PE and Sport (Institute National de Sport et Education Physique, INSEP). ENSEPS had considerable influence on schools because it supplied all the specialist staff and was responsible for any new professional initiatives. INSEP still influences the schools but now has a broader impact on research and sporting development in general. PE teachers are trained at special units attached to universities (Unites d'Education de Reserche de l'Education Physique et Sports, UEREPS – University Research Units for Sport and Physical Education).

The French equivalent to sports schools are called **sports study sections**. They consist of special classes for talented children but these are not allowed to interfere with academic study. Schools specialise in certain sports and children are selected to attend them. Some centres cater for excellence in one sport, but others are multisport centres. Expert staff are appointed and facilities are well above average. These sections are on the increase and, though they are regionally based, they are centrally controlled.

The extent to which the traditional secondary school curriculum is dominated by academic study and the policy of school sport is linked with the community largely explains why French sports

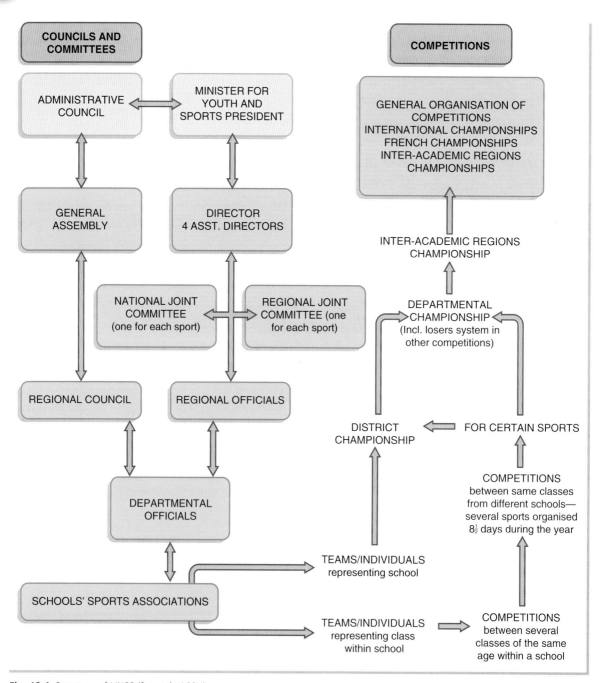

Fig. 18.4 Structure of UNSS (formerly ASSU).

schools have developed in the primary sector. Significantly, however, there are a number of specialist international schools in France where, for instance, circus schools are attracting children from a variety of countries.

Review question

1. Explain the role of the UNSS school sports afternoon in France.

(See Section 21.5 for cross-cultural review and exam-style questions on physical education.)

18.3 The administration of sport in France

The sports movement is made up of two networks – **Federation** and **Olympic**.

The basic unit in French sport is the club and for the most part clubs are affiliated to federations (Figure 18.5). The point to be made is that this network has been built from the clubs up to the federations, very much as in Britain. These federations determine the technical and ethical rules in their respective sports. They are delegated by the Minister of Sport to organise competitions at which international, national and provincial titles are awarded. The federations issue licences to each registered performer. This makes it very much easier to obtain accurate statistics on regular participation and ensure medical care.

There are four types of federation: **Sports Olympiques** (Olympic federations); **Sports Non-Olympiques** (non-Olympic federations); **Multisports** (associated federations); and **Scholaires & Universitaires** (school and university federations). These four bodies make up four 'colleges' within the French National Olympic and Sports Committee.

The Olympic network has been built the opposite way (that is, from the top down), where the **National Olympic Committee** represents and promotes French sport and includes members from all the sports federations. This process of finding and promoting talented performers is achieved through **regional** and **departmental** (county) **committees**.

Financial aid is controlled by the **French National Olympic and Sports Committee** in equal partnership with the state. This is divided into two sections: top-class sport at national level and Sport for All at regional level.

Sport currently comes under the **Ministry of Youth and Sport**. Regional and county directorates of youth and sport exist, but mainly to fulfil the objectives of the Ministry. A level of decentralisation has been taking place since 1982, with the establishment of regional and departmental councils which have the power to finance local sports facilities. This suggests that there is an increasing similarity with the regional and local sports advisory committees in Britain.

The latest development is for the government to set up three cooperative associations: the **National Council of Sport and Physical Activity**; a **National Committee for Research and Technology**; and a top-class **Sports Commission**.

There are a number of national centres of excellence, such as the **National Institute of Sports and Physical Education (INSEP)** (Figure 18.6), the **National Yachting School**, the **National Riding School** and the **Regional Sports and Physical Education Centres**. They all assist the Ministry in training officials and preparing athletes for top-class competition. The new British high performance centres are very much a reflection of the latter.

Ethnic sports in the provinces are very popular (Figures 18.7, 18.8). These range from a variety of folk activities in the Pays Basque to Breton wrestling and the ever-popular street bowls (boules/petanque).

'Sport pour Tous' (Sport for All)

Within everyone's reach; need to be physically active; a noble lifestyle; mass participation in a wide range of activities; encourage multisport development; socialisation of the family and community through sport; instil a love of the open air; a new approach as an alternative to elitism; part of the new image of the sports federations; and spontaneity as against the constrictions of professional sports.

(Free translation from *Le Sport pour Tous. Une Dimension Nouvelle*, 1976)

Review questions

1. Describe the role the Tour de France plays in French professional sport.

2. Explain the place of ethnic sport in French Basque society.

(See Section 21.5 for cross-cultural review and exam-style questions on sport.)

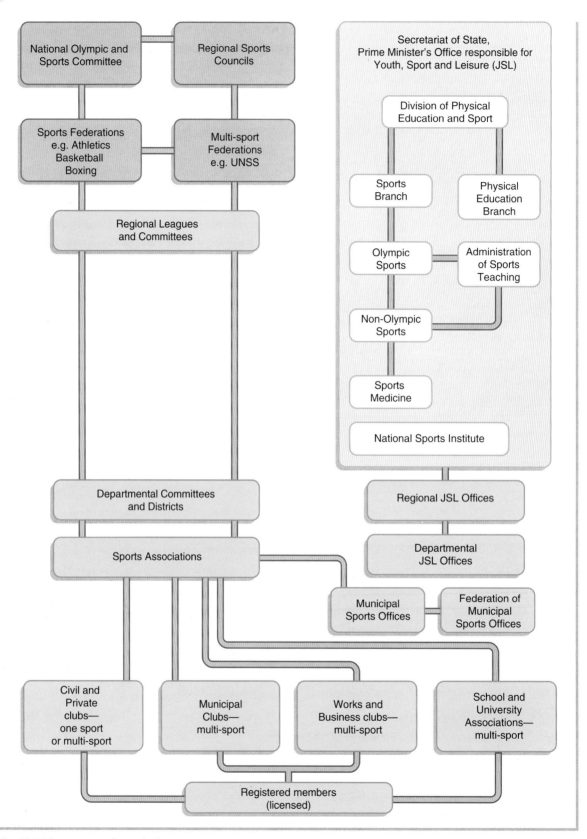

Fig. 18.5 The structure of sport in France.

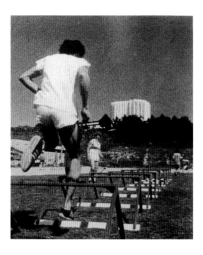

Fig. 18.6 INSEP lies in Vincennes Park on the outskirts of Paris.

- Its facilities include: six covered tennis courts, two swimming pools, outdoor track and field stadium, two straight tracks and a sprinter's track, one cycling track, two gymnasiums, football and rugby pitches, two fencing halls and the biggest judo hall in Europe
- Europe's biggest research laboratory specialising in various fields: physiology, biomechanics, measuring instruments for anthropometrical tests, muscle-building methods, computers to assist training and instruments to test and classify sports equipment
- An audiovisual department and library containing video equipment and publications, some of which are in English, Spanish and Arabic

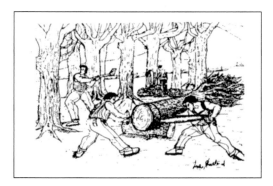

Fig. 18.7 Scieurs de Long.

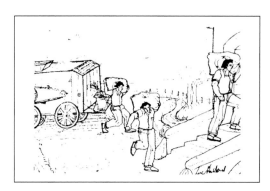

Fig. 18.8 Course au Sac en Relais.

18.4 The organisation of outdoor recreation and outdoor education in France

Similar to the United Kingdom, French **outdoor recreation** is taken to mean recreational activities in the natural environment. While it is fundamentally concerned with enjoying and appreciating natural scenery, there is an element of escape in that many outdoor recreationists are 'getting away from' the urban environment. There is also a concern for conservation, with environmentalists reminding us that abuse and excessive use of the countryside can lead to pollution and erosion.

When different ways of exploring the natural environment are considered, we are studying the area of **outdoor pursuits**. At the most recreational level, this can simply be the use of skills like canoeing or climbing to travel and reach places or it can mean engaging in the challenge of nature and the elements, through canoeing on wild water or attempting classified rock climbs. Finally, there is the sporting dimension, evident in sailing and canoeing, where contests are held on fixed courses.

The use of the term **outdoor education** implies the inculcation of educational values in the natural environment and may involve physical, personal and social development, as well as learning more about the natural environment.

The whole concept of French outdoor recreation is expressed in the phrase *le plein air*. Historically linked with twin European traditions of the **spa movement** and **naturalism**, it has become a campaign to remove the young from the corrupting influence of the inner cities and to introduce them to the simple pleasures of life in the countryside. However, French

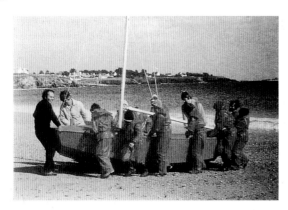

Fig. 18.9 Sea school in Brittany. Why are water sports so popular in France?

administrators recognise that fresh air may not be enough and so they include physical exercise and strive to re-establish the '**rustic simplicity**' of being able to make the most of the natural environment.

A number of key variables need to be taken into account when looking at the French development of outdoor recreation.

The amount of open countryside and the range of climatic and topographical types give the French people greater opportunities than those available in Britain. They can ski in the Alps, walk in the Massif Central, bathe in the Mediterranean, fish and canoe on the many waterways and sail on the extensive coastal waters (Figure 18.9).

The British have chosen to spread holidays over a 3-month period to offset crowding but the French still cling to traditional holiday periods, which means that in the first week of August workers 'down tools' and start a grand exodus to the countryside. Inevitably, this concentration causes crowding in the more popular areas but, as with British excursion trips, many holiday-makers appear to enjoy the bustle and social conviviality. At the centre of this ritual there is *le camping français*. Families swarm out of the cities and head for the sun, taking miniature homes along with them. Alternatively, the trains are filled to capacity twice a year to take skiers to the Alps at Easter and families to the sea in August, where 'beaches boil with Gallic bodies'.

The French family has changed a great deal since the Second World War (1939–1945). The Mazeaud Act (1976) was based on the suggestion that, with working wives and fewer children, spare time was becoming increasingly precious and parents were looking for more free time to pursue their own interests. This led local authorities and firms to sponsor holiday centres for children, **centres de vacances**. One example, the **colonie de vacances**, a rural institution, has much in common with the American camp school. In addition to freeing the parents, these 'colonies' are designed to take children out of the towns and, originally, many of the local authority centres made special efforts to cater for underprivileged children. Traditionally, wealthier children have tended to take private or commercial alternatives.

The programme in these residential centres includes educational, social and cultural elements as well as outdoor pursuits, with emphasis on promoting *le plein air*, a love of the open air. Children can stay at these residential centres for the whole summer holiday and are then returned to their parents.

Although reference has been made to residential *colonies de vacances*, there are many different types of leisure centre frequented by young people, some small and local, others of national significance, where outdoor pursuits are taught to a high level. For example, **Le Centre National des Sports de Plein Air** at Vallon-Pont-D'Arc is equivalent to Britain's Plas y Brenin and there is a famous mountain school at Chamonix.

Alternatively, in the Nantes district, for example, there are leisure centres available for children to use on Wednesday afternoons; there are 10 or more local centres spread throughout the town for children aged 4–15 to use in the holidays; there are adventure playgrounds situated at various points; and, on a larger scale, there is a *village de vacances*, which is a permanent holiday complex for children and an urban equivalent of a *colonie de vacances*.

If these are holiday opportunities for French children, then the classes are outdoor experiences promoted as part of the school programme (Figures 18.10 and 18.11). As early as 1953 snow classes were started, where children were taken out of the towns to stay in the mountains for about a month under the supervision of their regular teachers, PE staff and qualified ski instructors. In addition to the snow classes, there are now classes in the countryside and sea schools and, as a result of government support and subsidies from municipal and general councils, there has been a steady increase in the number of children involved. As early as in 1984, for example, some 120 000 children attended a total of 4600 classes.

The full title of the programme is *Les Classes Transplantées: La Ville à la Campagne* and the key to understanding its intention lies in the word 'transplanting'. Children are taken from the town to a country location in another region. It is an attempt to broaden children's experience and knowledge

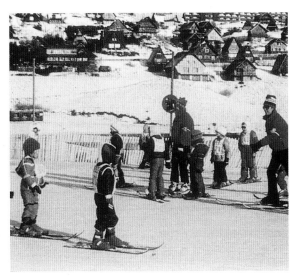

Fig. 18.10 Snow school in the Auvergne. Why has the French government poured money into snow schools?

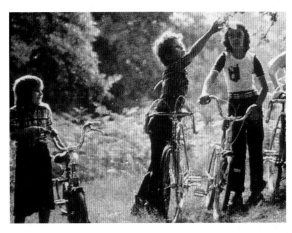

Fig. 18.11 Class de vert. How does this compare with English environment studies?

about the natural environment but also to take them to another part of France where traditions and customs may be different. It is a formal educational experience as parents have to be convinced that academic standards and health will not suffer as a result of a month away from formal schooling.

The Outward Bound movement, though focused on the UK and Commonwealth countries, has been developed in Belgium and was started in France in 1986 under the title **Hors Limites – Outward Bound**. Its first centre was constructed in 1993 at Banassac in the Canourgue in southern France. The scheme was initiated by Alain Kerjean, who envisaged something like the British Outward Bound, but it is already taking its own cultural shape. This is probably because as many Belgian instructors were used as British to train the French **formateurs**, but the French commitment to their own national philosophies and the ideology of **rural simplicity** means that Rousseau's ideas on education in the natural environment are having more influence than Kurt Hahn's philosophy of character building.

Consequently, there is already an emphasis on personal development in the outdoors as a form of therapy, rather than as a self-testing adventure experience. However, there is a wide variety of programmes for schools and universities (as well as those organised by the social services) and management and professional development training courses.

It is important to recognise the difference between the holiday and the school programmes. There are critics who believe that much of *le plein air* concept is lost in the formality of the *classes*; that it can be truly expressed only through a family holiday or as a leisure experience at a *centre de vacances*. There are others who see the value of the *classes* as the richest school experience, pointing to the social awareness of being taught in the natural environment. In both cases it would seem that the British outdoor education programme does not match up to the opportunities available to the average French child.

Review question

1. Explain the French '*classes transplantées*' in the context of their cultural and educational function.

(See Section 21.5 for cross-cultural review and exam-style questions on outdoor recreation.)

Reference

1. Whitaker J & Sons 2004 Whitaker's Almanack. A & C Black, London
2. Mermet G 1987 Francoscopie. Larousse, Paris

Further reading

Geographical influences

Lane H V (ed) 1986 *The world almanac*. Newspaper Enterprise Association, London

Paxton J (ed) 1991 *The statesman's year book*, 1988–89, 127e, Macmillan, Basingstoke

Whitaker J & Sons 2004 *Whitaker's Almanack*. A & C Black, London

Historical influences

Baker W J 1988 *Sports in the Western world*. University of Illinois, Urbana, Illinois

Holt R 1981 *Sport and society in modern France*. Macmillan, Basingstoke

Socio-economic factors

Cook M (ed) 1993 *French culture since 1945*. In: Greaves A (ed) Sport in France. Longman, London

Houlihan B 1994 *Sport and international politics*. Harvester Wheatsheaf, London

Rigby F 1978 *The place of PE and sport in a centralized system – France*. PE Review 1: 53–58

Organisation of outdoor recreation and education

Cook M 1993 *French culture since 1945*. In: Greaves A (Ed) Sport in France, Longman, London

French Embassy 1985 *Sports in France*. France Information, Paris

Hantrais L 1982 *Leisure and the family in contemporary France*. Leisure Studies 1(1), Polytechnic of North London, London

Holt R 1981 *Sport and society in modern France*. Macmillan, Basingstoke

Le Sport pour Tous 1976 *Une dimension nouvelle*. Ministry of Youth and Sport, Paris

Mairie de Paris 1991 *Sports et jeunesse: 10 ans d'action municipale*. 25 Boulevard Bourdon, Paris

Mairie de Paris 1992 *La direction de la jeunesse et des sports en chiffres*. 25 Boulevard Bourdon, Paris

Platt J 1973 *The development of sport exchange*. Outdoors 3(4), London

Rigby F 1978 *The place of PE and sport in a centralized educational system – France*. PE Review Spring NWCPEA, Driffield, N. Humberside

Roscoe D A, Roscoe J V, Honeybourne J, Davis R, Galligan F 2003 *Physical education and sports studies AS/A2 level student revision guide*, 3rd edn. Jan Roscoe Publications, Widnes

Smith P 1998 *The French experience*. Bulletin of Physical Education 34(3): 212–217

Physical education and sport in Commonwealth countries with particular reference to Australia

Learning objectives

On completion of this section, you will be able to:

1. Develop a Commonwealth perspective through a detailed review of physical education and sport in Australia.

2. Understand the cultural variables which exist in Australia.

3. Be aware of the structure and function of physical and sport education in Australian schools.

4. Understand the innovative policy and programme of sport in Australia.

5. Appreciate patterns of outdoor recreation in the natural environment of Australia.

Major Commonwealth countries including Australia, Canada, New Zealand and South Africa are of great global significance. Traditional colonial ties may no longer exist, but there is a commonality of language and transmitted culture which gives them a great deal in common with the United Kingdom. This is particularly the case in physical education where international schools have promoted the ethic of English public school athleticism for well over a century and the extension of this into rational recreation has resulted in regular Test matches and competition in the Olympic and Commonwealth Games.

These human influences may have sufficient similarities to make a comparison worthwhile but the size and population of the United Kingdom give rise to tremendous differences which might make cultural borrowing a hazardous pursuit.

It is not feasible to look at all these countries and so Australia has been selected because there is a considerable amount of contact at the moment as Britain aspires to follow their example in the development of sport.

19.1 The social setting of physical education and sport in Australia

We need to have a knowledge of the **cultural background** before we can hope to understand how organised physical activity functions in different societies. We will call these influences **cultural determinants** and look at them under three main headings: **geographical**, **historical** and **socio-economic**.

Geographical influences on physical education and sport in Australia

Geography is a very broad field of study but is limited in the analysis here to comments on population, land area, topography, climate, urbanisation and communications in the context of sport and physical education.

Population

The population growth for Australia since 1901 is shown in Table 19.1. On 31 December 2001, the population was over 19 million and in 1986, 91% of the population was urban. By 2004 the population had risen to approximately 20 million and some Australian politicians suggested that a near maximum population had been reached.

Table 19.1 Australian population growth								
Year	1901	1921	1947	1961	1981	1991	1997	2004
Population (millions)	4	5	8	11	15	16.9	18.3	20

2001 census figures recorded some 400 000 Aboriginal or native Australians. They have only been included in population statistics since 1967, which reflects their limited political status. Almost all native Australians now have mixed blood, but it is presumed that the statistics refer to those who identify with the Aboriginal culture.

For comparison, on 31 March 1993, New Zealand had a population of 3 494 000 and the Polynesian minority (mainly Maori) represented 18% of the population.

Before 1945 Australians were almost exclusively of British or Irish descent but by 1980 there was a 30% non-British minority. This was the result of two policies: a recognition of Asia as a market rather than Europe; and the need to populate or perish.

The expansion policy was entirely racially based. In the 1940s and 1950s Britons were preferred but displaced Europeans were accepted; in the 1960s people from the Middle East were accepted; and in the 1970s, Asians were admitted. This marked the end of the White Australia policy, which had been established against the so-called 'yellow peril'. These controlled phases of expansion have influenced racial stratification in much the same way as similar policies in the USA.

The 1994–1995 quota for new settlers was 86 000 and was strictly observed.

Size

The area of Australia is 2 966 151 square miles. The population in terms of different individual states in 1980 is given in Table 19.2 (ACT is the Federal Australian Capital Territory of Canberra, similar to Washington DC in the USA). Figures 19.1 and 19.2 are useful for comparative purposes.

In comparative terms, Australia is a similar size to the USA if Alaska is excluded. The five Australian states are much larger than any of the 50 American states. Western Australia is four times larger than Texas; New South Wales is as large as France and the UK combined; and Tasmania is as large as England.

Topography

There are three broad zones. First, three-quarters of Australia is a great flat plain, which is largely desert and unpopulated. Australians commonly refer to this as the Red Centre, consisting as it does of outcrops of exposed rock that has sacred significance to Aboriginal culture.

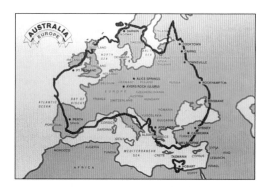

Fig. 19.1 Australia superimposed on Europe.

Table 19.2 Australian state population figures		
State	Area (nearest 1000 sq. miles)	Population (nearest 100)
New South Wales	300 000	6 025 500
Victoria	180 000	4 468 300
Queensland	680 000	3 155 400
South Australia	394 000	1 467 500
Western Australia	971 000	1 687 300
Tasmania	67 800	427 500
Northern Territories	518 000	170 500
ACT	800	299 400
(New Zealand	175 000	3 494 400)

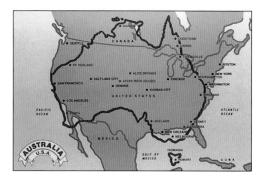

Fig. 19.2 Australia superimposed on the USA.

Secondly, running North–South from the Kimberley Mountains in the Northern Territory to the Eyre Peninsula in South Australia, there is a swathe of grassland that separates deserts to the West and East.

Third, there is the Great Dividing Range running down the East of the country, with its foothills running down to the Eastern coastal plain and round the South coast of Victoria as far as Adelaide in South Australia.

Climate

The significance of Australia being in the Southern hemisphere is that seasonal sports can be played all the year if international players have the money to travel. This is particularly relevant to professional sports such as cricket and, more recently, athletics and rugby and for sports of the wealthy, such as skiing and tennis.

The sheer size of the land mass is such that North Queensland is within 10° of the equator and experiences a *tropical* climate which includes summer monsoons and dry winters.

The Southern belt of Victoria and Tasmania is in the Westerly wind belt and is well into the *cool temperate zone* with cold winters and heavy rainfall, but hardly any of this rain reaches the interior. High precipitation just inland has produced large areas of temperate rain forest, where protected gullies have examples of ancient tropical vegetation. In the arid interior, however, the only saviour is the underground water of the Great Artesian Basin.

The climate down the East coast reflects its latitude, with *subtropical* in the North and *warm temperate* in the South.

The coast is influenced by the usual wind variables and the rising slopes of the Great Dividing Range have considerable rainfall as well as rapidly decreasing temperatures with altitude. It is reputed that within an hour of surfing in Pacific breakers, it is possible to be skiing in the Southern Alps.

Urbanisation

The population density of Australia is lower than that of any other major country and far below the other four countries studied herein. The 3 per square mile density has little meaning, however, as 84% of all Australians are urbanised, leaving vast tracts of emptiness in the Red Centre. The cities of Sydney, Melbourne, Brisbane and Adelaide have a total of 9 million inhabitants and Perth is the only other city with a million inhabitants.

Additionally, a map of Australian towns shows a whole string close to the Pacific Highway, from Brisbane South to Cape Horn on the Tasman Sea. It is significant that, despite its size, some economists suggest that Australia cannot successfully support a much higher population than it already has.

Communications

Road communication is dominated by a series of superb freeways on the American pattern. They link the major cities, which means that most are along the East coast. The size of Australia is best appreciated when it is realised that it can take 2 days to drive from Melbourne to Sydney, even on the freeways. The Red Centre has a few cross-continental freeways, but consists of mainly dirt roads. Rail travel is more popular and there are similarities with the Trans-Siberian Railway in Central Russia. However, the distances are such that air travel is preferred by the business community and tourists so, as with the USA, each major town has its own civil airport with regular internal flights. Significantly, the recently opened railway line from Adelaide to Darwin could revolutionise trade routes from Australia to South East Asia.

Review questions

1. Explain the contradiction that, despite the low average population of Australia, it is normally described as an urbanised society.
2. Explain the significance of the frontier spirit in Australia in the context of Wilderness.
3. Compare links between the size of a country, communications and sport in Australia.

Historical influences on physical education and sport in Australia

Aboriginal tribes probably entered Australia during the last Ice Age via land bridges and a short stretch of water from South-East Asia, some 30 000 years ago. Over this period tribal societies developed, with different languages and dialects evolving across Australia. Aboriginal society was highly organised, extremely well disciplined and spiritually rich, with territorial boundaries respected despite their semi-nomadic existence as hunters. Many of these features are still evident in the Northern Territory and Western Australia, despite exploitation by European colonialists. To legitimise European occupation of Aboriginal land, a 'legal fiction', known as *terra nullius* (empty land), presumed that the country was unoccupied before colonisation; this has remained a foundation of Australian law and even today there are doubts about the legality of Aboriginal land claims.

Much is made of Australia's initial function as a penal colony from 1788. Indeed, in 1830, 90% of the population of New South Wales (NSW) and Van Diemen's Land (Tasmania) were convicts, former convicts or relatives. However, by 1840, with transportation abolished, free settlements were flourishing and Anglo-Scottish Protestants worked alongside ex-convicts and Irish Catholic labourers.

The rest of the century was dominated by three themes. First, there was migration expansion and economic growth arising from a series of 'gold rushes', especially in Victoria, which resulted in a rapid urbanisation process. It is suggested that by 1891 Australia was the most urbanised country in the world and with this came a very powerful middle class.

The second theme was the expansion of responsible democratic government, with a spirit of independence from Britain, such that, by the 1850s, most of the states had separate constitutions that included wide adult male franchise. The negative experience of the American War of Independence may have convinced the UK not to resist this trend.

Third, there was a major attempt to invent and popularise a distinctive Australian nationalism. It is probable that the sporting ethic, which started at this time, was part of this movement and was called 'our sporting obsession' by Keith Dunstan.[1] He goes on to recognise three factors that bind Australia as a nation: Federation, the tragic loss of life at Gallipoli and cricket. The last is a reminder of the roots of the people's game and the incentive to beat the 'old enemy'. In 1877, 24 years before the Federation, the divided Australian colonies combined to play the first match against England as the 'Australian' team. The English immigrants had brought the game with them and there was a cricket club in Sydney as early as 1826. The All-England XI, which had done so much for cricket in the English counties, toured Australia in 1861 and had a similar stimulating impact.

The 20th century saw the rise of swimming as a national sport (Figure 19.3). The three main causal factors were probably the climate and beaches of the South Pacific coast; urbanisation, the emergent middle class and their views on cleanliness and athleticism; and the invention of the 'Australian crawl', which revolutionised speed swimming. The emergence of lawn tennis as an elite game had similar supportive elements, where Anglo-Saxon status was expressed through this urbanised game in an ideal climate, but

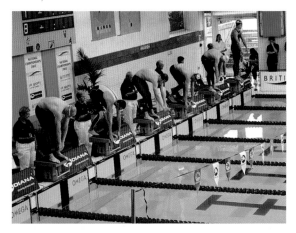

Fig. 19.3 One of Australia's finest sports. Photographer Helen Roscoe

there is also the role-model effect of such great champions as Hoad, Rosewall and Laver. There have always been strong female swimmers and in tennis the feminist cause was expressed through Margaret Court and, even more significantly, Evonne Goolagong, an Aboriginal women's world champion. Kathy Freeman has become the latest Australian sports star who has used her success to highlight feminist and Aboriginal causes.

Of all sports, only football divides Australia, but the exclusivity of different codes makes this a world issue.

New South Wales and Queensland are dominated by rugby league and rugby union, while Victoria, South Australia and Western Australia have a preference for 'Aussie' Rules football. Significantly, the game of association football did not develop as it had in Britain, probably because of the relative absence of industrialisation, but more recently Italian and Greek immigrants have brought soccer to Australia, complete with its spectator hooligan tendencies. In historical terms, colonial links with Rugby School and Melbourne Cricket Club led to the birth of the handling game but Celtic links may account for the eventual adoption of Aussie Rules with its similarity to Gaelic football. Meanwhile, the development of the rugby code around Sydney and Brisbane probably owes much to the high proportion of settlers from England and Wales in these areas.

The history of sport in Australia, therefore, reflects developments in the UK but middle-class developments remained dominant because there was hardly any industrial working-class influence. Private clubs stimulated by school athleticism produced a decentralised sporting system with state teams dominant and minimal Federal support. Test matches and the Olympic movement stimulated nationalism but Federal involvement was delayed until the 1970s.

Australia's failure at the Montreal Olympics (one silver and four bronze medals) led to widespread criticism and a review of the national administrative structure and Federal funding. Particular note was made of the successes of East European and Soviet state sponsorship and the selection and the training methods of their sporting elite. Significantly, it also became a political instrument of the Australian Labour Party.

1. Explain the extent to which Australian sport has been influenced by colonialism.

Socio-economic factors influencing sport and physical education in Australia

Centralised Federal influence on devolved state civil administrations

A decentralised civil administration at state level continues to resist centralised Federal dominance. As with the USA, Australia is a young country, with a population that is increasingly pluralistic, seeking to establish a national identity.

As a colonial country that denied Aboriginal culture, Australia developed a British pattern of democratic government, but generally of a more radical nature after dominion status had been achieved. This was evident in a Liberal dominance from 1949 to 1972. The growth of the Labour Party was influenced by concern over Communist involvement and religious friction involving a large Irish Roman Catholic minority. Since 1972 Labour has become the leading party and by 1990 had held power in five states and won three Federal elections, 1984, 1987 and 1990, but it lost power in 1996. The ex-Labour Prime Minister, Paul Keating, considers that nationalism is essentially linked with republicanism.

The Labour government reforms in 1972 led to a centralised policy, with national planning coming from the Australian Sports Commission and extensive Federal funding. However, the high level of independence maintained by individual states is reflected in the structure of their sport. Each state has its own sports organisation at elite and mass participation levels, which should not be seen as just an extension

of the Federal Australian Institute of Sport but as standing in its own right. This appears to mirror the pattern found in the USA and is even more evident in the independent republics that had been part of the Soviet Union.

In terms of Australian attitudes to national and state sport, Dunstan[1] quoted Mrs Ed Clark, the wife of a former American Ambassador: 'Living in Australia is like living in a gymnasium – there's always somebody practising something'.

In similar vein, Saturday radio in Australia has continuous sport on all four channels and there are regularly 25 hours of sport televised each week. There are obvious similarities here with the American sporting ethic but it is also important to recognise that counter-cultures exist in both countries.

1. How has Australia used sport to help establish a national identity?

Internationalism

Britain and Australia have a bond forged by common roots and the sacrifices of two world wars; this is enhanced by the regular opportunity to compete against each other in sport.

Despite moves towards republicanism, the Commonwealth Games does much to bind countries in 'friendly' competition and it is probable that the new centralised policy for sport in Australia is a copy of the Canadian approach. However, in economic terms, the past few years have seen Australia forming increased links with South-East Asia and the degree of Americanisation is evident from the amount of TV basketball. Finally, there is no doubt that Olympic success is a major national objective and the high level of sponsorship, together with the sporting obsession of the people, gives Australia a level of success far above their demographic expectations.

International boycotts

The principle of political boycott in international sport is nowhere more evident than in links with South Africa. All Communist and non-white countries exercised a total boycott but, though the majority of white countries would not send national teams, individuals could still play in South Africa from choice in certain sports.

The political reforms taken by the South African government, symbolised by the release of Nelson Mandela and his appointment as President, together with the steps taken by governing bodies of sport in the country to make their activities multiracial, have resulted in the international boycott being called off and South Africa being readmitted to the Olympics.

> ### Review question
>
> 1. Explain the notion of 'shop window' and sport in Australia.

Political

An apparently rich country in material wealth and positive attitudes, Australia has two permanent problems of a high rate of unemployment and a huge foreign debt. Underneath the surface is the danger of arousing racial hatreds and ethnic tensions in a pluralist society reaching the end of Anglo-Celtic dominance.

Unlike the UK, Australia owes little to industrialialisation. Its export of wool, meat and wheat to Britain has declined since the development of the European market and competition in South-East Asia is against countries with cheaper labour.

Australia is well endowed with energy resources, being a major exporter of coal, and is almost self-sufficient in petroleum. A century ago Australia had a gold rush similar to that in America and minerals remain an important source of income.

Australian political success over the last decade has been the reverse of the United Kingdom, with Labour being replaced by a Liberal Coalition. However, it would seem that the impact of media moguls like Kerry Packer and Richard Murdoch has revolutionised the status of professional sport in Australia to the extent that politics is often relegated to second place. However, Olympic sports have been advanced by a French and Soviet-style centralised funding policy in a determined attempt to produce elite performers in a wide range of activities. It is worth noting that the £49 000 000 budget of the British Sports Council with a 56 million population pales alongside the Aus$63 363 000 contribution by the Australian government in 1993–1994 for a mere 17 million citizens (the exchange rate in 1996 was approximately $2 to the pound).

The Tattersalls Lottery has a weekly top prize of approximately Aus$8 000 000, half that of the UK Lottery, but reflects the level of gambling in a country with a much smaller population. There are also additional state and private lotteries, as well as a major casino industry, all of which rival Tattersalls.

> ### Review question
>
> 1. Discuss the influence of government aid on sport in Australia.

Discrimination

Cultural variables have inevitably led to certain groups being discriminated against in a specific community and in a society. Normally, whatever form this takes, it is reflected in a country's sport.

Regional

The arid plateau of central Australia is the centre of Aboriginal culture and there is still poverty in these areas. The heart of the problem lies in European colonialisation in which, as in the USA, white settlers considered existing tribal cultures to be hostile and inferior. The native Americans and the Aborigines were shot indiscriminately, dispossessed of their land and denied franchise. In fact, Aborigines have only been included in Australian population statistics since 1967 and the Native Title Act that set up a system for assessing land claims only came into effect in 1994, but the failure of some recent claims suggests that there are ways round it. As with North America, these ancient tribes are in resurgence but a typical example is the tourist abuse of Ayers Rock, Uluru. This is a sacred place in Aboriginal culture and yet, despite appeals from Aboriginal leaders, white tourists insist on the right to climb over it.

Class

The total dominance of British settlers for nearly 200 years has led to a variation of the English class system being adopted. This does not include an upper class of landowners, nor an industrial working class, but there is a very strong conservative rural society and a powerful urban middle-class liberal society. Finally, there is the caricatured brash, chauvinist, lower class 'Bruce' who makes for a very boisterous spectator at cricket or football and is mentally and physically tough as a competitor.

Gender

Australia and the USA have a great deal in common in the context of the status of women. The Anglo-

- One hundred and twenty female administrators, players and coaches attended the 'Focus on Marketing and Management' seminar series conducted in Queensland, the Australian Capital Territory and Western Australia and with softball and basketball administrators.
- Eleven NSOs initiated activities or conducted planning seminars specifically targeted at increasing the involvement of women and girls in their sport under the Gender Equity Planning Program.
- The Active Girls Triathlon Series was extended from 21 events in 1992–1993 to 29 events in 1993–1994.
- The 3rd annual Prime Ministerial Women and Sport Awards was conducted to acknowledge special initiatives taken to encourage greater involvement of women and girls in sport, including those with special needs.
- Resource materials including four issues of the national magazine Active were produced to provide a communication vehicle for women's sport and greater recognition of women's sporting achievements.
- The ASC participated in the first international conference on women and sport, conducted in the UK, which agreed to an international set of principles aimed at developing a sporting culture that enables and values the full involvement of women in every aspect of sport. These were endorsed by 280 delegates from 82 countries.

Fig. 19.4 Women and sport, Australia (ASC Programme Performance, 1993).

Saxon core, with its Victorian ethic of the dependent female, is combined with the 'frontier' attitudes of a dynamic young country to produce a chauvinistic Australian male stereotype.

Predictably, sport has been a male preserve, which is still reflected in the dominance of male professional sports and the media coverage of them. Any breakthroughs by females have been influenced by cosmetic as well as athletic factors, by the independence of middle-class women and by the occasional irresistible talent of individuals like Kathy Freeman.

There is a very strong feminist counter-culture in Australia, with considerable publicity being given to women in sport at Federal and state levels (Figure 19.4). In the case of Kathy Freeman and Evonne Goolagong, it is also important to recognise that they were fighting for Aboriginal culture as well as gender identity.

Religion

The White Australia policy limited religious friction to the Protestant and Catholic divide and, as in the USA, the WASP hegemony prevails, a product of the English middle classes compared with the Catholic influence of Irish and Italian communities. The divide has been emphasised by political association, reflecting Anglo-Protestant Liberals and a Labour Party with a strong Irish Catholic minority supporting republicanism. The admission of Middle East and Asian communities has further increased the religious mix and has led to state education becoming secular.

Race

The White Australia policy was an Anglo-Celtic creation to keep Australia safe from the so-called 'yellow peril'. Its colonial base also served to keep other Europeans out and it was not until the 1950s that large groups of displaced persons were accepted from mainland Europe. Given an expansionist policy and a relatively low response from this source, the migration policy was extended in the 1960s to people from the Middle East and to Asians in the 1970s. The result is a pluralist society, similar to that in the USA but produced in a small fraction of the time. Class remains the major form of stratification, but there is racial ranking that generally reflects the changing migration policy. As in the USA, non-British Europeans are rapidly building themselves a place in the social order, but there are racial concerns over non-integrated Aboriginal Australians existing as a submerged class, while oriental communities, encouraged to settle on economic grounds, are resented by some conservative elements.

Attempts are being made to give Aboriginal Australians more status and their lifestyle, including their ethnic sports, is receiving recognition but the dominance of certain sports is linked with racial identity, reflected by the Anglo-Celtic games of cricket, rugby and Aussie Rules. The proportion of Aboriginal professional players, for example, in no way matches the Maori involvement in New Zealand. Association football, on the other hand, is strongest in the Italian and Greek communities. As in the UK, laws exist

- The ASC completed an examination of its role in funding and supporting disabled sport in Australia.
- Two additional Coaching Athletes with Disabilities (CAD) manuals were completed, bringing the total number of finalised manuals to six. Sport-specific coaching resources for the disabled (videos, manuals and courses) were developed in consultation with swimming, athletics, gymnastics and tennis coaches.
- Sixteen Level One coaching courses were conducted, and mainstream sports continued to include CAD material in the Level One coaching curriculum.
- Twenty-three elite athletes with disabilities were granted AIS Scholarships and training camps were held for swimming, athletics, weightlifting and basketball.

Fig. 19.5 People with disabilities – Aussie Able Program (ASC Programme Performance, 1993).

to prevent racism but even in sport, wealth and traditional rivalries cause elements of exclusivity and dissension.

Age

The notion of being a young, dynamic country bodes well for youth culture, as reflected in the support given to young athletes at Federal and state levels. This includes a careful monitoring of young athletes so that there is less commercial exploitation of young people than in the USA.

Alternatively, one might have expected the aged to be ignored in sport terms but the strength of the Healthy Outdoor Australian ethic is a lifetime obsession, one which only the recent fear of skin cancer has curbed. Private bowls, tennis and golf clubs abound in urban areas, where space still does not seem to be a problem, and every small town has

similar facilities, with organised walking trails. All these facilities are widely used by the elderly.

Disabled

As with Britain, a great deal was learned about physical disability as a result of wartime injuries and this, in combination with the Australian concern for health and activity, has resulted in, predictably, a major integrated adaptive programme in education. The Aussie Able Program (Figure 19.5) is a well-developed sports programme in most urban areas.

Review question

1. How does media coverage of sport reflect the status of women performers in Australian netball and swimming?

19.2 The administration of physical education in Australia

School system

As a British colony the 19th-century education system in Australia was dominated by a parallel development of English public schools at a time when **muscular Christianity** and athleticism were at their height. This culminated in the bravery, horror and human sacrifice of the 1914–1918 World War, epitomised by Australians at Gallipoli.

The diplomatic and commercial influence of upper middle-class English gentlemen and the development of schools for their children resulted in the formation of elite 'public' and preparatory schools. To quote G M Hibbins, 'The Melbourne public schools varied not one whit from the English public schools in the growing passion for games'. In identifying the birth

of Aussie Rules football in Melbourne, Hibbins pointed to the joint roots of Trinity College Cambridge and Trinity College Dublin, particularly as they were linked with Scotch College and Melbourne Grammar School in the 1850s. Without doubt, here is one factor which contributed to the Australian obsession with sport today.

The contemporary educational structure has been dramatically changed to a comprehensive national high school system but, unlike in the UK, fee-paying independent, private schools are now almost entirely religious foundations. This secularisation of government schools is similar to that in France, but the high school system tends to resemble its American counterpart. These government schools outnumber private schools by seven to one, but both sections

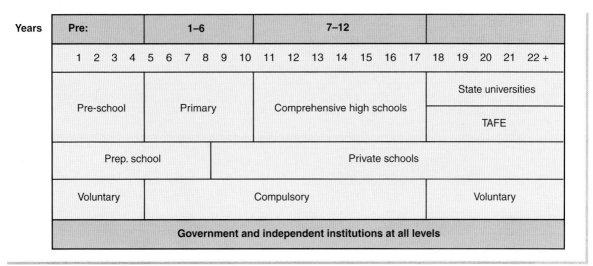

Fig. 19.6 Australian school system.

Notes: 1. Mainstream route is for children to attend preschooling.
     2. All children attend primary school, mainly co-education, years 1–6.
     3. Compulsory secondary education, years 7–10 with HSC years 11–12.

receive Federal grants. Despite this centralising influence, the administration of the educational system is controlled by individual states, where each is responsible for policy and operation, resulting in many variables between them.

It is important to establish that the private school system is very strong. Although it has a religious affiliation, it also has tradition and academic stringency that attract middle-class parents who are prepared to pay for what they consider to be an advantaged education for their children.

The structure of government schooling is normally co-educational and is compulsory between the ages of 6 and 15 years (Figure 19.6). Preschooling is popular but voluntary and mainstream schools are divided into primary and secondary, similar to the English model. After Year 10 (15+), continued schooling is optional as children with ambitions to enter higher education commence a 2-year higher school certificate (HSC) programme. Federal government operates a **Secondary Allowance Scheme** whereby grants, subject to a means test, are given to children to stay at school for their final 2 years to complete their HSC. In an attempt to meet regional needs, this national examination is now administered at state level; for example, Victorians now sit a Victoria Certificate of Education (VCE) which is set and assessed at state level. The size of Australia also makes it necessary for a special programme called the **Isolated Child Allowance Scheme** to help children with travel expenses and to assist with financial

support for using privately owned hostels. Other attempts to alleviate the distance problem are correspondence schools and schools of the air.

As with the UK, further education is also available for young people who do not follow the main academic route in the form of 250 technical and further educational institutions (TAFEs).

Higher education institutes have degree and diploma courses that last from 3 to 6 years. Fees were abolished in 1974 and full-time students have allowances subject to means tests. The Australians have followed the line of the British system by merging the three main units, universities, colleges of technology and teacher education colleges, into a single system of university higher education. Started in 1989, this is an ongoing process, as is a recent trend to start a private university system. In both Britain and Australia, these trends seem to be linked with the USA system and privatisation. In the Melbourne area, for example, there are four traditional universities, Melbourne, Deakin, La Trope and Monash, and two new universities, formerly the Royal Melbourne Institute of Technology (RMIT) and Victoria University of Technology (VUT), which had been polytechnics.

Physical education

Physical education has a traditional place on the curriculum that arises from the colonial system of 19th-century public school athleticism and elementary

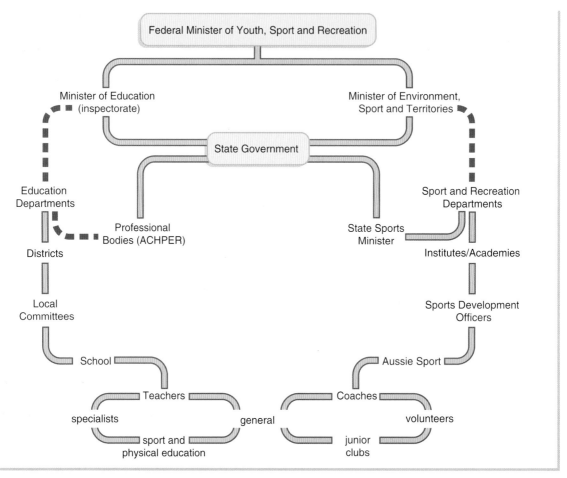

Fig. 19.7 Australian administration system for physical education and junior sport.

school physical training. In addition, although there are national bodies that promote PE and Federal funding to support it, policy and programming are decentralised to state level and thence down to district and local school boards (Figure 19.7), similar to the system in the USA.

The period from 1945 to 1972 matched the expansion of educational principles of **movement education** seen in Britain and part of this trend was the setting up of colleges of higher education that specialised in physical education. This also marked an extension of the facilities in schools and the diversity of activities taught in PE. The next decade (1973–1982) marked a high point in physical education with the appointment of a PE inspectorate and a policy of training specialist teachers for primary and secondary schools. As in the UK, this also marked the emergence of a graduate profession. At this time a wide range of curriculum ideas came from the Ministry of Education and the professional PE Association (Australian Council

for Health, Physical Education and Recreation; ACHPER).

Victoria was particularly progressive in education and physical education, but even this state found difficulty in sustaining a **daily physical education programme** for all primary children which was recommended in 1982 and supported by ACHPER. This was an attempt to establish a daily 30-minute PE lesson and to encourage teachers to use equipment and apparatus to increase children's games skills.

Unfortunately, this positive approach by physical educators was jeopardised in 1983 by general economic constraints and political reorganisation, including the closing of the PE branch of the Ministry and a series of in-service cutbacks. This led to a decline in the morale of physical educators, which was increased by the 1986 decision of the Federal government to put its weight behind an **Aussie Sport** policy promoted by the Australian Sports Commission (ASC) (Figure 19.8). This particular programme was designed to

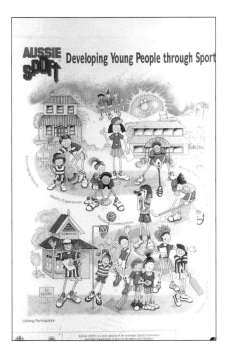

Fig. 19.8 Aussie sport: its place in school and community.

overcome the apparent lack of games skills among primary children and was initially directed towards the final three grades of primary schooling. Prior to this, sport in schools had reflected the British tradition of optional extracurricular groups and teams, with skill learning as part of the PE curriculum.

Federal government funds for the Aussie Sport scheme were to be distributed through state administrations and presented with a set of objectives which were largely acceptable to physical educators. However, the operation of the scheme was linked with sport outcomes rather than personal development, even though the general aim was to offer every primary child in Australia the opportunity to realise his or her physical and personal potential. In 1988, as an extension of this project, the ASC suggested modified forms of netball, hockey, soccer, baseball and rugby with the major objective of improving the 'quality, quantity and variety of sports available to Australian children'.

As with the USA, it is important to separate Federal and state initiatives as well as discrepancies between policies and enactment in schools. With Federal funding on offer, state legislators looked very carefully at the Aussie Sport project; for example, the Victorian Ministry of Education made an initial statement on sport education as early as 1987 and a survey was made

in 1989 to establish how much time should be given to physical activities in primary and secondary schools.

Also in 1989, an additional Aus$12.3 million was provided from the Federal budget to expand Aussie Sport over a period of 4 years and to introduce a new programme, **Youth Sports**, for young people between the ages of 13 and 18 years.

In Victoria the Youth Sports initiative has been effectively implemented with an extension of the Aussie Sport programme to cover all school-age children.

However, these sport initiatives tended to reduce the status of curriculum physical education, closely reflecting the American emphasis on school sport and appeared to be the Australian answer to the European sports school policy.

There were some initial problems with adopting Aussie Sport in Victorian schools, because educators were afraid of win ethic objectives being applied by overzealous coaches and of focusing on a young sporting elite, so in 1992 a committee was set up to review **physical and sport education** (PSE). This was associated with a Federal policy called the **School Education and Physical Education Project** (SEPEP).

SEPEP and PSE, though closely associated, do not have the same fundamental objectives. SEPEP is focused on the diversity of roles a young person can usefully adopt in sport. Not just a player and captain, but also as a coach, referee, organiser or administrator. This general experience, a process fashioned in English public schools, had been largely replaced by teacher domination in the United Kingdom. The PSE review was published and put into operation in 1993 and the focus of this programme was on basic motor skill development for young children, followed by more advanced specific sports skills and fitness programmes. Both projects function in Victoria and supportive programmes are run for general teachers. A committee was set up by the Directorate of School Education and the rationale included a sound fusion of educational and sporting objectives for all children aged 5–16 years. Not all age groups were accommodated initially, but the scheme has become fully operational since 1995 (Figure 19.9).

The intention is to give sport approximately one-third of the time allocated to physical activity on the curriculum. Though coaches may be used, every attempt is being made to qualify the teachers in a variety of sports to enable them to focus on specific sports skills in **sport education** and general personal development in the **physical education** lessons. Emphasis on codes of behaviour throughout reflects the general educational intention of the combined

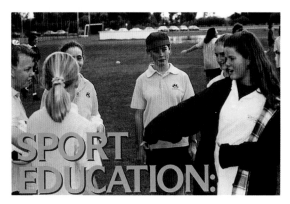

Fig. 19.9 Sport education.

programme. The recommended time allocation is 60 minutes' sport and 120 minutes' physical education per week in primary schools and 100 minutes' sport and 100 minutes' physical education in secondary school for Years 7–10. The overall objective at both levels is to achieve a daily lesson in either sport or PE and, though this is permissive legislation, every effort is being made to implement these intentions and make PSE part of the core curriculum with the full support of the Directorate of School Education.

Evidence to date suggests that additional sports funding has succeeded in the attainment of a daily physical activity session, where the educational criteria of ACHPER had failed in 1982.

To some extent these trends have been mirrored in the UK with the rivalry between PE teachers and sports coaches arising out of political support for sportscoach UK, but in England and Wales physical education gained some initiative through physical education becoming a core subject in an imposed national curriculum, increased credibility through key stage testing and increased status through the expansion of GCSE and GCE examinations in physical education. The recent tension between teachers and coaches regarding the John Major Initiative on School Sport, however, is a political strategy which might take Britain towards the PSE school policy, but successful implementation will depend on adequate additional funding and rationalisation.

Another similarity lies in the expansion of **sport science**. In both countries this is largely a higher education development which directly enhances the effective coaching and development of sport, but the funding in Australia was considerably higher than that in Britain, despite its smaller population. One outcome seems certain and that is the call for specialist PE teachers at primary and secondary level in both countries, either by increasing the proportion of physical educators in schools or by retraining teachers through coaching schemes in the Australian manner.

Years 11 and 12 are the optional examination years and, given that the Australian school year commences at the end of January, most children take this examination while they are still 17 years old. As a result the standards are acceptably lower than the English and Welsh A-Level. The Australian HSC was a national examination which is now in the hands of state departments of education and presented by a board of studies.

In the case of Victoria the examination is the VCE and physical education is a subject which can be taken. Its aims are to:

- understand the social, cultural, environmental and biological factors which influence participation in physical activity
- analyse the processes associated with skill development in the performance of physical activity
- examine the relationships between social, cultural, environmental and biological influences on participation in physical activity
- develop a critical perspective on physical activity.

There is a great deal of common ground between the VCE PE and the OCR, AQA and EDEXCEL syllabuses in terms of rationale, content and assessment, as well as in support documentation, where the VCE publishes common assessment tasks (CATs) which match the in-set material and answer schemes at GCE.

At a higher education level the **Australian College of Sports Education** (ACSE) is a joint venture involving the University of Canberra and the Australian Sports Commission. There are courses in sports administration, sports management, strength and conditioning, sports coaching and sports law. Facilities are at least equal to those of Springfield, Massachusetts, the Lesgaft Institute, St Petersburg, and the Paris INSEP and generally superior to those of any British institution, particularly in the context of sport science. It is important to note that the British development of high performance centres, which are normally associated with universities, are very similar to the AIS and its links with the ACSE in Canberra. With eight HPCs planned in England, there is also a similarity with the Australian Outreach AIS centres in each state capital.

As with the UK, admission to university is on a grading system but the Australian composite score is much more tightly structured according to specific subject requirements and, because VCE PE lacks some credibility, potential PE undergraduates may be disadvantaged.

State universities appear to focus on different programmes rather than compete with each other, as in the UK. In Victoria, for example, RMIT has a major Sport Science undergraduate and postgraduate programme; Deakin University has Bachelor of Applied Science degrees in Human Movement and Sport Coaching and Administration; and Melbourne University has a BEd (Primary) programme that produces specialist PE teachers.

In terms of undergraduate sport, intermural and intercollegiate sport is almost entirely a social experience. Distance might be a cause but, as in the UK, tutorial staff are not usually involved and coaches are employed by the Student Union sports associations. When student teams are needed for major competitions the administration is usually in the hands of elite sport institutions.

Given the British tradition of autonomous governing bodies of individual sports, the National Sporting Associations (NSAs) continue to have a major influence on Australian sport and the wealthier and more progressive governing bodies have established **junior development programmes** to match the Federal initiatives. For example, in 1984, the Australian Athletic Union launched its **Athletics towards 2000 Junior Development Programme** which involved the formation of a national commission and the selection of a junior squad and junior events coaches, similar in many ways to the English FA initiative at Lilleshall. To clarify that this is a governing body programme rather than a Federal one, there was funding in 2000 of Aus$50 000 from the ASC with Aus$250 000 from the Australian Sugar Industry as a direct sponsor of Australian athletics.

Review question

1. Describe the programme which links physical and sport education on the curriculum in Australian secondary schools.

(See Section 21.5 for cross-cultural review and exam-style questions on school physical education.)

19.3 The administration of sport in Australia

In 1975 the **Department of Tourism and Recreation** made initial moves to establish a Federal involvement in sport. Until that time sport was largely controlled by autonomous governing bodies known as **National Sporting Organisations** (NSOs) and received no direct Federal funding. At that time the annual budget for the Tourism and Recreation Department was only Aus$8 million per annum.

Federal involvement led to the formation of the **Sports Advisory Council**, which had a similar brief to that of the British Sports Council. Failures at the Montreal Olympic Games (1976) undoubtedly led to political pressure to establish the **Australian Institute of Sport** (AIS) in 1980. A **National Outdoor Stadium** had been built in 1977 for the Pacific Conference Games. This was the first step, to be followed in 1981 with the foundation of the **AIS** in Canberra as the administrative body to provide first-class coaching and training facilities for promising athletes. The initial programme catered for eight sports: basketball, swimming, weight lifting, track and field, gymnastics, netball, soccer and tennis, all of which had residential programmes at the Canberra centre.

Funding for the AIS came from Federal sources, administered through the reformed **Department of Sport, Tourism and Recreation**, and the budget was increased to Aus$24 million in 1982. The following year momentum for a **National Sports Plan** came to a head following a major newspaper campaign. Strongly nationalistic, it called for a centralised Federal administration and increased funding to establish an Australian sporting elite.

By 1989 the sport administration had been absorbed into a new ministry, the **Department of the Environment, Sport and the Territories**, which, as its first major act, established the **Australian Sports Commission**. Here was the start of a massive expansion in Federal funding.

The Australian Sports Commission, Canberra (ASC)

The ASC is governed by a Board of 12 Commissioners appointed by the responsible Minister. Its dual objectives are to increase participation in sport and sports activities by Australians and to establish excellence in sports performance. Its headquarters are in Canberra but it has administrative offices in the different states.

In addition, the Sports Development Division of the ASC is responsible for **Aussie Sport** and **Youth Sport Programmes** as well as the **Australian Coaching Council** (ACC) and the **Australian College of Sport Education**.

National Australian Institute of Sport, Canberra (AIS)

Athletes receive scholarships to cover board and other expenses, including travel to sporting venues and coaching. An excellent sports science and medicine support service was also set up. No expense was spared in building this national facility for elite sport at a cost of Aus$100 million and it is ranked among the world's best training facilities. In addition, the AIS has Aus$11 million a year to cover administration costs and a further Aus$2.2 million to run the facilities. The Federal government pays 95% of this with the remainder coming from commercial sponsorship.

As with the British National Centres of Excellence and High Performance Centres, there is a clause in the constitution of the AIS that the sports facilities are also available for use by individuals, community sports clubs and state and national sporting organisations. The common question is the extent to which the facilities are actually available to the public, given bookings by the resident elite groups as well as high fees.

By 1994 the scope of the AIS had been expanded to 20 sports, with scholarships for 500 athletes and a support team of some 70 coaches. To illustrate this from the sport of swimming, there were 37 full-time scholarships on 1-year programmes in 1986. They were serviced by coaches, masseurs and physiotherapists, with support from sports science psychologists and physiologists, with education available for any young swimmers. In addition, the swimming unit had some 270 visiting scholarship holders on weekly visits and some 66 visiting coaches under the same arrangement.

The AIS has a basic function of supplementing and refining coaching in Australia, but also functions as a scientific research centre where performers are tested in an attempt to improve coaching effectiveness.

As a reflection of the size of Australia and as a gesture to federalism, the AIS established outreach centres in different major cities (Figure 19.10) where specific national squads were based and trained. The AIS Tennis Centre in Melbourne is a typical example (Figure 19.11).

Australian Institute of Sport.

Canberra: gymnastics, basketball, netball (f), road cycling (m), road and track cycling (f), rowing, soccer (m), swimming and polo, track and field.

AIS Regional Units

Adelaide: cycling, cricket

Brisbane: squash, diving, rugby union, softball

Gold Coast: sprint canoeing

Melbourne: golf, tennis

Perth: hockey, volleyball (f),

Sydney: volleyball (m), baseball

State Institutes / Academies of Sport.

ACT, Queensland, Northern Territory, NSW, S. Australian, Tasmanian, Victorian, W. Australian.

Fig. 19.10 AIS academies and associated sports (f = female only; m = male only).

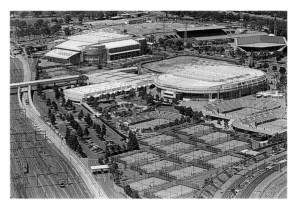

Fig. 19.11 Melbourne Tennis Centre. To what extent is this a successful part of an outreach strategy by the AIS?

Established in 1988, the **Cricket Academy** in Adelaide is probably the best known outreach institution, largely because over the past few years Australia has produced an outstanding national team; in their 1997 tour, nine of their test team were products of the Academy. A policy has been maintained that around 14 of Australia's best young cricketers are on full-time scholarships, which includes professional coaching as well as access to sophisticated sport science technology.

When the British Minister of Sport visited Adelaide in January 1995, he commented that he was impressed with the specialisation and the scholarship system. He also hinted that lottery money might be used in Britain to follow this example. As a result, the English Cricket Board and County Associations have regularly sponsored young cricketers to attend the Adelaide Cricket Academy, thus supplementing its income. However, they have now gone one step farther and appointed Rod Marsh, ex-director of the Adelaide Academy, to run the English Institute of Sport Cricket School at the HPC in Loughborough.

There is also an **intensive training centre** (ITC) programme in Australia, which provides decentralised sport opportunities for elite and potentially elite athletes. These programmes are often in smaller towns, supplementing the academies and acting as feeder programmes for AIS scholarships. ITC is a vehicle for recognising promising talent and is supported by a full-time professional coaching system.

The **Australian Athlete Scholarship Scheme** (AASS) is the equivalent to the World Class Performance Plan and the World Class Performance Potential Plan in the UK. The aim of the AASS is to provide direct and timely financial assistance to elite Australian athletes. Scholarships are awarded to acknowledge the expenses and hardship elite athletes incur in the pursuit of excellence. The **national sporting bodies** (equivalent to the UK governing bodies) nominate athletes for scholarships, but they normally also have high national and/or international rankings. The money is paid directly to the athlete for individual activities and to the sporting body for team games.

There is also a parallel scholarship programme for coaches. In its second year, in 1995 the **National Coaching Scholarship** (NCS) programme had 37 coaches involved.

The **Australian Coaching Council** (ACC) is a programme of the Australian Sports Commission and is sponsored from the Federal budget. A centralised professional system, it also has state and territorial centres with sub-offices at regional level. Its major function is to service the **National Coaching Accreditation Scheme**, a programme which is similar to the sportscoach UK scheme (Figure 19.12).

Level	Course Format	Course Duration (minimum suggested)	Experience Required as a Practising Coach
0	Coaching principles and sport-specific practical	6 hours	This is a non-accreditation orientated course
1	Coaching principles Sport-specific theory and practice	4 hours 10 hours } 14 hours	1 season (or equivalent— at least 30 hours— decided by National Sporting Organisation)
2	Coaching principles Sport-specific theory and practice	30 hours 30 hours } 60 hours	2 seasons (or equivalent— at least 60 hours—decided by National Sporting Organisation) in addition to Level 1
3	Advance sport-specific information on the theory and practice of coaching	100 hours	3 seasons (or equivalent— at least 100 hours—decided by National Sporting Organisation) in addition to Level 2
High Performance	Individualised sport - specific programme to augment existing high performance coaching abilities	Determined by ACC and National Sporting Organisation (generally 2–3 years depending on coaching commitments)	Must be coaching high performance athletes and be Level 3 (if available) qualified
Up-dating	Following accreditation under the NCAS, coaches are required to fulfil updating requirements over a four-year period as set down by their national sporting organisation in order to keep their accreditation.		

Fig. 19.12 National Coaching Accreditation Scheme in Australia.

The ASC, with its agency the AIS, engages in research and reform policies. Having established the schemes to accommodate athlete sponsorship and coaching, focus has now moved on to specific issues which influence sport in the context of Australian society.

SportsLEAP is a national programme, with organisation at state level, which helps elite athletes in the areas of employment, education and personal development and helps them balance these long-term objectives with their immediate sport commitments. Part of this is to support athletes with their careers as their sporting opportunities decline.

Equal opportunity for **Women in Sport** (see Figure 19.4) is a worldwide issue but has a particularly high profile in Australia, as it does in the USA, because of the male dominance of sport in a society where a macho image has stimulated a radical feminist movement. There is no doubt that Australian women's swimming, athletics, tennis and netball are world class and the male preserves of cricket, rugby and squash are being pressurised by successful women performers.

Each state has its own Women and Sport promotional schemes, complete with publications stating their case. An example of success arising from this progressive ASC policy is the central funding available for women's water polo, which helped to make them world champions in 1994 and 1995.

The **Aussie Able Program** (see Figure 19.5) is equally positive as it strives to give people with disabilities equal opportunity for sport. This scheme is very similar to the American Adaptive programme and may well reflect the shared attitudes of young, successful, sophisticated democracies as they try to broaden the opportunities of disadvantaged groups.

The **National Aboriginal Sport Foundation** is an organisation within the ASC. It has been responsible for the founding of the **Aboriginal Sport and Recreation Programme**, which employs some 24 development officers. The revival of Aboriginal culture is a flagship of the liberal Australian society, much the same as the Native American movement in the USA. In both cases it has become a political device; however, in sport, where ability rather than social status is the primary motive, talented individual Aborigines are able to socially and financially advance themselves and the Aboriginal cause as a result of success in international sport – Lionel Rose MBE, predictably in professional boxing; Evonne Goolagong MBE, an Aboriginal world tennis champion in a middle-class game; and now Kathy Freeman, an international

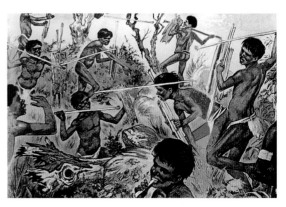
Fig. 19.13 Aboriginal children playing war games.

sprinter and Olympic gold medallist, with the education and will to use her status in sport to promote Aboriginal causes. It is essential that the lifestyle of urban Aboriginals is differentiated from tribal communities living in the 'outback'. Figure 19.13 reflects a reinforcement of old tribal activities and values, where children are role playing the serious activities of their ancestors, as hunters and fighters.

Drugs and sport is a world issue and it is significant that the UK, Canada and Australia are at the forefront of athlete education in this problem. The **Australian Sports Drug Agency** is very active and the AIS and academies, with their emphasis on sports science, are committed to promoting ethical and medical explanations for the exclusion of drugs in sport.

The administration of Federal sport in Australia

In addition to the AIS outreach centres working under the control of Canberra, there is an autonomous sports administration promoted by each state (Figure 19.14); it would be inaccurate to regard this as a direct extension of a 'performance pyramid'. Stemming from a reaction to the Montreal Olympics in 1976, individual states introduced programmes, with the South Australian Institute being set up in 1982, Western Australia in 1984, New South Wales in 1985, Tasmania in 1987, ACT in 1988, Victoria in 1990 and Queensland in 1991. Their executive officers meet as the **National Elite Sports Council** (NESC), which includes AIS representatives.

In addition to the significance of autonomy, out-of-state programmes were seen to be a major problem, particularly for young performers, and there were also concerns that the AIS was a little too elitist. In

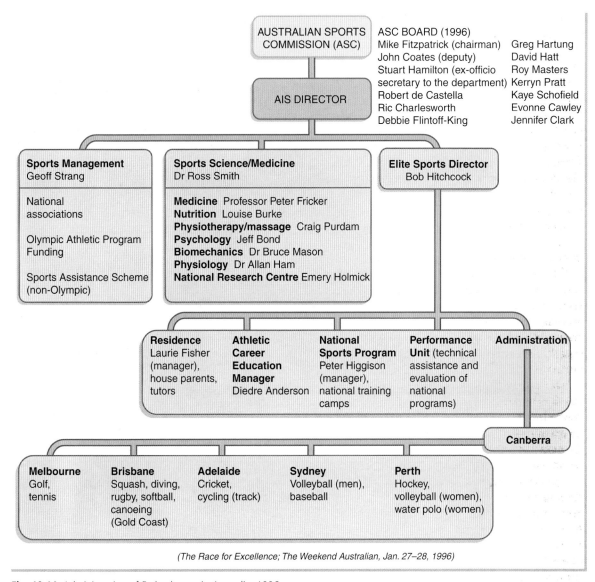

(The Race for Excellence; The Weekend Australian, Jan. 27–28, 1996)

Fig. 19.14 Administration of Federal sport in Australia, 1996.

reality, Canberra also had a very active **Federal (Commonwealth) Department for Recreation Development** in Canberra, but Sport for All objectives are best administered at a regional level, even if the state efforts are to some extent coordinated and financed nationally.

The result is that Victoria, for example, has its own **Department of Sport and Recreation** (SRV), largely funded by state and commercial sponsorship, which is part of the **Department of Arts, Sport and Tourism** (Figure 19.15). The SRV administers and financially supports sporting associations, major sports facilities and recreation camps in the state and provides documentary information as well as a comprehensive coaching service.

At an elite level, the **Victorian Institute of Sport** (VIS) was established in 1990 to assist the most promising performers in Victoria. Its guidelines are to enable access to advanced coaching, to supply a service in sports science and sports medicine, to facilitate competitive opportunities and to assist career development. It is jointly financed by government aid and private sponsorship, where once again the Commonwealth Bank is the main contributor, and as such the individual centres of excellence are justifiably called academies. In 1996 the VIS operated a major

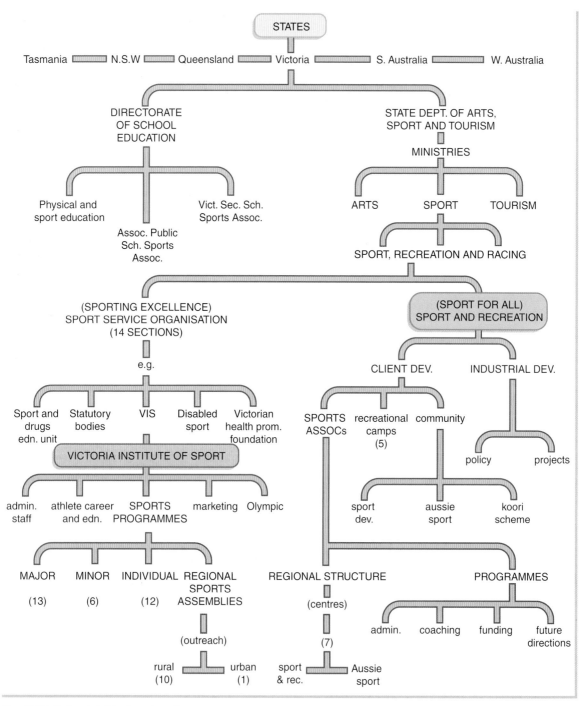

Fig. 19.15 State administration of sport.

programme involving 13 different sports and run from various facilities in the state by a head coach on a 2- or 3-year basis. In addition, there are six minor programmes of 1 year's duration and individual scholarships in 11 minority sports and 10 sports for disabled athletes.

Professional sport

The main professional sports bodies are business enterprises and represent the highest standard of performance in cricket, together with the four codes of football. Significantly, football is very much associated with certain states. Aussie Rules is centred on Melbourne (Victoria) but includes teams from Western and South Australia; rugby union and rugby league are centred on Sydney (NSW) but are also major games in Queensland. They are all controlled by professional league administrations but the unsuccessful attempt to prevent a super league commencing in rugby league reflects the power of the existing clubs and media moguls such as Packer and Murdoch.

Over the last few years, there has been a geographical expansion of both Aussie Rules and rugby union. There are now very successful Aussie Rules teams in Sydney and Brisbane and rugby is now very strong in Melbourne.

Soccer is making rapid progress as a professional game and the latest developments are to reduce its ethnic associations. The development of basketball as a major American promotion is growing in popularity as a result of extensive TV publicity, but baseball and/or softball tend to be limited to the Sydney area. Other activities which tend to ignore the 'pro-am' variable, such as tennis and golf, exist at the highest level in each state.

The **draft system**, which is part of the American professional selection process, has existed in Aussie Rules and rugby league but the draft has been made illegal in rugby league on human rights grounds since 1993.

Two specifically Australian features are worthy of mention. The **Brownlow Medal** is given annually in Aussie Rules for the 'Best and Fairest'. This is one of the most violent games being played and it is very 'British' to associate fair play with ability at a professional level (Figure 19.16). The second feature is the **state of origin games**. In both Aussie Rules and rugby league, the premier matches of the season have formed a series in which professionals play for their own state rather than the home state of their club. This gives the poorer states a chance to use players who have moved to bigger clubs. The only

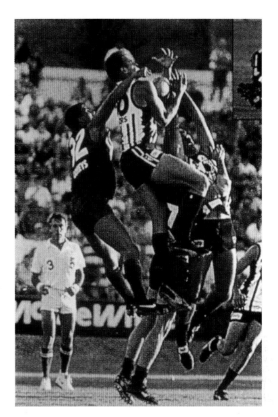

Fig. 19.16 Aussie Rules football.

criticism of a series which draws the biggest crowds in Australian sport is the decision to calculate the state of origin from the player's residence at 15 years of age rather than their birthplace.

Review question

1. Explain the extent to which Aussie Rules can be said to be an ethnic sport in Australia.

(See Section 21.5 for cross-cultural review and exam-style questions on sport.)

19.4 The organisation of outdoor recreation and outdoor education in Australia

Outdoor recreation is taken to mean recreational activities in the natural environment. While it is fundamentally concerned with enjoying and appreciating natural scenery, there is an element of escape in that many outdoor recreationists are 'getting away from' the urban environment. It is important to recognise, however, that cities like Melbourne and Adelaide are carefully laid-out garden cities with considerable parkland space even in the city centres.

There is also a general concern for conservation, with environmentalists reminding the Australian public that abuse and excessive use of the countryside can lead to pollution and erosion.

When different ways of exploring the natural environment are considered, we are studying the area of **outdoor pursuits**. At the most recreational level, this can simply be the use of skills like canoeing or climbing to travel and reach places or it can mean engaging in the challenge of nature and the elements, through canoeing on wild water or attempting classified rock climbs. Finally, there is the sporting dimension, evident in sailing and canoeing, where contests are held on fixed courses.

The use of the term **outdoor education** implies the inculcation of educational values in the natural environment and may involve physical, personal and social development, as well as learning more about the natural environment.

In Australia, the terms **outdoor recreation** and **outdoor education** have exactly the same connotations as in the UK, where they refer to positive physical experiences in the natural environment. At an administrative level, control in Australia is centralised through the Federal Department for the Arts, Sport, the Environment, Tourism and the Territories, with the Ministry of Education retaining responsibility for outdoor education as a part of physical education.

The size of Australia, with its variety of topographical and climatic conditions, makes it comparable with the USA, but because the population is so small and because the bulk of it is urbanised on the East coast plain, there are huge tracts of wilderness which have literally no townships and as such are readily comparable with central Russia.

In terms of attitude, there are many apparent similarities with the USA in so far as Australia is a young striving society with past links with Britain, but an increasingly pluralist society. Both the USA and Australia have come through a process of emigration and rolling back frontiers, with all the spirit of adventure linked with this.

As a young multicultural society, Australia is also striving to establish an identity which cannot be readily linked with historical roots and as a Federation it is difficult, politically, to bring a country together as a national unit. This need has already been linked with the significance of sport in Australia and the extent to which the Australian government is prepared to fund sport but, as with the USA, there is the potential to build national pride in the natural beauty of the Australian countryside.

Much is known worldwide about the beautiful beaches and awareness of the interior has increased due to the *Crocodile Dundee* films, but the Australian Federal government has now engaged in a comprehensive programme of promoting international tourism on a large scale to attract Japanese, European and American visitors. This has been sponsored at Federal level but is organised by individual state departments and run by the National Parks and Wildlife Service.

It is important to understand that although Australia has national parks, the term is really a misnomer as they are run by individual states and are not controlled at Federal level, as in the USA. Certainly, a similar process to that enacted by Theodore Roosevelt in America has happened in Australia and establishments like **Uluru Park**, which includes Ayers Rock (Figure 19.17), **Kakadu Park** in the Northern Territory and the **Barrier Reef** are world famous.

The stringent USA grading of outdoor recreation sites from urban picnic areas to wilderness has not yet been achieved in Australia. The British notion of freedom and romanticism has meant that provision is often very sparse off the beaten track and Australians have reserved the Aboriginal idea of 'going walkabout', where bushwalking is far less sophisticated than the backpacking American model. If you understand that huge areas of Australia are virtually wilderness country of the most hostile kind, with few or no marked roads off the superhighways, you can appreciate that a genuine frontier adventure situation still exists in Australia – indeed, places like the **Simpson Desert** and the **Kimberley Mountains** are barely mapped.

There is a wide variety of natural facilities extending outward from each large city; these can take the adventurer into the wilderness in less than 100 miles. Managed by **State Departments of Conservation, Forest and Lands**, the largest areas tend to be called national parks, with state parks covering an intermediate area and smaller regional parks being of about a 5-mile radius. In the Darwin Region of the Northern Territory, for example, there are open country picnic sites within and beyond the city limits; within

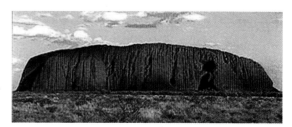

Fig. 19.17 Ayers Rock (Uluru), Australia. Photographer Helen Roscoe

Rowing has long been a tradition in the older cities and remains part of the independent school sector, with Australian scullers among the world's best and, farther inland, there are numerous graded rivers which have encouraged various types of canoe racing and rafting. Also the mountains, particularly the Southern Alps, have allowed mountaineering clubs to flourish and numerous ski resorts to be opened up. On a massive land mass, it is not surprising to find cycle road racing high on the Australian sports agenda with academies in Canberra for men and women.

In a young country with so many natural hazards, it is reasonable to expect **outdoor education** to be high on the school physical education agenda, if only to prevent unnecessary loss of life through uninitiated individuals and groups becoming lost or injured in the bush. It would appear that the urgency of this educational programme on safety, conservation and recreation grounds has not reached the levels found in the USA or France, but there has been a long-held colonial tradition of valuing the outdoors, even if this has been couched in terms of the freedom of the individual to 'do their own thing'.

Consequently, the older programmes in Australian schools have hinged on knowing about the outdoors in the nature study sense, rather than an experiential level involving physical activity. As new teaching styles evolved, so did the notion that first-hand experience in environmental studies was valuable and in 1980 the **Australian Curriculum Development Centre** produced a set of aims for **environmental education** which encouraged taking young people into the natural environment.

Parallel to this, there was a strong movement in the 1980s to encourage **education for leisure**, a campaign which had evolved in the UK a decade earlier; a major part of this was **leisure in the outdoors**. This movement was pioneered by ACT where, for example, the **Australian College of Education**, Canberra, started undergraduate programmes in leisure studies and schools in ACT were encouraged to develop leisure and outdoor education programmes.

In this way the work being done by physical educationists as part of their broad curriculum, where **education in the outdoors** included mountain and water activities, was reinforced by a central policy arising from this new awareness of the significance of leisure education. The physical education notion of field trips giving rise to greater understanding of the natural environment and the development of personal and social skills, which was part of the public school ethic, had not been entirely lost but until the 1980s

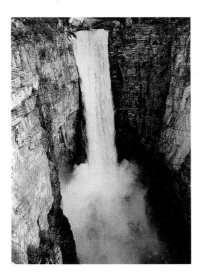

Fig. 19.18 Kakadu National Park, Australia.

30 miles there are nature parks which encourage rambling, mountain biking and horse riding; intermediate bushwalking and adventure environments at Litchfield Park and the Katherine Gorge National Park, some 50 miles away; and extreme wilderness conditions in the huge Kakadu National Park (Figure 19.18).

A difficult concept to understand is the attitude of the majority of Australians to their own beautiful, if frightening, outback. The vast majority of Australians are city dwellers, with the affluence of an economically advanced society and the creature comforts of modern urban living. Some young people regard bushwalking as a necessary life experience but many Australians prefer urban sports and Channel 6. It is this love affair of Australians for the rigours of sport which physical recreationists and environmentalists hope to expand into the adventure and national pride dimensions of the Australian wilderness. At the moment, for example, many Australians have four-wheel drive vehicles but very few take them onto the dirt roads of the outback.

The extremes of the natural environment, combined with the emphasis on competitive sport, have led to outdoor pursuit enthusiasts reaching international standards. As the first non-American winners of the Americas' Cup for ocean yachting, the Australians broke a stranglehold Britain had not been able to break for well over 100 years. The Eastern seaboard of Australia displays its wealth through its yachting community, but a beach society also excels at surfing and wind surfing as well as well-drilled beach rescue teams. Polynesian and East Asian influences have also led to the popularity of outrigger and dragon racing.

the majority of Australian physical educationists chose not to teach outdoor education. Today, however, given that the bulk of the school population lives within easy reach of the sea, you will find school minibuses ferrying children for scuba-diving and canoeing lessons.

The character-building notion imparted by public schools in Britain has continued in many of the Australian independent schools, the most famous of which is **Timbertop**. Founded in 1952, it is a branch of Geelong Grammar School, one of Australia's foremost independent schools. It is a forested mountain campus in the Victorian Alps, some 3 hours' drive from Melbourne.

In 1966 Prince Charles spent a year there as a teenager, while attending **Gordonstoun**. The reason for the extended visit may have been political but it demonstrated the similar philosophy and curriculum operated by Gordonstoun and Timbertop. Though Gordonstoun's site on the Scottish coast results in a greater emphasis on water activities, they are both adventure schools and both independent and both expound the philosophy of Kurt Hahn.

Timbertop has self-contained living quarters for some 200 boys and girls who spend their ninth year at school (14–15 year olds) in this mountain environment without telephone, television, video or CD provision. They live collectively in units of 16, adopting a spartan existence that requires personal responsibility and group cooperation. Furthermore, for a year the competitive sports they pursued at Geelong, such as cricket, rugby and football, are replaced by bushwalking, rock climbing, abseilling, cross-country skiing, canoeing and orienteering. There are additional physical education classes, but focus is on cooperation rather than competition and gender integration through aerobics, weight training and recreative volleyball.

Though research on the long-term effects on students is limited, claims are made that notions of self-esteem and a sense of community are instilled and recorded responses by the young people suggest that after the initial acclimatisation problems, the year is seen to have been a valuable experience. The authorities of the school make three strong points.

- That every decent Australian child must be interested in competitive sport is an idiocy which has caused a lot of unnecessary unhappiness to a number of children.
- Australia is one of the most urbanised societies in the world. It needed a protest and Timbertop supplied it.

- In the year in the bush a boy learns to know his capacity and discovers that it is much greater than he expected. He also perhaps learns his limitations when faced with the natural world, and this is also a good thing.

(Taken from Montgomery & Darling,[2] the apparent gender bias being explained by girls not being included until 1975.)

The whole concept is identifiable in the support for adventure education in Britain, France and the USA, but is also recognisably a counter-culture movement supporting cooperation as opposed to competition that is the dominant ethic in Australia and the USA.

There is evidence[3] that this 'experiment' continues to be very popular with school authorities and pupils. Normal academic schooling continues successfully in this environment and evaluation of the adventure experience continues to be based on cooperative attitudes, initiative and leadership and the safe application of skills in the natural environment.

There is little doubt that, in both Britain and Australia, the public school sector has the financial means to maintain outdoor education as a major feature of schooling, whereas state schools in both countries work on restricted budgets and limited aspirations of urban teachers. The inclusion of **adventure education** in the physical education core elements in Britain has been paralleled by directives from the Curriculum Development Centre in Australia, which has led to the funding of residential centres in an attempt to give all Australian children a taste of outdoor education through organised field studies. These appear to exist at four levels.

1. **Centres as extensions of classrooms**. These are outdoor schools designed to facilitate a first-hand experience of the natural environment; for example, the outdoor school at Arbury Park in the Adelaide Hills.
2. **Environmental centres**. These exist throughout Australia and focus on environmental studies rather than adventure education.
3. **Outdoor pursuit centres**. This is the largest group of field centres; they are outdoor activity centres mainly staffed by physical education teachers. In New South Wales, for example, McRae[4] identified 12 sport and recreation centres and five 'under canvas' sites.
4. **Outdoor leisure and environmental centres**. These have a broader input than the outdoor pursuits centres, in that they also include environmental studies as part of an integrated

study approach to the natural environment and its preservation.

It is easy to trace a similar range of centres in Britain and the level of successful uptake is similar, depending on local government support and the initiative of staff from specific schools. On the other hand, the Australian system lacks the organisational stringency, diversity and funding found in the USA and France, with their purposeful political, educational and domestic support for outdoor education. Similarly, although private camps exist, they have nothing like the uptake of the American summer camp system, although, as in the UK, many Australian students act as counsellors in American summer camps.

The **Outward Bound Trust** has existed in Australia since the 1960s, with the Outward Bound School at Tharwa in ACT (Figure 19.19); there has been an active research programme operating since 1972. The latter is typical of the Australian focus on sound scientific principles being developed in the educational and sport fields and is an ongoing research programme on staff training, programme design and implementation.

As an independent, non-profit-making educational organisation, its objectives are the same as the parent organisation in Britain, designed to promote self-discovery and social awareness in the natural environment. The following courses are run at Tharwa.

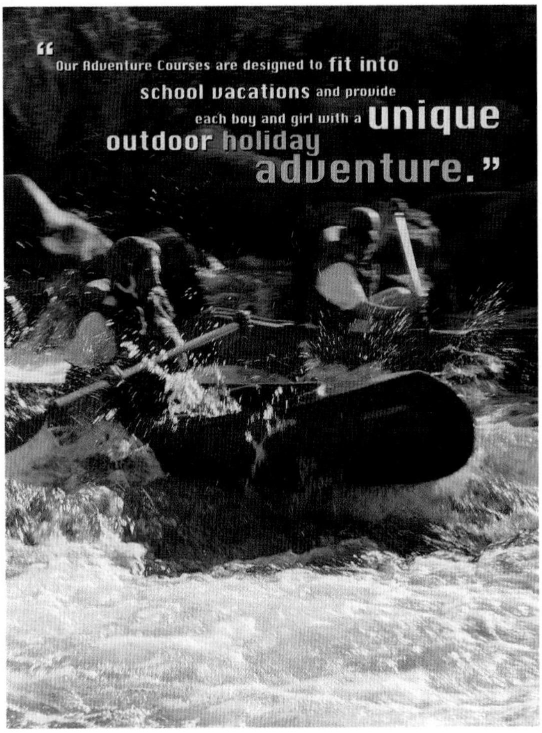

- **Challenge courses**. 22–28 days' duration – basic wilderness skills; community project; group discussion; solo periods of solitude and reflection. Includes Classic and Ultimate Challenge; Marine and Ski Classic Challenge. Involves canoeing, climbing and expedition skills in hazardous environments.
- **Adult courses**. 9 days' duration – a chance to get away from urban living; includes mixed and women-only courses; and marine, skiing and horse-riding courses.
- **Adventure courses**. 8 days' duration – children aged 12–16 years; a fun and unique experience programme, linking in with the Duke of Edinburgh Award. Includes pack and paddle courses; horse adventure courses; and sailing adventure courses.
- **Courses for past participants**. 9 days' duration – children aged 14–16 years; involving horse expeditions, marine and ski expeditions.
- **Family courses**. 9 days' duration – for families of four; designed to strengthen family bonds.
- **Discovery courses**. 9 days' duration – including disabled and able-bodied courses; intellectually disabled courses; and customised discovery courses of 1–22 days' duration.
- **Special needs programmes**. 10–12 days' duration – for young people with behavioural problems.
- **Wilderness first aid courses**. 7 days' duration – a Leadership Wilderness programme.
- **Schools and educational programme**. 5–12 days' duration – with values which closely relate to British outdoor schools and includes programmes for schoolchildren and university students and related programmes for educators and parents.
- **Management and corporate training programme**. 1–16 days' duration – designed as a partnership between staff and client representatives to develop individual and team initiatives.

Like it? That would be one of the biggest understatements around. It's been one of the most incredible experiences I've ever had. Things that I'd never really contemplated doing before; here I was in the middle of the Snowy River. I just couldn't believe it!

Fig. 19.19 Tharwa Outward Bound Adventure Course.

(Discovery course participant)

(See Section 21.5 for cross-cultural and exam-style questions.)

References

1. Dunstan K 1973 *Sports*. Cassell Australia, Sydney
2. Montgomery E M, Darling J 1967 *Timbertop*. F. W. Cheshire, Sydney
3. McArthur A, Priest S 1993 *Timbertop*. Adventure Education 10(1):20-26
4. McRae K 1986 *Outdoor education 'down under'; diversity, direction*. Adventure Education 3(3):25–27

Further reading

Geographical influences

Regional Surveys of the World 1994 *The Far East and Australasia*, 25e. Europa, London

Historical influences

Adair D, Vamplew R 1977 *Sport in Australian history*, Oxford University Press, Oxford
Cashman J 1996 *Paradise of sport*. Oxford University Press, Oxford
Dunstan K 1973 *Sports*. Cassell Australia, Melbourne, Victoria
Howell R, Howell M 1987 *A history of Australian sport*. Shakespeare Head Press, Drummoyne, New South Wales
Vamplew R 1994 *Sport in Australia*. Cambridge University Press, Cambridge

Socio-economic factors

Booth D, Tatz C 2003 *One-Eyed: A View of Australian Sport*. Allen & Unwin, St. Leonards, NSW
Cashman J 1996 *Paradise of sport*. Oxford University Press, Oxford
Clark R 1999 *Fixing the Olympics*. Information Australia, Melbourne

Daly J A 1991 *The quest for excellence*. Australian Government Publishing Service, Canberra
Davis D et al 1986 *Physical education: theory and practice*. Macmillan, South Yarra, Australia
Dunstan K 1973 *Sports*. Cassell Australia, Sydney
Houlihan B 1994 *Sport and international politics*. Harvester Wheatsheaf, London
Roscoe D A, Roscoe J V, Honeybourne J, Davis R, Galligan F 2003 *Physical education and sports studies AS/A2 level student revision guide*, 3rd edn. Jan Roscoe Publications, Widnes
Vamplew W, Stoddart B 1992 *Sport in Australia: a social history*. Melbourne, Victoria

Outdoor recreation and education

Australian Sports Commission 1995 *Fact sheets and brochures on specific academies*, Aussie sport, women in sport, etc. ASC, Belconnen, ACT 2616
Cheshire F W, Neill J 1997 *Outward Bound Australia*. Tharwa Outward Bound School, ACT 2620
Daly J 1991 *The quest for excellence*. ASC, Belconnen, ACT 2616
ISCPES 1991 *Sport for All. Into the 90s*, vol 7. Meyer and Meyer Verlag, Berlin

Physical education and sport in North America with particular reference to the United States

20

Learning objectives

On completion of this section, you will be able to:

1. Develop global awareness through the study of the USA as part of North America, but also as a superpower.

2. Understand the cultural variables which exist in the United States as a capitalist society.

3. Become aware of the structure and function of school physical education and interschool sport in the United States.

4. Understand the basis of the policy, administration and practice of sport in the USA.

5. Appreciate the development and organisation of outdoor recreation in the diverse natural environment of the United States.

In studying the United States there is a need to take the more global view of North America, particularly in the geographical sense of it being a single land mass, but also developmentally in that there has been particular interaction between Canada and the States, both sharing a common heritage, but also to a lesser extent the relationship between the US and Mexico as an emergent neighbour.

20.1 The social setting of physical education and sport in the United States of America

We need to have a knowledge of the **cultural background** before we can hope to understand how organised physical activity functions in different societies. We will continue to call these influences **cultural determinants** and look at them under three main headings: **geographical**, **historical** and **socio-economic**.

Geographical influences on physical education and sport in the United States

Geography is a very broad field of study, but is limited in the analysis here to comments on population, land area, topography, climate, urbanisation and communications in the context of sport and physical education.

Population

The population growth for the USA from 1930 to 2001 is shown in Table 20.1. In 2001, this had risen to circa 281 million with approximately 80% Caucasians.

Table 20.1 US population growth

Year	1930	1950	1960	1980	1988	1998	2001
Population (millions)	106	151	179	227	245.8	270.3	281

Size

The area of the USA is 3 539 289 square miles. In terms of different individual states:

- Texas has area of 262 000 square miles
- California has area of 156 000 square miles
- New England has an area of 63 000 square miles.

In comparative terms, the UK is about two-thirds the size of California, but has well over twice the population; France is four-fifths the size of Texas but with over four times the population. Geographically, therefore, each state is equivalent to a European country.

Topography

Every type of terrain occurs, from wide plain and deserts to the high mountains of the Rockies. There are wide expanses of 'frontier country', with backpacking and winter sport provision, and extensive coastal waters, with New England being the centre of ocean sailing.

Climate

There are ten climatic zones.

1. Pacific coast, ranging from polar to warm temperate to desert in the South
2. Mountain states, with relief and latitude factors
3. High plains, cold continental, ranging from blizzards to dust bowls
4. Central plains, temperate continental and high rainfall
5. Mid-West, continental with hot summers and cold winters
6. Great Lakes, similar to the plains, but very cold winters
7. Appalachian Mountains, with cool temperate moving South to warm temperate, but very high rainfall
8. Gulf coast, subtropical
9. Atlantic coast, temperate maritime (similar to UK)
10. New England, cool temperate with severe winters and warm summers.

All sports and recreational pastimes are possible with such a complex pattern of climate, but distance can be a problem.

Urbanisation

Population density is circa 66 per square mile. Massive areas are virtually unpopulated, while some areas, such as parts of California, have huge urban sprawls and air pollution problems.

Communications

Sophisticated interstate air travel and transcontinental railways, with complex freeways and Greyhound coach services. There is extensive car use, with a custom of travelling long distances compared to Europeans.

Review questions

1. Explain the significance of the frontier spirit in the USA in the context of Wilderness.
2. Compare links between the size of the country, communications and sport in the USA.

Historical influences on sport and physical education in the United States

In the 18th century, only the Eastern seaboard had been settled by Europeans, but a primitive version of lacrosse (baggataway) was already being played by a variety of Indian tribes. European culture steadily took over and, according to Baker,[1] the geography of colonial sports reflected the varied origins of the settlers. In the English colonies, courtly activities such as hunting and horse racing were evident, as well as popular festivals; and international cricket matches were being played by 1751.

As in Europe, many of the popular recreations suffered at the hands of Puritanism. Following the War of Independence, field sports continued in the East but the phrase 'frontier sport' reflected the spirit of survival and individualism through such festivals as 'barn raisings'.

The Civil War took American society yet another step away from the 'courtly mould' of the English gentry and sport became a key element in the emergence of an American identity. Both codes of English football were played at American universities in the 1870s, but it was the rugby style at McGill and Harvard that became more popular. At Princeton in 1879, 'guarding the runner' marked the first step towards the Grid Iron game. Amateur rowing and athletics were also part of a collegiate input that established the tradition of collegiate sport.

Alternatively, the American national game of baseball was well established by the 1860s, with the National Association of Professional Baseball Players coming into being in 1871, marking the popular replacement of cricket (Figure 20.1).

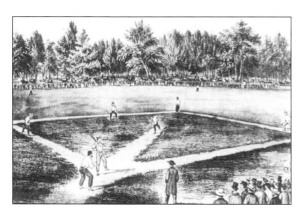

Fig. 20.1 The American national game of baseball. A print by Currier and Ives dating from 1866.

The great John L Sullivan and Jack Johnson made USA the centre of world professional boxing, a status it still retains.

Although American sport was extremely masculine, the traditional role of the female was less entrenched than in Europe and so lawn tennis, croquet and cycling were popular among middle-class women, with bloomers and rational dress accepted much earlier than in England.

The influence of the Young Men's Christian Association (YMCA) was also considerable and the combination of James B Naismith and the Springfield YMCA University led to the birth of basketball in 1891, followed by volleyball in 1895. Significantly, women were encouraged to play both games from the beginning.

Gymnastics and physical training were very popular among German and Scandinavian ethnic communities, to the extent that both activities were well established in Massachusetts by the 1820s, with fully qualified civilian instructors. However, such was the significance of sport in the universities and high schools that it was games rather than gymnastics which emerged triumphant, epitomised by the American cry of 'health and sport' as against 'health through physical education!'.

The frontier was a reality until 1918, personified by the dynamic lifestyle of President Theodore Roosevelt. When it finally disappeared, the rugged scenery became the vehicle whereby national pride was sustained through backpacking in wilderness environments, with well-administered national and state parks.

Review question

1. The development of sport in the USA reflects a nation adapting games to meet its cultural needs. Discuss.

Socio-economic factors influencing sport and physical education in the United States

Nationalism

The USA has a 'pluralist' policy, unlike Britain and France, whose policies are 'assimilative'. This means that every cultural group living in the USA is encouraged to keep its ethnic identity, on the grounds that this is one of the basic freedoms in the 'Land of the Free'. The various racial groups retain a cultural identity; they seem to dominate certain geographical areas and vary considerably in terms of economic wealth and social status. The biggest change over the last decade has been the size of the Afro-American group being over taken by the Hispanic group.

Generally speaking, the last group to enter the country has the lowest status. Consequently, Caucasians tend to have a higher status than members of the black community, but they in turn are higher up the social ladder than the Puerto Ricans, Mexicans and Vietnamese. Each of these racial groups has been identified with particular sports; for example, there have always been strong links between the Italian community and baseball and there are a disproportionate number of black professional basketballers. To some extent this may reflect the social exclusivity of certain sports; for example, track and field has a very broad racial input but the majority of top golfers and tennis players are white.

The autonomy of the 50 states is another obstacle to a national identity. Federal control is resented and the diversity of lifestyles is such that a state identity is far more relevant than a generalised national character, which tends to be meaningless except in international affairs. It can be seen, therefore, that national pride is not easily established in a young country, particularly one which has a decentralised administration and is practising pluralism.

Yet another problem has been the country's history of isolationist policies. However, the post-Second World War role of America as the champion of the Western world has brought the country into the international arena.

Sport most certainly plays its part in all these facets of nationalism. In addition to being a vehicle for ethnic and racial identity, activities such as professional boxing have allowed individuals to climb out of the social gutter. American football, baseball and basketball are uniquely 'American', culturally fashioned to meet the needs of a confident, get-up-and-go society and endowed with a status that makes sport one of the unifying features in a country where competitiveness is an esteemed quality and where the mass media is the main conforming agency.

The extent to which the honour of citizenship is respected and the ritual associated with the Oath of Allegiance and the Star-spangled Banner reflect a country that is striving to achieve the American Dream.

It is important to recognise that loyalty functions on a continuum from support for the local community to concern for the starving world. For example, New Yorkers can choose to support either the Jets or the Giants but when one of them plays any other football team the whole city rallies behind them. Probably, if this happens to be a game against a Californian team, they will gain not only the support of the state of New York but of the whole East coast. Should they reach the Super Bowl, they are now representing a conference, in other words half the American football public (Figure 20.2). As for the rest of the world, the game is a spectacle of excitement and athleticism; a mixture of showbiz and gladiatorial combat. Like Hollywood, it is a dream rather than a reality: symbolising American competitiveness and commercial enterprise but not necessarily reflecting the conscience of the American people.

Review question

1. How have the USA and Australia used sport to help establish a national identity?

Internationalism

As the major power in the North American subcontinent, the USA has attempted to keep an economic and political hold on the other countries. This is particularly true of Mexico and Central America, but their policy suffered a considerable setback when Fidel Castro gained control of Cuba.

The international political status of the USA has meant that it has had to defend its reputation on the sports field.

In terms of games, the greatest threat in ice hockey and basketball until the recent past came from the Soviet Union. For Americans, to be beaten in games which they originated has always been the bitterest of pills to swallow. The same attitude has applied to Cuban and Soviet successes in track and field athletics, boxing and volleyball.

International boycotts

When the USA and the Soviet Union boycotted each other's Olympic Games they were using sport as a pawn in international politics. That the boycotts were made in the context of the Olympic Games, a festival which supposedly involves individuals rather than nations, is a sad reflection on both the USA and the USSR and its satellites. In Britain and France athletes were allowed to choose in each case.

The principle of political boycott in international sport is nowhere more evident than in links with South Africa. All communist and non-white countries exercised a total boycott but, though the majority of white countries would not send national teams, individuals could still play in South Africa from choice in certain sports.

The political reforms taken by the South African government, symbolised by the release of Nelson Mandela and his appointment as President, together with the steps taken by governing bodies of sport

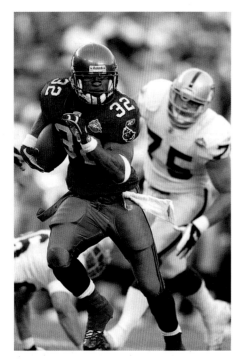

Fig. 20.2 Tampa Bay Buccaneers 48 versus Oakland Raiders 21, Super Bowl XXXVII, Quakomm Stadium, San Diego.

in the country to make their activities multiracial, have resulted in the international boycott being called off and South Africa being readmitted to the Olympics.

Review question

1. Explain the notion of 'the American Dream' and sport in the USA.

Political

The US is a republic with an elected president and two elected Houses, the Senate and the Representatives. There is a two-party system with the Democrats and Republicans, both on the political right. Socialism remains a political taboo in a strongly capitalist economy.

State legislation is highly significant, with the state governor having as much power as most national leaders in Europe.

As a relatively young society, the USA is still striving for an identity. It continues to admire the 'macho' image and has romantic associations with the 'frontier spirit of the Wild West' (Figure 20.3), much as the English warm to the notion of 'Merrie England' at the time of Shakespeare. This promotes an energy in America to forge a modern, unified nation from a melting-pot of exiles and immigrants.

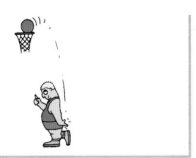

Fig. 20.3 Playing the American way.

Review question

1. Briefly describe the impact of capitalism on sport in the USA.

Finance and resources

The capitalist economy is based on the self-made man who has risen 'from rags to riches'. This is a key

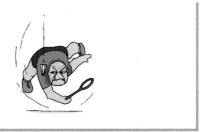

Fig. 20.4 'A winner never quits, a quitter never wins' (Anon).

factor in American competitiveness, tying in closely with the 'win-at-all-costs' philosophy (Figure 20.4).

Winning isn't the most important thing – it's the only thing.

(Vince Lombardi, professional football coach)

How can you be proud of a losing team?

(Jim Tatum, college football coach)

If it's under W for Won, nobody asks you how.

(Leo Durocher, professional baseball manager)

A team that won't be beaten can't be beaten.

(Bill Roper, college football coach)

Some American sports slogans taken from *Nice guys finish last.*[2]

Advanced technology and material wealth give the USA the confidence to accept its role as the major world power, with the demise of the Soviet Union. It also takes its responsibility as a benevolent society seriously through aid to the Third World and American support for the Voluntary Service Overseas.

Affluence is also evident in the extent to which Americans travel abroad on business and tourist visits. Europe is a major attraction for many Americans as they attempt to find their roots.

Review question

1. How has a market economy determined the funding of sport in the USA and what is the likely influence of sport in Russia following the 1991 reforms?

Discrimination

Regional

The historical division of America is North–South and the racial variable remains much more evident in the South. However, there is also a major differential East–West, in which the Eastern seaboard has a much greater affinity with Europe.

The most important regional comment is that there is no such thing as an American view, only a Californian or a New Yorker view, suggesting that it is always dangerous to generalise whenever you comment on American attitudes and traditions.

The underprivileged group varies according to the region, in that it is the Mexican in California but the Puerto Rican in New York. The general principle is that the latest immigrant group finds itself at the bottom of the social ladder.

Class

There is no clearly defined class element in the USA, but early English settlers took the concept to the Eastern seaboard. There is a clear meritocracy based on wealth and this is also linked with old families such as the Dutch families of New Amsterdam (New York) and the Irish families around Boston.

Gender

Feminism is strong in the USA. The frontier spirit gave the American woman a more dynamic role, but it also produced a society with chauvinistic tendencies, epitomised in the masculine sports scene. Women's rights have been fought for at political and educational levels, but it is the extent to which women have inherited wealth that has made some commentators suggest that America is a matriarchal society. There is less traditional separation of the sexes in terms of occupations and community games. Lapchick[3] and others have analysed the feminine image in America where, in the major games, girls appear to accept the limited role of cheerleaders.

Title IX of the Education Amendment Act of 1972 stated:

No person in the United States, shall, on the basis of sex, be excluded from participation in, be denied the benefits of, or be subjected to discrimination under any education program or activity receiving federal financial assistance.

Where competitive women's sport existed in the early 1970s, it was often financed with a budget of less than 1% of the men's athletic programmes. Title IX required equality of opportunity, facilities, practice time, coaching and travel, though it is important to recognise that private organisations can opt out.

Religion

In a pluralist society, with so many religious minorities, decisions are left to the communities themselves, sometimes resulting in individuals losing various freedoms for religious reasons.

Race

The subjugation of the Native American (Red Indian) and the slavery of black Americans have resulted in a form of racial inequality, which continues to exist despite legislation. Wealth, education and sport have helped to break this down but there are very few black quarterbacks at top level. The most significant break-through has been in the middle class game of tennis, where the Williams sisters continue to dominate (Figure 20.5), and Tiger Woods as the world's best golfer. On the other hand, there is a black dominance in basketball, athletics and positions in American football other than quarterback. This suggests that freedom of opportunity is still being denied in certain privileged sporting situations.

A considerable amount of research is being carried out in this area. There are two basic hypotheses being tested. One is concerned with **centrality**: that the dominant male WASP (white Anglo-Saxon Protestant) society tends to control all the central and/or decision-making playing positions in professional football and baseball. This research is also being undertaken in England in the context of rugby, soccer and cricket. The second research area is concerned with **stacking**: that certain playing positions are directly linked with promotional prospects, on the grounds that, as decision-making positions, the successful player has a capacity for

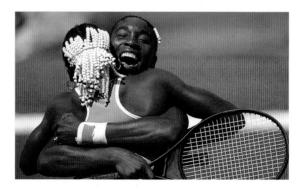

Fig. 20.5 Sarena and Venus Williams after winning the Ladies Doubles, French Open, Roland Garos 2003. Photographer Philippe Millereau/Action Plus

management. This would appear to hold for American football, baseball and basketball at a professional level. The vast majority of players in these privileged positions are white and so this limits the prospects of ethnic minorities reaching coaching or management status.

Finally, the views of Professor Harry Edwards are worth noting. He suggests that, in any discriminatory situation, there are three groups of people: a small group of conservatives who do not want change and therefore seek to retain the dominance of one minority group; the reformists at the other end of the scale who actively seek equal opportunity; and the mass of people in the middle who, apathetically, go along with the existing system as a self-prophesying admission of their own inadequacies.

Age

Though undoubtedly America is the wealthiest country, with the highest level of recreational provision, the highest standard of performance and the largest Olympic team, television news coverage has shown a New York scene of young black boys tumbling on old mattresses in a derelict building site. Without wishing to make too much of a spontaneous street activity, it would seem that a self-help policy inevitably means that the most talented and the wealthiest gain most. The plight of the loser in a the competitive society, identified by Arthur Miller in *Death of a salesman,* could also be referring to a social administration that pays little attention in recreative terms to the underprivileged, except as a law and order issue or as a source of potential commercial profit. A similar criticism could be levelled at Britain.

Disabled

America has a very active physical activity policy for disabled people, particularly in education. They call it an adaptive programme on the grounds that they are helping those with special needs to adapt to and cope with their particular disability, but also to alert able-bodied people to the needs of others. There is an active programme of assimilation, but also an awareness that special needs sometimes need special attention.

Review questions

1. Racial stratification still exists in the USA. Compare the chance of reaching the top in sport with obtaining a top career.
2. Discuss the exploitation of young sports stars in the United States.

20.2 The administration of physical education in the United States

American education and physical education are **decentralised**, but not to the same extent as in Britain (Figure 20.6).

It is very important for a European to recognise that each American state is comparable to a European country and that Federal action by the American government is rather like a confederation of European states agreeing to a unifying policy and constitutional foundations.

The size and population, together with a tradition of state autonomy, has resulted in each of the 50 states of America being responsible for the jurisdiction and general administration of their own education. However, the pluralistic, community-centred tradition means that control is administered at local board level.

Given these variables, it is always dangerous to generalise. Certainly, each state is different and the relative affluence of a state determines the quality of its educational system. This also applies to the local school boards, some of which are in wealthy neighbourhoods while others are impoverished. In addition, some urban school boards are responsible for hundreds of schools, while some rural boards are responsible for just two or three.

American education has a private and a public sector, where the private sector is self-supporting and often associated with church groups. Though it tends to cater for a more affluent section of the community, this is more apparent at college level than in the schools. The American school system is outlined in Figure 20.7.

If we look at the school as the primary unit, there is a very important difference between an American school and the British equivalent. The American teacher responsible for physical education in the school does not produce his/her own programme. This is presented by the superintendent employed by the school board for the area. The teacher simply

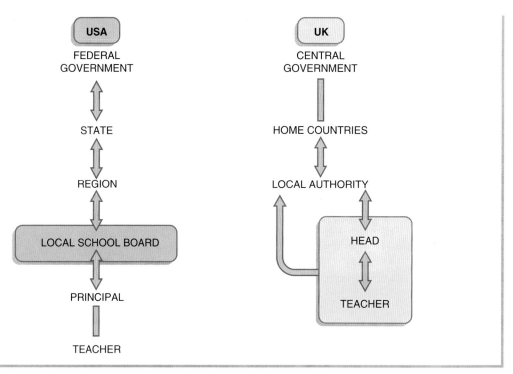

Fig. 20.6 Diagrammatic comparison of decision making in the USA and the UK.

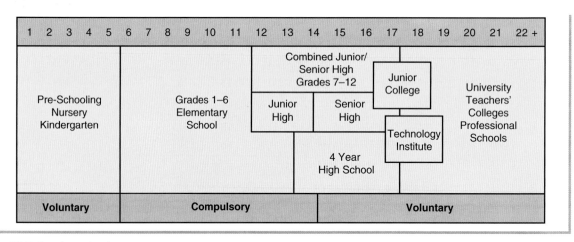

Fig. 20.7 American school system.
Notes: 1. Mainstream route is for children to attend preschooling.
2. All children attend elementary school, normally progressing from Grade 1 to 6.
3. Most children attend junior high school (equivalent to the UK middle school), followed by senior high school, graduating from Grade 12.
4. At 17 years old, approximately one-third leaves school, one-third goes to junior college (about half of whom progress to university) and one-third goes straight to university.

works through this set programme, much as the French teacher has to. The value of this approach is a guarantee of minimal content and planned progression; however, it tends to remove the elements of spontaneity and creativity evident among better

teachers in the British system. It would also seem to promote an instructional approach, in that the heuristic style identified in **movement education** is not easily written into a fixed programme. Given that most of the teaching content is in fitness programmes and direct skill learning, it is not possible to write a programme of progressions, so the American system is flexible enough to allow individual differences, human and physical, to be recognised. Unlike the French and English syllabuses, the American programmes are localised, allowing for community variables. Additionally, there are avenues for review, where teachers can approach the superintendent and work towards innovation.

A programme exists for elementary and high school children and specialist teachers teach the subject at both levels. Elementary schools average three 50-minute periods each week, but the larger high schools often work on a tri-semester basis limited to five subjects per semester. In the event, physical education may be taught daily for two terms, but excluded from the third term.

It is also important to recognise that the top-quality high school facilities are used extensively. An example of the use of an ice rink in Minneapolis high school is:

- 4.30am: individual ice hockey coaching
- 7.25am: six 1-hour PE lessons start
- 2.30pm: ice hockey coaching recommences.

In Minneapolis, for example, the school day and bus travel are closely interrelated. The early start at the high school reflects the fact that the oldest children catch the first bus, followed by the junior high and then the elementary age group. The seniors are picked up first, followed by the others, to give each type of school an equal-length day.

The advantage of the early finish in the senior high school is that it allows for the implementation of not only a major athletics programme, but also programmes in drama, dance and other subject areas.

Federal administrative structure of education

Each of the 50 states is responsible for the establishment and maintenance of a system of free public education. Each state is responsible for the general instructional programme, the certification of teachers, building standards and financial support (Figures 20.8, 20.9).

If we are looking for a set of objectives for American PE, four patterns are most common.

1. The traditional importance of sport in American society makes interscholastic athletics (in the general American sense of the term) by far the most powerful local objective, encouraged by

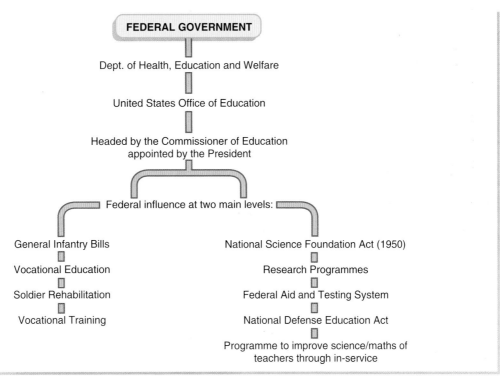

Fig. 20.8 Federal administrative structure of education in the USA.

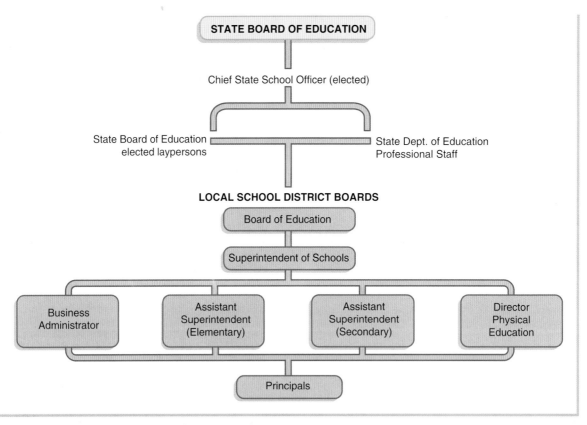

Fig. 20.9 State administrative structure of education in the USA.

ambitious parents and reflecting the commercial competitiveness of American society. This promotes skill-centred programmes and may result in an elitist programme, where the physically able will have greater opportunities with better staff.

2. Certainly since the Kennedy administration, great importance has been placed on physical fitness and particularly measurements of this. Once again, in a society where accountability is significant, physical educators look for a measurable facet of their subject. An awareness of health-related fitness is also very popular in Britain, but one must always consider the value of the experience on the one hand and the time taken measuring temporary outcomes on the other.

3. Educators who follow the Dewey tradition and who are aware of trends in Europe have introduced **movement education**, where task-orientated programmes encourage students to engage in decision-making situations. This approach has been adopted more readily by females, at least partly because they are not as

committed to the competitive sports tradition. It is because the **movement** or **heuristic** approach is seen to conflict with the competitive ethic that there are relatively few examples of this 'counter-culture' approach in boys' programmes, despite the number of books written on it.

4. The basis of American schooling is traditionally social education – the bringing together of pluralistic communities into harmonious, patriotic units. It also stresses the individuality of the American citizen, his/her ability to cope and his/her desire to make good. The more aggressive qualities fit well within the competitive sports concept but many of the progress reports in high schools also include gradings for social attitudes such as cooperation, sportsmanship and leadership.

If we look at the specific objectives of certain schools, we can see the extent to which they identify with these suggested patterns (Figure 20.10).

The importance of the extracurricular athletics programme cannot be overstated. The boys aspire to make one of the interscholastic squads; children

Orange County School District (Benning, 1978) **Objectives of PE programme:** • Maximum motor development, commensurate with their physical abilities. • Move with ease, confidence and a sense of well-being. • Movement utilised as a means of self-expression. • Develop and maintain a high level of physical fitness. • Desirable social growth and development. • Utilise motor skills in worthwhile leisure activities.	**California State Board of Education (Benning, 1980)** **PE goals:** • Motor skills. • Physical fitness. • Self-image. • Social behaviour. • Recreational interests.

Fig. 20.10 Objectives of elementary school (Grades 1–6) and state pattern.

compete to be part of the cheerleader support group; the reputation of the school and community rests on athletic success; and parents, in addition to the kudos gained, realise that success can mean a sports scholarship place in higher education.

There is some conflict between feminists and the role of girls in the male athletics arena. Certainly, **Title IX** (legislation which requires state educational institutions receiving Federal money to fund and staff boys' and girls' programmes equally) has dramatically increased the quantity and quality of girls' physical education and sport participation.

In the context of girls and the athletics programme, there has been a tremendous increase in the number of programmes in traditionally female sports and the national reputation of women's athletics, swimming, basketball and volleyball has led to scholarship potential in higher education for girls as well as boys. However, in many senior high schools girls would still rather be selected for one of the cheerleader teams than actually participate as performers in their own right. Certainly, cheerleaders work extremely hard and the number of girls involved is considerable, given that each competitive team in the major sports has its own cheerleader group. It may well be that more girls should be actively involved in school athletics as performers on the field of play, rather than playing a supporting role as entertainers confined to the sidelines. However, the admittedly limited possibilities of creative dance in schools allow at least some girls expression at a performance level.

Physical education is required to be taught co-educationally; while this prevents some of the more aggressive athletic sports being played on the curriculum, it tends to make instructional method even less suitable, given the diversity of the class.

A similar comment might be made about the **adaptive programme**. A great deal of money has been spent on the education of children with special needs. They are given special help, but every attempt is also made to integrate them into the class and the community. While this objective is admirable, it is questionable whether an instructional approach from a formal programme with mixed groups is the most effective teaching style.

Europe has no equivalent to the American senior high school athletics programme, which makes a considerable amount of money from spectator support and is thus self-sustaining. It pays for the building of outstanding facilities, which are also available for curriculum classes, and pays the salary of coaches in each of the major sports. The Director of Coaching has a highly responsible post and usually a far higher salary than the PE teachers in the school. He is responsible for his team of coaches and for the administration of public occasions and may also teach PE part time (Figure 20.11). However, his appointment, as is the case with all the coaches, depends very much on results.

The advantages to physical education of the status of sport in the high school have already been outlined, but there are also disadvantages. Inevitably, the objectives and the programmes in PE tend to be obscured by the pressure to build successful squads in the leading interscholastic sports. This leads to a focus on physical objectives rather than humanistic ones. This may be one reason why **testing** and **measuring** play such a vital part in American PE.

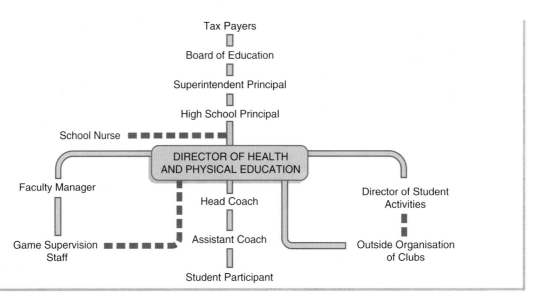

Fig. 20.11 Organisation of athletes.

Another problem which tends to reduce the significance of physical education, as Europeans perceive it, is the misfortune that the profession is an ageing one, largely because a huge enrolment programme after the Second World War has resulted in a large number of teachers of pensionable age, in a profession which is far less mobile than the British equivalent. Full pension rights require 30 years minimum in the same state; the more outgoing teachers make it in coaching and teaching a fixed programme can inhibit job satisfaction.

It is also important to remember, however, that the Kennedy administration promoted a major fitness programme that was one of the few Federal projects that directly influenced physical education. This includes programmes for children with special needs and concerns over the problem of obesity among young people.

Review question

1. Explain the significance of testing and measuring in physical education in US senior high schools.

(See Section 21.5 for cross-cultural review and exam-style questions on physical education.)

20.3 The administration of sport in the United States

Three ethics appear to co-exist in American sport.

1. The **Lombardian ethic**: winning is everything. The end-result justifies the means of achievement.
2. The **radical ethic**: the excellence of outcome is important, but more important is the way it is achieved.
3. The **counter-culture ethic**: the process is more important than the result. A strongly anti-competitive view, with eco-sport as an extreme example.

Structure and function exist within these conflicting ethics and remain sufficiently fluid to accommodate them.

It is important to remember that in America **athletics** is a term used to describe high-level sport and is often associated with professionalism and the Lombardian ethic. The term **lifetime sport** is associated with the European 'Sport for All' concept and tends to reflect the radical ethic; it is regularly associated with the intramural sports scene in educational institutions. The term **eco-sport** has been used to reflect sport which is healthy, fun and environmentally based, rather than competitive, and reflects the counter-culture ethic.

The structural basis of American competitive sport, athletics, lies in the specific club unit within an institution or a community. It is invariably private, in the sense that members subscribe to it, but at higher amateur and professional levels it is subsidised by sponsorship and gate money.

There are four main levels at which this administration functions: high school, collegiate university, amateur and professional (Figure 20.12).

The **National Federation of State High School Athletic Associations** (SHSAA) is a national advisory body which has branches in each of the states and controls interscholastic competition. Very little Federal money finds its way directly into sport. The exception is the sponsorship of the Olympic team. These individual organisations have met over many years and produced associations which act as governing bodies to maintain rules, regulations and competitions.

At the collegiate and university level, there are two organisations in operation. The **National Collegiate Athletic Association** (NCAA) is responsible for the interscholastic athletic programmes at larger institutions and the **National Association of Intercollegiate Athletics** (NAIA) controls the athletic competitions between smaller colleges.

The surge of feminism in American colleges and the increase in the number of women athletes as a result of Title IX seems to have resulted in a counter-productive administrational move, where in 1981 the independent Association of Intercollegiate Athletics for Women (AIAW), which had been responsible for female athletic programmes, lost control and the male-dominated NCAA took over responsibility for all athletics. In addition to scholastic institutions, religious associations, like the YMCA, and larger industrial

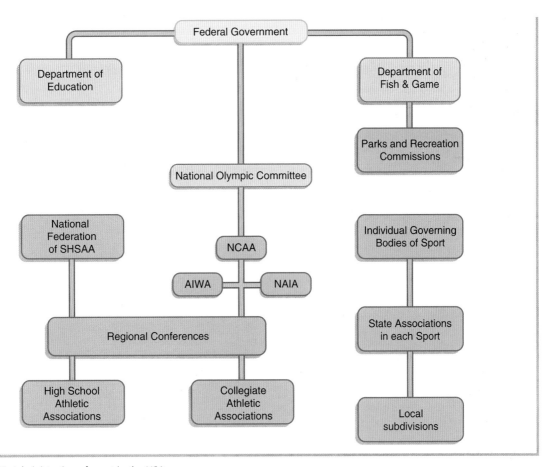

Fig. 20.12 Administration of sport in the USA.

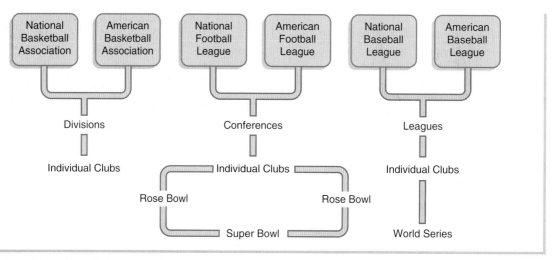

Fig. 20.13 Professional associations in the USA.

companies and trade unions have had considerable influence in the promotion of sport.

At a third level, there are the **individual governing bodies** of American amateur sport. As a result of the President's Commission on Olympic Sport (1977) and the subsequent Amateur Sports Act (1978), the powerful **Amateur Athletic Union** (AAU) was replaced by the creation of individual governing bodies of sport, for example **The Athletic Congress** (TAC) for track and field athletics, the **United States Gymnastic Federation** (USGF), the **United States Amateur Swimming** (USAS), etc. The rivalry between the NCAA and the AAU has thus been removed by legislation.

At a fourth level there is the professional scene. Each major professional sport has a separate controlling body or bodies (Figure 20.13). Such is the place of sport in America that to achieve success as a professional sportsperson is to be almost guaranteed heroic and financial status for life.

Formation of the United States Olympic Committee (USOC), 1950

The various Olympic developmental programmes – sports club based in Western Europe, sports school in Russia and Eastern Europe and armed services in developing countries – contrast sharply with the system of non-government involvement somewhat unique to the USA.

(Johnson W. 1974 Secondary school sports. *Gymnasion* XI(1))

Children's sport in the community exists very much on the same lines as English 'lads and dads' soccer. Parents and ex-players coach teams to play in leagues. The criticism is sometimes levelled that professional attitudes are encouraged at a time when recreational and educational values would be better. **Pop Warner Football** and **Little League Baseball** are the two best-known organisations (Figure 20.14) and to young Americans this may be the start of the glory trail to the Super Bowl or the World Series.

The huge commercial enterprise of collegiate football and basketball not only pays for the scholarships and seasonal costs of the whole athletic and

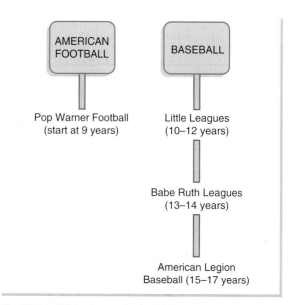

Fig. 20.14 Children's sport in the USA.

intramural programmes, but also subsidises other college projects (Figures 20.15–20.18). The American 'alumni' or 'old students' are a constant source of patronage, but it is often a successful athletic programme which motivates their generosity. There are criticisms at intervals from 'academics' against the 'jocks', but such is the public and alumni commitment that there seems little likelihood that this tradition

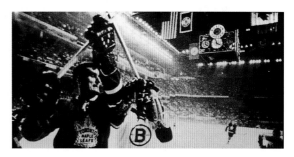

Fig. 20.18 Can you account for the high level of violence in some American games, but the low level of spectator violence?

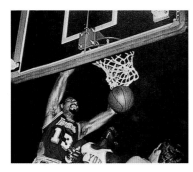

Fig. 20.15 Why are high-scoring games attractive to the American public?

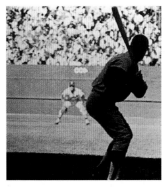

Fig. 20.16 Why baseball and not cricket in America?

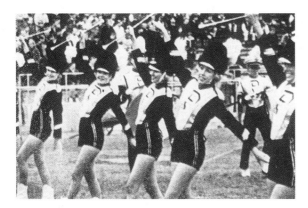

Fig. 20.17 Can you explain why American females accept this role in sport?

could be seriously threatened by any counter-culture revolution. Sports scholarship students should not always be blamed for their apparent lack of interest in academic studies. Often the commitment required by the coaching staff prevents even the well-intentioned athlete having enough time to study as well as train.

There are now some scholarships for women, but by far the biggest growth area is in female soccer. As a game it does not suffer from the gender rivalry found in Europe and so the female game is expanding rapidly in the USA at school, collegiate and national level.

The college athletes in the major sports have sports scholarships which give them a free higher education, as long as they fulfil the requirements of the coach in their particular sport. Baseball tends to have been an exception here, in that it has been very much the inner-city game and numerous community leagues exist to act as a proving ground for those aspiring to reach the professional ranks. However, such is the huge payment of top players that there is now considerable university involvement.

At a professional level, by far the largest amount of money is made through television and, as with any advertising franchise, this income is a direct reflection of success. Huge crowds attend professional American football games, but the facilities are of such a high standard that violence seldom breaks out. Baseball is again an exception here. The crowd is more volatile and the players are given to occasional fist-fights, suggesting some parallels with European soccer. It is also important to recognise that the distances travelled for away games result in most American professional games being played in front of home crowds.

Such is the pressure on winning at collegiate and professional athletics that coaches have a highly paid but a very insecure, job. Reference is often made to 'hire and fire' policy. This means that, as with European soccer managers, you are retained only as long as you win regularly.

Amateur sport is very strong in the USA, possibly because of the status of professional sport, but also because to many Americans sport is the last frontier. The Americans consistently furnish one of the largest Olympic teams and invariably finish in the top three medal winners. The strength of American amateur sport reflects the quality and variety of collegiate athletics. With around 50% of 18 year olds going into higher education and with a far higher proportion of promising athletes taking advantage of enthusiastic athletics departments, the American Olympic Committee has a ready-made selection process. Such is the intensity of competition between universities that there are also numerous sports scholarship places for promising athletes from Europe and Africa, to enable colleges to boast a winning team.

America differs markedly from Europe in that it does not have a strong private sports club system. This may be the result of the strong collegiate representation, which supplies quality athletes. However, this results in a rapid reduction in sports participation after college, except for the few who are good enough for the professional ranks.

The pro-draft system exists for American football and basketball. Well over 700 college football players are drafted into the professional ranks each year. This still represents less than one in a thousand college players making the professional game. The procedure is for the draft to be ranked and the lowest placed professional club has first choice. This system is not absolute, as wealthier clubs can break the draft by offering highly lucrative private deals with the clubs who have an early draft choice.

To some extent this frustrates the Sport for All idea and, even with exceptions like tennis and golf, many of the facilities for these two games are associated with country clubs where membership is very expensive. More recently, European soccer and rugby have become popular and clubs are springing up. It would be wrong to say that Americans have no sporting amenities for the less wealthy adult, but these tend to be recreationally based ice rinks and swimming pools or outside basketball courts.

Review question

1. Comment on the place of ethnic sports in the United States.

(See Section 21.5 for cross-cultural review and exam-style questions on sport.)

20.4 The organisation of outdoor recreation and outdoor education in the United States

Outdoor recreation is taken to mean recreational activities in the natural environment. While it is fundamentally concerned with enjoying and appreciating natural scenery, there is an element of escape in that many outdoor recreationists are 'getting away from' the urban environment. There is also a concern for conservation, with environmentalists reminding us that abuse and excessive use of the countryside can lead to pollution and erosion.

When different ways of exploring the natural environment are considered, we are studying the area of **outdoor pursuits**. At the most recreational level, this can simply be the use of skills like canoeing or climbing to travel and reach places or it can mean engaging in the challenge of nature and the elements, through canoeing on wild water or attempting classified rock climbs. Finally, there is the sporting dimension, evident in sailing and canoeing, where contests are held on fixed courses.

The use of the term **outdoor education** implies the inculcation of educational values in the natural environment and may involve physical, personal and social development, as well as learning more about the natural environment.

The size and beauty of the USA's natural resources are sufficient in themselves to make outdoor recreation one of the most rewarding elements in American culture, but there is also the legacy of Theodore (Teddy) Roosevelt. Acknowledged to have been one of the country's greatest presidents, 'TR' established a tradition of conservation and national pride in America's unspoilt wilderness. By 1909 he had set aside some 230 million acres of national forest, more than 50 Federal wildlife refuges and doubled the number of national parks. Despite tragic economic setbacks like the 'Dustbowl' in the 1930s, this pride in the 'Great Outdoors' has remained part of the American Dream, nurtured no doubt by the heritage of the 'Frontier Spirit' which went with it.

In 1965, the Land and Water Conservation Fund Act ensured that the 'dream' could be a financial possibility, when the **Bureau of Outdoor Recreation**, as part of the **Department of the Interior**, was given the power to administer a fund for state, local and Federal outdoor education purposes (Figure 20.19). As a result, all states now have park systems and every **State Highways Department** has to maintain roads into recreational areas.

Given the status and scope of these natural parks, it has been necessary for the Bureau to produce a coordinated administration. It is difficult for Europeans to conceive wilderness areas so vast that, without a stringent organisation, many hikers could become lost and die. Necessary regulations take away some of the freedom of action expected by hikers in Britain, but are essential to ensure safety standards. One method used to enlighten the public is through a classification of areas (Figure 20.20).

Wilson[4] suggested that in the 1970s there was a major expansion in what was called 'wilderness sport participation' and research indicated that the two main reasons were a desire to escape from the

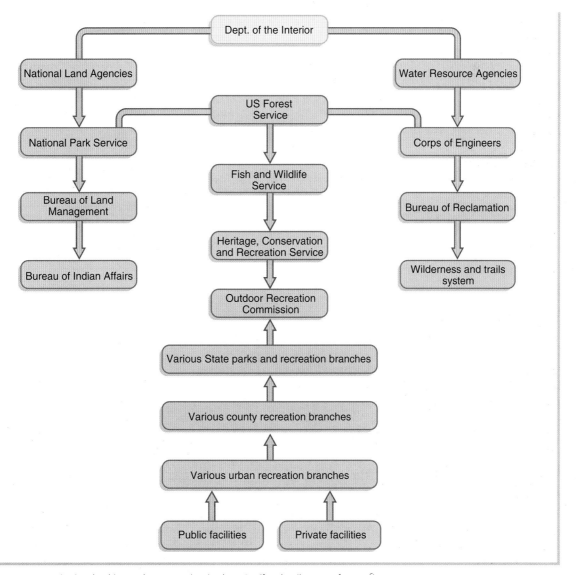

Fig. 20.19 Agencies involved in outdoor receation in the USA (for details, see reference[6]).

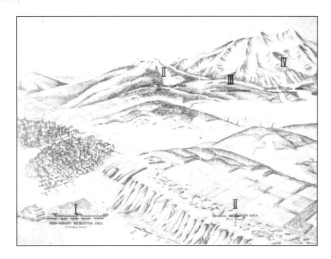

Fig. 20.20 Classification of national park areas.

- Class I: areas intensively developed near towns and designed for extensive use.
- Class II: areas with substantial development for a variety of recreational uses.
- Class III: areas which are suitable for recreational use in a natural environment, but which are within easy reach of habitation.
- Class IV: areas of outstanding scenic beauty some distance from civilisation.
- Class V: undisturbed, roadless areas, characterised by natural, wild conditions, including 'wilderness areas'.
- Class VI: historical and cultural sites.

technology and urbanisation of modern living and a desire to achieve a greater sense of self-awareness. These related attitudes were shared by mountaineers, backpackers, cross-country skiers and cyclists alike and were also found by the national park and forest services, as well as state park authorities.

Outdoor education has developed since the Second World War as part of an 'alternative' form of education. Very much in line with the philosophies of William James and John Dewey, it represented an experiential approach to learning and was readily associated with nature study and inter-disciplinary study. Jensen & Young[5] claimed that there were four main categories of outdoor education – personal growth programmes, inter-disciplinary studies, socialising agencies and recreational education.

In Britain, France and the USA there has been a desire to broaden the experience of urban children but in America there is also a 'counter-culture'

element operating, as an escape from the elitism and commercialism of the professional sports scene.

The **American Outward Bound Association** is an extension of the British Outward Bound Trust. It is a non-profit-making educational organisation and has the support of many senior high schools, where credit is given for attendance. Programmes range from standard 21–26-day experiences in the wilderness to shorter intensive adventure experiences; there are also courses in leadership skills and for potential business executives. These courses also include a variety of snow experiences, canoeing and backpacking, rock climbing and cycling, all with the intention of testing the resilience of the individual in an alien environment and group coordination in challenging situations (Figures 20.21, 20.22). In 1991 there were six centres: Dartmouth, Colorado, Hurricane Island, North Carolina, North-West and South-West. They are all situated in areas of natural beauty with wilderness characteristics.

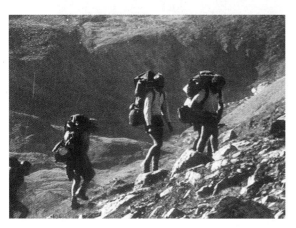
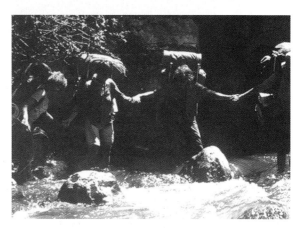

Figs 20.21 and 20.22 What characteristics of the Outward Bound movement do these photographs illustrate?

In addition to outdoor education as a direct extension of schooling and Outward Bound as an intensive adventure experience for those over 16 years of age, there is a wide-ranging provision of summer camps. As with the French system, it is important to distinguish between programmes with an educational basis and those with a recreational-vacational function. Examples of American children's camps go back to the 19th century; most of these were associated with taking impoverished children out of their depressed urban environment.

Since the Second World War camp schools have mushroomed in all the more scenic areas, particularly where there is a large supporting population within a convenient distance. These are essentially holiday experiences and there is a strong tradition of American children spending at least part of their long summer vacation in a residential camp school (Figures 20.23, 20.24). These permanent institutions are run by a variety of groups and ownership tends to dictate the type of child involved. Many camps are run by the state or individual civic authorities; these tend to be heavily subsidised to allow poorer children to 'escape' to the countryside. Then, there are camp schools which are sponsored by firms, ethnic groups and religious bodies and finally, there are commercial camps, where the reputation of the centre tends to dictate cost and, consequently, the clientele. In all cases, the children are on holiday and every effort is made to give them a good time, but also a safe time.

Traditionally, there are numerous challenges designed to encourage personal growth, socialisation and a love of the natural environment, combined with 'camp fire' and patriotic ritual.

There is little doubt that, as in France, there is a tendency for American parents to go on separate holidays while the children are under careful supervision at camp school. From the children's point of view, many make lasting friendships, particularly when they return to the same camp year after year.

A number of organisations, like Camp America and BUNAC, have the franchise to appoint staff from various countries and many British students work as counsellors over the 6–8 week period.

Review question

1. Compare the American summer camps with Outward Bound schools in the US.

(See Section 21.5 for cross-cultural review and exam-style questions on outdoor recreation.)

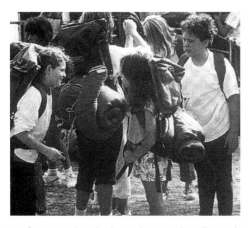 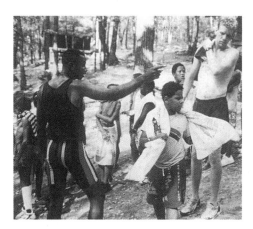

Figs 20.23 and 20.24 What do these photographs tell you about an American school camp?

References

1. Baker W J 1988 *Sports in the Western World*. University of Illinois, Urbana, Illinois
2. Gardner P 1974 *Nice guys finish last*. Allen Lane, New York
3. Lapchick R E (ed) 1996 *Sport in society*. Sage, London
4. Wilson W 1977 *Social discontent and the growth of wilderness*. Sport Quest Winter 27:
5. Jensen M, Young A B 1981 *Alternatives for outdoor education programming*. Journal of Physical Education, Recreation and Dance 52:
6. Weiskopf D C 1982 *Recreation and leisure*. Allyn and Bacon, New York

Further reading

Geographical influences

Bale J 1982 *Sport and place*. Hurst, London

Lane H V (ed) 1986 *The world almanac*. Newspaper Enterprise Association, London

Paxton J (ed) 1991 *The statesman's year book*, 1988–89, 127e. Macmillan, Basingstoke

Historical influences

Lucas J A, Smith R A 1978 *Saga of American sport*. Lea and Febiger, Philadelphia

Swanson R A, Spears B 1995 *History of sport. Physical education in the United States*. McGraw Hill, Boston, Massachusetts

Socio-economic factors

Calhoun D W (ed) 1987 *Sport, culture and personality*. Human Kinetics, Champaign, Illinois

Edwards H 1973 *Sociology of sport*. Dorsey Press, Homewood, Illinois

Houlihan B 1994 *Sport and international politics*. Harvester Wheatsheaf, London

McPherson B D et al 1989 *The social significance of sport*. Human Kinetics, Champaign, Illinois

Miller A 1977 *Death of a salesman*. Viking, New York

Sage G H (ed) 1990 *Power and ideology in American sport*. Human Kinetics, Champaign, Illinois

Roscoe D A, Roscoe J V, Honeybourne J, Davis R, Galligan F 2003 *Physical education and sport studies AS/A2 level student revision guide*. 3rd edn. Jan Roscoe Publications, Widnes

Wiggins D K 1995 *Sport in America*. Human Kinetics, Champaign, Illinois

Outdoor recreation and education

Bucher C A et al 1970 *Secondary school physical education*. Mosby, St Louis

Calhoun D W 1987 *Sport, culture and personality*. Human Kinetics, Champaign, Illinois

Ewart A 1989 *The history of outdoor adventure programming*. Journal of Adventure, Education and Outdoor Leadership 6(4): 10–15

Hellison D R 1985 *Goals and strategies for teaching PE*. Human Kinetics, Champaign, Illinois

McPherson B D et al 1989 *The social significance of sport*. Human Kinetics, Champaign, Illinois

Sage G H 1998 *Power and ideology in American sport*, 2nd edn. Human Kinetics, Champaign, Illinois

Physical education and sport in Communist and post-Communist countries with particular reference to the Soviet Union (Russia)

Learning objectives

On completion of this section, you will be able to:

1. Develop a global perspective of Communist countries where sport and politics are intertwined.

2. Understand the shared and specific cultural variables in Communist countries, but particularly those applying to the Soviet Union.

3. Be aware of the structure and function of physical education in Soviet schools.

4. Understand the role of sport in Soviet society.

5. Appreciate the basis of 'tourism' in the Soviet Union with particular reference to the natural environment.

6. Be aware of post-reform trends as they concern physical culture, sport and tourism in Russia.

21.1 The social setting of physical education and sport in the Soviet Union and post-reform Russia

Following the 1939–45 World War, the USSR engaged in a process of expanding the Communist world. This took immediate effect with the European countries behind the 'Iron Curtain'; with the emergence of Red China; successful campaigns in Africa and South-East Asia; and the revolution in Cuba. The disproportionate funding of sport by these countries as a political vehicle had a dramatic effect on the status of sport and physical education worldwide. Today, many of these countries have chosen to end their authoritarian, Communist regimes and adopt various levels of market economy. Nevertheless, the impact of establishing sport as a political shop window has left these countries with an infrastructure and commitment to sport which continues to bring them success, making a study of their approach a valuable global dimension.

We need to have a knowledge of the **cultural background** before we can hope to understand how organised physical activity functions in at least one of these countries and so the focus will be on the USSR as a Communist society and later as post-reform Russia. We will call these influences **cultural determinants** and look at them under three main headings: **geographical**, **historical** and **sociocultural**.

Geographical influences on physical education and sport

Geography is a very broad field of study, but is limited in the analysis here to comments on population, land area, topography, climate, urbanisation and communications in the context of sport and physical education.

Table 21.1 Former Soviet Union population growth				
Year	1970	1979	1983	1989
Population (millions)	242	262	273	286.7

Population

The population growth for the former Soviet Union since 1970 is shown in Table 21.1. The most important 'ethnic' comment is the former Soviet policy of encouraging Russians to settle in all the other republics.

Size

The area of the former Soviet Union was 8 649 490 square miles. Before its dramatic disintegration, the Soviet Union consisted of 15 republics, each of which might be compared with an American state or European country. West of the Ural Mountains is much more technically developed, with a more rapidly expanding population than on the East, or oriental, side of the Urals, which remains rural and underdeveloped.

With the break-up of the Union in 1991, it is important to provide data for at least some of the individual republics.

- Russia – a population of 146.1 million (2001) with an area of 7 625 000 square miles
- Ukraine – 51.7 million with an area of 174 412 square miles
- Georgia – 5.5 million with an area of 26 611 square miles
- Lithuania – 3.7 million with an area of approximately 26 000 square miles.

In comparative terms, Russia covers seven-eighths of the old Soviet Union but has about only half its population. It is over twice the size of the USA with around two-thirds the population. The Ukraine is about the same size as California, but has similar population figures to France or the UK.

Topography

Covering one-sixth of the Earth's land surface, Russia has a full range of land features, similar to that in the USA but with a limited seaboard, mainly in the Arctic Circle.

Climate

There is a range of climates but no tropical conditions. Mainly, it is very much continental, giving cold winters and hot summers, but with large areas in the colder latitudes making winter sports a central feature. The Steppes have a traditional reputation for equestrianism and wrestling is very popular in certain Southern republics (Georgia, etc.). The extreme cold of the Siberian winter delayed development until the advent of the 'Sunshine Cities' policy in the 1970s.

Urbanisation

Population density is 31 per square mile (half that of the USA but with more uninhabitable areas). Major cities are in the west, with St Petersburg (Leningrad) and Moscow, and there is a large population on the Black Sea, where many of the tourist resorts are situated.

Communications

There are complex road and rail networks in the European republics, but only two trans-continental rail links to the East coast. Air travel is the only hope for speedy communication. Many of the Asian republics are isolated by distance and primitive roads.

Review questions

1. Explain the significance of the frontier spirit in the former Soviet Union in the context of wilderness.
2. Compare links between the size of a country, communications and sport in the USSR.

Historical influences on sport and physical education

Whereas the UK had an industrial revolution in the 19th century, Russia was very much a feudal society until the October Revolution in 1917. This meant that there were nobles who pursued the 'courtly' activities of field sports and horse racing and the peasants who retained their occasional festivals. These folk activities were tribal, with examples of horse riding on the Steppes, troika in the Arctic Circle and wrestling as far apart as Georgia and Siberia.

The emergence of rational recreation was restricted to a wealthy elite, except in a few industrial towns such as St Petersburg.[1] Gymnastics and drill did develop as a part of the European movement, with Swedish influences from 1835 and the Czech Sokol movement from 1870. It was soon after this that Lesgaft introduced a system of drill gymnastics, which was adopted in most grammar schools by the 1880s.

The second phase of development followed the 1917 Bolshevik Revolution, but sporting developments were limited because of the poverty of the people, the political focus on education, industrialisation and militarism and the ravages of a civil war which continued until 1921.

Lesgaft became a cult figure and the Sokol movement was encouraged because of its social basis. Lenin recognised the need for 'improved health for the young' and in 1920 the Supreme Soviet of Physical Culture was established. This led to the formation of the Pioneer movement in 1927 and the Preparation for Labour and Defence (GTO) in 1931. Meanwhile, the trade union movement had started to encourage sport for the workers and sports clubs were formed by such societies as Dynamo, Locomotiv and Spartak.

The first Moscow Spartakiad (sports festival) was held in 1928 and school spartakiads were established from 1935. It was around this time that Sportsmen's Awards were introduced.

Alongside the GTO and sport, there was a strong military component and the encouragement of ethnic sports (Figure 21.1).

All this was internal and designed to be politically conforming as well as to bring the republics together in friendly competition. After the Second World War, Moscow Dynamo Football Club toured Britain and in 1956 the Soviet Union felt ready to compete in the Olympic Games for the first time since 1908.

This process of nation building and the formal political and economic integration of the 15 republics continued until the appointment of Mikhail Gorbachev as General Secretary of the Soviet Communist Party in 1985. Though apparently a confirmed Communist, he was unhappy with the old-style authoritarian form of government and concerned about the Soviet

economy. By 1989, two words symbolised the reforms he started to enact. *Glasnost* reflected a policy of public frankness and accountability and *perestroika* was a policy whereby Soviet institutions and the economy were modernised and Westernised.

The political consequences were that after nearly 70 years of authoritarianism, free speech was encouraged among groups of people, the newspapers and the media. At republican level, this released all the old nationalist and racist hates held in check by the Communist regime, resulting in calls for independence by different republics. The Baltic states of Latvia, Lithuania and Estonia led this fight for political freedom and, though there was pressure from Gorbachev to subdue this nationalism by force, he eventually allowed them to achieve independence.

It was only a very short time before all the remaining republics called for levels of independence, so the Supreme Soviet ceased to be the centralised controlling body. Gorbachev tried to keep this revolutionary trend in check by establishing an elected Soviet president to hold the various republics together, while allowing the individual republics to make their own decisions on how far down the democratic path they wished to go. However, the emergence of nationalist leaders, such as Boris Yeltsin of Russia, led to the removal of Gorbachev and the emergence of individual presidents for each republic. By 1996 no single, stable politic pattern had emerged as the Liberals competed with the old-style Communists in the battle for power.

There is little doubt that democratic policies would have had the support of the majority in the old Soviet Union in the name of *glasnost* but *perestroika* which is now meeting opposition because linking liberal politics and racial enmity with a market economy is causing some hardship. (This pattern can be seen at its worst in the former Yugoslavia, with its combination of racial hatred, territorial bitterness and religious bigotry.) The same thing could easily happen in a number of the old-style Soviet republics, resulting in civil war and the abhorrent 'policy' of ethnic cleansing.

The end of authoritarian rule by the Supreme Soviet was welcomed as a step towards democracy, but there was a security in the old regime where decisions were made for you in an atmosphere of full employment. Many initial enthusiasts for the reforms are now looking for a return to that security, having witnessed an increase in crime, unemployment and food shortages and a rise in national dissent. There might yet be a reversion to an authoritarian form of socialism, run by 'reformed' Communists and

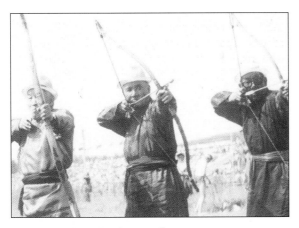

Fig. 21.1 Traditional archery is still seen.

supported by an older generation, or a disenchanted youth might be attracted to right-wing political groups.

Sociocultural factors influencing sport and physical education in the Soviet Union

Nationalism

The former Soviet Union was faced with even greater problems of national identity. Many of the 15 republics that constituted the Union had been independent countries previously. It was acknowledged that within these republics there were at least 100 distinct nationalities and 180 spoken languages. In literacy terms, 60 of these were taught in schools, there were 65 newspaper languages and books were published in 76 languages.

The political uniformity and authoritarianism of the Soviet Union did tend to cement relations between the constitutionally autonomous republics, but attempts had also been made to establish a cultural unity through the policy of making the Russian language compulsory in schools. Inevitably, this 'Russianisation' programme met with a great deal of opposition from the various republics.

Most of Eastern Europe has in recent years moved dramatically from single-party Communist authoritarianism to multi-party democracies, a process which has been part of the break-up of the Soviet Union. With the three Baltic states leaving the 'Union', the remaining 12 republics were tied only temporarily by trade agreements and specific treaties. As a result, the centralised civil administration between the republics no longer exists in a formal sense, but various arrangements, such as the Commonwealth of Independent States (CIS) grouping for the 1992 Olympic Games, were in place in the interim. Several of these republics are now entering international competitions as individual states. However, there is little likelihood that the administration of sport and physical education within each republic will become decentralised in the short term. On the one hand, they have more pressing issues to occupy them and on the other, former Soviet sport is changing to a nationally based system as found in Russia and the Ukraine.

Howell[2] used the phrase 'sport and politics intertwined', which expressed the dual role of sport to reinforce a Soviet identity on the one hand and to allow continued ethnic expression on the other. The significance of ethnic minorities remains in the independent republics, but politics is being taken out

of sport as nationalism overtakes communism. The association between sporting excellence and communism may yet cause a backlash, in which the replacement of authoritarianism by 'people power' may also lead to an emphasis on popular and ethnic sport.

The nationalistic significance of excellence in sport, evident in France and Germany, is developing in Russia and the other republics. An excellent infrastructure already exists and so it depends on the strength of nation building, integrational intentions and parental ambitions.

Review question

1. How has sport in the former Soviet Union helped to establish a national identity?

Internationalism

The former Soviet Union supported international communism and used sport as a vehicle to promote accord, but also to allow nationalistic rivalries to be released in the relatively harmless sporting arena. This was achieved through contests against Eastern bloc countries.

The Soviets also poured money and coaching expertise into Cuba to beat the Americans on their own doorstep. Cuba remains a Communist power at the moment but from 1992 has, of course, had to retain its political stance as well as its sporting excellence without money from 'Mother Russia'. It may well be that several of the old-style 'Soviet' republics will remain Communist and continue to use sport as a shop window or perhaps, like China, try to embrace a market economy without relaxing Communist control.

International boycotts

When the USA and the Soviet Union boycotted each other's Olympic Games they were using sport as a pawn in international politics. That the boycotts were made in the context of the Olympic Games, a festival which supposedly involves individuals rather than nations, is a sad reflection on both the USA and the USSR and its satellites. In Britain and France athletes were allowed to choose in each case.

Review question

1. Explain the notion of 'shop window' and sport in the former USSR and Russia today.

Political

Politics was intertwined with sport in the Soviet Union and was responsible for the USSR not sending a team to the Los Angeles Olympic Games.

Tsarist elements ended with the 1917 Revolution. Until the break-up of the Soviet Union, Marxist ideology ruled, implemented by Lenin on the basis of socialism working towards communism. Being an egalitarian society, mass participation in sport was central and part of a 'collective' system. It is still too early to say whether communism is finished in the independent states that once formed the Soviet Union. It is likely that the old-style authoritarianism has become outmoded, but various forms of 'socialism' might well emerge in some states while others might revert to a form of democratic socialism, having found the market economy and capitalism unpalatable.

If it is unlikely that single-party politics will reappear, some of the Marxist precepts may survive, including man as a social animal; working for the state; living in a changing world; and the spread of international 'socialism'. The old protectionist consumer-based society is being replaced in Russia and the Ukraine by a market economy that idealises the entrepreneur and a supply-based society. Whether this can be maintained in the face of efforts to slow down the change or even initiate a counter reform has yet to be settled.

What has now to be decided is whether the image of the manual worker or the bourgeois intellectual is going to dominate Russian thinking and whether sport will continue to be the shop window (Figure 21.2). Much depends on whether sporting excellence is linked with the old order or as a symbol of a new national identity in a market economy.

Review question

1. Explain the phrase that sport and politics are intertwined in the former USSR.

Finance and resources

This was a socialist economy in which the source of money was the state, with the bulk of its distribution through work and trade unions. Wealth did not lie in the hands of the individual or private enterprise, but not all workers had the same wages. The industrialisation of the European USSR led to population growth in towns and increased wealth; hopefully this trend will not only continue but will spread to the Eastern republics.

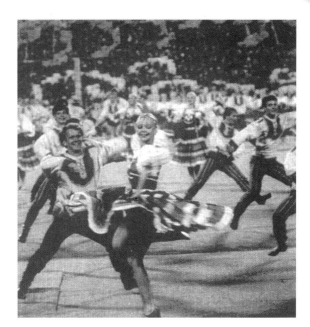

Fig. 21.2 Traditional dancing.

Raw materials are abundant in the Urals and elsewhere. The amazing speed at which industrialisation took place was the result of authoritarian, directed labour policy emanating from the Stalin era. Sputnik and the success of the USSR in space demonstrated a technological advance which at the time shocked the USA.

Considerable sporting and tourist developments were sponsored by the trade unions through the factories and collective farms. Each union had its own holiday camps and sports facilities, where workers were rewarded with holidays which reflected their level of productivity. The economic reforms will probably mean that the factory owners or management panels will take over organisation and sponsorship, given that state and union money is no longer available. The principle of rewards for working hard, however, could still apply as an incentive.

In the past, every Soviet citizen who wanted to take up a sport had to pay a token 30 kopecks admission fee to use the local facility. Any representative expenses were paid by the sports society or the USSR Sports Committee. This is standard procedure in all advanced countries, but there will certainly be some difficult times still to come as the transition continues and before adequate commercial money can be negotiated, given the state of the economy that still persists despite the de-unification of the Union.

The opportunities made available to Soviet citizens produced an even spread of popularity across five sports: track and field athletics, volleyball, skiing, soccer and basketball.

Some commercial money has already become available within Soviet sport, from gate receipts, the sale of sports goods and publications and the promotion of various lotteries. It is likely that these lotteries will continue, given that the rest of the Western world has now followed the Soviet example.

One can also expect an extension of the American win-at-all-costs philosophy as Russia and the Ukraine change to adopt professionalism and the commercialism attached to television advertising.

Review question

1. What is the likely influence of a market economy on sport in Russia following the 1991 reforms?

Discrimination

Cultural variables have inevitably led to certain groups being discriminated against in a specific community and in a society. Normally, whatever form this takes, it is reflected in a country's sport.

Regional

The standard of living in the European republics was higher than that in the East, but this is more a case of emergence than discrimination.

Class

The presumption is that, with the Bolshevik Revolution in 1917, the class system was destroyed. Such is the nature of humans that the ambition to get on and do the best for your children inevitably leads to an undercurrent of meritocracy. This was called the 'white collar cult' in the Soviet Union. Party policy was directed against this in the past but the new era of *glasnost* may change this. Sport was one of the few areas where individualism was encouraged, but even here the rewards of success tended to be wrapped up in social benefits.

Physical aptitude was the key factor in sporting achievement. Societal status came as a result of this and was not a prerequisite.

In a political system based on economics, the value of an individual lay in his/her contribution as a worker.

Unions had a range of holiday camps and choice was linked with effort.

> Soviet trade unions show particular concern for the organisation of holiday activities for working people and their children. In the summer of 1983, for example, nearly 14 million children spent their holidays in 68,000 Young Pioneer camps. The cost of maintaining a child at a camp for one shift (26 days) is 100 roubles. But half the accommodations at Young Pioneer camps is free, for the other half parents pay only 20% of the actual cost. The past few years have seen an expansion of facilities for the summer holidays and recreation of parents with their children. In 1985, trade union-sponsored holiday homes and hotels have three times more accommodation for families than ten years ago.
>
> (Novosti Press 1985)

It is inevitable that, if Russia and the Ukraine continue to introduce a market economy, the old infrastructure of full employment and a narrow differential between rich and poor will be eroded. The Soviet Union had already built up a wealthy class of high-ranking party officials, but the reforms are producing a new class of rich entrepreneurs. However, in the long term, the old 'white collar tradition' will probably re-emerge. The consequence of these trends may be a widening of the wealth continuum; also, if jobs become scarce there may be a backlash associated with the ethnic minorities, similar to events in Britain and France.

Gender

The Soviet Union attempted to adopt universal female equality. In a society based on both parents working there was no differential and, therefore, no discrimination. To some extent this accounted for the success of Soviet and East European female athletes. They were not handicapped by traditional myths and roles as is the case in Western democracies.

However, having quoted Articles 34 and 35 of the Soviet Constitution on sexual equality, the text *Women in the USSR*[3] went on to explain that: 'Unlike several Western countries, such popular men's sports as football, judo and boxing are not cultivated'. This was supposedly on health grounds, but the suggestion was made that women had many other alternatives. To some extent, this was cultural pressure to deter women from taking part in these activities and it may well be that there was more freedom for women to play soccer in Britain than in the Soviet Union.

There is certainly more freedom for girls to play soccer in the USA than anywhere else in the world and liberal trends in Russia has made women's soccer acceptable.

Religion

There was a political policy of atheism, but it was based on education rather than a destruction of churches. It was hoped that religion would die with the older generations, but a strong Christian and Moslem minority still exists and *glasnost* has allowed more religious freedom in Russia and the Ukraine.

Race

There has been a level of discrimination against the Jewish community. This was partly because they were accused of putting their race and religion before 'socialism', but also because the Soviets feared a 'brain-drain' to Israel. *Perestroika* has allowed Jews to go to Israel, but the future may yet bring a re-emergence of anti-Semitism in Russia and the Ukraine.

Even in the case of the Jewish problem, there was no question of discrimination influencing sporting opportunity. The desire to maintain the economy and to produce champions was far too strong to allow racial discrimination to exist in sport.

It might be argued that individuals who were not party members lost some of the advantages associated with pioneer palaces and workers' camps, but even in this context appeasement was a vital factor in an authoritarian society and recreation was regarded as a conforming instrument.

Age

> *Every Soviet child, regardless of the financial state of its family, enjoys equal opportunities for physical and intellectual development. Apart from free medical care and universal free education, the state fully finances the development of the interests and abilities of every child at art studios, music and sport schools, young technicians' and young naturalists' centres, etc.*

> (Novosti Press 1985)

The Soviet Union was politically aware that the future of its community ideology lay in the hands of its children. From a very early age, therefore, the state was presented as a benefactor. Children's groups from the Octobrists (young children) to the Pioneers (adolescents) were given the best possible facilities, complete with a high level of political education. The Komsomol, which represented the politically active youth of the country, had considerable influence on impressionable young people.

With both parents employed, the state recognised the need to keep children occupied in a positive way and sports palaces and outdoor camps were very popular inducements to keep young people 'off the streets', complete with a reward system of competitive 'pins' and prestige camps available for those who tried hardest.

Finally, the 'Olympic Reserve' policy encouraged the identification and promotion of young talent in sport, with a view to selection and special treatment – an attraction to children and parents alike.

It is important to recognise that this appealed to the politically committed citizen and also to ambitious parents who saw a chance of using the system for their own ends.

Perestroika has removed the political indoctrination motives and this, together with the end of funding, has led to a breakdown in organisations for young people. In time, there may be a re-emergence of Scouts and Guides, but in the meantime children are increasingly being left on the streets, encouraging deviance and lawlessness. It will be a tragedy if the superb pioneer palaces for young people fall into disrepair before an alternative programme can be implemented. However, it is important to recognise that the children and competitors who were brought up in an atmosphere of *masterstvo* (a creaming process to produce excellence) are now the teachers and coaches and their commitment is resulting in a new generation of elite performers.

Disability

In the dark days of the Cold War, the Soviet authorities would not have admitted to the existence of a handicapped group in their society. However, *glasnost* has shown that this is just as big a problem in Russia and the Ukraine as it is in the rest of Europe. The problem is that if these 'new' republics continue to descend into economic depression, the less able are likely to suffer most.

Review question

1. Discuss the possible exploitation of young gymnasts in the former Soviet Union.

21.2 The administration of physical education in the USSR (Russia)

In the former Soviet Union education was free, universal and administered by the state after the 1917 Revolution. As a union of so many different republics and cultures and as a conformist, authoritarian society, the Soviet Union had a centralised system of education, where the school was regarded as one of the most important agencies for the retention and promotion of Marxism. The break-up of the Soviet Union has led to each republic becoming the highest level of government, but Russian education continues to be centralised and part of a 'socialist' if not a Marxist political regime.

Physical culture was considered to be of great importance in a society which emphasised the role of the manual worker as against the part played by the intellectual. Physical education was a small part of this broad concept and referred to directed activities on the school and university curriculum.

A shortage of schools and teachers to keep pace with the rise in population has remained a problem in some republics and has resulted in a 'split-shift' system of schooling, requiring an early start for one group and an afternoon start for the other. This allows widespread use of some of the palaces, clubs and sports schools for the other half of the day.

There has also been an important educational role for extra-mural establishments like **Young Pioneer Palaces**, schoolchildren's clubs and centres for young technicians, naturalists and tourists. In 1985 there were some 5000 pioneer palaces and 6700 children's sports schools. The political and economic crisis has resulted in the palaces losing not only their political justification, but also their automatic state funding. Their continued existence now depends on local sponsorship and the efforts of parents and teachers.

Physical education continues to be a compulsory subject with a stipulated 2 hours per week. The general Soviet philosophy of exercise breaks also applied to schools and on occasions short exercise sessions were held between lessons. Exercise breaks are also practised by the Japanese and so the political changes may not affect these programmes if production rather than political motives are adopted. In addition, an emergent Russia will probably give health as well as production a high profile, retaining the status of regular exercise. The Soviet schools worked to a general syllabus, which was also the case in physical education. Speak & Ambler,[4] after a visit to several schools, commented that the common syllabus was not only recommended

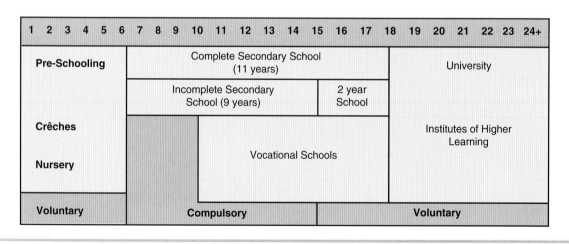

Fig. 21.3 The Soviet school system.
Comments:
1. A primary objective of literacy, a fear of intellectualism, a need for economic advancement and a desire to lead the world for the sake of Communism are intentions which do not easily co-exist.
2. The intention continues to be to give free schooling for all through an egalitarian, polytechnic education.
3. Preschooling is still widespread, part of a policy to enable both parents to work.
4. The last 2 years of schooling are designed to link with industry and higher education.
5. Vocational schools continue to be of many kinds and include various types of sports schools.

but observed. The Soviet school system and central administration are outlined in Figures 21.3 and 21.4.

A journal, *Physical Culture at School*, had been published monthly by the Ministry of Education, which contained articles on methodology, skill learning analysis and lists of GTO (preparation for labour and defence) standards around the country. Speak & Ambler[4] were impressed with the quality of the articles and the value of the publication to practising teachers.

There continues to be a policy of co-education, at least up to the age of 15 years, with male and female staff involvement. The content of the syllabuses has regional alternatives to account for climate, but in the main the term 'physical education' refers to a wide variety of gymnastics, games and athletics.

As with France and America, the existence of a set of instructions tends to result in direct teaching of specific skills, but all the work had an underlying political component. This political indoctrination is no

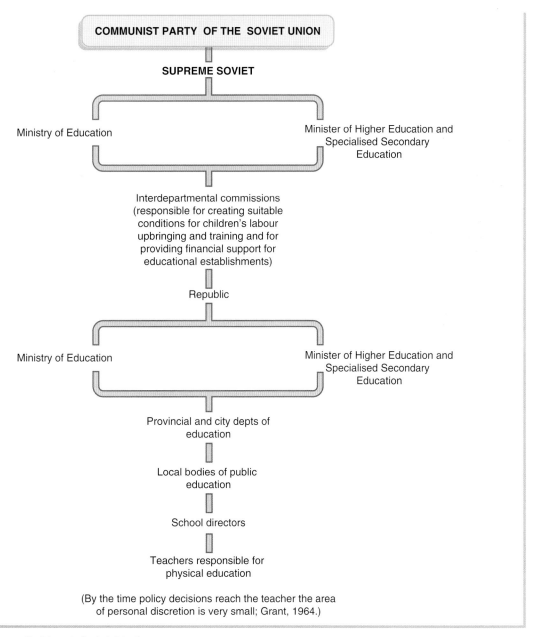

Fig. 21.4 Former Soviet central administration.

longer a part of the educational system, but it will take some time before a new set of values is established; however, it is likely that in the foreseeable future the major concern will continue to be with exercise and basic levels of fitness.

The GTO award system (preparation for labour and defence)

The GTO classification was centrally organised and given priority in all schools. It catered for the young, through to middle age, and it was meant to encourage mass participation and not just record-hunting. It was a graded system of physical exercise which promoted health, ensured medical supervision and provided a unified system. The tables (see Figure 21.5) were revised regularly and the content was changed to match changes in political attitudes.

Though it was designed and categorised for all age groups, there were three sections for children of school age: boys and girls aged 10–13, 14–15 and 16–18 years.

There was some criticism that the tests exercised a time-consuming constraint on actual teaching, a problem which exists in most countries where assessment becomes more important than learning. Information coming out of Russia in 1993 suggested that the GTO is no longer operating. It was always likely to be interpreted as 'political' by reformers and it may be some time before a substitute fitness programme is put into effect and when this happens, it is much more likely to be linked with fitness for sport.

In 1975, the quality of school facilities was poor, but in the intervening years there may have been improvements. The reason for the limited school provision reflected the importance of sporting facilities in the factories and community, leaving PE as a minimal health and social control provision. Once again there are parallels here with America, but in the Soviet Union the extra-curricular programme was often away from the general school. This view was substantiated by Speak & Ambler,[4] who found hardly any interschool sport but some school teams working towards knock-out tournaments which would lead to **spartakiads** at specific times of the year.

There was a major increase in the number of sports schools in the Soviet Union: figures for 1971 showed 4079 junior sports schools, whereas it was claimed that there were 6700 in 1985. However, these figures are no longer relevant in the context of post-reform Russia, given changes in political policy and current economic problems. Their function has been to search

for and develop talent and they have been the key to Soviet athletic success. Administrators have referred to them as 'our Olympic reserve'. Their aim was for pupils to obtain their school-leaving certificate with proficiency to 'Master of Sport' level in their chosen sport. An example of facilities is given in Figure 21.6.

The junior sports schools normally recruited 11 year olds, but the age was lower in the case of some sports, e.g. swimming (7–8 year olds) and gymnastics (9 year old girls and 10 year old boys). There were also youth sports schools with a 4-year programme for 15–20 year olds. While there has been specialisation, a wide range of activities continued to be covered at a low level and academic schooling has not been interfered with.

Riordan[1] refers to 'children's and young people's sports schools'. These would seem to be facilities which have been open to most enthusiastic children, maybe as part of a school, a factory provision or a pioneer palace, and making sports coaching available outside normal school. Different centres specialise, but they tend not to be exclusive. Riordan goes on to identify **sports proficiency schools** and **higher sports proficiency schools**. At these selective day schools talented children were given the best coaching available.

Finally, there continues to be a large number of **special sports boarding schools**, where the very best young performers are given a special educational programme in ideal surroundings. There is little evidence of pressure being applied by the authorities to recruit. On the contrary, parents and children work hard for selection and while teachers and coaches gain recognition for finding talent, many are reluctant to part with their most promising athletes. There is likely to have been at least a temporary breakdown in local sports schools, although there is evidence that factories are sponsoring local sports facilities. It would also seem that the prestigious sports boarding schools are too good to be abandoned by a society used to picking up Olympic medals.

In higher education, there continues to be two separate but cooperating bodies: the **Faculty of Physical Culture and Sport**, with the objectives of preparing students for the GTO and promoting *massovost* sport (mass participation); and the **Burevestnik** or university students sports society, which caters for elite sport. With the GTO now defunct, it is likely that the Faculty of Physical Culture will focus on mass participation, similar to the intra-mural programmes in the USA.

The Moscow University Faculty of PC and Sport has around 100 staff belonging to eight departments or commissions. Facilities include 10 sports halls,

'Handgrenadier' Strength & Courage for Youths & Girls 16–18 years			

Requirements: (pass examination)

1. Knowledge about physical culture and sport in Soviet Union.
2. Knowledge & carrying out of rules of personal and public hygiene.
3. Master programme of elementary battle-training, including section on defence against weapons of mass-striking-power and to remain one hour in a gas-mask, or to take a course on programmes of training specialist in organisation–DOSAAF–or to have one of the practical technical specialities (for youths). For girls, to know the basic rules of civil defence and stay in a gas-mask for one hour.
4. To be able to explain meaning of and carry out the set of exercises relating to morning hygienic gymnastics.

Exercises & Standards.

Kinds of exercise	BOYS		GIRLS	
	for silver badge	for gold badge	for silver badge	for gold badge
1. Running 100 m (sec.)	14.2	13.5	16.2	15.4
2. Cross-country				
500 m (min. sec.)	—	—	2.00	1.50
1000 m (min. sec.)	3.30	3.20	—	—
OR				
Skating (ordinary skates)				
500 m (min. sec.)	1.25	1.15	1.30	1.20
3. Long jump (cm)	440	480	340	375
OR				
High jump (cm)	125	135	105	115
4. Grenade throwing weight				
500 gram (m)	—	—	21	25
700 gram (m)	35	40	—	—
OR				
Putting the shot weight				
4 kg (m)	—	—	6.00	6.80
5 kg (m)	8	10	—	—
5. Ski racing				
3 km (min.)	—	—	20	18
5 km (min.)	27	25		
OR				
10 km (min.)	57	52		

Kinds of exercise	Youths		Girls	
	for silver badge	for gold badge	for silver badge	for gold badge
In snowless regions				
Forced march 3 km (min.)	—	—	20	18
5 km (min.)	35	32		
Cross-country cycling				
10 km (min.)	—	—	30	27
20 km (min.)	50	46		
6. Swimming 100 m (min.sec.)	2.00	1.45	2.15	2.00
or without timing (m)	200	—	100	
7. Pulling-up on horizontal bar (no. of times)	8	12		
Lifting from a hand and holding by rolling* over or by strength. (*revolution)	3	4		
Arms supported on gym bench, bend and straighten (no. of times)	—	—	10	12
Shooting small calibre rifle at 25 m (points)	33	40	30	37
OR				
at 50 m (points)	30	37	27	34
Shooting with battle-weapons: elementary exercises according to programme of elementary military training on assessment	satis-factory	good	satis-factory	good
9. A hike and test of hiking skills and ability to find one's bearings	1 hike of 20 km or 2 hikes of 12 km	1 hike of 25 km or 2 hikes of 15 km	1 hike of 20 km or 2 hikes of 12 km	1 hike of 25 km or 2 hikes of 15 km
10. Sport rating for: Motorcar, outboard motor, motorbike, glider, parachute, aeroplane, helicopter, under-water sport, all round sea-sport, modern pentathlon, machine-gun firing, radio, scouting (finding one's bearings), wrestling (all kinds), boxing		III		III
11. Any other kind of sport		II		II

Fig. 21.5 The GTO awards, USSR – ready for labour and defence. Sample table.
Note: for the gold badge it was necessary to fulfil not less than seven standards at the level established, including a temporary swimming and two standards at silver badge level (excluding the tenth standard). Girls who passed a course for 'combatant medical orderly' were considered to have passed a tenth standard gold badge test.

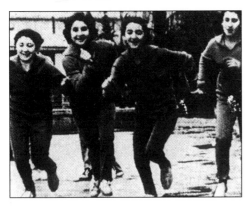

Fig 21.6 Vocational School No. 68 in Baku is frequently called a sports school. It has 12 sports clubs in which activities are run by volunteer trainers – instructors and foremen employed at the school. Future cooks, sales assistants and other specialists in the services successfully participate in city competitions in various sports.

a swimming bath, indoor athletics track, eight open-air basketball courts, eight volleyball courts, a special soccer pitch and two practice pitches.

The premier institute of physical culture is the Lesgaft Institute in St Petersburg. It trains some 5000 students in physical culture with a specialist staff of 325 lecturers. For a decade following the reforms, staff continued with reduced pay and privileges, but as Russia has succeeded in becoming a member of the G8 advanced group of nations, so expertise is being recognised and facilities modernised.

Review question

1. Describe the Soviet GTO system and explain its function before the reforms and suggest its possible future.

(See Section 21.5 for cross-cultural questions.)

21.3 The administration of sport in the USSR (Russia)

Nowhere has there been a better example of the so-called **sport pyramid** (Figure 21.7) than in the former Soviet Union. The idea that the **participation** base and the **diversity** base should be **universal** is still at the **ought** stage, but it is well beyond the Sport for All campaigns in the Western world. Our participation plans, though now well advanced as a result of improved facilities and marketing, could not cope if there was a sudden increase in participation percentages. The UK has now identified target groups who are not participating, but Britain is still faced with a variety of social constraints. There will continue to be a diversity in terms of opportunity in all sports until certain traditional social barriers are broken down.

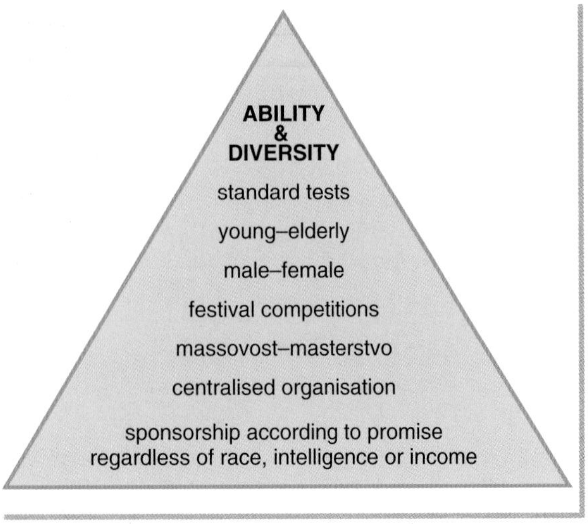

The reforms in Russia may have had a temporary adverse effect on the status of sport and on equal opportunity for sport in the different republics. Economic constraints and the emergence of a market economy may result in a re-emergence of social inequalities, but if the reforms are 'people led' then the sporting infrastructure is in place to retain the high status of sport.

The narrowing of the pyramid should be delayed as long as possible; marketing this means keeping the public active in sport as long as possible. We have seen that the major sports in America are for the youthful and outstanding. Britain has many sports clubs which extend the period of participation, but the Soviet Union progressed further with the principle of sport for life by encouraging a range of strategies to keep the public interested.

The programmes that encouraged participation for life included the GTO scheme (Figure 21.8), which had classified fitness and achievement figures for male and female adults, who were also graduated according to age. There were also classified sports rankings that allowed athletes to set personal targets of achievement and for the better performers, there were national

ABILITY
&
DIVERSITY

standard tests

young–elderly

male–female

festival competitions

massovost–masterstvo

centralised organisation

sponsorship according to promise
regardless of race, intelligence or income

Fig. 21.7 A sport pyramid.

GTO Badge Holders	Sports Rankings:		Titles
1. Men, 40–60; Women, 35–55;	I		Merited Master of Sport
2. Men, 19–39; Women, 19–34;	II	Adult Rankings	Master of Sport (International Class)
3. Boys and Girls, 16–18;	III		
4. Boys and Girls, 14–15;			Master of Sport (of the USSR)
5. Boys and Girls, 10–13.	I		Candidate Master of Sport
	II	Junior Rankings (15–18 yrs)	
	III		**State Honorific Award:** Order of Lenin

Fig. 21.8 The GTO award scheme, ranking and titles.

awards of athletic proficiency, rising through Masters of Sport to the Order of Lenin for services to sport. Though the politically orientated GTO is now defunct, it is probable that the sports rankings will undergo only a temporary collapse as they are features of all top sporting countries. However, the reform movement will no doubt re-label the top awards, allowing role status and financial endorsement to replace political meritocracy.

The narrowing of the pyramid in the Soviet Union towards sporting excellence was not accidental but rather a carefully constructed stairway where every help was offered to allow athletes to achieve their optimum potential. Certainly, there was an ulterior political motive, but individual sportspersons gained from this state endorsement. Sporting excellence in a huge range of activities appears to have been promoted; a policy of delaying work commitments for the vital periods of training was established and a circular process of development was encouraged whereby achievement and knowledge were fed back into the sport programme.

We are looking at a pyramid which still appears to be intact in most of the independent republics, where a base called **massovost** encourages all citizens to participate in sport, regardless of age, sex or race. With sport regarded as a purposeful institution in Soviet society, there is the organisation – a wide range of sporting festivals and standardisation programmes – to stimulate and maintain participatory interest. The point of the pyramid representsa 'creaming' process to produce excellence, called **masterstvo.**

The opportunity to participate has been the key to all Sport for All campaigns. The frequency of provision varies from one republic to another, but the Supreme Soviet was committed to a policy of state sponsorship. This could be seen in the number of factory sports units; the diversity of voluntary sports clubs; the availability of pioneer palaces; and the convenient placing of 'sandlot' facilities in built-up areas. All these facilities have been available to members of the public on the payment of a small annual subscription of 30 kopecks (less than a pound or a US dollar). Although financial aid is no longer available from the Supreme Soviet, it is possible that, if a market economy is widely introduced, some republics will continue to give state aid, as in France, while others will look for a mixture of public and private funding.

Spartakiads, or sports festivals, were held by all the voluntary clubs and urban units. They brought competitors together in competition but were also structured on a knock-out basis, so that success could take an athlete to a higher level of competition. The ultimate spartakiad was the National Games, which were held annually. However, the break-up of the Union has meant that the highest internal competitions are now the individual republic spartakiads but, given peaceful co-existence in the future, many of the republics will still want to compete together to test their relative athletic strengths.

The organisational structure of Soviet sport (Figure 21.9) was **centralised** with administrative and financial control maintained by the **Supreme Soviet Sports Committee.**

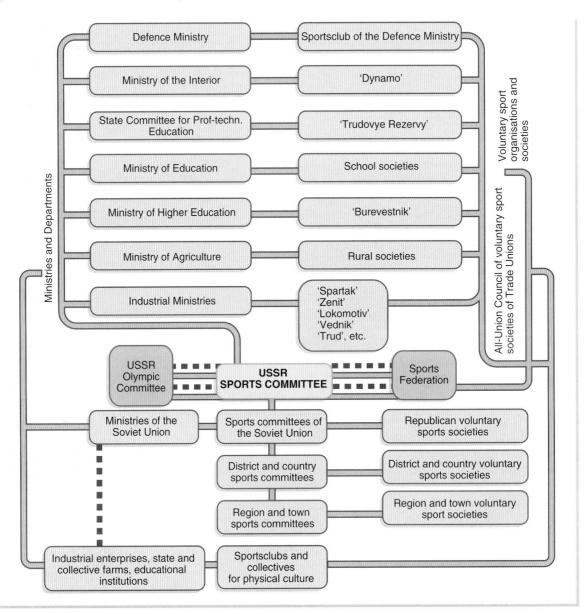

Fig. 21.9 Organisation and structure of sport in the former Soviet Union.[4]

At a second level, there was a tripartite control by three central committees: the Union of Sports Societies and Organisations Committee; the Sports Federations Committee; and the Soviet Olympic Committee. At a third level, these committees had branches in each of the 15 republics. Within each of these republics, which are the size and population of most European countries, there were regional committees responsible for major cities and rural areas. There is no reason why the internal structure of sport in the republics should have changed, unless there were major financial problems to overcome.

Finally, there are the local organisations and clubs known as **kollectivs**. The majority of these were factory linked and sponsored by the trade unions. Their own working committees had lines of communication through to the central committees. Even if some of the republics remain 'socialist', it is unlikely that all funding will continue through the unions, although unions are likely to continue to support their own workers as they do in the West. However, there is already evidence that the management of various factories and businesses is channelling money into leisure provision to retain the quality of life for the community.

The importance of *massovost* and *masterstvo* in Soviet society was reflected in the amount of financial expenditure and the kudos of sport in the community and internationally and also by the quality and availability of coaches to encourage standards of performance. The status of coach was always a very honoured one in Soviet society, the job often being awarded as a reward for services as a performer, and has proved an 'advantaged' career opportunity. With the reforms, job security has disappeared from coaching and many have been attracted by good financial offers from abroad. Their expertise is acknowledged by leading athletic nations and so the best are in great demand. Though this is good for world standards, the exodus will eventually undermine performance in the ex-Soviet republics.

The Soviet sports scene was subdivided into four groups: **Olympic**, **non-Olympic**, **ethnic**, and **technical**. Each fitted into seasonal and team or individual variables and some had climatic constraints operating.

The greatest effort was made in the Olympic activities, mainly because this was where success would receive the most recognition, but also because it was the public arena where amateur competition could be promoted worldwide. It may be a coincidence but the reforms in the Soviet Union occurred at the same time as the Olympic movement entered a phase where professional performers were allowed to compete. This suggests that the older Soviet motives of displaying amateur qualities as a political image will now move across to presenting a nationalistic and commercial image by producing Russian or Ukrainian champions as the world's best performers (Figure 21.10).

The role of ethnic sport in the former USSR was vital, as it was so racially and culturally diverse, but it is just as important in the separate republics, as they are also multi-racial; to prevent conflict it is important to encourage cultural activities which allow harmless tribal expression (Figure 21.11).

Non-Olympic activities continue to be encouraged because they extend the diversity of sporting experience. Rugby football is a typical activity in this context and field sports, like hunting and shooting, are carried on without social exclusivity.

Finally, technical activities such as parachuting, biathlon and motor racing were the least universal in the Soviet Union, tending to be the preserve of military personnel. If they are to continue, given the

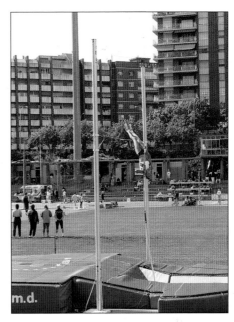

Fig. 21.10 Why is Russia so good at technical events such as pole vaulting? Photographer Helen Roscoe.

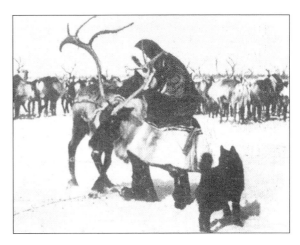

Fig. 21.11 A lassoo thrower catching reindeer at an area competition for reindeer drivers, hunters, fishermen and geologists in Naryan Mar, capital of the Jamalo-Nenets Autonomous Area. Other national sports, such as reindeer and dog-sled racing, jumping over sleighs and hatchet throwing are also popular there.

new market economies they will need the commercial sponsorship of international companies and will probably be the first activities to become exclusive.

The Soviet Union was contemplating the establishment of professional soccer teams to compete on equal terms with the rest of Europe and South America. This trend was overtaken by the reforms and now all the major football clubs are being organised on a professional basis. With the authoritarian regime at an end, there is also the opportunity for the best players to join other European clubs but, while this is very good for the players and their families, it may undermine the quality of the game in the republics. This is a complete break with the Marxist tradition, because the concept of professionalism in the gladiatorial sense of American football, and the 'opium of the masses' sense of British football, can hardly be justified in a 'socialist' society. It may well be that amateurism is moving so fast along the path of fully sponsored training and playing time, that there is just as little future for the old concept of professionalism as there is for amateurism. With social inequalities ostensibly removed, it may be possible for all athletes to strive for world champion status and receive rewards commensurate with their ability. If this is the case and there is an opportunity to excel, with a parallel career base for those who fail, together with an efficient

feedback into the sport, the republics may be on the road to a far more socially desirable system.

It is important to recognise that many of the features the Soviet Union initiated in sport, albeit politically orchestrated, have now been adapted by France, Australia and Britain. These include sports schools, urban facilities, centres of excellence and the use of lottery money. As they make an economic recovery, there seems little doubt that these advances in sport provision will once again become flagships of a successful society in Russia and the Ukraine.

Review question

1. How has the professional status of the elite performer changed since the cultural reforms in Russia?

(See Section 21.5 for cross-cultural questions.)

21.4 Tourism in the Soviet Union and post-reform Russia

As the Soviet Union considered itself to be an emergent 'socialist' society, it is important to recognise that recreation had bourgeois connotations and consequently the term **tourism** was more regularly in use.

The struggle for literacy and military preparedness meant that more dynamic aspects of physical culture had priority in the early years and that tourism became a priority only after 1968.

The term **tourism** implied a raising of the cultural and political awareness of the Soviet people. A major part of this cultural awareness concerned the natural environment but, with such a diverse and ancient country, there was also a considerable interest in the country's heritage. Pride in Mother Russia was framed in a political acknowledgement that, without communism, there would be no culture worth visiting. In the context of the reforms it is difficult to justify the continued use of the term 'tourism', as it has had so many political connotations, but its broad basis remains conceptually attractive. However, it is likely that, with progress towards a market economy, the label and concept of 'recreation' will become a part of the new order, hopefully without the negative characteristics of discrimination.

As a country which has become industrialised over the last century, working-class free time was many

years behind the Western model. A 5-day, 40-hour week was not broadly established until after 1972 and, up to 1968, 15 days 'prescribed leave' was the annual holiday for the majority. In 1972, however, a legal minimum of 15 days was established and an upper limit of 26 days. This led to a dramatic change in lifestyle, the weekend becoming a major leisure period, achieving a significance not unlike that of European countries. There was an inevitable shift of interest from explosive sports and spectatorism in the cities to a pattern of weekend excursions, where rural centres with a variety of sporting facilities were built.

In terms of the natural environment, the 15 republics have the same diversity as the USA but with at least twice the area of wilderness. However, the administration of the Soviet Union was totally different, with central control emanating from the **Supreme Soviet** and policy exacted through a series of master plans. These were transmitted to the various republics, the regions within the republics and down to individual districts. In addition, all Soviet republics had their own voluntary nature protection societies with a reputed membership of one in five of the population. With the republics now independent, it is unlikely that the administrative structure within each has changed in the short term but it is likely that national interests will be more adequately served, even though there may be a halt in the expansion of recreational programmes until the respective economies are on a more sound footing.

It would seem that national support for conservation will continue. The **State (National) Forestry Committee**, for example, is not only responsible for all logging and felling but it also controls the woodworking industry as a whole and is responsible for the protection of forests. At a rough estimate, almost a third of the old Soviet Union is forested, with timber reserves put at 82 000 million cubic metres in 1977. Very much the same is true of nature reserves in terms of conservation, but also the provision of facilities and communications to encourage tourism, sport and camps.

Given the importance of sport and active leisure, every opportunity was made to turn natural resources into outdoor pursuit facilities; most of these were administered and sponsored by individual factories. Parts of the old Soviet Union are naturally suited to specific outdoor pursuits: the Carpathian Mountains have numerous skiing centres; the Black Sea is famous for aquatics and sailing; and the Pamir Peaks are excellent for mountaineering and rock climbing.

The **tourism** aspect of **physical culture** made giant strides forward as a result of the National Economic Plan (1971–1975), when children's **Excursion-Tourist Stations** were set up, tourist sections were encouraged in the various sports clubs and tourist centres were built throughout the Soviet Union, rather than just in the traditional holiday centres of the Black Sea and the Caucasus.

Though well behind the USA in the development of national parks, there is a trend in this direction, as witnessed by the Armenian National Park.

Angling is very popular, as in all European countries, and major efforts have been made to reduce the levels of river pollution in industrialised areas.

Soviet holiday categories before the reforms

There were four main categories.

1. The majority of workers applied to attend camps run by their factory trade union. Normally, with the larger firms and farm collectives, a trade union had access to a number of camps of varying standards and the selection process involved an assessment of the worker's contribution to the firm over the year. In this way, a pass to a Black Sea resort was used as a work incentive. It is probable that factories will continue to sponsor these holiday camps, but it is more likely that the management or a joint committee will take on the funding. However, if the industries need money they might well sell these assets to entrepreneurs.

2. **Independent holidays** represent an increasing trend among the better off urban white collar workers. Although it would seem to be a political contradiction, there has been a strong tradition of financially secure families having a holiday home or *dacha*, which would be visited at weekends and holidays. It seems probable that with the increased freedom of *perestroika* more and more families will be hoping to organise their own holidays around hotels and *dachas*.

3. **The Communist Youth League (Komsomol)** – a political youth organisation for 15–26 year olds – organised holidays called **operational camps** (Figure 21.12). These involved a sizeable group of student volunteers working on major projects during the summer vacation. The largest was assisted in the building of the Baikal–Amur Railway (BAH), resulting in an alternative route to Siberia being established which opened up huge areas for population expansion. The break-up of the Soviet Union resulted in the Communist Party, and its youth wing, the Komsomol, losing most of their influence. The principle of encouraging young people to help develop major projects is a sound one but with the removal of authoritarianism any new programme is more

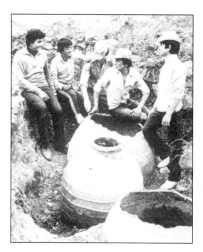

Fig. 21.12 Operational tourism. These youngsters spent their summer holidays at operational camps, helping archaeologists carry out excavations of ancient settlements.

likely to be on the lines of the Voluntary Service Overseas which operates in the Western world.

4. **Children's holidays**. As with the other countries discussed, there are two concepts operating – **outdoor education** and **holidays** in the outdoors. However, under the Soviet dictum of purposeful leisure, it was difficult to separate the two, all children's leisure having been to an extent educational, even if it was only a form of political education. Schools in the different republics have clubs, which they call circles, and some of these involve outdoor activities. The pioneer palaces, which are community facilities for children, also have circles.

It is important at this point to identify the main children's organisations operating before the 1992 reforms. We have already mentioned the **Komsomol**, which was a highly political youth group that now exercises little power. There were two younger groups. The **Pioneers** (Figure 21.13) were boys and girls aged 7–17 years and the **Octobrists** (after the October Revolution) were under 7 years old. These political youth groups are now in disarray with their funding cut off and their political function rejected. However, care for the well-being of children is deeply rooted in Russian society and so families will probably promote a 'Scouting' equivalent in the near future.

The Pioneers were much more politically orientated than Scouts or Guides but shared several common features. These included a desire to reinforce a strong moral code; encouraging a sound understanding of the natural environment; performing tasks for the community; and instilling a sense of national pride. They wore a uniform and had organised activities at school and in the community palaces. Though centralised, their organisation tended to work from the republic down through regional committees to district level and there was a direct link with political organisations at each level. Soviet children were not obliged to be Pioneers and many attended the Pioneer palaces and camps without being members, suggesting that if a new source of funding could be found these excellent facilities could be utilised by the new outdoor education organisations.

Prior to the break-up of the Soviet Union, the majority of Soviet children attended a summer camp which had much in common with the American summer camp system. However, none of the Soviet examples were profit making; they all had very close ties with the Komsomol and Pioneer organisations; they were run on much more authoritarian lines; and they were mainly sponsored and managed by trade union societies. Normally, parents had to pay about 30% of the cost, with the trade union covering the balance. Camps lasted for 6 weeks during the long summer vacation and most catered for about 400 children. Quality varied and schools were able to recommend their best pupils as a reward for effort. The most famous children's camp was probably Artek on the Black Sea (Fig. 21.14).

The programme at the camp included some related school subjects, such as environmental studies, and

1. A Pioneer loves his Motherland and the Communist Party of the Soviet Union.
2. A Pioneer prepares himself to enter the Komsomol organisation.
3. A Pioneer honours the memory of those who gave their lives in the struggle for freedom and for the prosperity of the Soviet Motherland.
4. A Pioneer is friendly to the children of all countries.
5. A Pioneer learns well.
6. A Pioneer is polite and well disciplined.
7. A Pioneer loves labour and is careful of public property.
8. A Pioneer is a good comrade: he cares for the young and helps the old.
9. A Pioneer is brave and unafraid of difficulties.
10. A Pioneer is honourable and values the honour of his detachment.
11. A Pioneer hardens himself, does physical exercises every day, and loves nature.

Fig. 21.13 Extract from the Pioneer Principles. How does this differ from the UK Guide or Scout movement?

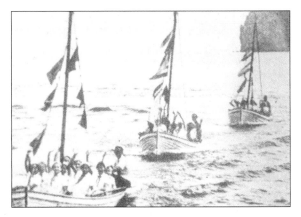

Fig. 21.14 Artek Pioneer camp on the Black Sea. Only children with outstanding 'merit marks' had a chance to attend this showpiece.

some political lessons, but most of the time was spent exploring the natural scenery or engaging in other outdoor activities. As with the American camps, there was much 'camp fire' ritual and numerous group challenges. However, most of the outdoor programme was structured to achieve the **Young Tourist Award** (children aged 12–15 years) and the **Tourist of the USSR Award** (those aged 16 years or more).

Finally, we must mention the historical features of tourism. Post-Revolution history was very important to the Soviet Union, particularly for the Russians; children were constantly reminded of the way the country had to struggle to achieve its status and of the bravery of its people, especially in the fight against Germany in the Second World War. With independence and *glasnost*, the history books may be rewritten, allowing the development of a free pluralist society that can grow to appreciate the natural environment without any political overtones being included.

Review question

1. Describe the links between the Soviet Pioneer movement and their camp schools and suggest likely changes as a result of the 1991 reforms.

(See Section 21.5 for cross-cultural questions.)

21.5 Cross-cultural review and exam-style questions

Review questions on physical education

1. **a.** Compare the systems of assessment in France, with their brevets and the Baccalaureat, with testing and measuring in senior high schools in the United States.
   b. Compare the systems of assessment in Australia with sports awards, key stage testing and general examinations in the UK.
2. Compare the latest developments in the preparation of high level school sport in the UK, with Australia's Sport Education and Physical Education policy (SEPEP); French UNSS and Sport Sections; and extra-mural sport in the American senior high schools.
3. Describe the place of the Soviet sports school prior to the reforms and suggest its possible future in the light of sports school/college programmes emerging in France and the UK.

Exam-style questions on physical education

1. Primary PE in France is dominated by a *tiers-temp* pedagogy but distance from Paris tends to determine the extent to which it operates.
   a. Briefly describe the *tiers-temp* pedagogy. (*2 marks*)
   b. What is implied in the comment about Paris? (*2 marks*)
   (*Total 4 marks*)
2. Compare sport in secondary schools in Australia or the USA with our own extra-curricular sport. (*7 marks*)
3. Teaching styles in primary PE vary according to the dominant ideology in the country concerned. Compare the different teaching methods you would be likely to find in Australian, French and former Soviet Union primary schools and explain these in the context of respective ideologies. (*10 marks*)

Review questions on sport

1. Compare the place of ethnic sports in each of the five countries.
2. How does the status of the professional performer vary in the five countries? Select sports to show how skill, gladiatorialism and commercialism determine the image of the top performer.
3. What are the similarities and differences between strategies to achieve excellence in sport in any two countries you have studied? What cultural factors determine these variables?
4. Sport for All is an international policy, but opportunity, provision and esteem vary from one country to another. Discuss.

Exam-style questions on sport

1. The escalation of violence in professional contact sports is an international problem

   a. Aussie Rules in Australia is one of the most explosive professional games in the world. Explain the features which lead to outbreaks of violence in this game. (*4 marks*)

   b. The Soviet Union has produced world-class ice hockey teams and players over the past two decades, but their game has been based on skill. Suggest ways in which this approach might have reflected the political system that dominated Soviet life before the 1991 reforms. What tendencies would you expect to emerge in Russia today? (*5 marks*)

   c. Analyse the cultural influences which may have caused American football to differ from the rugby code which came from England. (*6 marks*)

   d. Association football has only recently become accepted in the USA.

      i. Explain why female soccer appears to be much more readily accepted in the USA than it is in England. (*4 marks*)

      ii. Discuss the causes of spectator hooliganism in British soccer and American baseball. (*6 marks*)

   (*Total 25 marks*)

Review questions on outdoor recreation

1. Compare the American summer camps with the French *colonies de vacances* and the Outward Bound movement which exists in both countries as well as in the UK and Australia.

2. How does the outdoor education programme in the UK compare with the '*classes transplantées*' in France?

3. Compare the development of national parks in England with that in Australia.

4. Describe the links between the Soviet Pioneer movement and their camp schools and suggest likely changes as a result of the 1991 reforms.

Exam-style questions on outdoor recreation

1. Scenery is a major factor in attracting tourists to national parks.

   a. What are the geographical similarities between the USA and Australia which might attract tourists to their national parks? (*3 marks*)

   b. Examine the conflict between recreation and conservation in the British Isles and explain why this is not such a problem in France. (*3 marks*)

   (*Total 6 marks*)

2. The structure and function of outdoor education is influenced by the dominant ideology of different cultures.

   a. Compare the Scout and Guide movement in the UK with the Pioneer movement in the Soviet Union in the context of their summer camps. (*4 marks*)

   b. What cultural similarities might account for the UK, France, the USA and Australia all having Outward Bound centres? (*4 marks*)

   c. The USA has summer camps and France has *classes transplantées* and the *colonies de vacances*. Comment on the differences between them and explain the factors which determine these differences. (*11 marks*)

   (*Total 19 marks*)

References

1. Riordan J 1977 *Sport in Soviet society*. Cambridge University Press, Cambridge
2. Howell R 1975 *The USSR: sport and politics intertwined*. Comparative Education 11(2): 137–145
3. *Women in the USSR*. 1976 Novosti Press, Moscow
4. Speak M A, Ambler V H 1976 *PE, recreation and sport in the USSR*. University of Lancaster, Lancaster

Further reading

Geographical influences

Bale J 1982 *Sport and place*. Hurst, London

Lane H V (ed) 1986 *The world almanac*. Newspaper Enterprise Association, London

Paxton J (ed) 1991 *The statesman's year book*, 1988–89, 127th edn. Macmillan, Basingstoke

Sociocultural factors

Calhoun D W (ed) 1987 *Sport, culture and personality*. Human Kinetics, Champaign, Illinois

Houlihan B 1994 *Sport and international politics*. Harvester Wheatsheaf, London

Maguire J 1999 *Global sport*. Polity Press, Oxford

Mangan J A 1999 *Sport in Europe – politics, class and gender*. Frank Cass, London

Roscoe D A, Roscoe J V, Honeybourne J, Davis R, Galligan F 2003 *Physical education and sport studies AS/A2 level student revision guide*. 3rd edn. Jan Roscoe Publications, Widnes

Tourism

Grant N 1964 *Soviet education*. Penguin, Harmondsworth

ISCPES 1986/7/8 *Comparative PE and sport*, vols 3/4/5. Human Kinetics, Champaign, Illinois

ISCPES 1991 *Sport for All. Into the 90s*, vol 7. Meyer and Meyer Verlag, Berlin

Glossary of terms

adaptive (USA) term used to describe programmes for people with special needs.

athletics (USA) high level sport reflecting excellence in performance, stringent administration and normally professionalisation.

Aussie Able (AUS) a programme directed to help people with special needs to participate in sport and as such is similar to Disabled Sport in the UK and Adaptive Sport in the USA.

Aussie sport (AUS) a Federally funded programme to improve the level of sporting activity among young children as a community venture. This is the result of fears by senior administrators that the young people of Australia are increasingly inactive.

brevets (FR) School tests, which are held at regular intervals and include physical education tests, similar to the key stage tests in the UK.

counter culture (USA) a term used to express a non-popularist view. In the case of sport, it is against the win ethic and the excessive competitiveness of professional sport, promoting instead the educational values of physical education, lifetime sport and eco-sport.

draft system (USA/AUS) designed to retain a degree of equality in professional leagues in the USA and in Aussie Rules in Aus. Promising performers are ranked and distributed in reverse order of the success of league clubs. Aus. rugby league no longer supports this process as a result of legal action on human rights grounds.

eco-sport (USA) a counter-culture approach to sport, which is minimally competitive and supports play in the natural environment.

exemplary schools (AUS) mainly secondary schools, which have shown particular qualities in physical education and sport and as a result have been given additional funding to improve facilities and staff expertise. They are similar to sports colleges in the UK.

frontier spirit (USA) reflects the spirit of the pioneer white settlers as they trekked West in the face of considerable hardship and loss of life. Today, although the notion is still reflected in gun laws and some rodeo festivals, the frontier is now more likely to be perceived as sport or space.

game occurrence (USA) phrase coined by John Loy, Jnr to describe low level sporting activity or physical recreation.

GTO (RUS) Preparation for Labour and Defence. This test programme is no longer in operation, but it represented an attempt to politically mobilise Soviet society into a fitness framework, which had sport, work and military connotations.

komsomol (RUS) a politically active youth corps which dominated the political and sporting development of young people during the communist period.

massovost (RUS) the name given to mass participation in sport as a socialist objective.

masterstvo (RUS) the name given to outstanding performers in sport which is supported by such classifications as Masters of Sport and the Order of Lenin.

native American (USA) refers to the original settlers in North America, alternatively known as Red Indians, but the latter is now regarded as politically incorrect.

Pioneers (RUS) young people aged between 11 and 15 who belonged to a politically active organisation, which had similarities with the UK Scout movement.

pluralism general term, normally applied to the USA, where minority cultures are allowed to retain their traditions.

rural (rustic) simplicity (FR) a feature of French ideology where the countryside has a central role in French life because of its perceived beauty, but also the tranquillity which acts as a counter culture to intellectualism.

shop window (RUS) a term often used to show a partial view of sports performance in a totalitarian society. It suggests that as an act of propaganda a small number of highly talented performers are shown to the world, with the political suggestion that these represent the wider success and status of sport in that country. It is a critical title in that it is presumed that these successful few are pawns in a policy to hide those who have failed to make it in sport and to satisfy the people in the country that socialist objectives are being achieved. As a result it brings hope to the people, but obscures the real picture.

spartakiade (RUS) festival games held at different levels from town gatherings to national championships.

stacking (USA) applies to societies where society is ranked on a discriminatory basis. In the USA this is very much a racial ladder where achievement is limited according to ethnic origins. Although this is a stratified societal ladder, it also applies to sport but because sport depends so much on ability and desire, less advantaged cultures use it as a vehicle for advancement. Even so, there are constraints on minorities breaking into such advantaged roles as management and ownership.

tier-temps pedagogique (FR) there is some misunderstanding about this term. It appears to suggest a primary school organisation where academic, social and physical education is given one-third of the time and focus. However, it is more likely that though the three areas have been identified, physical education comes a distinct third in rank order. Whichever definition applies, there is a change taking place as sport becomes more important to the French and as primary sports schools are being developed.

Timbertop (AUS) an elite school which focuses on adventure education in the natural environment. Very similar to Gordonstoun in the UK.

title IX (USA) significant Federal legislation, giving females equal funding with males in federally funded institutions.

transplantées, classes (FR) are attempts by the State to take children into different natural environments and improve their awareness of the natural world and their love of France.

tourism (RUS) a term used to describe outdoor recreation, but including the cultural aspects of a community in terms of traditions, buildings and hardships.

UNSS (FR) are initials for a national organisation which caters for children's sport outside school. It encourages regular sport participation in local community facilities with a high level of coaching expertise available and where the licensing system can be initiated.

wilderness (USA/AUS) hazardous open country that is so extensive that individuals cannot readily walk out of it to major roads and settlements. Both America and Australia have huge tracts of land which fit this heading, most of them now part of a national park organisation.

zero-sum (USA) means all or nothing and reflects the win-at-all-costs ethic, which is often applied to American professional sport, particularly by zealous coaches.

Historical perspectives and popular recreation

22

Learning objectives

On completion of this section, you will be able to:

1. Develop a historical perspective so that in understanding the past, you better understand the present.

2. Understand the main characteristics of preindustrial Britain as a social setting for sports and pastimes of that period.

3. Have knowledge of a variety of sports as they fit into a number of profiles.

4. Be aware of the main characteristics of these activities as shared and different features.

5. Understand the organisation of these activities and the dominant attitudes of the players and public who were associated with them.[LOX]

22.1 Historical perspectives

Henry Ford suggested that all history is bunk, but then cars devalue more quickly than culture!

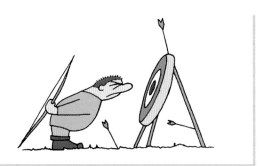

Fig. 22.1 Looking at the past helps us to understand the present and to do something about the future.

An approach to historical study

The study of sports history can stand on its own as it increases the knowledge and understanding of people and situations in the past. It can be based on different sports or socially based on different sectors of society at a particular time. In each case the intention is to establish what happened as objectively as possible, attempting not to allow our present situation to affect our judgement.

We would like to suggest that history comes to life when we attempt to interpret the intentions and attitudes of people, as well as their recorded actions. However, we must be careful not to find what we are looking for rather than what really happened. Remember, we want to understand history, not change it. For example, it is thrilling to think that

Webb Ellis picked up the ball and in so doing invented the game of rugby football ... but it wasn't quite as simple as that!

The focus of this book is on **contemporary physical education and sport**, but we need to look at the past as part of a **continuum of change**, where understanding how things have developed may give us the keys to the present. It is important to recognise that synoptic questioning requires you to be able to link these causative factors from the past with modern concepts, sports administration and contemporary issues.

So how can I become a historian?

The basic approach is to establish a **descriptive record** of events. Look through *Wisden* or some contemporary narrative accounts. The value of this knowledge lies entirely in its accuracy, but be careful – we know from modern reports that they can be biased.

The second level takes us into the **interpretation of relationships**.

You might want to know the links between games in the 19th-century public school and the authority of the headmaster or between football in a community and the local factory. In this situation, the historian tries to build as complete a picture as possible, providing a greater understanding of the human experience in a social setting.

The objective work of Joseph Strutt in *Sports and pastimes of the people of England*[1] helps us to understand what popular recreations were like before the 19th century.

Sometimes, even fiction can be helpful in this context. Thomas Hughes, in *Tom Brown's school days* (1857), may have exaggerated reality but his romantic style has given us a valuable insight into public school life through a fictional adventure.

The historian is interested not only in one time and place but in the influence of one situation or experience on another. Thomas Hughes' book may have been inaccurate but it was believed by generations of schoolboys and almost certainly was the single greatest influence on trends in public school athleticism.

Third, some historians think they can identify causation factors. I suppose I've just done it in the case of *Tom Brown's school days*. They try to recognise patterns of development and identify the cultural determinants which influenced sport and reflected society. Bailey looked at sport and the middle classes;[2] Cunningham studied the industrial working classes in the context of leisure;[3] and Newsome attempted the even more difficult task of linking sport, education and religion.[4] It is useful for you to read extracts from books like these.

How do I know certain things really happened?

Some historians put up hypotheses just like scientists, but the majority ask questions and look for answers in the **evidence** available. This leads to the tricky point that if you don't ask the right questions, you won't find out what really happened.

Equally important, if your evidence is inaccurate, your conclusions are worthless. Still, let's not give up but rather look at **types of evidence**.

Primary evidence is taken to be information reported by a person who was a witness to the event as a direct experience and could be presented in written or oral form. Written material is more permanent but changes every time it is rewritten and oral evidence changes every time it is recalled or retold. For this reason maps, pictures, authentic documents and supported testimonies are most valuable on accuracy grounds and oral evidence tends to be suspect without support.

Once that evidence is copied or retold, it becomes secondary evidence and that much less reliable.

Try to go to a county record office or local history study centre and look at some primary evidence. Most libraries have documents and photographs, they keep old papers and periodicals and they have books written at the time of the event. Then you can re-approach your contemporary histories to confirm their level of accuracy. A good historian always looks for cross-references.

Finally, take your tape recorder to the oldest people you know and ask them to recall 'the old days'. They'll probably love to talk to you and what they get wrong will, in many cases, be more than compensated for by the insights they will give you into events which would otherwise never be recorded.

Investigation 22.1 Let's test out some evidence

1. The painting in Figure 22.2 was exhibited at the Royal Academy in 1839.

   a. Is this a primary or secondary source?

   b. How would you justify the claim that this is a valid piece of evidence on the development of football?

   c. Interpret the structure of the game from this painting.

   d. How does the painting reflect the society of the day?

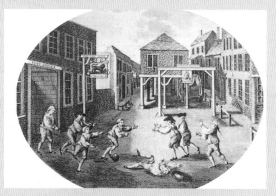

Fig. 22.2 Football played in the marketplace, Barnet. Drawn and engraved by Bowles and Carver, c. 1740.

2. The following extract is from a booklet at the Black Country Museum on the Tipton Slasher.

   Sayers was a small man, a middleweight, about 11 stone in weight and five feet eight inches tall. Perry announced that this fight was to be his last and the experts all agreed with him that Sayers would be slashed to ribbons within a few rounds.

   Noah Hingley, who had been born a nailmaker, and in 1857 was a thriving industrialist with chain and cable works already established at Netherton, warned the Slasher not to risk his all on the fight.

   'Yoh bay gettin' no younger,' he said. 'You're a fighter and yoh con lose – I'm a skamer [schemer] and I con win. Why don't you invest some money with me for a rainy day.'

   The Slasher was a stubborn man and he thought he could not lose. Noah Hingley's advice was unheeded. His all was spread amongst the bookmakers at 2 to 1 on. £400 was deposited as stake money.

   On the 16th June, 1857, the ring was pitched on the Isle of Grain. Tass Parker and Jack MacDonald, a hideously disfigured old pug who had been a chopping block for many better men, were the Slasher's seconds. Sayers' seconds were Bill Hayes and Nat Langham. Langham was a recently retired fighter, now publican, who had defeated Sayers some years earlier. Tom had been forced to retire blinded in this fight, but there had been no permanent damage to his sight.

   This was indeed the Slasher's last fight. He entered the ring at the apparent peak of fitness for he had trained hard, and he left it a broken, half blind and mentally impaired man. Early in the fight Sayers struck the Slasher a violent blow on the temple.

   The Slasher went down like a load of wet cement and his seconds had to work very hard on him to bring him to the scratch.

   I believe that the Slasher had a brain injury when he entered the ring and this chance blow activated it, for after this he fought a brainless battle. His skill and ring craft had gone and from

   the way in which he struck and missed he could not have been focussing properly. The contest lasted for one hour and forty-two minutes, and one of the rounds lasted fifty minutes, a record never likely to be surpassed.

   Owen Swift, the Slasher's principal backer, was sickened by the slaughter and stopped the fight in favour of Sayers. The blinded Slasher, who would not surrender, was held down by the four seconds whilst the sponge was thrown in.

   Twice during the contest his black eyes had been nicked and the blood sucked from them by Parker and MacDonald. This is an eye witness description of the Slasher at the end of the fight.

   'Perry's face had long since lost its humanity. A hideous gash stretched from his lip to beneath his right eye. His right ear was hanging in ribbons and the blood fell copiously on to his chest. He was as mad as a baited bull. Striking the thin air where Sayers was not. For his eyes no longer saw. Where they should have been were two black swellings oozing blood.'

   a. i. Is this fact or fiction?

      ii. What is the level of objectivity?

      iii. Is it primary or secondary evidence?

   b. What phrases give you an insight into the prize ring?

   c. What does it tell us about the attitudes and opinion of the people involved?

   d. To what extent is this a commentary on Black Country life?

   e. Where might you go from here, if you were a social historian interested in this topic?

22.2 Factors underlying the origins of sport

We need to know only a little about the origin of some of our older sports and the cultures they grew up in to set the scene.

Tribal

We have been invaded by numerous races in the distant past and each one has brought its own cultural activities with it. Some of our sports can be traced back to the Celts, Romans and, particularly, the Normans.

Ritual

Most sports and pastimes had religious and ceremonial associations, both pagan and Christian. These were joyful festival occasions held on special days. We only need to look at events associated with Shrove Tuesday and May Day to recognise this.

Survival

Many ancient sports have their origin in fitness to survive in dangerous surroundings, the ability to obtain food and military efficiency with a weapon. Often there has been an interesting transition from functional to recreative in activities linked with survival.

Recreative

In all societies children copy adults in their play. Similarly, all civilisations seem to reach a point where the level of maturity is measured in the recreative pursuits of their leading citizens and the violent activities of the lower orders.

Review question

1. Without presuming that an activity necessarily belongs in only one category, explain the placement of the following activities.
   - Stag hunting
   - Mob football
   - Archery
   - Pancake races
   - Real tennis

22.3 The pattern of popular recreation in Great Britain

The term **popular recreation** is used to describe natural, often violent, sports and pastimes (Figure 22.3), which were part of an ancient feudal right to recreation, claimed by all branches of the rural community.

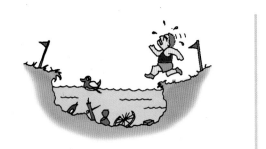

Fig. 22.3 Popular recreation: the right to participate regardless of personal risk.

Some landmarks you ought to know about

You should be aware of the Tailteann Games. Watman[5] tells us they originated around 2000 BC in County Meath, Eire, and continued until 1168 AD with the Norman Conquest of Ireland. It is probable that similar Celtic games existed in Britain at least until the Roman Conquest.

Now to the Romans. Read this extract to form a picture of Roman Britain.

It is unlikely that these sports ever included athletics meetings on the Greek pattern. The nearest point to Britain at which such meetings are known to have been held is Vienne, in the Rhône valley near Lyons. The athletics festivals in this city, established by a bequest in the will of a citizen, were abolished about AD 100 by a magistrate, and on appeal to the Emperor his decision was upheld. The reason for the abolition was that the meetings constituted a danger to the morals of the citizens; such was the reputation of Greek professional athletes in the Roman world at this time. If Greek sport was on the retreat in this way in a part of Gaul where, owing to the influence of the Greek cities of Marseilles, Nice and Antibes, it had earlier been strong, it is highly improbable that it would have crossed the Channel into Britain.

On the other hand, it is certain that the exhibitions in the arena were available in Britain. A dozen amphitheatres have been identified in the province. Two of them are well known, Maumbury Rings at Dorchester in Wessex and the arena of the legionary fortress at Caerleon. These do not compare in size with the vast structures on the Continent. The oval arena of each is roughly half the size of a soccer pitch; the amphitheatre of the small fort at Tomen-y-Mûr, beautifully situated among the hills of Merioneth, would hardly accommodate a tennis court. There is little direct evidence of the entertainment provided in these places, but there is no reason to suppose that in this respect Britain differed from other parts of the Empire. A vase in Colchester Museum depicts gladiators and bear-baiting; it was almost certainly made in East Anglia, and this suggests a familiarity with these subjects in the province. The smaller arenas may well have exhibited cock-fighting, a popular pursuit among the Romans.

The same degree of uncertainty hovers over the question whether the provincials of Roman Britain were able to enjoy chariot racing. A mosaic found in a Roman villa at Horkstow in Lincolnshire and now in the British Museum depicts a chariot race. This of course merely shows that the owner of the villa was interested in racing; it does not prove that the racing took place in Britain.[6]

Compare this with the following extract which refers to the contribution made by the Saxons in sporting terms.

Indeed, it is not by any means surprising, under the Saxon government, when the times were generally very turbulent, and the existence of peace exceedingly precarious, and when the personal exertions of the opulent were so often necessary for the preservation of their lives and property, that such exercises as inured the body to fatigue, and biased the mind to military pursuits, should have constituted the chief part of a young nobleman's education: accordingly, we find that hunting, hawking, leaping, running, wrestling, casting of darts, and other pastimes which necessarily required great exertions of bodily strength, were taught them in their adolescence. These amusements engrossed the whole of their attention, every one striving to excel his fellow; for hardiness, strength, and valour, out-balanced, in the public estimation, the accomplishments of the mind; and therefore literature, which flourishes best in tranquillity and retirement, was considered as a pursuit unworthy the notice of a soldier, and only requisite in the gloomy recesses of the cloister.

Among the vices of the Anglo-Saxons may be reckoned their propensity to gaming, and especially with the dice, which they derived from their ancestors.[1]

Investigation 22.2   Popular recreation precepts

1. Try to explain the following **popular recreation precepts** (this may require you to read extracts from Brailsford,[7] Ford[8] or Malcolmson[9]).

   a. Feudal basis of the **courtly** and the **popular**: courtly with courtesy and high culture; **popular** with peasant vulgarity and low culture.

   b. Both an inherent part of the **Merrie England** concept.

   c. **Conservatism** of the **rural gentry** not wishing to change the natural order of country life, with the **escapism** of the **peasant class**.

   d. Attacked by the **clergy** as decadent and irreligious; by the **middle classes** because it offended their sense of decency; and by the **industrialists** because they needed a disciplined **work force**.

   e. **Popular recreation** against the **Protestant work ethic**.

   ▶

2. The second step is to link these **precepts** with the **social groups** and **activities** shown in Figure 22.4 and explain why certain **reforms** took place.

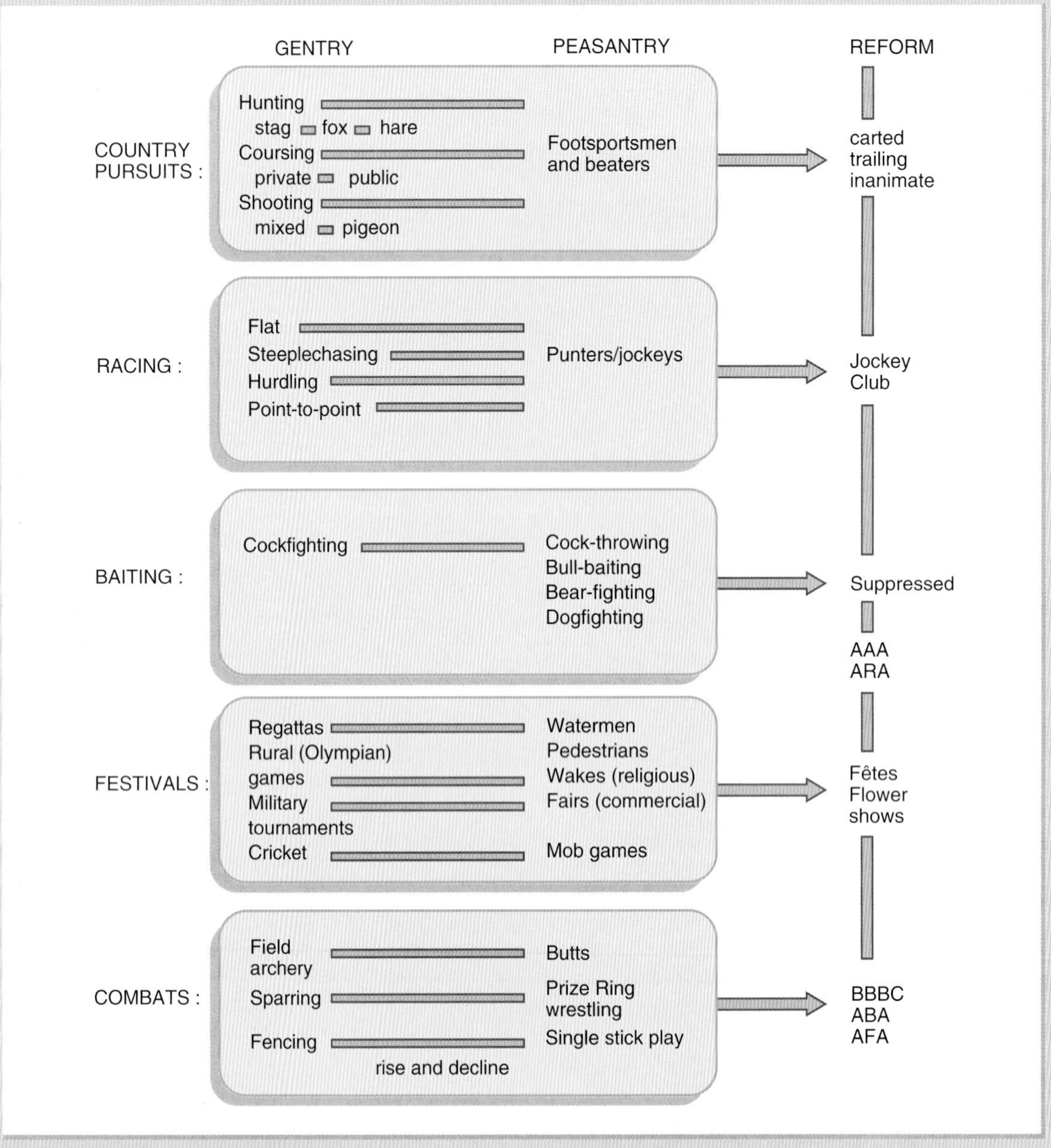

Fig. 22.4 The reform of sporting games.

By the 15th century, pagan and Christian recreations were hopelessly intertwined within the concept of **Merrie England**. Another extract from Strutt[1] should set the scene.

May Day festivals

This custom, no doubt, is a relic of one more ancient, practised by the Heathens, who observed the last four days in April, and the first of May, in honour of the goddess Flora. An old Romish calendar, cited by Mr. Brand, says, on the 30th of April the boys go out to seek May-trees, 'Maii arbores a pueris exquirunter'. Some consider the May-pole as a relic of Druidism; but I cannot find any solid foundation for such an opinion.

It should be observed, that the May-games were not always celebrated upon the first day of the month; and to this we may add the following extract from Stow: 'In the month of May the citizens of London of all estates, generally in every parish, and in some instances two or three parishes joining together, had their several mayings, and did fetch their may-poles with divers warlike shows; with good archers, morrice-dancers, and other devices for pastime, all day long; and towards evening they had stage-plays and bonfires in the streets. These great mayings and may-games were made by the governors and masters of the city, together with the triumphant setting up of the great shaft or principal may-pole in Cornhill.

This is the first of a number of pictures which are useful for interpretation purposes; they serve to stimulate discussion and they help to develop analysis techniques. However, there is not the space to explain more than a selection of these illustrations in the text.

Figure 22.5 is an excellent picture to clarify the development of sport in this country. There are three combative situations which need to be rationalised. The central one is the serious, noble pursuit of

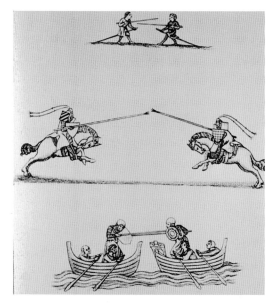

Fig. 22.5 Jousting.

jousting. It involves two knights and it is not clear whether this is a battle scene or a tournament event. Either way, it is training for war by an elite, who presumed the existence of physical components necessary for a successful combat, but also a code of chivalry which eventually emerged into fair play in a sporting situation. It seems, therefore, that the source of this activity is military and limited to the ruling class and associated with their survival and status.

If we look at the top combat, it seems that this represents children at play, copying the ruling class. They are making do with sticks to represent horses and lances, but are nevertheless 'mastering reality' in the relative safety of a pretend game. This suggests that combats did not have their origin in play, but in serious survival situations, where playing at the activity came later. This is another useful generalisation: that the origin of most sports was serious and functional. As an observed copy, however, it is questionable whether the children's play included an awareness of the chivalric code as they would have been 'playing out' their own values through the observable features of the activity. However, children's fantasies tend to clearly define 'goodies' and 'baddies' and as such values are identified and even polarised.

The bottom combat is on the water in boats. It involves the notion of team, because the rowers are part of the combat, but the seriousness of the situation is reduced because the approach speed of the antagonists is much slower and the consequence of a good strike is a ducking for the other person. Here we have an example of a quintain. The noble activity of jousting has been corrupted into a frivolous festival activity, where the crowd has a good laugh and the winners get a prize. The extent to which fair play operated would probably depend on festival regulations. This is still a high-risk activity, where the rigour of life was acted out in the ritual of the folk festival.

This debasement of serious activities was common in medieval England, where the peasantry 'took a rise' out of the ruling class in their rural festivals. However, the message is that non-serious merry-making often arose out of serious forms of activity and even these frivolous events had serious cathartic and community-building functions.

Further extracts also illustrate the idea.

Bull-running in Stamford

Bull-running was a prominent diversion in Tutbury, Staffordshire, Stamford, Lincolnshire, and perhaps one or two other towns. The bull-running in Stamford, held on the 13th of November, was a major festive occasion for the town and its surrounding countryside which attracted each year hundreds of spectators and participants. The sport was essentially a free-for-all bull-fight without weapons, or at best with only sticks and heavy staffs; it seems to have been much like some of the bull-runnings recently (or still) found in parts of France and Spain, and it was characterized by a similar sort of carnival atmosphere. On the morning of the 13th the entrances to the main streets were barricaded, shops were shut up, and at eleven o'clock, with the bells of St Mary's tolling his arrival, a bull was released from a stable to the swarms of onlookers and participants (called 'bullards') who packed the street. The excitement was provided by the ensuing confusion and disorder, and by displays of daring in tormenting the bull – by throwing irritants at him, perhaps, or by baiting him with a red effigy and then manoeuvring out of his way. A talented bullard might pack himself in an open-ended barrel and roll it at the bull: the objective here was to provoke him to toss the barrel, and yet at the same time to avoid getting dislodged or mauled. 'If he be tame,' wrote a hostile observer in 1819, 'he is soon surrounded by the canaille, and loaded, as the bullards express it; that is, some have hold of his horns, and others his ears, some are beating his sides with bludgeons, and others are hanging at his tail.' A man in trouble would be aided by diversionary antics from his friends. Sometimes the bull was stormed by groups, and often he was simply chased through the streets. After an intermission for lunch the bull was again let loose, but this time he was driven towards the main bridge spanning the Welland River. The bullards surrounded him on the bridge and together lifted him over the parapet and into the water: this was known as 'brigging' the bull. He would shortly make his way to the adjacent meadow where a few dogs might be set upon him (though he was not tied down), and where bullards would give chase for a while around the muddy lowland. In late afternoon he was escorted back to town, frustrated and fatigued no doubt, but not usually mutilated. He was then slaughtered and sometimes the meat was sold cheaply to the poor or served up in the public houses. The odd bull which had refused to be 'brigged' was spared his life.[9]

Festival wakes

The inhabitants of Stone, Staffordshire, where the church was dedicated to St. Michael and All Angels, celebrated their patronal festival with bull-baiting, bear-baiting, dog-fighting and cock-fighting.[7]

Investigation 22.3   Past sporting events

1. Can you now describe the atmosphere at Stamford on 13th November 1819?
2. Can you explain what is meant by a wake?
3. Do you understand the ritual associated with medieval festivals?
4. We know that the Norman Conquest led to the establishment of our present nobility. It also led to the development of the **tournament** and the clear division of sports into **courtly** and **popular**. Use Figure 22.5 to describe this class divide through an explanation of the **joust** as against the **quintain**.

You need to know something about the Tudor dynasty and athleticism. Henry VIII was a champion of most sports, but he also restricted certain activities to the nobility. Figure 22.6 shows Henry throwing the hammer, but he was also a great horseman and a champion real tennis player.

The blackest time for sports in English history was during and after the Civil War (1649). The country

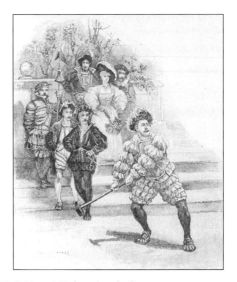

Fig. 22.6 Henry VIII throwing the hammer.

was divided into two complex groups. The Royalists tended to be gentry, rural and High Church, while the Parliamentarians or Roundheads were largely merchant class, urban and Low Church. The success of Cromwell led to the imposition of a Puritan lifestyle which continued as an ethic for the lower classes for many years after the Restoration.

Popular recreation was criticised on religious grounds as well as being identified with the King's Book of Sports.

Some of the cruellest popular recreations were not revived. Cock throwing, which involved throwing sticks or stones at a tethered cockerel, was banned but cockfighting continued. Bear baiting became less popular, even though bull baiting continued.

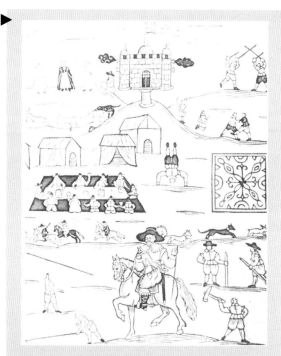

Fig. 22.7 The Dover Games were revived after the restoration of Charles II. Shown are the types of activities that were reintroduced.

Investigation 22.4   Popular recreation before the Civil War

Read the following.

And as for Our good people's lawfull Recreation, Our pleasure likewise is, That, after the end of Divine Service, Our good people be not disturbed, letted, or discouraged from any lawful recreation, Such as dancing, either of men or women, Archery for men, leaping, vaulting, or any other such harmless Recreation, nor from having of May Games, Whitson Ales, and Morris-dances, and the setting up of Maypoles, and other sports therewith used, so as the same be had in due and convenient time, without impediment or neglect of Divine Service: And that women shall have leave to carry rushes to the Church for the decoring of it, according to their old custom. But withal we doe here account still as prohibited all unlawful games to bee used upon Sundayes onely, as Beare and Bullbaitings, Interludes, and at all times, in the meaner sort of people, by law prohibited. Bowling: And likewise we barre from this benefit and liberty, all such knowne recusants, either men or women, as will abstaine from comming to Church or Divine Service, that will not first come to the Church and serve God: Prohibiting, in like sort, the said Recreations to any that, though conform in Religion, are not present in the Church at the Service of God, before their going to the said Recreations.[10]

Investigation 22.5   The Dover Games

1. In Figure 22.7, how many activities can you name?

2. To what extent were the old 'courtly' and 'popular' concepts also revived?

A country in transition

The Puritan ethic of the 17th century gave way to the Protestant ethic in the 1700s, marking the birth of Britain as an industrial nation, as a world power and as a centre of evangelism. If these three forces were not enough, the conservatism of rural England was shaken by the emergence of a Regency clientele, with high living in fashionable spa surroundings, architectural genius and the Fancy dominating upper-class life. The Fancy was a mixed group of 'sportsmen' who were preoccupied with horse racing, cockfighting and the prize ring, totally consumed by the blood, sweat and wager of the contest.

The date which is often used to identify these seeds of change is 1760. Let's look in a little more detail at the three major 'revolutions'.

The **Industrial Revolution** began with the increased use of coal in smelting and led to factories and industrialists taking over from the ancient cottage industry controlled by independent craftsmen.

This machine age came to the countryside, reducing labour intensity at the same time that enclosure marked a reduction in common land. This was an agrarian revolution which forced countless farm labourers to take their families to the towns in search of work. It is also important to recognise that the prospect of industrial wages attracted the more ambitious farm workers to the towns.

With machine-operated factories, an expanding capitalist economy and abundant cheap labour, the industrial towns grew at a tremendous rate, a phenomenon which has been called an **urban revolution**. Though this is often identified as a working-class population expansion, it also marked the emergence of a powerful, respectable, urban middle class.

In older towns, this led to many of the old slums being cleared and fashionable shopping centres being built. Each major town became a corporation and built its own town hall, free library, cottage hospital and public swimming baths.

In the heavily industrialised towns, factories and smoke replaced green fields and tightly packed, back-to-back, terraced houses were built as near to the factory as possible. From 6 a.m. to 6 p.m. for 6 days a week, men, women and children worked in the 'satanic mills'.

Country life

We now need to consider the impact of these changes on popular recreation. Let's look at **country pursuits** first. Despite the growth of towns, country life continued much as before, particularly as it concerned the **landed gentry**.

Investigation 22.6 Country sports

1. Figure 22.8 shows the older sport of **otter hunting**. Today, the otter is protected and most people regard it as a loveable creature. In the 19th century, it was hunted and killed mercilessly. Try to explain the Victorian attitude to otter hunting and why we feel differently today.

2. Fox hunting (Figure 22.9), on the other hand, is still very popular in many parts of the country, although there is an increasingly vociferous lobby against it, manifested most vividly by the activities of the hunt saboteurs. Can you identify the attractions of fox hunting to the landed gentry in the 19th century, covering, for example, the athleticism required?

3. This ancient sport (Figure 22.10) was very popular in rural England throughout the 19th century. Hares were 'flushed' out of 'cover' and two greyhounds were 'unleashed' by the 'slipper' and the dog which made the 'pussy' deviate the most times won the 'course'. Can you interpret this statement and also establish the attractions of such an event at that time?

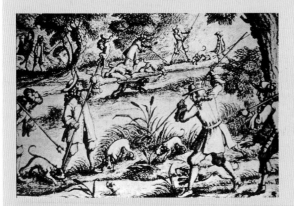

Fig. 22.8 Otter hunting.

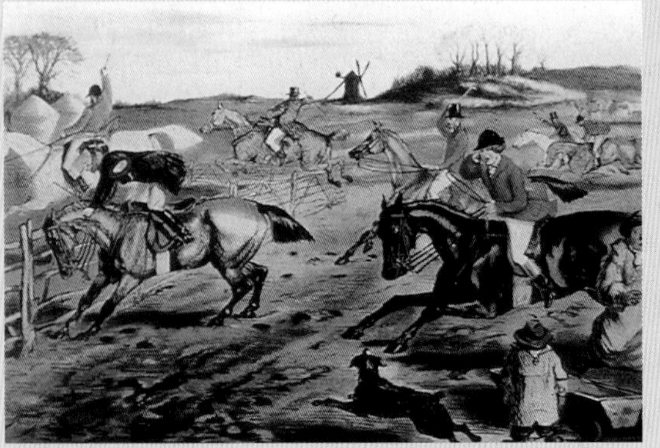

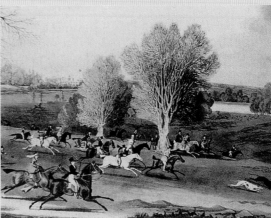

Fig. 22.9 Fox hunting.

Fig. 22.10 Coursing.

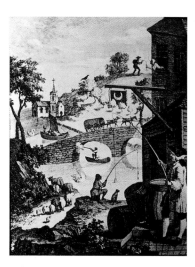

Fig. 22.11 Fishing and fowling in a village.

Rural villages and market towns

Figure 22.11 is an excellent general interpretive medium, reflecting life in a rural village or market town.

It is possible to draw inferences from the placement of a settlement at a river crossing but also at a secure site in a meander. As such, the river acted as a defence, as a source of sanitation, as a communication route and as a recreational facility. In terms of communication, it is important to recognise commerce along the river as well as access across it, at a ford or bridging point.

Our focus is on recreation and so it is important to see the river as a washing and bathing place, where competitions could develop, but also as a riverbank facility, where flooding prevented houses being built on the water meadows. The function-based origins of many sports can also be established from the illustration, where commercial boating and sailing may have given rise to canoeing, rowing and sailing for pleasure. Fishing might have been an occupation or a means of supplementing diet, but became a regular pastime and the same applied to shooting. The ownership of a gun or rod was one of the ambitions of all young males, including labourers, the only restriction being the game laws.

From this notion of a river town, with the festival occasion in the form of a regatta, it is easy to progress to the notion of market towns and the links between markets, fairs and sportive festivals. This leads on to the more sophisticated developments which occurred in the county towns, which became the focus of such major events as horse racing, county cricket and prize fighting, where major venues were normally on the water meadows.

Finally, it is also important to register the significance of the seasons, more particularly the summer months, with the attraction of bathing, and the cold spells, when the frozen surfaces provided popular skating venues as well as ice fairs.

Investigation 22.7 The reflective and sporting pastime of angling

Izaak Walton identified a sport for every man, but 19th-century work patterns and pollution resulted in a class divide for 'game' and 'coarse' fishing. Explain this statement in the context of the 'revolutions' we discussed earlier.

Investigation 22.8 Shooting

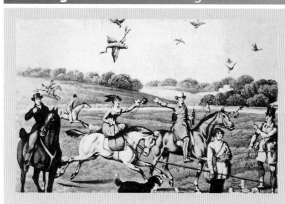

1. You may have seen the film *Kes*. It was about the relationship between a boy and a kestrel. Can you examine this and other elements in the sport of falconry (Figure 22.12)?

Fig. 22.12 Falconry.

2. **Mixed shooting** also had a similar attachment, this time between a man and his gundog (Figure 22.13). Though falconry as a sport is no longer acceptable, pheasant and grouse shooting still are. How do you account for this? Is it due to social privilege, marksmanship, food for the table or something else?

3. **Pigeon shooting** (Figure 22.14) was equally popular, with birds sprung from traps for marksmen to shoot at, but now society has changed this to **clay pigeon shooting**. Why was pigeon shooting curtailed while mixed shooting survived?

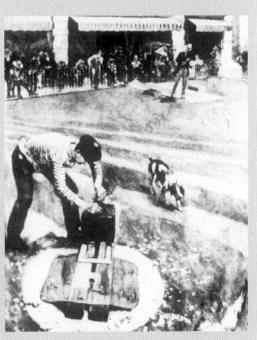

Fig. 22.14 Pigeon shooting.

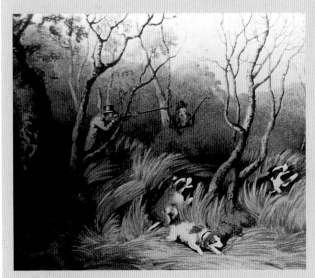

Fig. 22.13 Mixed shooting.

Horse racing and blood sports: the traditional festival occasions

Horse racing (Figure 22.15) is as old as horse riding. It is human nature to make a contest in any unpredictable situation which allows the measurement of one person's competence against another. Horse racing had two distinct phases of development. The first took place in the reign of Queen Anne when three Arabian stallions were used to start bloodstock breeding in Britain. The second came when the railways allowed horses and crowds access to different racing centres, resulting in a well-organised **racing calendar**.

The development of the hunt and horse racing is an important chapter in the development of 19th-century gentry lifestyle. The hunt, with its athleticism and ritual, reflected the significance of physical endeavour among male and female members of the upper class. The horse was at once a symbol of wealth, a vehicle that increased spatial freedom, a possession which brought pleasure and challenge and reinforced the gentry's affinity with the countryside.

The athleticism of a day in the hunting field should not be underestimated. Riding over rough country for distances of over 60 miles held tremendous risks for the riders and required great courage and skill. The challenge element was enhanced by the decision

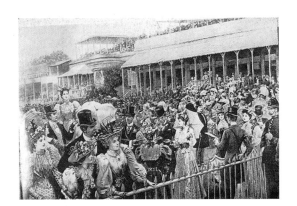

Fig. 22.15 The Epsom Races.

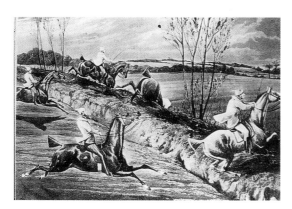

Fig. 22.16 Steeplechasing.

to hunt the most able adversary in its natural environment, resulting in a personal test in a sporting environment, where the quarry had every chance to escape from ineffective riders and hounds. Here is a re-emergence of the tournament duality of physical endeavour and chivalrous conduct, which has become the essence of rational sport.

Such was the momentum of this athleticism that, after a day's hunting and feasting, the gentry often saddled up in the evening to engage in a friendly, but often wagered, steeplechase as shown in Figure 22.16. The eventual professionalisation of the steeplechase as a result of the improvement of bloodstock, the love of the wager and the development of horse racing as a major festival occasion led to regular race meetings and professional jockeys controlled by the Jockey Club, a governing body which was copied by all later sports bodies.

This evolution led to lower-class jockeys being employed, as a servant class, but the athletic commitment of the gentry continued through amateur point-to-point racing organised by individual hunt clubs.

> ### Investigation 22.9 Horse racing and steeplechasing
>
> 1. Use Figure 22.15 to explain the level of organisation in flat racing after 1870.
> 2. Figure 22.16 gives clues as to the development of steeplechasing. Use this visual evidence to explain what might have happened.

Blood sports were relics of an earlier period. They were extremely cruel but arguably reflected a cruel society, where the function of animals was either to work or entertain. **Cockfighting** went hand-in-glove with the **races. Bull baiting** could always be guaranteed to attract a crowd.

> ### Investigation 22.10 Blood sports
>
> 1. Figure 22.17 shows two fighting cocks, with an apparently respectable crowd. The birds will fight to the death, there will be blood and feathers everywhere and money will change hands – but not until the cock has crowed. Can you appreciate the attraction at a time when a person was hanged for stealing a sheep?
> 2. Can you apply the attractions of the cockfight to bull baiting (Figure 22.18), thus explaining its popularity at that time?

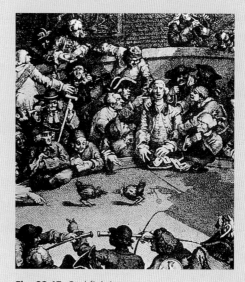

Fig. 22.17 Cockfighting.

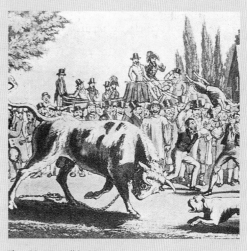

Fig. 22.18 Bull baiting.

3. Can you link this with refrigeration and beating a steak before cooking it?
4. Can you explain why in the UK bulls are no longer baited and yet bullfighting is still acceptable in some countries?
5. Can you link this analysis with shooting, where the gundog has been replaced by the bull terrier, but the man/woman has a similar chance to test his/her training and breeding skills and put money on them?

Popular sporting festivals and pedestrianism

The term **pedestrian** referred to a group of lower-class individuals who earned part of their living by competing in certain sports for money. It was a forerunner of the term **professional**. One of the earliest examples of this was in sculling. Thames watermen competed for the Doggett Coat and Badge on 1st August annually from 1715 (Figure 22.19). The competition arose from the idea of wager boats. Small boats ferried passengers across the Thames and wagers were struck to see who could get across first.

A similar situation existed on the roads, in that the upper class employed footmen on their coaches, who took part in wager foot races. These developed into challenge events over long distances with wagers being made on the result or on the 'walker' completing his self-imposed task. One of the most famous occasions of this type occurred in 1800 when Captain Barclay completed 1000 miles in 1000 hours for 1000 guineas.

These events became very popular, attracting huge crowds on the major horse-race courses. The best-known competitors were two Americans: Deerfoot who toured Britain in the 1860s, accepting challenges at all distances; and Weston, who walked 2000 miles in 2000 hours around Britain in the 1870s and gave a lecture on 'abstinence' each evening.

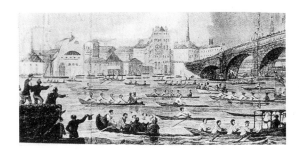

Fig. 22.19 The Doggett race.

Early **cricket professionals** fitted much the same mould. They were paid wages to keep the ground in order, coach gentlemen players and play when wager matches were arranged.

Investigation 22.11   The development of cricket

1. What aspects of Figure 22.20 lead you to think it is an 18th-century example of cricket?

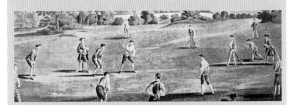

Fig. 22.20 Marylebone Fields in 1748.

2. Figure 22.21 shows a women's county cricket match in 1811. Can you recognise similar characteristics to the men's game and note the freedom of female opportunity prior to Victorian constraints?

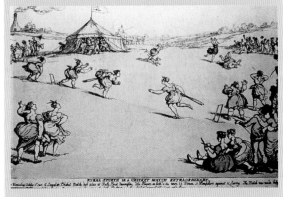

Fig. 22.21 Hampshire v. Surrey.

Having written in depth about the gentry and their values, the illustration of pedestrianism can help us to interpret the popular and courtly cultures. The lower class pedestrian, competing for money, is using his talents to earn a living in a more pleasant environment and with the likelihood of making much more money if he is good enough and is able to use his winnings shrewdly. The question of athleticism is not in doubt, but the need to win may jeopardise any values of looking for a challenge; being able to afford, and therefore prepared, to lose; and being willing to cheat.

If we identify the other competitor as a gentleman amateur who represents courtly values, the suggestion is that his athleticism is based on the testing of self against others and the elements as a personal challenge and that the behaviour code which arises from this is that the challenge is a test of temperament and to cheat is to cheat yourself.

The notion of cheating may be an ethical principle in the case of the gentleman performer and adjudged the act of a blackguard and unacceptable, but the notion of cheating by a pedestrian is more likely to hinge on the expedient possibility of being caught and barred from competition. It is too simplistic to presume that principle and expediency are culturally exclusive, but it is easy to see that a pedestrian who competes for money to feed himself and his family may not have the advantage of adopting 'high-culture' ethics when those around him 'play the game'.

It is this apparent stigma of the professional which is at the basis of amateur–professional antagonism. At its most exaggerated in the mid 19th century, even the notion of training was seen to be a debased practice by amateurs as it did not help them to achieve their goal of being able to accept the challenge of any eventuality as a consequence of their natural physi-

cality and temperament. Part of this was rooted in the separateness of feudal society, but also in the amateur notion of the all-rounder as against the specialist or gladiator.

The survival of folk games

Folk games were occasional contests between different groups in a community and often involved considerable violence (Figures 22.23 and 22.24). By the 19th century many of them had been suppressed, but some survived as an annual event in more isolated towns. You may have heard of the **Ashbourne Football**, the **Haxey Hood Game**, **Lutterworth Mob Hockey**, the **Hallaton Bottle Game** and mob football at **Atherstone** and **Derby**.

Dunning & Sheard[11] produced a framework to show the structural properties of these folk games (Figure 22.25).

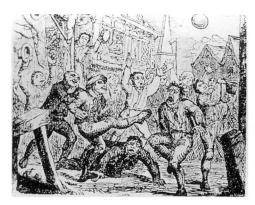

Fig. 22.23 Town mob football.

Investigation 22.12   Pedestrian and gentleman amateur

Figure 22.22 shows a 'ped' and a 'gent'. Can you list their motives for competing?

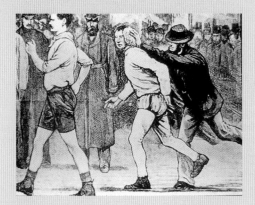

Fig. 22.22 Pedestrianism.

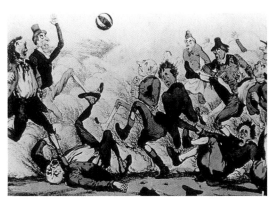

Fig. 22.24 Rural mob football.

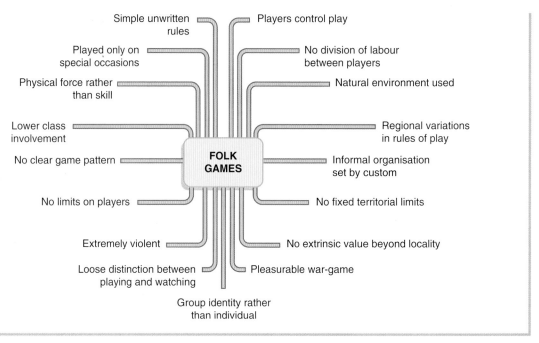

Fig. 22.25 Structural properties of folk games.

Investigation 22.13   Mob games

1. Can you set up a mob game situation, such as mat-ball, and compare it with a modern game such as volleyball, using a simplified version of the Dunning & Sheard framework (Figure 22.25)?

2. The following is an account of the Derby game given by Glover in his *History of Derbyshire*, published in 1829. How does this description match up with the folk game framework?

The contest lies between the parishes of St. Peter's and All Saints, and the goals to which the ball is taken are 'Nun's Mill' for the latter and the Gallows balk on the Normanton Road for the former. None of the other parishes in the borough take any direct part in the contest, but the inhabitants of all join in the sport, together with persons from all parts of the adjacent country. The players are young men from eighteen to thirty or upwards, married as well as single, and many veterans who retain a relish for the sport are occasionally seen in the very heat of the conflict. The game commences in the market-place, where the partisans of each parish are drawn up on each side, and about noon a large ball is tossed up in the midst of them. This is seized upon by some of the strongest and most active men of each party. The rest of the players immediately close in upon them and a solid mass is formed. It then becomes the object of each party to impel the course of the crowd towards their particular goal. The struggle to obtain the ball, which is carried in the arms of those who have possessed themselves of it, is then violent, and the motion of the human tide heaving to and fro without the least regard to consequences is tremendous. Broken shins, broken heads, torn coats, and lost hats are amongst the minor accidents of this fearful contest, and it frequently happens that persons fall owing to the intensity of the pressure, fainting and bleeding beneath the feet of the surrounding mob. But it would be difficult to give an adequate idea of this ruthless sport. A Frenchman passing through Derby remarked, that if Englishmen called this playing, it would be impossible to say what they would call fighting. Still the crowd is encouraged by respectable persons attached to each party, who take a surprising interest in the result of the day's sport, urging on the players with shouts, and even handing to those who are exhausted oranges and other refreshment. The object of the St. Peter's party is to get the ball into the water down the Morledge brook into the Derwent as soon as they can, while the All Saints party endeavour to prevent this and to urge the ball westward. The St. Peter players are considered to be equal to the best water spaniels, and it is certainly curious to see two or three hundred men up to their chins in the Derwent continually ducking each other. The numbers engaged on both sides exceed a thousand, and the streets are crowded with lookers-on. The shops are closed, and the town presents the aspect of a place suddenly taken by storm.[12]

Here is a modern description of the Haxey Hood Game.

There is, for instance, the Haxey Hood Game in Leicestershire, in which tightly rolled lengths of sacking are used. There is, perhaps, something sinister about the ritualistic method of play, which it has been suggested could be symbolic of the struggle between winter and summer. However, the legend behind the game does not support this theory of the struggle between the seasons. It is said that sometime in the 13th century, while riding on the Isle of Axeholme, Lady Mowbray lost her hood. It was found and returned by 12 peasants from the village of Haxey. As a reward she gave to the village a piece of land, thence called the Hoodland, the rent from which had to be used to buy hoods each year to be played for by 12 villagers. The game is also thought to have been played at Epworth on the Isle of Axeholme.

On the Eve of St. John (23 June) each year at Haxey a committee is elected consisting of 12 Boggons – sometimes called Boggans or Boggins – one King Boggon and a Fool.

On the following day at 2 p.m., to the pealing of the church bells, the committee meet dressed in scarlet jerkins and tall hats, except for the Fool who wears a grotesque costume; he has his face blacked and smeared with red ochre and is dressed in trousers of sackcloth with coloured patches and a red shirt. On his head he wears a tall hat with a goose's wing and red flowers adorning it. He carries a short-stocked whip on the end of which is a sock filled with bran.

The boggons then go up to the top of Haxey Hill. There, on the village boundary, they form a circle with the King Boggon in the centre holding 13 hoods. The King Boggon throws a hood and if someone other than a Boggon catches it he tries to run to a nearby public house while the Boggons attempt to stop him. If he succeeds in reaching the pub he demands a shilling. If, on the other hand, he is caught by a Boggon, the hood is returned, to be thrown up again. On the 13th hood throwing, a part of the game known as the sway begins. Hundreds of people join in and attempt to force the hood into a public house. If successful, drinks on the house are called for and the hood is kept on the premises for the following year.[13]

The Haxey Hood Game doesn't involve a ball and the Hallaton Game starts with a scramble for hare pies and concludes with a 'bottle' kicking game. Yes, and they are still being played today! Little wonder every attempt was made to stop these activities. In the Middle Ages various kings pronounced edicts and later, local corporations established bylaws banning street football. We should also recognise the changing times which produced more effective policing, a breakdown of the old rural traditions and the growth of middle-class respectability.

There were as many alternatives involving the use of a small ball and often a stick, each culture seeming to have its own version. The Scots played shinty, the Irish hurley, the Cornish hurling and the English 'bandy', a game normally played on ice.

Investigation 22.14   Mob stick games

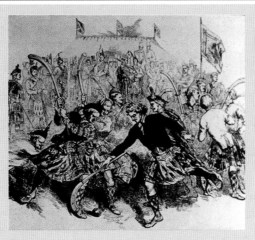

Fig. 22.26 Shinty at Blackheath.

1. Can you pick out the characteristics of this game of shinty (Figure 22.26) and find out why it was being played at Blackheath in London?

2. How many of the mob characteristics are evident in Figure 22.27?

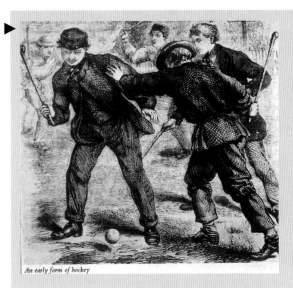

An early form of hockey

3. Find out if your own local area had a mob game. It would be a worthwhile school or college project to produce a picture of it. For example, if you find yourself in Gloucester Cathedral, look at the mob game carving on one of the misericords and a stained glass window of a 'golfer'.

Fig. 22.27 One of the most famous mob hockey games was held annually at Lutterworth in Leicestershire.

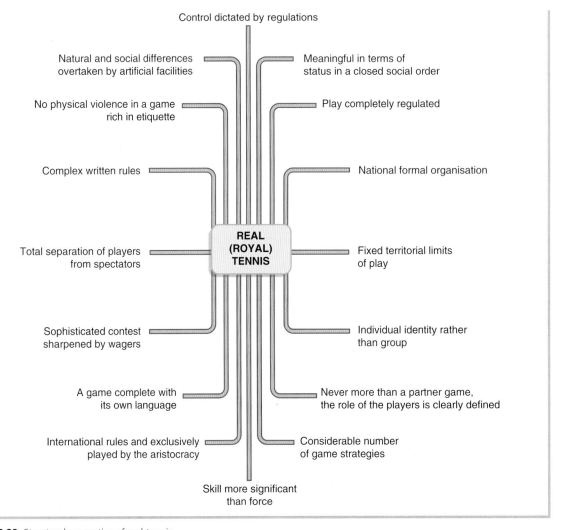

Control dictated by regulations

Natural and social differences overtaken by artificial facilities

Meaningful in terms of status in a closed social order

No physical violence in a game rich in etiquette

Play completely regulated

Complex written rules

National formal organisation

REAL (ROYAL) TENNIS

Total separation of players from spectators

Fixed territorial limits of play

Sophisticated contest sharpened by wagers

Individual identity rather than group

A game complete with its own language

Never more than a partner game, the role of the players is clearly defined

International rules and exclusively played by the aristocracy

Considerable number of game strategies

Skill more significant than force

Fig. 22.28 Structural properties of real tennis.

'Courtly' games

The **sophisticated exclusivity** of **real tennis** was the exact opposite to the **rustic simplicity** of **folk games**. Here was a 'courtly' game borrowed from France and developed as a reflection of high culture in Tudor England. By the 18th and 19th centuries, the game had become the exclusive property of the nobility, supported by a servant class of professionals in the cricket mould.

If we use the Dunning & Sheard[11] framework we now have a completely different set of characteristics (Figure 22.28).

With the rise in popularity of rackets and lawn tennis, an exclusive clientele continued to regard real tennis as the ultimate game (Figures 22.29 and 22.30). The courts at Lord's, Queen's Club, Hampton Court and Royal Leamington Spa served simply to reflect its 'Royal' status.

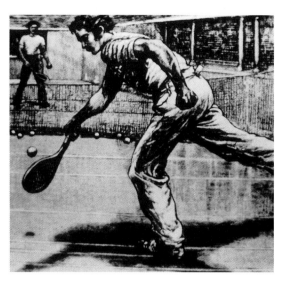

Fig. 22.30 This picture of the Honourable Arthur Lyttleton playing real tennis is another key to the status of the game. A member of the nobility and a famous diplomat, he was one of England's greatest 'Corinthians'. He was an amateur tennis champion; played cricket for England; was an outstanding soccer player, athlete and golfer; and was also a leading yachtsman.

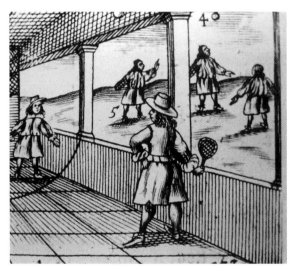

Fig. 22.29 Even from this early picture of real tennis, you should be able to establish why it was so exclusive but it is important to recognise what is happening outside the court of play.

The rise and decline of contests

Archery and **fencing** share a similar history. They both involved weapons of war and so had great importance, until gunpowder made them obsolete. They would have completely disappeared but for a dedicated band of followers who first of all valued the ceremonial role of both activities and then built each into a sophisticated sport in its own right.

Investigation 22.15   Archery

1. Can you think of reasons why a churchyard (Figure 22.31) might have been used for this occasion?

2. To what extent does Figure 22.31 tell you whether this is military training or a sport?

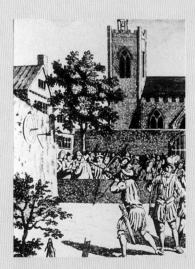

Fig. 22.31 An early picture of archery in an English churchyard.

3. How does Figure 22.32 express the social elitism of archery?

4. Why was it acceptable for these women to take part?

5. Use Figure 22.33 to explain the transition of an activity from a military training exercise to a sport?

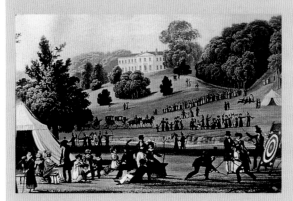

Fig. 22.32 When archery was revived in the late 18th century it was part of the Regency movement, an expression of the most exclusive members of society.

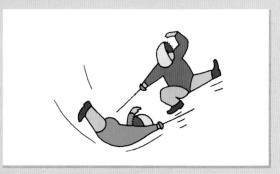

Fig. 22.33 Military sports – when does the idea of training for war change to training for sports?

Unlike archery, swordplay cut across society. There was a lower class version of backswords or single sticks and a 'courtly' version of fencing which owed its status to the duel.

Single stick play (Figure 22.34) was very much part of the rural festival and the intention was to hold contests, where the winner was the first to draw blood.

Fencing (Figure 22.35), on the other hand, was retained after the sword had lost its military function, with the rapier being carried as a ceremonial weapon and used for duelling if a gentleman's honour was questioned.

Prizefighting dates back to the 13th century when there were 'gladiatorial' schools preparing individuals to defend themselves and compete if they wished in 'sword and buckle' contests. In Henry VIII's time these so-called professors of defence had formed a company entitled Masters of Defence. This was the cradle of the Noble Art of Self Defence which came to prominence in the 18th century, led by James Figg

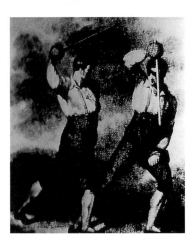

Fig. 22.34 Single sticks.

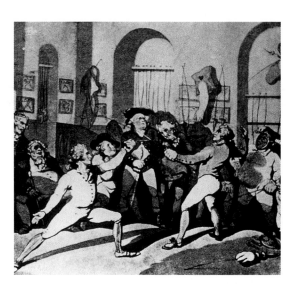

Fig. 22.35 Fencing practice at Angelo's Academy in London. Once duelling was banned, fencing declined, only to re-emerge at the end of the 19th century as part of physical training, alongside gymnastics.

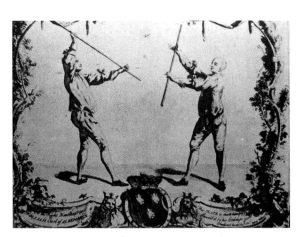

Fig. 22.36 Figg on the 'stage' ready to accept any challenger. As a Master of Defence he had to be able to defend himself against all comers at swordplay, cudgels, quarterstaff and grappling. He was also employed as a tutor to 'fashionable dandies' who wished to test their skill and this occasionally included ladies.

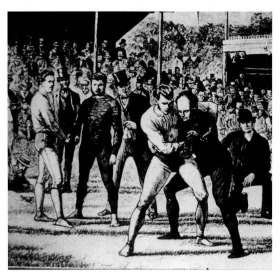

Fig. 22.38 Cumberland wrestling.

(Figure 22.36) who opened the Academy of Boxing in London in 1718.

Figure 22.37 shows Figg being beaten by his pupil Jack Broughton. Broughton had already won the Doggett Coat and Badge and went on to become famous by changing the rules of the prize ring and establishing the birth of **pugilism**. He excluded weaponry and wrestling, limiting the contest to bare-knuckle punching and throws. The tradition of teaching the gentry to defend themselves continued and it was as a result of 'sparring' that 'mufflers' were used – yes, boxing gloves!

Unfortunately, when Broughton unexpectedly lost to Jack Slack in 1750, the Duke of Cumberland, his patron, took it badly (largely because he lost a wager of £10 000) and used his influence to drive the prize ring underground. From this time the Fancy had to run the gauntlet of the police and magistrates but when good champions came along they still attracted the crowds and huge sums of money changed hands.

When grappling was removed from the prize ring, **wrestling** lost much of its popularity. For many years it only survived in isolated areas, such as Cumberland (Figure 22.38) and Devon, where individual styles were retained. This pattern changed when professional wrestling became part of the music hall and when amateur wrestling was included in the revival of the Olympic Games in 1896.

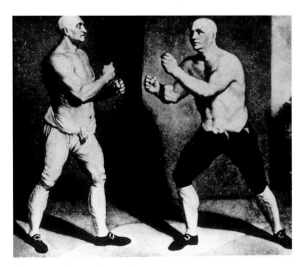

Fig. 22.37 Figg and Broughton.

Investigation 22.16

As a final task, it is important to be able to put activities into a social setting. For example, using the prize ring (Figure 22.39A) and a mob game (Figure 22.39B), you should be able to take a popular recreation characteristic (Figure 22.39C, Column A) and explain why it existed using the societal influences of the time (Figure 22.39C, Column B).

▶

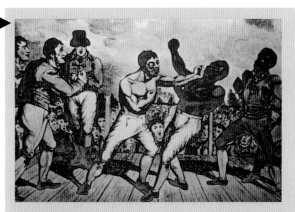

Fig. 22.39A Prize ring.

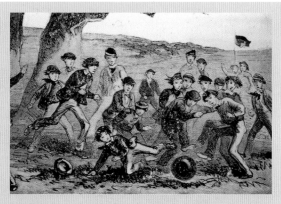

Fig. 22.39B Mob game.

Column A	Column B
POPULAR RECREATION CHARACTERISTICS	PRE-INDUSTRIAL CULT DETERMINANTS
Courtly/Popular	Feudal Society
Localised	Minimal Communications
Occupational	Agricultural and Cottage Industry
Rural	Village, Market and Country Town Life and London
Occasional	Limited Free Time
Cruel/Violent	Harsh society with law and order problems
Ritual/Festival	Pagan/Early Church support Puritan/Protestant constraints
Limited Local Codification	Poor Media Communications
Wagering	Rags to Riches?

Fig. 22.39C

Conclusion

In synoptic terms it is important to recognise that popular recreational patterns were carried into the public schools by boys attending these schools; that there was a gradual but incomplete transition from popular to rational recreation, linking the two inseparably; and that popular recreation persisted in many working class communities, particularly in the play forms of young children and so associations remained with the development of drill and physical training for school children. Less obviously, it was often the popular recreations which were carried abroad by immigrants when they went to the United States and Australia and so there is also a synoptic strand between popular recreation and the development of colonial sport.

Exam-style questions

1. Outline some aspects of early festivals in Britain, considering their links with wakes and fairs. (*5 marks*)

2. Use Figure 22.22 to discuss the background and aspirations in a 19th-century walking race of:

   a. a **gentleman amateur** and

   b. a **pedestrian**.

   (*5 marks*)

3. The prize ring consists of the fighters and their patrons. Explain the status and the function of both groups. (*5 marks*)

4. It has been suggested that a game has many of the characteristics of the cultural group who play it. Figures 22.27 and 22.29 show examples of mob hockey and real tennis. Describe the characteristics of each game and discuss the extent to which this reflected the class of people who played them. (*10 marks*)

References

1. Strutt J 1801 *Sports and pastimes of the people of England*. White, London
2. Bailey P 1978 *Leisure and class in Victorian England*. Routledge and Kegan Paul, London
3. Cunningham H 1980 *Leisure in the industrial society*. Croom Helm, London
4. Newsome D 1961 *Godliness and good learning*. Murray, London
5. Watman M F 1968 *History of British athletics*. Hale, London
6. Harris H A 1975 *Sport in Britain*. Stanley Paul, London
7. Brailsford D 1969 *Sport in society*. Routledge and Kegan Paul, London
8. Ford J 1977 *Prizefighting*. David and Charles, Newton Abbot
9. Malcolmson R W 1973 *Popular recreations in English society*. Cambridge University Press, Cambridge
10. Govett L A 1890 *King's book of sports*. Elliot Stock, London
11. Dunning E, Sheard K 1979 *Barbarians, gentlemen and players*. New York University Press, New York
12. Shearman M 1887 *Athletics and football*. Badminton Library series. Longman, Green, London
13. Jewell B 1977 *Sports and games*. Midas, Tunbridge Wells
14. Whitfield C 1962 *Robert Dover and the Cotswold Games*. Evesham Journal, Evesham, Worcester

Further reading

Baker W J 1982 *Sport in the Western world*. University of Illinois, Urbana, Illinois
Birley D 1993 *Sport and the making of Britain*. Manchester University Press, Manchester
Birley D 1995 *Land of sport and glory: sport and British society 1887–1910*. Manchester University Press, Manchester
Birley D 1995 *Playing the game: sport and British society 1910–45*. Manchester University Press, Manchester
Brailsford D 1992 *British sport: a social history*. Butterworth Press, Cambridge
Brailsford D 1999 *A taste for diversions: sport in Georgian England*. Butterworth Press, Cambridge
Brasch R 1986 *How did sport begin?* Tyron Press, Dumfriesshire
Davis R J 1997 *Popular recreation*. Teacher's guide, Privately published. Pershaw, Worcs
Holt R 1989 *Sport and the British*. OUP, Oxford

Polley M 1998 *Moving the goalposts*. Routledge, London
Wigglesworth N 1996 *The evolution of English sport*. Frank Cass, London

Multimedia

Video

The history of sport series. 1992 DD video, Middlesex

CD-ROMs

Davis R J 2003 *Individual Activities and Games*. Privately published. Pershaw, Worcs
Roscoe D A, Roscoe J V, Honeybourne J, Davis R, Galligan F 2003 *Physical education and sport studies AS/A2 level student revision guide*. 3rd edn. Jan Roscoe Publications, Widnes

Athleticism in 19th-century English public schools

Learning objectives

On completion of this section, you will be able to:

1. Develop a historical perspective of developments which have occurred in the educational system of England.

2. Understand the main characteristics of public school education from the end of the 18th century to the beginning of the First World War in 1914.

3. Use *Tom Brown's school days* as a fictional portrayal of life in public schools during this extended period.

4. Be aware of the 'boy culture' which took popular recreations into the public schools.

5. Be aware of the extension of this into a social control vehicle as a result of the impact of liberal heads.

6. Understand the full expression of athleticism in a variety of public schools, including the values related to it.

7. Be aware of the initial impact of public school athleticism on society through the emergence of rational recreation.

23.1 Background to public school development

The European Renaissance, which marked the rebirth of Greek 'idealism' in a Christian context, reached England during the 16th century. Our main interest lies in the re-emergence of Olympism and the associated importance of 'Man of Action' and the oft-quoted phrase *mens sana in corpore sano* (a healthy mind in a healthy body). It is important to recognise that these values came to England at the time of the great Tudor dynasty and so had all the more impact because Henry VIII championed athleticism as well as nationalism and intellectualism.

The education of the ruling class at this time was through tutors who imparted knowledge but also leadership qualities. The influence of Roger Ascham on the education of Queen Elizabeth I was considerable, particularly as it concerned his belief that archery reflected a model lifestyle. It was at this time that the Age of Chivalry was changing to the Age of Courtesy, where men like Elyot suggested that sporting pastimes made man stronger and more valiant, without the need for life to be endangered.

Monastic schools had existed prior to the Tudors but the Reformation led to their dissolution, leaving an educational void which was filled by the endowment of 'free' grammar schools by various monarchs (free in this context means free from church control). It was around this time that Mulcaster became Master of Merchant Taylors School and recognised the value of healthy exercise for boys at the school. Unfortunately, these endowed grammar schools were very small, seldom having more than 30 boys; they were mainly local day schools and most of the boys left school at 16 years of age. With such small schools, controlled by one 'master' and consisting of only a schoolroom, there was little likelihood of anything more than mob games being played and even this was frowned upon by masters committed to the Puritan ethic.

If you want to know more about the roots of our education system, Brailsford[1] is a very good source of information.

23.2 The structural basis of the English public school system

Definitions

An endowed place of education of old standing to which the sons of gentlemen resort in considerable numbers and where they reside from eight or nine to eighteen years of age.[2]

The only important addition to this is the factor that the children tended to be 'non-local'. It is a useful exercise for readers to find out what they can about one public school and then test their knowledge against the key definitive words identified in Figure 23.1.

The word **athleticism** (Figure 23.2) is less straightforward to define, because it was a developmental word and the full expression of public school athleticism was not achieved until the 1850s. It had fundamental links with the **muscular Christian view of manliness** reflecting **physical endeavour and moral integrity**. It is important that you should be able to

explain these values in the context of your favourite sport a 100 years ago and today.

If you feel you need to know more about the meaning of these terms in a 19th-century context, read some of Newsome[3] or Percival.[4]

From around 1860, many changes occurred which led to an exploitation of the English gentleman's love of sport. In modern phraseology, there was almost a 'sports school' situation. This led Smith[5] to suggest that **athleticism** became 'the exaltation and disproportionate regard for games, which often resulted in the denigration of academic work and in anti-intellectualism'.

With so many old and new schools involved, the problem lies in deciding whether this '**cult of athleticism**' actually led to a lowering of academic standards. You need to study a number of different public schools to assess the extent to which this might have been the case.

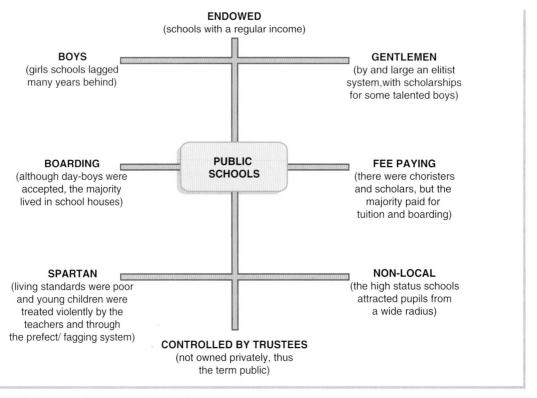

ENDOWED
(schools with a regular income)

BOYS
(girls schools lagged many years behind)

GENTLEMEN
(by and large an elitist system,with scholarships for some talented boys)

BOARDING
(although day-boys were accepted, the majority lived in school houses)

PUBLIC SCHOOLS

FEE PAYING
(there were choristers and scholars, but the majority paid for tuition and boarding)

SPARTAN
(living standards were poor and young children were treated violently by the teachers and through the prefect/ fagging system)

NON-LOCAL
(the high status schools attracted pupils from a wide radius)

CONTROLLED BY TRUSTEES
(not owned privately, thus the term public)

Fig. 23.1 Key definitive words for English public schools.

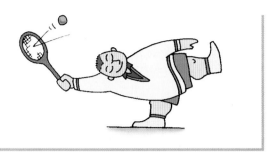

Fig. 23.2 Athleticism – playing according to the letter and spirit of the game.

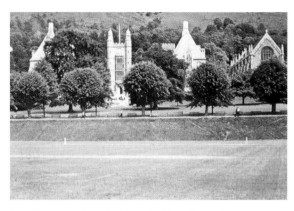

Fig. 23.3 This view of Malvern College shows the impressive school buildings facing the playing fields.

Types of public school in the 19th century

If you have managed to look at athletic developments in a number of public schools, you can categorise your examples using the following list and then look around for a local example of each type of school.

Clarendon schools

Examined in the 1864 Clarendon Report, these were nine exclusive boys' schools. They were Eton, Harrow, Rugby, Shrewsbury, Charterhouse, Westminster, Winchester, St Paul's and Merchant Taylors. Each had expanded to take over 300 pupils at the end of the 18th century and the first seven were predominantly non-local and boarding. Matthew Arnold called them 'Barbarian' schools because they maintained the gentry tradition.

Ladies' academies

Finishing schools for the daughters of the gentry, these were normally small and more concerned with elegance and etiquette than with academic learning.

Proprietary colleges

These were middle-class copies of the gentry schools. They were built with outstanding facilities to attract wealthy clients and eventually broke the monopoly held by the few elite schools. Cheltenham College (1841) was the first to be opened, with other famous colleges at Clifton, Marlborough and Malvern (Figure 23.3). Matthew Arnold called these proprietary schools 'Philistines' because he claimed they were simply materialistic copies of the traditional gentry schools.

Cheltenham Ladies' College (1854) was the first proprietary school for girls but by the end of the 19th century almost every major town had a middle-class girls' high school.

Denominational schools

Cathedral schools at such county towns as Canterbury, York and Worcester were ancient foundations which became King's schools after the Reformation, but they remained small until the 1870s.

Towards the end of the 19th century, the Church of England built some new boarding schools to educate the sons and daughters of the **clergy**. Lancing College is the best known of these 'Woodard' schools.

Endowed grammar schools

Almost every town in England had its own 'free' grammar school for boys, named after the king or queen who endowed it. Some of these schools built up a reputation in the mid-19th century and became major public schools. The most famous of these are Uppingham, Repton and King Edward's, Birmingham. However, the majority remained small until the 1880s, when there was an expansion of secondary education for boys from the commercial classes.

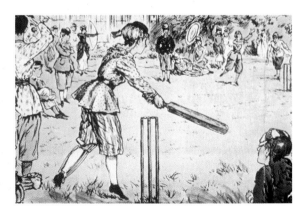

Fig. 23.4 Although this picture is called The Ladies' Cricket Club, it looks as if the club could be operating from within a private girls' school or ladies' academy.

In general, girls' grammar schools did not appear until the 20th century.

Private schools
These were owned by individuals or families. The quality of education varied considerably but some of them, for example Malvern Girls' College, eventually became exclusive public schools. Many of these better schools had excellent sporting facilities to attract an upper-class clientele (Figure 23.4).

23.3 The technical development of sports in the public schools

Though this was a gradual development over a period of 50 years, it is easier to review it in three stages and limit comment to gentry schools for boys, middle-class schools for boys and middle-class girls' schools.

Stage one: schoolboys and popular recreation

The traditional gentry schools expanded at the end of the 18th century, resulting in a considerable increase in income, which led to improved facilities and staffing. This started a spiral which in turn led to a small number of schools becoming exclusive and being able to charge higher fees.

Boarding gave the boys a great deal of time together outside the classroom and in their free time they played the games they had learnt at home. These were entirely organised by the boys and ranged from the relative sedateness of cricket to the violence of mob football; from illegal poaching to organised hare and hounds; from casual boating to rackets in the 'quad'.

In *Tom Brown's school days*, Thomas Hughes writes about the sports Tom experienced at home.

The great times for back-swords came round once a year in each village, at the feast. The Vale 'veasts' were not the common statute feasts, but much more ancient business. They are literally, so far as one can ascertain, feasts of the dedication, i.e. they were first established in the churchyard on the day on which the village church was opened for public worship, which was on the wake or festival of the patron Saint, and have been held on the same day in every year since that time.

In fact the only reason why this is not the case still, is that gentlefolk and farmers have taken to other amusements, and have, as usual, forgotten the poor. They don't attend the feasts themselves, and call them disreputable, whereupon the steadiest of the poor leave them also, and they become what they are called.

Class amusements, be they for dukes or plough-boys, always become nuisances and curses to a country. The true charm of cricket and hunting is, that they are still more or less sociable and universal; there's a place for every man who will come and take his part.

Investigation 23.1   Popular sports in schools

1. Upper-class boys took various popular sports to the schools. How does Hughes, in *Tom Brown's school days*, offset the values of rural sports against the intolerance of authorities?

2. Take any example of a primitive game in a public school and explain why it developed its unique qualities.

Some headmasters did their best to stop the more violent activities taking place in school. You will probably know the famous phrase by Butler of Shrewsbury, 'Football is only suitable for butchers' boys', but at the same time he condoned cricket and was only critical of rowing because of the danger of drowning. Meanwhile, there seems to have been support for cricket and rowing at Eton and Westminster before the 19th century and the Harrow authorities did not attempt to curtail archery or rackets (Figure 23.6).

In reality, the early headmasters were powerless to stop any of these activities, particularly when they took place away from the school. Flogging was the normal punishment for any kind of disobedience but occasionally, there were cases of rioting in the schools and then it was necessary for the militia to be brought in.

Most of the problems arose when boys went into the town or travelled to other schools. There was invariably a great deal of drunkenness and riotous behaviour. Some of the rural sports carried with them

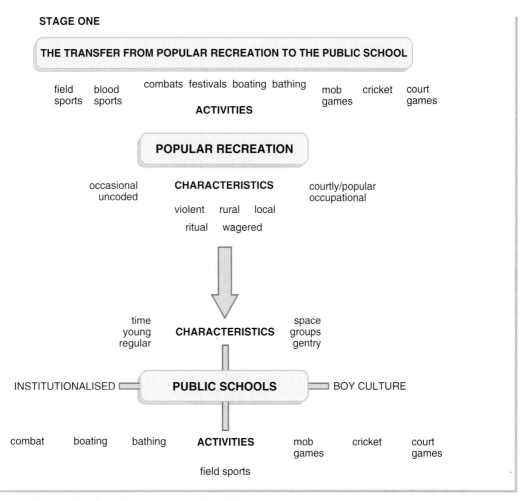

STAGE ONE

THE TRANSFER FROM POPULAR RECREATION TO THE PUBLIC SCHOOL

field   blood   combats festivals boating bathing   mob   cricket   court
sports   sports   games   games

ACTIVITIES

POPULAR RECREATION

occasional   **CHARACTERISTICS**   courtly/popular
uncoded   occupational

violent   rural   local

ritual   wagered

time   space
young   **CHARACTERISTICS**   groups
regular   gentry

INSTITUTIONALISED   **PUBLIC SCHOOLS**   BOY CULTURE

combat   boating   bathing   **ACTIVITIES**   mob   cricket   court
                                                          games   games

field sports

Fig. 23.5 Stage one. The transfer of popular recreation to the public schools.

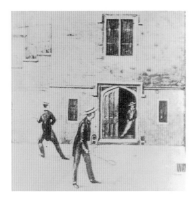

Fig. 23.6 Racket ball being played in the cloisters at Harrow School.

a tradition of drinking and gambling, which the boys were only too keen to include in their school life.

A number of key features are associated with this initial phase of school sport. The boys brought the games into the schools and were responsible for their organisation. They had the opportunity to play them regularly and so the occasional popular recreations became part of a continuous season of play and this had a major impact on the regularisation of rules. Some sports were already socially acceptable and these were encouraged by the school authorities and with regular play possible, standards of performance improved dramatically.

Where the sports lacked existing rules, the facilities available at the school determined the developmental

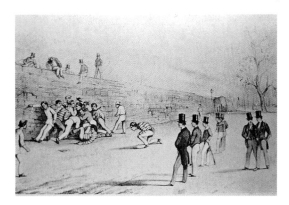

Fig. 23.7 The Eton wall game.

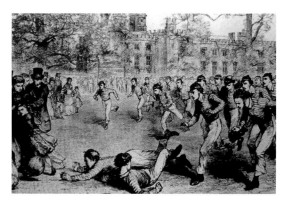

Fig. 23.8 Rugby at Rugby School. Dr Arnold was watching this game with a Royal visitor, something he would hardly have done if he had been against the game.

form of the activity: for example: the 'Close' at Rugby with its soft turf; the 'Quad' at Charterhouse, where the 'dribbling' game emerged; and the unique version of mob football found at Eton, where the 'wall game' was instituted (Figure 23.7).

Stage two: Arnoldian influence and the role of a Christian gentleman

In 1828, Dr Thomas Arnold was appointed head of Rugby School; he died in office 14 years later. For well over a century he has been regarded as the father of public school athleticism, largely as a result of the impact of *Tom Brown's school days* published in 1857 (Figure 23.8).

Many modern writers, including McIntosh,[6] Ogilvie,[7] Bamford[8] and Percival,[4] recognised that Arnold was one of a number of progressive headmasters who established an environment which eventually stimulated athleticism (Figure 23.9). It is important that you recognise the modern change of emphasis. For example, McIntosh suggested that:

While it is probable that Arnold's reforms at Rugby indirectly encouraged the growth of athleticism, both there and in other schools, it is improbable that he was immediately responsible for the change of attitude or that he himself approved of athleticism.

Also, it was Dr Thomas James (1778–1794), who initially expanded Rugby School and it is now felt that many of Arnold's ideas came from the reforms he had seen operating at Winchester School under Dr W S Goodall. It has been successfully argued that Arnold was much more concerned with moral reform – a desire to produce **Christian gentlemen** – than to promote a **muscular Christian** tradition. He

believed in a form of 'manly piety' which was moral, intellectual and social rather than physical.

The safest analysis is to recognise that the athletic momentum came from the boys and Arnold was astute enough to use this enthusiasm to achieve a range of moral reforms which hinged on the boys being given responsibility. Even this level of intention was questioned by Bamford[8] when he suggested that Arnold's reputation was the consequence of nostalgic staff loyalty, the enthusiasm of some Old Rugbeians and a 'train of fortuitous circumstances' in which the emergence of rugby football as a national game had particular relevance.

Having identified the supposed 'accident' of events, it is important to mention Wymer,[9] who had access to Arnold's family records. He suggests that Thomas Arnold loved cricket to the degree of having his children tutored in the game; that his lifelong friendship with William Wordsworth reflected his love of the Lake District and mountain walking; and that his enjoyment of swimming, shooting, sailing and riding suggested that he had a high regard for healthy physical activity.

However, there was a direct conflict between Arnold's moral stance and some of the field sports pursued in the school. He was not prepared to allow poaching, fishing or any activity which involved trespass, on the grounds that it caused friction between the school and the community. On the other hand, he made no attempt to interfere with cricket or football. In addition to the two extracts about the cricket match against the MCC and Tom's playground fight against Slogger (Investigation 23.2), you should also try to read about Tom's adventures with the gamekeeper, when he goes fishing; the problems

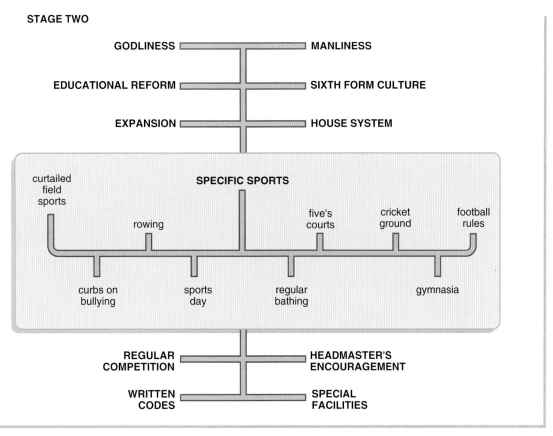

Fig. 23.9 Stage two. The influence of liberal heads on public school sporting activities.

met by Tom, East and Arthur when they try to enter the Hare and Hounds; and the famous description of the football match, where Tom decides that his help is needed to save the game (Figure 23.10).

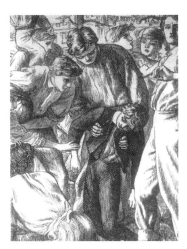

Fig. 23.10 Tom's exploits at football.

Investigation 23.2   Sporting incidents

Tom Brown's school days may be romantic recollections of someone's childhood but there is much to be learnt from reading some of the sporting incidents.

1. Read this extract on a cricket match and see if you can identify the values that the game is presumed to have.

    '*Come, none of your irony, Brown,' answers the master. 'I'm beginning to understand the game scientifically. What a noble game it is, too!'*

    '*Isn't it? But it's more than a game. It's an institution,' said Tom.*

    '*Yes' said Arthur, 'the birthright of British boys old and young, as habeas corpus and trial by jury are of British men.'*

    '*The discipline and reliance on one another which it teaches is so valuable, I think,' went on the master, 'it ought to be such an unselfish game. It merges the individual in the eleven; he doesn't play that he may win, but that his side may.'*

'That's very true,' said Tom, 'and that's why football and cricket, now one comes to think of it, are such much better games than fives' or hare-and-hounds, or any others where the object is to come in first or to win for oneself, and not that one's side may win.'

'And then the Captain of the eleven!' said the master, 'what a post is his in our School-world! Almost as hard as the Doctor's; requiring skill and gentleness and firmness, and I know not what other rare qualities.'...

'I am surprised to see Arthur in the eleven,' said the master, as they stood together in front of the dense crowd, which was now closing in round the ground.

'Well, I'm not quite sure that he ought to be in for his play,' said Tom, 'but I couldn't help putting him in. It will do him so much good, and you can't think what I owe him.'...

'I think I shall make a hand of him though,' said Tom, smiling, 'say what you will. There's something about him, every now and then, which shows me he's got pluck somewhere in him. That's the only thing after all that'll wash, ain't it ...'

Finally, if Thomas Hughes is to be believed, there is a lot to be learnt about the Doctor and the role of the Sixth Form in the following extract about a fight (Figure 23.11).

2. What do you gather from this extract and what is to be gained from letting the fight continue?

Meantime East is freshing up Tom with the sponges for the next round and has set two other boys to rub his hands.

'Tom, old boy,' whispers he, 'this may be fun for you, but it's death to me. He'll hit all the fight out of you in another five minutes, and then I shall go and drown myself in the island ditch. Feint him – use your legs! Draw him about! He'll lose his wind then in no time, and you can go into him. Hit at

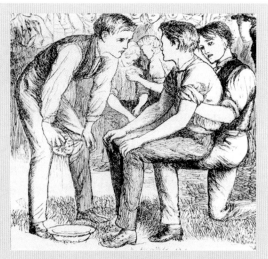

Fig. 23.11 The fight from *Tom Brown's school days.*

his body too; we'll take care of his frontispiece by and by.'...

'Ha! Brooke. I am surprised to see you here. Don't you know that I expect the sixth to stop fighting?'

Brooke felt much more uncomfortable than he had expected, but he was rather a favourite with the Doctor for his openness and plainness of speech; so blurted out, as he walked by the Doctor's side, who had already turned back –

'Yes, sir, generally. But I thought you wished us to exercise a discretion in the matter too – not to interfere too soon.'

'But they have been fighting this half-hour and more,' said the Doctor.

'Yes, sir; but neither was hurt. And they're the sort of boys who'll be all the better friends now, which they wouldn't have been if they had been stopped any earlier – before it was so equal.'

In all five extracts, it is valuable to identify the technical changes which have occurred; to establish the different social relationships which exist; and to recognise the ethics which Thomas Hughes is promoting in this romantic portrait of public school life.

It would be wrong to assume that Thomas Arnold was alone in this process of educational reform. Kennedy of Shrewsbury, Moberly of Winchester, Wordsworth of Harrow and Hawtry of Eton were all 'new brooms' sweeping away a decadent system of thrashings and classics for a new wave of moral and social education, where athleticism was becoming an instrument for the promotion of a new set of values

(Figure 23.12). In sporting terms, the technical changes which occurred between 1830 and 1850 hinged on the regularity of play and the responsibility of the Sixth Form to organise fixtures. In the later schools, the boarding house became an important social feature and one of the roles of the house master was to see that the boys were usefully organised and this was often achieved through sporting competitions. The desire to get rid of antisocial elements such as gambling, blood sports and poaching was commonplace and this was achieved by attempting to limit activities to the playing fields, where Arnold felt that boys learnt to make their own moral decisions.

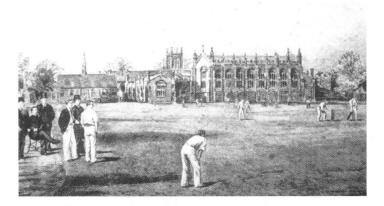

Fig. 23.12 This picture of Cheltenham College and its 'Playground' was typical of the second phase of sports development, in which governors and trustees were prepared to recognise the importance of sport in the life of the public schoolboy.

Stage three: athleticism and the Corinthian spirit

The influence of the first generation of progressive headmasters on the pupils was so great that these young disciples carried their interpretation forward to Oxford and Cambridge. It was in the **'melting pot'** of these universities that athleticism became the all-important catalyst and the Oxford–Cambridge competitions in a wide range of sports served to identify the most talented performers. Many of these **'blues'** became assistant masters and not only coached the boys but played for the school team when required.

It was in the 20 years following Arnold that most of the new proprietary colleges were opened and the headships were awarded to assistant masters from the gentry schools. Men like Cotton of Marlborough, Percival of Clifton and Jex-Blake of Cheltenham were typical of a new breed of headmaster who were enthusiastically in favour of athleticism as an educative medium. In human terms, therefore, the staff were now actively supporting sport in school rather than merely condoning it.

It was this second generation of teachers who carried athleticism into the 'muscular Christian' era. Expansion in the size, significance and number of schools led to a massive building programme which invariably included a gymnasium and extensive playing fields. The school day included morning academic studies, afternoon games and evenings involved in prep (homework) and house activities. The time spent on playing a particular game could be up to 5 hours a day, with **professional coaches** and **'blues'** producing a standard of play which raised the quality of amateur performance throughout the country (Figure 23.13).

It was in the public schools that the first football rules were written and it was the fixtures between these schools, and matches with gentlemen's clubs, that started regular organised **rational recreation**. Nor was it simply a technical development. The term 'rational recreation' implies a moral component.

With some additional reading you should now be able to describe the technical changes which occurred in public school sport from 1800 to 1870. The Clarendon Report (1864) gave considerable recognition to the development of athleticism in the nine elite gentry schools and the Taunton Commission Report was published in 1868, having gathered information on 782 other public schools and colleges.

Cheltenham Ladies' College was included in the Taunton Commission Report and by 1868 they had afternoon games and a wide programme, which included callisthenics, swimming and horse riding. Miss Beale, the headmistress, was not too keen on 'aggressive games' on the grounds that they were not lady-like, but she allowed tennis and rackets and the School Council eventually persuaded her that a hockey field was also a necessity. A study of specific school histories will help you to see that despite initial opposition, all the girls' high schools had an extensive athletics programme by the turn of the 19th century and were largely responsible for the growth of female athleticism in society at large.

Social control through physical activity in the public schools

In looking at technical development, we have been concerned with **recreative** and **sporting** changes. A second level of analysis lies in the way various authorities used athleticism as a vehicle to control themselves and others. The area of social control through school sport is initially a case of interaction between individual players; the team and its captain; relationships with opposing teams and schools; and the influence of the teacher developing these games.

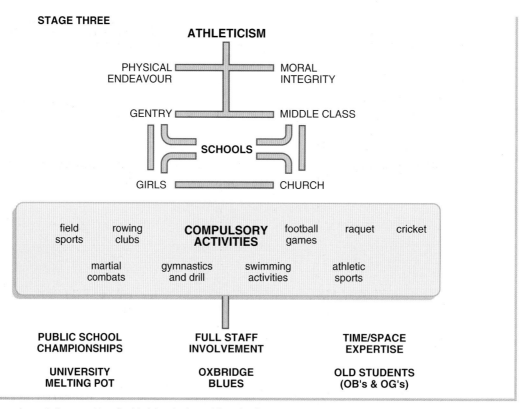

STAGE THREE

ATHLETICISM

PHYSICAL ENDEAVOUR — MORAL INTEGRITY

GENTRY — MIDDLE CLASS

SCHOOLS

GIRLS — CHURCH

| field sports | rowing clubs | **COMPULSORY ACTIVITIES** | football games | raquet | cricket |

| martial combats | gymnastics and drill | swimming activities | athletic sports |

PUBLIC SCHOOL CHAMPIONSHIPS   **FULL STAFF INVOLVEMENT**   **TIME/SPACE EXPERTISE**

UNIVERSITY MELTING POT   **OXBRIDGE BLUES**   **OLD STUDENTS (OB's & OG's)**

Fig. 23.13 Stage three. Full expression of athleticism in the public schools.

In an institution with a defined code of behaviour, these relationships were conditioned by the rules of the school and the attitude of the authorities. There would seem to be links betwen the decline of bullying and beatings and the growth of athleticism in these schools. Consequently, when analysing the levels at which social control operated in public school sport, it is important to use instances which involved peer groups, house allegiances, influences from assistant teachers, decisions by the head and even influences from the governors and public on special sporting occasions. Evidence of attitudes and values influenced in this way can come from specific school histories, but the extracts from *Tom Brown's school days* are most useful, if you look at the social affinity between Tom, East and Arthur; the dominance of Brooke as football captain; the decision making by Brown as captain of cricket; and the respect given to Dr Arnold in terms of what he encouraged or rejected in school sport at Rugby School. Finally, it is important to recognise the permanent impact of these socialising features in that the loyalty of old boys and girls was reflected in the way they supported and funded their school in later life; the way values attributed to sport were carried into life; and the huge change from popular to rational recreation, which was predominantly the influence of ex-public school boys establishing sports clubs and redefining amateurism.

Investigation 23.3   The moral component of rational recreation

1. What moral elements might be promoted as a result of this rowing fixture (Figure 23.14) between Eton and Westminster?

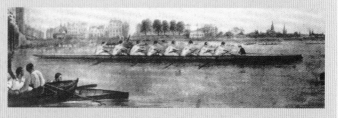

Fig. 23.14 Interschool rowing.

▶ **2.** Explain the changing role of people in Figure 23.15, as school sport evolved. Comment on such things as individual and group status, discipline and leadership opportunities.

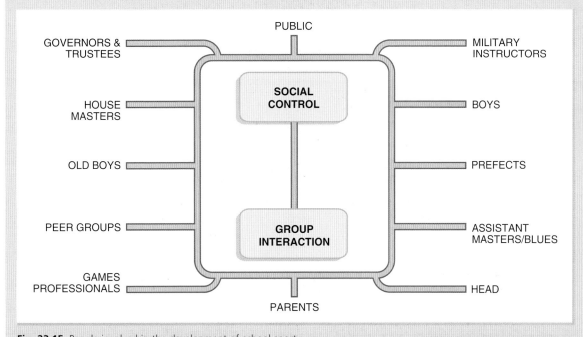

Fig. 23.15 People involved in the development of school sport.

23.4 Athleticism and character development

Probably the most significant feature of public school athleticism was the belief that school sport was not only a vehicle for personal development, but the essence of education itself, representing a model lifestyle. It consisted of a fundamental link being made between **manliness** and **godliness** in what has been called **muscular Christianity** – an educational experience involving **physical endeavour** and **moral integrity**.

You may have read Henry Newbolt's poem:
There's a breathless hush in the Close tonight
Ten to make and the match to win –
A bumping pitch and a blinding light,
An hour to play and the last man in.

The verse ends with the well-known line:

Play up! Play up! and play the game.

It is easy for us to link this with a game we've played with all the tensions of a close finish but the poet is writing about more than cricket here. He goes on to say:

The river of death has brimmed its banks
And England's far and Honour a name,
But the voice of a schoolboy rallies the ranks:
Play up! Play up! and play the game.

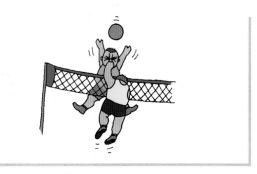

Fig. 23.16 Play up! Play up! And play the game!

Can you see the importance of the game and the way you play it, if it is preparing you for life and the battlefield? In such a game, to win gracefully and to lose with honour is so much more meaningful and to do your best could mean being willing to give your life. Honour, bravery, brotherhood, leadership – these are the values the public schools saw in the games they played and they believed that through them, these qualities became a permanent part of the player and also of the person.

Investigation 23.4 The relevance of athleticism

Figure 23.17 shows an outline of the main values which the public schools linked with athleticism. Comment on the relevance of each of these today:

1. in the context of physical education
2. in the extent to which they exist in professional sport.

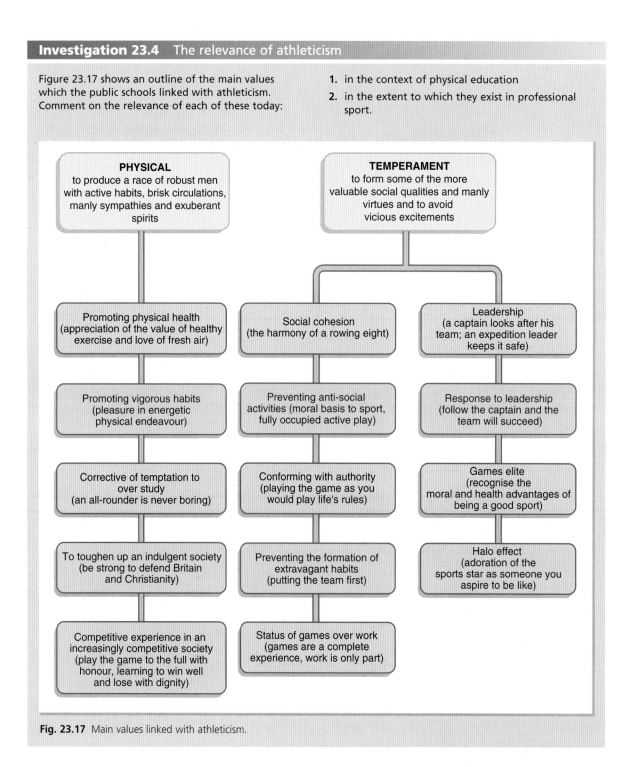

PHYSICAL
to produce a race of robust men with active habits, brisk circulations, manly sympathies and exuberant spirits

TEMPERAMENT
to form some of the more valuable social qualities and manly virtues and to avoid vicious excitements

Promoting physical health (appreciation of the value of healthy exercise and love of fresh air)

Social cohesion (the harmony of a rowing eight)

Leadership (a captain looks after his team; an expedition leader keeps it safe)

Promoting vigorous habits (pleasure in energetic physical endeavour)

Preventing anti-social activities (moral basis to sport, fully occupied active play)

Response to leadership (follow the captain and the team will succeed)

Corrective of temptation to over study (an all-rounder is never boring)

Conforming with authority (playing the game as you would play life's rules)

Games elite (recognise the moral and health advantages of being a good sport)

To toughen up an indulgent society (be strong to defend Britain and Christianity)

Preventing the formation of extravagant habits (putting the team first)

Halo effect (adoration of the sports star as someone you aspire to be like)

Competitive experience in an increasingly competitive society (play the game to the full with honour, learning to win well and lose with dignity)

Status of games over work (games are a complete experience, work is only part)

Fig. 23.17 Main values linked with athleticism.

23.5 The influence of public school athleticism on sport in society

Popular recreation was in decline in the last quarter of the 19th century and was being replaced by **rational recreation**. It is probable that the development of athleticism in public schools had more influence on this trend than any other social factor. Figures 23.18 and 23.19 show the various ways in which this happened. It is important that you compare these with the present links between physical education in school and sport in society.

It would also be worth your while to obtain a detailed knowledge of one particular public school (there are history texts written on most of them) and also be able to take one of the major sets of activities –

cricket, rowing, football, racket games, etc. – through the technical changes.

Finally, not a great deal of reference has been made so far to girls' public schools. Mangan & Park[10] and/or Fletcher[11] are the best published works in this field, but most of the girls' public schools and older high schools have published histories.

The existence of academies for young ladies at the beginning of the 19th century tells us that the girls in upper-class families were educated and that this reflected the important role played by the wife on major estates. Their husbands were often away on political or business affairs and at these times the

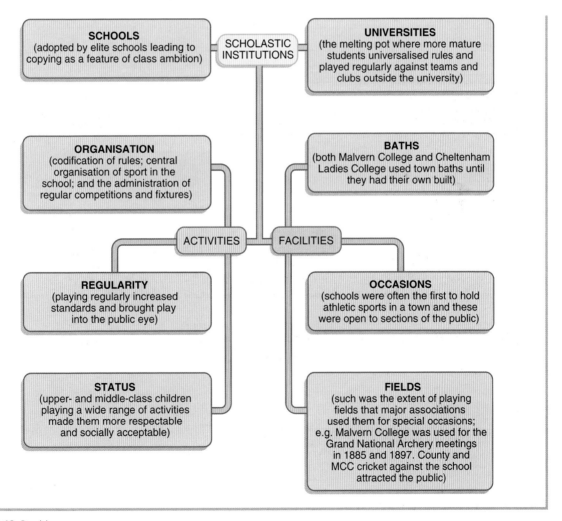

Fig. 23.18 Provision.

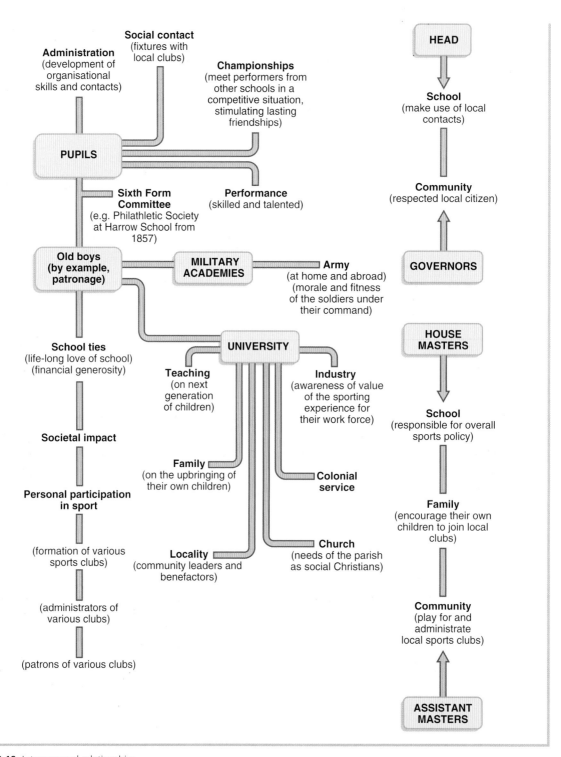

Fig. 23.19 Interpersonal relationships.

responsibility of running the household was extended to the estate. Their wealth, free time, privacy and privilege also led to an active life of hunting, shooting and archery and so their education, though focusing on deportment and etiquette, was not limited to this. It is also important to recognise that a gentry family which endorsed games for the boys also resulted in the girls taking part. The Foster family at Malvern College, for example, not only produced outstanding sportsmen but the daughters led the development of sport at Alice Ottley School, Worcester.

It is easy to see why high schools for girls were delayed, but also why they were late in developing sport, if you recall the impact of the role of women in Victorian England. The expansion of the middle classes on the grounds that the successful businessman 'kept' his wife, together with the expected dress code, delayed the development of athleticism in girls' schools, limiting it to callisthenics. However, with the development of lawn tennis as a useful social accomplishment, the game spread from a pastime for young teachers to the inclusion of the Sixth Form and

as cleanliness because a pillar of respectability, so schools like Cheltenham Ladies' College encouraged regular, organised visits to the town swimming baths. Meanwhile, an expansion of Malvern College for Girls included an indoor swimming bath, which was still in regular use in the 1990s. This was also the period when alpinism and romanticism in the Lake District were at their height and so girls were encouraged to go on vigorous excursions in the countryside.

However, it was a second generation of schools like St. Leonards and Roedean in Sussex which broke the barrier by allowing lawn tennis throughout their schools; hockey as a mob game, before young teachers fashioned the rules; and cricket, at least for younger girls. It is important to recognise that many of the high schools were day schools and so this dramatically reduced the time available to develop games, but by the 1890s all reputable girls' high schools had a games programme and as a result of Swedish drill becoming important, many had specialist PE teachers who had been trained at Dartford and other ladies colleges.

Review questions

1. What were the technical developments that occurred in public school sport during the 19th century?
2. How did social control vary in relation to athleticism?
3. What were the main values that the sporting experience was supposed to be giving young people?
4. What was the impact of certain headmasters and other staff on the development of athleticism?
5. Why did the Old Boys have such a large influence on the development of athleticism in their own schools and in society at large?

Exam-style questions

1. Explain the initial changes that occurred when boys took popular recreations into the gentry public schools at the beginning of the 19th century. (*5 marks*)
2. In *Tom Brown's school days*, Tom fights Slogger because he bullied 'Little Arthur' (see Figure 23.11). Explain the attitudes shown by the different people involved in that episode. (*5 marks*)
3. What were the major influences of the universities on the expansion of athleticism in the public schools and society at large? (*5 marks*)
4. Discuss the technical developments that had occurred in public schools by the 1870s and the extent to which these demonstrate links between athleticism and character building. (*10 marks*)

References

1. Brailsford D 1969 *Sport and society*. Routledge and Kegan Paul, London
2. Smith S 1952 Edinburgh review. In: McIntosh P C (ed) *Physical education in England since 1800*. Bell, London
3. Newsome D 1961 *Godliness and good learning*. Murray, London
4. Percival A C 1973 *Very superior men*. Knight, London
5. Smith W D 1974 *Stretching their bodies*. David and Charles, Newton Abbot
6. McIntosh P C 1952 *Physical education in England since 1800*. Bell, London
7. Ogilvie V 1957 *The English public school*. Batsford, London

8. Bamford T W 1967 *The rise of the public schools*. Nelson, Windsor
9. Wymer N 1953 *Dr Arnold of Rugby*. Hale, London
10. Mangan J A, Park R J 1987 *From 'fair sex' to feminism*. Frank Cass, London

11. Fletcher S 1984 *Women first: the female tradition in English physical education*. Athlone Press, London

Further reading

N.B. Many of these books are out of print, but are obtainable through lending libraries. Similarly, old schools and local archival centres have copies of school magazines which give some tremendous insights into the place of sport as far as the boys and girls of the school were concerned.

Davis R J *Athleticism in 19th-century public schools*. Teachers' Guide. Privately published. Pershore, Worcs

Dunning E, Sheard K 1979 *Barbarians, gentlemen and players*. New York University Press, New York

Hughes T 1857 *Tom Brown's school days*. Various publishers

Money T 1997 *Manly and muscular diversions*. Duckworth and Co, London

Simon B, Bradley I 1975 *The Victorian public school*. Gill and Macmillan, Dublin

Roscoe D A, Roscoe J V, Honeybourne J, Davis R, Galligan F 2003 *Physical education and sport studies AS/A2 level student revision guide*. 3rd edn. Jan Roscoe Publications, Widnes

Walvin J 1978 *Leisure and society*. Longman, London

Multimedia

Video

Tom Brown's school days. 1992 Leisure View Videos, London

The pattern of rational recreation in 19th-century Britain

24

Learning objectives

On completion of this section, you will be able to:

1. Develop a historical perspective of the recent past on the present.

2. Understand the main characteristics of industrial Britain as a social setting for sports and pastimes of that period.

3. Have a knowledge about a variety of sports as they fit into a number of profiles.

4. Be aware of the main characteristics of these activities as shared and different features.

5. Understand the organisation of these activities and the dominant attitudes of the players and public who were associated with them.

6. Understand the place of amateurism and professionalism in rationalised sport.

A new form of physical recreation began to emerge in Britain around the 1850s. It consisted of a formal, morally based presentation of contests, individual activities, games and outdoor pursuits, by respectable members of the community, in a form which no longer contained the excesses evident in popular recreation. It stemmed from the gentry and gentry schools and was enthusiastically taken up by the middle classes and their schools. As a product of social Christianity and liberalism, these sporting opportunities were gradually made available to the working classes, together with a respectable form of professional sport to accommodate a new form of spectatorism.

Elias & Dunning[1] called this process the 'genesis of sport', suggesting that primitive sports associated with popular recreation had little or nothing in common with this **rational recreation** (Figure 24.1) as a sophisticated reflection of an industrialised society: that sport as we know it was born in the mid-19th century. This is an interesting theory but it has loopholes, some of which are explored by Cunningham.[2]

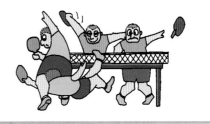

Fig. 24.1 Rational recreation – the test of temperament and physical competence.

24.1 Social factors influencing the development of rational recreation in Britain

Urbanisation and population expansion

The size of towns determined the recreative needs of a community. Old towns had medieval slums which were gradually cleared to make shopping and commercial centres. The larger the town, the greater the distance to the countryside and natural recreative provision. The rate of growth, particularly of the lower class, meant that population outstripped recreative provision. There was a gradual improvement in facilities towards the end of the 19th century with public parks being opened and public baths being built.

Communications and travel

The distance an individual could travel was dependent on the free time available and the cost. An increase in the speed of transport allowed people to travel further in the same time (Figure 24.2). Travel had two basic links with sport:

- as a means of getting to a sporting venue, in the transport sense
- the process itself was recreative or sporting.

It is possible to link river communications with angling, bathing, fowling and boating. With roads, there was the growth of pedestrianism and walking race horses, followed later by the impact of the cycle. Finally, the railways opened up the countryside and the seaside resorts. They allowed fixtures to be made in different towns and stimulated spectatorism (Figure 24.3).

Communication and literacy

The printed word was a positive influence on sport. The evolution of the free press, the promotion of literacy, the mechanisation of the printing industry, cheaper production of weekly newspapers and the publication of pocket editions led to an informed public. This permanent record was also achieved by artists who recorded major sporting events and in the 1890s photography played a considerable part in promoting and reflecting sport, particularly once pictorial supplements were published by the weekly press.

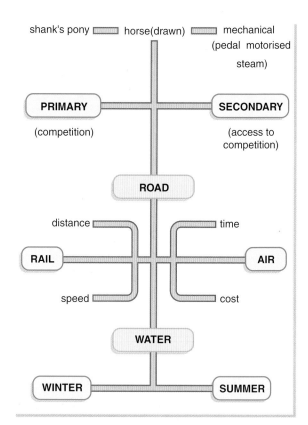

Fig. 24.3 Communications, transport and sport.

Religious and secular institutions

You have already read about the negative influences of religion on popular recreation. The picture changed completely when **muscular Christianity** and **rational recreation** came together. Young curates, fresh from public school and university, joined parishes and promoted athleticism for their parishioners. The YMCA, in particular, became an athletic as well as a religious centre (Figure 24.4) and it encouraged young clerks to engage in a variety of rational sports (Figure 24.5).

Similarly, there were mechanics institutes and working men's clubs which tried to wean the lower-class male away from drink and popular recreation by offering social amenities, literary classes and rational recreations.

The working classes and industrial provision

While cottage industries existed, the workers were able to select their own time for recreation but

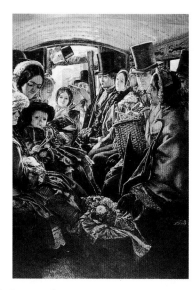

Fig. 24.2 An excursion to Epsom Down.

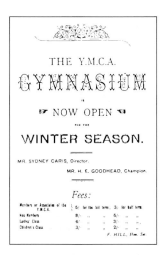

Fig. 24.4 Source: Burton-on-Trent YMCA, 1884–1885.

factories changed this. Machines determined working hours and pay reflected profits and sales. It was commonplace for men to be working for 72 hours a week for one pound.

A major breakthrough came with the **Saturday half-day**. Clerks and skilled workers achieved this by the 1870s, semi-skilled workers in the 1880s and most labourers by the 1890s, resulting in most working-class males doing a 57-hour week by the end of the 19th century.

Working-class opportunities for sport must be seen in the context of the squalor of the industrial slums, the poverty of those out of work (Figure 24.6) and low wages, which caused a family man to work overtime (Figure 24.7).

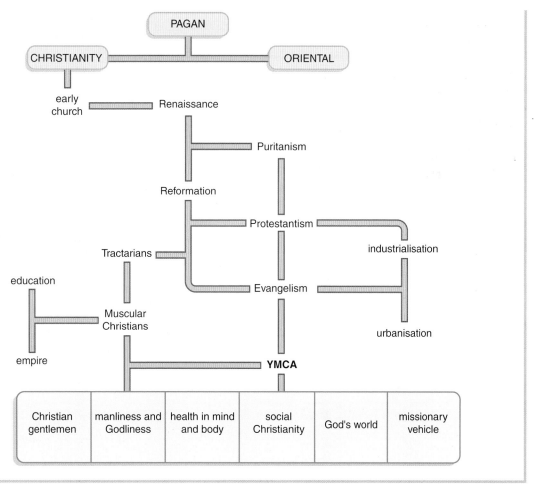

Fig. 24.5 Religion and sport.

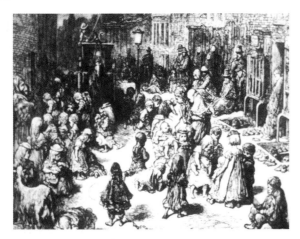

Fig. 24.6 Poverty on the streets.

The sons of industrialists brought athleticism to the factories and started sports clubs. Initially, this only involved the salaried staff, but gradually facilities were built for shop-floor workers in the belief that it would improve health, morale and loyalty. An older form of patronage continued to exist where an annual feast or excursion was paid for by the owners. With larger firms this often involved a day trip to the seaside, with all expenses paid (see Figure 24.2).

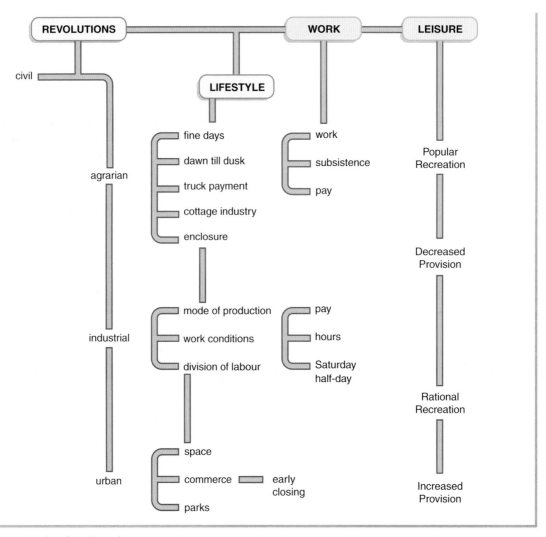

Fig. 24.7 Sport and work in the 19th century.

24.2 The rational development of activities and games

Swimming, athletics and gymnastics

Swimming and bathing

Recreational bathing

When it was hot, the natural thing to do in river towns was to go bathing. The trouble was it was dangerous and the sight of naked urchins upset respectable citizens. As a result, bathing stations were built on the river bank.

Spa and sea bathing

'Taking the waters' became a Regency fashion and led to spa towns being built with extensive bathing facilities. The fashion then switched to the seaside which led to seaside bathing.

Public baths

The Wash-house Acts (1846) led to many industrial towns building public baths to clean up the labouring classes. They were called 'penny baths' because there was a fixed limit on charges for the second-class facilities.

Competitive swimming

Most of the middle-class swimming clubs were formed in the private Turkish baths. The first national championships were held in 1874 with the formation of the Swimming Association of Great Britain (SAGB) and the Amateur Swimming Association (ASA) was formed in 1884. Water polo mainly developed in the public baths and was codified in 1885. The Amateur Diving Association was not formed until 1901.

Athletics and cross-country

University athletics

Public schools had sports days which formalised the old rural sports. The Old Boys took this idea to Oxford and Cambridge, with the Exeter College Autumn Meeting (1850) being the first amateur athletics meeting. It was run like a horse-race meeting.

The Wenlock Olympian Games

Meanwhile, Dr Penny Brookes re-established an old rural sports at Much Wenlock in a rational form. In 1865 the National Olympian Association (NOA) was formed as a governing body and they defined amateurism.

Amateur athletics

The Amateur Athletic Club (AAC) was formed in 1866 by ex-Oxbridge gentlemen athletes. They also defined amateurism but excluded the working class. They were rivals of the NOA and set up their own National Championships in 1866. In 1880, the Amateur Athletics Association (AAA) was formed; the 'exclusive' clause was removed and 'no financial gain' became the central amateur criterion.

Cross-country running

Almost like the poor man's hunting, many harrier athletic clubs were formed in the 1880s with 'hare and hound races' and 'paper chases'. These clubs also held summer sports meetings, which led to the British tradition of middle-distance running.

Gymnastics

Archibald Maclaren, an intellectual friend of Ruskin and Morris, was a versatile sportsman. An outstanding oarsman, he built a gymnasium at Oxford (1850) and one at Aldershot for the Army (1861). He published texts on gymnastics and the public schools and urban clubs used his approach rather than Continental methods.

Muscular Christianity and the YMCA

Gymnastics was recognised as a non-competitive instrument for increasing respect for the human body. Liverpool and Manchester YMCAs had a great influence on developments.

Investigation 24.1 The development of rational recreation

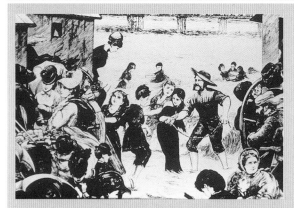

Fig. 24.8 Bathing huts at the seaside.

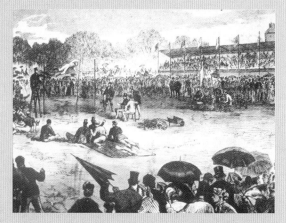

Fig. 24.9 Athletic sports meeting.

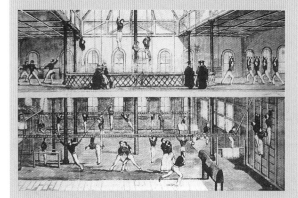

Fig. 24.10 Maclaren's gymnasium.

1. What does Figure 24.8 tell you about bathing and Victorian morality?

2. Use Figure 24.9 as a basis to explain the development of amateur athletic sports meetings.

3. Describe English gymnastics from Figure 24.10.

Invasion games

The classification of an **invasion game** in modern times is a territorially fluid team game with goal targets and involving free play of the ball with variations of body contact.

In rational recreation terms, they were rule based with a 'spirit' and 'letter' of play; they were highly organised, with governing bodies and affiliated clubs, and played regularly with fixtures, officials and club colours in fixed seasons.

Association football

The public schools changed the mob games into respectable, regular games. Eton, Harrow and Charterhouse promoted a 'dribbling' game which was played under the Cambridge Rules from 1856. Old Boys' teams helped form the Football Association (FA) in 1863. There were 10 clubs in 1867 rising to 50 by 1871. By 1905 there were 10 000 clubs, with 272 in the FA Cup.

Professionalism was legalised in 1885 and the Football League was formed in 1888. At the opposite end of the scale the Corinthian Club had gentlemen as members and only played friendly games. The game spread to all sections of society with leading clubs being formed from:

- **Old Boys' teams**, e.g. Leicester City from the Old Wyggestonians
- **street teams**, e.g. Rotherham (1884) was formed under a street lamp
- **employees' teams**, e.g. Manchester City from the Lancs & Yorks Railway Club (1885)
- **church teams**, e.g. Everton (1878) was a Sunday School team
- and various other sources, e.g. Sheffield Wednesday was an Early Closers' team.

Rugby football

This code was initially limited to Old Rugbeians. They founded Guy's Hospital Club (1843) and Blackheath (1862). In 1871, Blackheath and 20 other clubs formed the Rugby Football Union (RFU) and in 1877 the game was restricted to 15 a side.

The 'broken time' debate led to a split between southern and northern clubs in 1895 on the subject of professionalism and this led to 22 clubs breaking away to form the Northern Union, which eventually became the Rugby League.

Hockey

There were initially two separate lines of development. Blackheath and Bristol rationalised the old mob game in a form which lasted until 1895.

Meanwhile, a number of cricket clubs in the Home Counties were experimenting with winter hockey. In 1871 there were clubs at Richmond, Teddington and Sutton. A Hockey Union was set up in 1876 to join the two codes, but they could not agree. In 1886 the Hockey Association was formed, based on the Teddington model, and the Blackheath game slowly disappeared.

Women's club hockey can be traced to an East Molesey Club in the 1880s. The Irish Ladies' Hockey Union was formed in 1894 and a year later the All-England Women's Hockey Association (AEWHA) was established to coincide with the first international fixture between Alexandra College, Dublin, and Newnham and Girton Colleges, Cambridge.

Investigation 24.2   The invasion games

1. Use Figure 24.11 to show how the rational game of Association football differs from mob football.

2. Use Figure 24.12 to show how the rational game of rugby football differs from mob football.

3. What qualities were the girls trying to promote through hockey (Figure 24.13)?

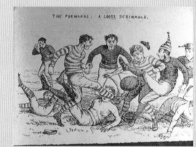

Fig. 24.12 Rugby football.

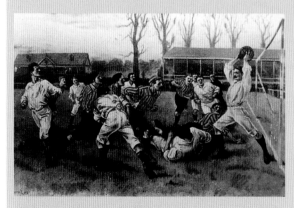

Fig. 24.11 Association football.

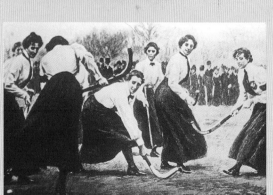

Fig. 24.13 Hockey.

Target games

The classification of a target game is that it involves a team or pair in a game which has targets such as wickets, skittles or holes. There is alternate play, which restricts body contact, and in team versions each team has a separate role to play, e.g. batting or fielding.

Many of the rational elements of these games developed much earlier because they were less violent. Strict rules of play, spirit and letter were observed and controlled by governing bodies. Though games tended to be on a friendly basis, championships involving amateurs and professionals had early developments.

Cricket

The tour of the All-England XI in the 1840s led to a growth of gentlemen's county cricket clubs. The old village clubs continued alongside these, while there was a massive growth in the number of urban middle-class clubs. (Croquet, rounders and baseball function within the same general classification.)

Regular fixtures at all levels led to increased competition at county level and so more artisan professionals were employed and middle-class amateurs started to play county cricket. Such was the belief in the value of cricket that church leaders, teachers and employers started to encourage the urban working class to play the game.

Women's cricket was limited by Victorian attitudes, but in the 1880s there was a revival of the 'ladies' game as the result of increased athleticism in the middle-class girls' schools.

Golf

This was always the Scottish equivalent of cricket. It suited a smaller population, uneven terrain and an inclement climate. It was also close to the other Scottish game of shinty.

Golf was normally played on 'links' (seaside) and St Andrews has always been the 'home' of the game. In Scotland, golf was a 'popular' game, but in England wealthy Scots introduced it to the upper class and it remained an elite game throughout the 19th century. There was always a lower-class version of the game, even in England, where an artisan club had use of the course in return for keeping it in good condition. Ladies used the men's courses until their numbers grew sufficiently to open their own.

Bowls

Skittles, bowls and quoits belonged to a group of games which were associated with taverns. This delayed their acceptability in respectable circles until middle-class clubs started to be formed and public parks started to provide greens for the lower classes. The Yorks & Lancs Crown Green Association (1888) and the Flat Green Association (1895) were the two governing bodies which coordinated fixtures and championships.

Quoiting was very popular in rural areas in the last quarter of the 19th century, but has almost disappeared today.

Investigation 24.3 The target games

1. Identify the changes in cricket from the 18th-century game (Figure 24.14).

2. Use your knowledge of female sport to establish why golf was acceptable for 'ladies' (Figure 24.15).

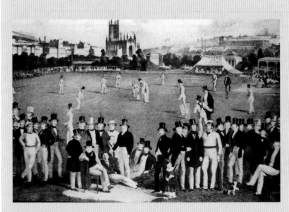

Fig. 24.14 Cricket.

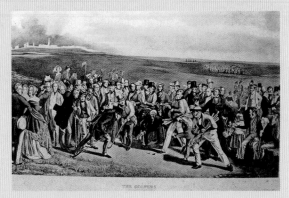

Fig. 24.15 Golf.

▶ **3.** Can you account for the advantages and disadvantages of skittles being associated with taverns (Figure 24.16)?

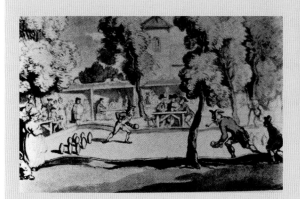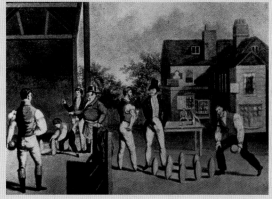

Fig. 24.16 Skittles.

Court games

The classification of these games is based on a court being used for play. There should be no body contact, with alternate play over a net or against a wall and points are scored; singles or pairs can play.

The rational game goes back to real tennis which, because of its exclusivity, was sophisticatedly codified from the 16th century. This game evolved into a variety of forms to suit different situations and conditions.

Rackets

Initially the poor man's version of real tennis, its popularity in public schools, alongside fives, led to clubs being set up throughout the country. The rational stage was achieved when 'open' courts with one wall were changed to indoor 'closed' courts. Prince's Club, and then Queen's from 1886, controlled the codification of the game. The 1880s also saw the introduction of a junior 'squashy' ball, which has led to the modern game of squash.

Badminton

This game had slightly different roots, because there was an ancient pastime called shuttlecock and battledore. It was still being played in gardens in the 19th century and legend has it that, on a wet day,

the family at Badminton House (Duke of Beaufort) took the game indoors.

The first rules were written in 1877 by members of the British Army and Diplomatic Corps in India. The Badminton Association was formed in 1893 and the championships were held at Wimbledon, alongside lawn tennis and croquet.

Lawn tennis

The modern game has three main roots. Major Gem introduced a game at Leamington in 1866 and the Leamington Club had written rules by 1870; J. H. Hales introduced Germain Tennis in 1873; and Major Wingfield patented a game called 'Sphairistike' in the same year. The modern rules of lawn tennis were codified by the MCC in 1875, with the All-England Croquet and Lawn Tennis Club being established at Wimbledon in 1876.

One reason why lawn tennis became so popular was the changing role of the middle-class female. In the privacy of their own gardens, it became acceptable for females to play this social game.

Initially exclusive, early tournaments were associated with county cricket. These tended to be played behind closed doors and it wasn't until 1884 that public championships were held for 'ladies' at Wimbledon.

Investigation 24.4   The court games

1. Can you find some explanations for rackets being played in Fleet Prison (Figure 24.17)?

2. Why do you think badminton did not have a governing body until the 1890s (Figure 24.18)?

3. Discuss the links between lawn tennis, athleticism and female participation in sport (Figure 24.19).

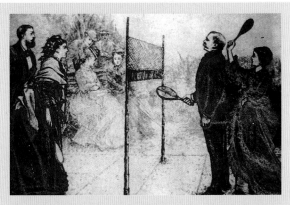

Fig. 24.18 Badminton.

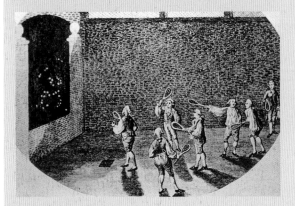

Fig. 24.17 Rackets.

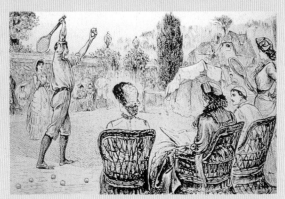

Fig. 24.19 Lawn tennis.

Aquatic activities

Rowing

So-called amateur regattas appeared around 1870. They tended to exclude the lower classes as they were run by clubs consisting of public school oarsmen.

The Amateur Rowing Association (ARA) controlled rowing on the Thames from 1879 and by 1885 became the national governing body. The 'exclusion clause' limited competitive rowing to public school boys. The National Amateur Rowing Association (NARA, 1890) was a rival body which permitted broader participation.

Canoeing

Canoe touring was popular in the last half of the 19th century, largely due to the exploits of John MacGregor and his book *A thousand miles by Rob Roy canoe*.

Sailing

Yachting was a sport of the aristocracy and the Royal Navy. The Duke of Cumberland Cup (1781) was the premier schooner race. Several clubs on the Isle of Wight were patronised by William IV and Queen Victoria.

The America's Cup was first held in 1851 as a challenge between British and American yachts. The winner chose the next venue and until recent times the Americans won every contest.

Dinghy sailing started with the Solent Classes in 1870. Middle-class clubs were formed at Southampton and Portsmouth and promoted races for 21-, 25- and 30-foot craft.

Skating

There were three main lines of development on ice. The oldest were the ice fairs, which were very similar to rural fairs.

Speed skating came from Holland and developed on the Fens. The National Skating Association (1879) controlled the amateur championships and there were also professional championships.

Figure skating developed with improved skates. The world centre was the Serpentine in London.

Difficulties were met when attempts were made to develop 'glacariums' and so roller skating rinks developed in the 1870s as an alternative.

Investigation 24.5   Aquatic activities

1. Can you explain the main characteristics of Henley (Figure 24.20)?

2. How many reasons can you find to explain why Britain has never won the America's Cup (Figure 24.21)?

3. Use Figure 24.22 to explain the many attractions of ice and roller skating.

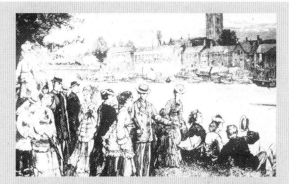

Fig. 24.20 Rowing.

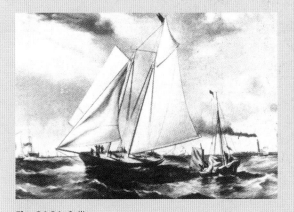

Fig. 24.21 Sailing.

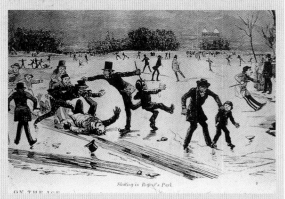

Fig. 24.22 Skating.

Climbing, skiing and cycling

Climbing

Life in the mountains initially hinged on shepherds and local people acting as guides. The Romantic Movement brought the gentry to the mountains, but it was the scenery rather than climbing which appealed to most of them. This love of mountain scenery extended to the Alps and snow climbing developed through the Alpine Club (1857). This led to the development of **mountaineering** – the art of reaching the summit.

Scientists looking for alpine plants opened up the Lake District and North Wales. W.P. Haskett-Smith at Wasdale Head and O. G. Jones at Pen-y-Gwryd were the most famous climbers. This led to **rock climbing** – the practice of finding the most difficult route up a crag. While mountaineering was very much an upper-class pursuit, rock climbing was taken up by the middle and working classes.

Skiing

The use of bone skates and snow shoes in Nordic countries is ancient but it was Arthur Lunn, an English alpinist, who first used wooden skis as a means of racing down hill on snow and, from the beginning, it was taken up as a pastime as much as a method of travelling on snow.

Cycling

An excellent sport to show social variables, cycling reflected the urban and industrial revolutions in that a machine was used as an urban substitute for a horse. The bicycle became the most common vehicle whereby people in towns managed to escape to the countryside. It was very much an urban, middle-class male preserve to begin with. The gentry despised it and the working class could not afford it. It started as a novelty fashion with the hobby horse and progressed, via France, to the boneshaker or velocipede. The inventiveness of English industrialists led to the Ordinary or Penny Farthing. The large wheel allowed increased speed and kept the person above the mud, but it was dangerous. A safer version, the tricycle, was developed and this was largely used by women and the elderly until the Rover safety and pneumatic tyres were invented.

There were three main branches of cycling. Track racing (British Cycling Union, BCU) was part of the athletic sports meeting; touring (Cycle Touring Club, CTC) became highly organised with consuls, guide books, repair shops and hotels; and, finally, there was the development of road racing. The problem with the latter was that mass starts were banned and so pursuit racing took its place in England. Mass starts were allowed on the Isle of Man and the Continent, which led to the Tour de France becoming the premier road-racing event.

In terms of social class development, the gentry, particularly ladies, took up cycle touring, following the lead of Queen Victoria's daughters. At the same time the second-hand cycle trade allowed poorer people to buy bicycles. Middle-class women followed the lead of the upper class and fashion became an important feature, first with 'bloomers' and later the 'rational dress' (divided skirt).

Investigation 24.6   Climbing and cycling

1. Why were there very few limits on women climbers (Figure 24.23)?

2. Explain the influence of cycling on female sporting opportunities (Figure 24.24).

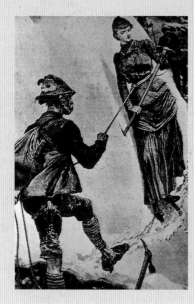

Fig. 24.23
Mountaineering.

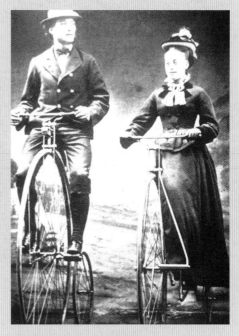

Fig. 24.24 Penny Farthing riders.

At the end of Chapter 22, activity characteristics were aligned with preindustrial cultural determinants (Investigation 22.16, with Figures 22.39 and 22.40).

The same approach can be applied to rational recreations in an industrialised society.

Investigation 24.7   Boxing by Queensberry Rules and Association football

1. Compare boxing by Queensberry Rules (Figure 24.25A) and Association football (Figure 24.25B) in the context of rational recreation characteristics (Figure 24.25C; column A) with postindustrial cultural determinants (Figure 24.25C; column B).

2. Compare your answers with those in Investigation 22.16.

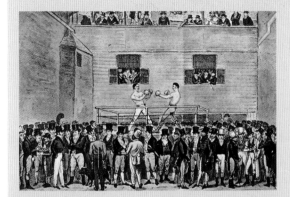

Fig. 24.25A Queensberry Rules boxing.

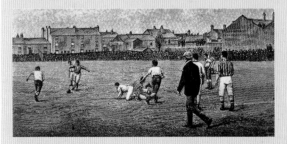

Fig. 24.25B Association football.

RATIONAL RECREATION CHARACTERISTICS	POST INDUSTRIAL CULTURAL DETERMINANTS
respectable	middle class emergence
rural/urban/ industrial sport	agrarian/urban/ industrial revolutions
stringent administration	business administration and commercial acumen
codified	increased literacy and the media
local/national/ international	travel and the railways improved roads
regularised	increased free time
fair play & channelled aggression	temperance & friendly societies muscular Christianity public school ethos
control of gambling	capitalist economy law and order
exclusive/ conciliation	social class and gender discrimination
amateur/professionalism	bread and circuses

Fig. 24.25C Rational recreation characteristics and postindustrial cultural determinants.

In synoptic terms it is important to recognise that just as popular recreations had a direct impact on the public schools, so athleticism in these schools established a dual set of values of physical endeavour and moral integrity which was directly translated into rational recreation in post-industrial society. However, it is important to recognise that vestiges of popular recreation, public school traditions and 19th-century athleticism, whilst presumed to be outmoded, still exist in modern society and therefore it is worthwhile to draw synoptic links between the past and the present.

Similarly, the spread of rational sport through Europe and the colonies has given it an international impact which creates global links in the past and present and these dimensions, too, justify a degree of synoptic evaluation.

Exam-style questions

1. **a.** Explain the characteristics of **rational recreation** as shown in Figures 24.11 and 24.25C. *(5 marks)*

   b. Describe the main influences on the development of bathing and swimming in the 19th century. *(5 marks)*

   c. Explain why cricket was more immediately acceptable as a respectable game. *(5 marks)*

   d. Use Figure 24.19 to explain the idea that lawn tennis was invented by the middle class and comment on the influence of the game on female participation in sport. *(10 marks)*

   (Total 25 marks)

2. **a.** If public schools initiated the development of respectable sport in Britain, it was the railway network which allowed it to spread so rapidly.

   i. How did transport limit the spread of sport before the railways were built? *(4 marks)*

   ii. How did the railways influence holiday patterns and the spread of games (Figure 24.3)? *(5 marks)*

   b. Describe the changing relationship between **sport** and **religion** in the UK (Figure 24.5). *(6 marks)*

   c. The Industrial Revolution took the control of work from the craftsman and gave it to the machine. How did the constraints on free time and wages influence working-class sport and how were conditions improved towards the end of the 19th century (Figure 24.7)? *(10 marks)*

   (Total 25 marks)

References

1. Elias N, Dunning E 1996 *Quest for excitement*. Blackwell, Oxford

2. Cunningham H 1980 *Leisure in the industrial society*. Croom Helm, London

Further reading

Bailey P 1978 *Leisure and class in Victorian England*. Routledge and Kegan Paul, London

Baker W J 1988 *Sports in the Western world*. University of Illinois, Illinois

Brailsford D 1992 *British sport: a social history*. Lutterworth, Leicester

Dunning E, Sheard K 1979 *Barbarians, gentlemen and players*. New York University Press, New York

Holt R 1989 *Sport and the British*. Clarendon, Oxford

Mason T 1980 *Association football and English society*. Harvester, Brighton

Mason T 1989 *Sport in Britain: a social history*. Cambridge University Press, Cambridge

Polley M 1998 *Moving the goalposts*. Routledge, London

Roscoe D A, Roscoe J V, Honeybourne J, Davis R, Galligan F 2003 *Physical education and sport studies AS/A2 level student revision guide*. 3rd edn. Jan Roscoe Publications, Widnes

Walvin J 1975 *The people's game*. Allen Lane, New York

Walvin J 1978 *Leisure and society*. Longman, London

Wigglesworth N 1996 *The evolution of English sport*. Frank Cass, London

Transitions in English elementary schools

25

Learning objectives

On completion of this section, you will be able to:

1. Develop a historical perspective of drill, physical training and physical education.

2. Understand the main characteristics of elementary state education at the beginning of the 20th century.

3. Be aware of the military drill approach in the 1902 Model Course.

4. Understand the progression into physical training and the reasons for these changes.

5. Appreciate the changes which occurred to establish physical education as a progressive school subject.

6. Appreciate the effect of various wars on development as well as other cultural influences.

25.1 19th-century drill and gymnastics

J.C.F. Guts Muths (1749–1839) was the 'father of European gymnastics'. He published *Gymnastics for the Young* and this was a source of subsequent developments in Sweden (P.H. Ling, 1776–1839), Germany (F.L. Jahn, 1778–1852), Denmark (F. Nachtegall, 1777–1847) and Britain (A. Maclaren, 1820–1884).

Maclaren used continental developments, but felt that many features were unsuitable for English students. He preferred apparatus work and a mixture of other activities, such as walking and riding, swimming and country pursuits.

Dr Mathias Roth was the leading supporter of the Swedish System in England and was a rival of Maclaren. He supported 'rational gymnastics' for medical and military reasons.

Elementary schooling prior to 1870 was dominated by two major organisations: the National Schools Society (1811), a Church of England association, and the British and Foreign Schools Society (1808), which was linked with non-conformism. Some of these schools had playgrounds and even playing fields, but many in the industrial towns had no playing facilities and could not cope with the massive population explosion, despite a great deal of absenteeism.

The 1870 Forster Education Act was an attempt to 'plug the gaps' in elementary schooling and led to the establishment of board schools. The Act ignored Roth's efforts and the 1871 Code of Regulations only introduced 'permissive' legislation:

> *Drill for boys only, if given under a competent instructor, for not more than two hours a week, and twenty weeks in the year, could be counted as school attendance.*

This consisted of marching, posture exercises and dummy arms drill and was taught by Army NCOs for sixpence a day and a penny a mile for marching, using the *Army Field Exercise Book* (1870). Girls were included in 1873, but the content remained 'free-standing' military drill.

Gymnastic apparatus was available in public schools and some open spaces, but the intention of the drill in working-class schools was to improve the fitness of Army recruits and to instil discipline.

In the 1890s the Education Department recommended the inclusion of some Swedish drill, largely as a result of Swedish-trained inspectors being appointed in London. There was also a trend for qualified teachers to take over the drill from the military instructors.

The Prize Day Programme for the Worcester board schools in 1894 (Figure 25.1) reflects this broader approach. Changing attitudes were also evident in a speech by the Rev. C.E. Hopton in Worcester in 1899:

> I hope that when the Transvaal War [Boer War] is over people will be able to say that those victories had been won on the playgrounds of the elementary schools of England. To teach boys to be brave, noble, honest and self-sacrificing, so that when they went out into the world, those characteristics would stick by them, and would fit them to be worthy citizens of this great country.

It would seem that at least one **muscular Christian** felt that the same qualities were achievable by poor children as well as by the rich.

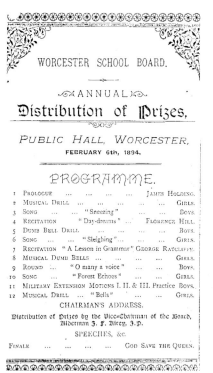

Fig. 25.1 Prize day programme.

25.2 The 1902 model course[1]

The Boer War (1899–1902) was fought between the British Empire and the Boers, South Africans of Dutch extraction. Great Britain lost a great deal of prestige because her large but ponderous army found it very difficult to defeat a small force of mobile guerrilla fighters.

Back in England, accusations were mainly that the working classes were unhealthy and ill prepared to fight and, as a scapegoat, politicians blamed the Swedish drill being taught by teachers in the elementary schools. As a result the Model Course was imposed in 1902 in all these schools. It was produced by the War Office and controlled by Colonel Fox of the Army Physical Training Corps (APTC). He was instructed to achieve two main objectives:

- to increase fitness for military service through acquaintance with the discipline of military drill
- to train children to 'withstand the hardships of combat and have familiarity with weapons'.

There was a directive that these lessons should replace Swedish drill and military instructors should be used. Boys and girls were involved in this programme up to the age of 12 years, but they were instructed as little soldiers, not children.

Investigation 25.1 The 1902 Course

It is important that you should have some idea of the content of this syllabus and the method of instruction and this is a very good opportunity for you to use role-play methods by going through a model lesson. Young people today are not used to the command–response of military drill and so you should find it an interesting experience.

Enact the following lesson (also see Figures 25.2–25.5), where teachers or students can take it in turns to act as instructors.

Note: — is a long cautionary word;

and ∪ is a short, sharp executive command.

▶

▶ **Lesson**

‾‾‾ ∪   ∪ ∪   ∪   ‾‾∪ ‾‾‾ ∪

1. *Right marker; in two ranks, fall in; right form.*

   (This means falling in on the marker's left, an arm's distance apart.)

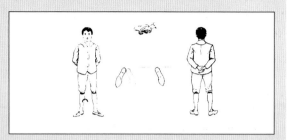

A. Stand at ease.

‾‾‾‾ ∪   ‾‾‾ ∪

2. *Stand at ease; atten-tion.*

   (Repeat this, looking for exact positions and moving together.)

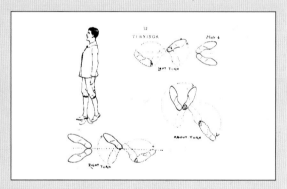

B. Attention.

‾‾‾ ∪ ∪ ∪ ‾‾‾‾‾‾ ‾‾‾ ∪

3. *Right turn, one; two; by the left, quick march;*
   ∪ ∪ ∪ ∪   ‾‾‾ ∪ ‾‾‾ ∪
   left, right, left, right (etc.). Squad halt; about turn;
   ‾‾‾ ∪ ‾‾‾ ∪ ‾‾‾ ∪ ‾‾‾‾ ∪
   quick march; squad halt; right turn; stand at ease.

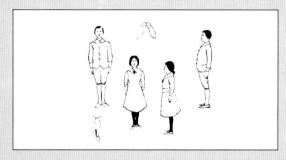

Fig. 25.3 Turning.

‾‾‾ ∪ ‾‾‾ ‾‾‾‾‾ ‾‾ ‾‾‾‾‾

4. *Atten-tion; arms bending and stretching,*
   ‾‾‾ ∪ ∪ ∪ ∪ ∪ ∪
   arms bend; out; bend; up; bend; down (repeat);
   ‾‾‾‾‾ ∪
   stand at ease.

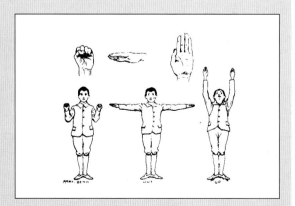

Fig. 25.2 Standing positions.

Fig. 25.4 Arm bending and stretching.

5. Exercise with staves (corner poles):

‾‾‾ ∪ ‾‾‾ ‾‾‾ ‾‾‾ ‾‾‾ ∪
Atten-tion; ready; astride with cross stave ready;

∪ ∪ ∪ ‾‾‾ ∪ ‾‾‾ ∪ ∪ ∪
one; two; three; and up; and forward; one; two;

∪ ‾‾‾ ∪ ‾‾‾ ∪ ‾‾‾ ∪
three; and up; and forward; stave ready;

‾‾‾ ∪ ‾‾‾ ∪
atten-tion; stand at ease.

‾‾‾ ‾‾‾ ‾‾ ‾‾‾ ∪ ∪ ∪ ‾‾ ∪
6. *Deep breathing by numbers; in; out; in; and out.*

‾‾‾ ‾‾ ‾ ‾‾ ‾ ∪ ∪ ∪
7. *Marching back to class, left turn; one; two;*

‾‾ ∪ ‾‾‾ ∪ ‾ ∪
quick march; squad halt; fall out (right turn).

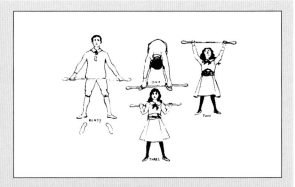

Fig. 25.5 Exercise with staves.

If you insist on this being done accurately and seriously, you will soon realise the difficulties of synchronised movement and you will be able to judge the degree of exercise you are achieving. You should also question the level of activity, skill and individuality.

25.3 Early syllabuses of physical training

The Model Course came under constant attack from inspectors and teachers and in 1904, the Board of Education set up two **interdepartmental committees**.

One committee examined the Model Course and criticised it on the grounds that there was no apparent intent to equate physical exercise with general education, it had a specific military function, it failed to recognise the need to cater for different ages and sexes and it caused a reduction of subject status through the use of military personnel rather than qualified teachers. The formal recommendation was that a new syllabus be produced which recognised different ages and sexes.

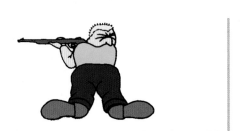

Fig. 25.6 Drill or physical education? A healthy mind in a healthy body means keeping your eyes on the target!

The second committee looked specifically at the 'physical deterioration among the working classes' and recommended that the male adolescent population should undergo training that would 'befit them to bear arms'.

By separating elementary school physical training from military training, the battle had been won to reinstate Swedish 'therapeutic' exercises.

The 1904 syllabus[2]

This was the first Board of Education syllabus and it set out to satisfy the recommendations of the relevant interdepartmental committee.

How the syllabus covered these intentions
At a **conceptual** level, it identified the **physical effect** – that is, the intention to improve health and physique, and the **educational effect** – that is, to develop qualities of alertness, decision making and the control of the mind over the body. This was 1904, but a modern PE lesson quite probably has similar intentions.

Now **how** did the committees expect to put these into practice? Their view of our subject started from a medical (physiological) base. They wanted to present a system of physical exercises which would improve respiration and circulation and stimulate nutrition. They envisaged things like play activities: the development of vital capacity through breathing exercises, corrective exercises to improve posture, exercises against resistance and control exercises involving skill learning. Once again, you might be surprised at the knowledge and 'vision'.

The problem lay in putting these theories into practice. They produced 109 tables, each consisting of a series of activities designed to systematically exercise the whole body. The structure of each **table** consisted of such exercises as: arms, balance, shoulders, head and trunk, marching, jumping and deep breathing.

A study of the syllabus shows that not all the military features were removed; for example, the students were still taught in lines with marching, commands were still formal and 'attention' was still 'pigeon chested'.

The authorities suggested that the class teacher should give two or three 20-minute lessons a week, but that there should also be daily 'recreative sessions to refresh the child for further study'.

Some of the **content** of the 1904 syllabus is shown in Figure 25.7 and you should be able to compare this with the exercises in the defunct Model Course.

What may not have become apparent is that in recognising age variations, the syllabus separated **infants** into a different category and, for children less than seven years old, play became an accepted part of the lesson. There was also considerable stress on the **open air** and the importance of having suitable clothing.

PLAY RUNNING OR MARCHING

Play or Running about.

The children should, for a minute or two, be allowed to move about as they please.

II PRELIMINARY POSITIONS AND MOVEMENTS

Attention.
Standing at Ease.
Hips Firm.
Feet Close.
Neck Rest.
Feet Astride.
Foot Outward Place.
Foot Forward Place.
Stepping Sideways.
Heels Raising.
Right Turn and Right Half Turn.
Left Turn and Left Half Turn.

III ARM FLEXIONS AND EXTENSIONS

Arms Downward Stretching.
Arms Forward Stretching.
Arms Sideways Stretching.
Arms Upward Stretching.

IV BALANCE EXERCISES

Heels Raising.
Knees Bending and Stretching.
Preparation for Jumping.
Heels Raising (Neck Rest).
Heels Raising (Astride, Hips Firm).
Heels Raising (Astride, Neck Rest).
Head Turning in Knees Bend Position.
Knees Bending and Stretching (Astride).
Leg Sideways Raising with Arms Sideways Raising.
Knee Raising.

V SHOULDER EXERCISES AND LUNGES

Arms Forward Raising.
Arms Sideways Raising.
Hands Turning.
Arms Flinging.
Arms Forward and Upward Raising.
Arms Sideways and Upward Raising.

VI TRUNK FORWARD AND BACKWARD BENDING

Head Backward Bending.
Trunk Forward Bending.
Trunk Backward Bending.
Trunk Forward Bending (Astride).
Trunk Backward Bending (Astride).

Note Exercises bracketed should be taken in succession

VII TRUNK TURNING AND SIDEWAYS BENDING

Head Turning.
Trunk Turning.
Trunk Turning (Astride, Neck Rest).
Trunk Turning (Feet Close, Neck Rest).
Trunk Sideways Bending.
Trunk Sideways Bending (Feet Close, Hips Firm).
Trunk Sideways Bending (Feet Close, Neck Rest).

VIII MARCHING

Marking Time (From the Halt).
Turnings while Marking Time.
Quick March.
Marking Time (From the March).
Changing Direction.

IX JUMPING

Preparation for Jumping.

Note Work from this Column should be omitted until the above exercise has been taught under IV.

X BREATHING EXERCISES

Breathing Exercises without Arm Movements.
With Deep Breathing, Arms Sideways Raising.

Fig. 25.7 1904 syllabus, HMSO.

Investigation 25.2 The 1904 syllabus

1. Explain the meaning and intentions underlying the following recommendations:
   a. 'exercises from many well-known systems'
   b. 'suitable for children of school age'
   c. 'without need of apparatus'
   d. 'no exercises likely to prove injurious'
   e. 'to be purposeful'
   f. 'as a minimum of exercises'.

2. You may like to repeat the role-play exercise of Investigation 25.1, emphasising the changes. Remember, you are now looking at teachers with children, rather than NCOs with little soldiers; there should be a more varied lesson, but still taught through action–response commands.

Major political and administrative changes occurred over the next few years. In 1906 the Education Act was particularly concerned with the welfare of working-class children and the Open Spaces Act improved urban leisure provision with the development of more public parks. The following year, under the radical Liberal government of Lloyd George, physical training was directly linked with the Medical Department of the Board of Education, with the appointment of Dr George Newman. An immediate administrative development was the appointment of Miss Rendal and Lt Commander Grenfell as staff inspectors, both with backgrounds in Swedish drill. Meanwhile, Colonel Malcolm Fox was sent to Sweden to learn more about their approach. These events led to a revised and expanded syllabus being published in 1909.

The 1909 syllabus[3]

In 1909 two new emphases arose. The first was an increase in therapeutic elements, probably directly due to Dr George Newman:

The purpose of physical training is not to produce gymnasts, but to promote and encourage the health and development of the body.

The second reflected a change in social attitude:

The value of organised games as an adjunct to physical training is very great, though they should not take the place of the regular lessons of physical exercise.

Three of the male associations linked with gymnastics objected to the first purpose and the Ling Association, largely representing female teachers, objected to the second, reflecting the gulf between men and women in the PE profession.

In terms of **content** the 1909 syllabus had 71 tables instead of 109, suggesting that there was a tightening up of alternatives. The work remained 'free standing' with unison response to commands, but Danish rhythmic swinging exercises were also included.

The 1919 syllabus[4]

This followed the First World War (1914–1918). It is important to recognise the tragedy of this war with so much loss of life, particularly as it virtually wiped out a generation of public school boys. Less well known was the huge number of additional deaths which occurred in a flu epidemic immediately after the war.

If there was a positive outcome, it was the improved status of women as a result of their contribution in schools and factories during the war. Blame for the low level of fitness among the working classes was once again levelled at school physical training, but Dr George Newman cleverly deflected this, claiming that remedial exercises and morale-boosting recreational activities in convalescent camps had helped to prepare the wounded for a full return to civilian life.

It was Newman's recognition of the 'recreational' which represented the most significant innovation in the 1919 syllabus.

The formal nature of the lesson has been reduced to a minimum and every effort has been made to render them enjoyable and recreative.

It was suggested that half of every lesson should be devoted to 'active free movements, including games and dancing' and the tables were remodelled to:

place increased responsibility upon the class teacher and to allow scope for personal initiative, freedom and enterprise.

However, particularly in the case of lessons for older children, the tables allowed the old-fashioned teacher to continue to use the old restrictive exercises. The theory that there was a need to:

consider happiness and enjoyment while accustoming the body and mind to external suggestions and stimuli was made possible for infant children by a complete restructuring of lessons for the under-7 year olds. The more serious intention of therapeutic exercise remained central for the older children. The whole class was still expected to work in unison in response to direct commands.

If we look outside the classroom at society, this obedience training and therapeutic focus reflected the rigid social class demarcation before the Second World War, where those in power were anxious to retain a clean, disciplined working class, who worked hard and accepted their 'place' in society.

The 1933 syllabus[5]

We have now reached a period in history which is within living memory of relatives and friends and so your first task should be to find out from them what life was like in the inter-war years and what they did in PE. They may remember the giddy years of the 1920s when the upper-class 'flappers' had their last fling; they might recall the business influence of the urban middle class, which was literally taking over our society; or they might remember the harsh reality of post-war Britain, where soldiers and sailors were demobilised, many of them with injuries, without any planning, little financial support or prospect of work. Never was the social class system more clearly defined, but the compulsory school-leaving age had risen to 14 and many secondary schools were being built for working-class children. All these new 'senior' and 'central' schools had playing fields and a gymnasium.

The industrial depression in the 1930s left the working class without jobs, but the crash of the stock exchange and the stagnation of industry also affected the middle classes. It was in the middle of this depression that the last Board of Education syllabus was produced, but it was a highly respected publication and 'has been recognised as the watershed between the best of the past and revolutionary developments yet to come'.

The concept of therapeutic exercise to produce a sound physique remained, but the recognition of gymnastic and games skills was a major step forward, reflecting both the Reference Books published in 1927 for secondary schools. Children were still taught by direct method, but elements of play were carried through into the lessons for older children.

Probably the most revolutionary change was the introduction of group work. All the other syllabuses had been class activities with everyone doing the same thing at the same time. The 1933 syllabus included a final phase in each lesson in which the class was divided into four or more sets or corners, where different activities were set for each group. This was the first vital step towards the decentralised lesson.

Figure 25.8 shows a table from the 1933 syllabus. The teacher would select items from each of the six sections, but Part I and Part II would be of about equal length. Where other pages are listed, the syllabus gave additional information on these pages. Look out for a copy of this syllabus in second-hand bookshops – there are still plenty around.

25.4 The effects of the Second World War (1939–1945)

The majority of male PE teachers were enlisted and many were engaged in training military personnel. This was an entirely different war from the previous one, in that there was a mobile rather than a static battle ground, civilians were much more at risk through bombing and training strategies were concerned with individual initiative and survival rather than the stoic obedience training of old. Large numbers of soldiers were taken prisoner and it was realised that recreative activity helped to maintain morale in the prisoner-of-war camps.

Finally, the threat of air raids led to the mass evacuation of children from industrial towns to the countryside, giving them a taste of rural life. The bombing itself, with the inevitable tragic loss of life, at least levelled many of the 19th-century slums and resulted in a massive rebuilding programme.

The 1944 Education Act was a progressive piece of legislation, which ensured every child a free education. The tripartite system of grammar, technical and modern schools tended to reflect the class system, but it was soon to be overtaken by a move towards comprehensive education.

These post-war years marked the emergence of a full expression of physical education. The theory behind the inter-war syllabuses had educative intentions, but

PART ONE

1

Introductory Activity

1. Free running, at signal, children run to 'homes' in teams. (Four or more marked homes in corners of playground.) All race round, passing outside all the homes, back to places and skip in team rings.
2. Free running, at signal all jump as high as possible and continue running. Brisk walking, finishing in open files, marking time with high knee raising.
3. Aeroplanes. (Following the leaders in teams.)

Rhythmic Jump

1. Skip jump on the spot, three low, three high (continuously) *(Low, 2, 3, high, 2, 3, etc.)*
2. Astride jump. Astride jumping—begin! 1, 2, 1, 2, etc. stop!
3. Skip jump, four on the spot, four turning round about (8 counts) and repeat turning the opposite way (8 counts)

2

a. (Astride [Long sitting].) Trunk bending downward to grasp ankles. Unroll. *(With a jump, feet astride—place [with straight legs—sit!]) Grasp the ankles—down! With unrolling, trunk upward—stretch! With a jump, feet together—place!*
b. (Astride [Astride long sitting].) Trunk bending downward to touch one foot with opposite hand.
c. (Feet close [Cross-legged sitting].) Head dropping forward and stretching upward. *(Feet—close!) Head forward—drop! Head upward—stretch! (Crouch.)* Knee stretching and bending. ('Angry Cats') *(Crouch position—down!) Knees— stretch! bend! up! down! etc. stand—up!*

3

a. As small as possible, as tall as possible. [(Crook sitting, Back to wall) Single arm swinging forward–upward to touch wall.] [(Crook sitting) Drumming with the feet, loud and soft.]
b. Single arm circling at a wall. (Run and stand with side to wall, nearest hand supported against wall about shoulder height. Circling with free arm. Turn about and repeat.)

4

a. Free running like a wooden man. Finish in open files in chain grasp. (One foot forward, heel level with the other toe.) Knee full bending and stretching with knees forward. (Several times. Move the back foot forward and repeat.) (Lean standing.) Hug the knee. [(Crook lying.) Hug the knees. (Lower the feet quietly.)]
b. Running in twos, change to skipping, finish in a double ring facing partner holding hands. Knees full bend. Knee springing. Hands on ground and jump up. Knees full bend ! *Knee springing—begin! 1, 2, 1, 2, etc. Stop!* Placing the hands on the ground, with a jump stand—up!
c. Form a ring. Gallop step left and right, at signal, run and stand with side to wall, nearest hand supported against wall (the other arm sideways). Kick the hand. (Turn about, or run to opposite wall and repeat several times with each leg.)

5

a. Brisk walking anywhere, change to walking on heels or toes, at signal run to open files facing partners. (Feet-close, Arms forward, Fists touching.) Trunk turning with single elbow bending. (Elbow raised and pulled back. 'Drawing the bow.') *(Feet—close! With fists touching, arms forward—raise!) With the right arm, draw the bow—pull! Let go! With the left arm—pull! Let go! etc. Arms—lower!*
b. Race to a wall and back to centre line and join right hand across with partner. Tug of war with one hand.
c. (Informal lunge with hand support.) Head and trunk turning with arm raising to point upward. *[Left (right) foot forward with knee bent and left (right) hand on knee (informal lunge)—ready!] With arm raising to point upward, head and trunk to the right, (left)—turn! With arm lowering, forward—turn! (Repeat several times.) With a jump, feet change!*

PART TWO

6

Class Activity

1. Running, jumping over a series of low ropes. (In ranks of six or eight in stream.)
2. Frog jump anywhere.
3. Free running or skipping, tossing up a ball and catching it. (A ball each. Who can make the greatest number of catches without missing?)

Group Practices

1. Running or galloping with a skipping rope. (A rope each.)
2. Running Circle Catch, with a player in the centre throwing, or bouncing and catching a ball.
3. Sideways jumping over a low rope, partner helping. (Partner astride rope, performer holding partner's hands does several preparatory skip jumps on the spot and then a high jump over the rope landing with knees bent and standing up again.)
4. In twos, crawling or crouch jump through a hoop, held by partner.

Game

Odd Man.
Free Touch with 6 or 7 'He's'. ('He's' carry a coloured braid or bean bag as distinguishing mark.)
Tom Tiddler.

7

Free walking, practising good position, lead into school.

Fig. 25.8 A table from the 1933 syllabus.

the 'practical' was predominantly physical training. There were probably four major areas of influence from within the subject.

1. F.J.C. Marshall and E. Major lectured at Carnegie College, Leeds, before the war, publishing several books. Though they continued to accept the 'tables' approach, they were part of a move to increase the importance of skill learning and the use of small apparatus. They were in the services during the war, but wrote a number of progressive articles for the *Journal of PE* suggesting changes towards contests, self-testing and initiative programmes. Perhaps the most important transitional phrase used was the suggestion that 'the child was more important than the system'.

2. Leading female physical educationists were also going into print. An article by Veronica Tyndale-Biscoe (1945) described the modern dance extension of Rudolf Laban's work, using phrases like 'the body as a medium of expression'. Similarly, Ruth Clark (1946) wrote about Austrian gymnastics, referring to movement in an educational medium and suggesting that 'working on apparatus at his own pace has particular value to the timid child, who gains courage through the discovery for himself of his own capabilities'.

3. **New apparatus**: C.E. Cooke, an organiser in Bristol, visited the Northern Command Physical Training School and saw commandos using scrambling nets and assault course equipment. She felt that young children would 'enjoy the skill and adventure provided by this apparatus' and published her adaptations. With the flush of post-war building, many local authorities introduced their own versions of frame and tubular apparatus in their primary schools and even old schools were given 'apparatus stations' (Figure 25.9).

4. **The Halifax Experiment**: Miss Dudgeon was working in a children's rehabilitation clinic during the war. The cornerstone of physical training had always been that all children should respond to a set

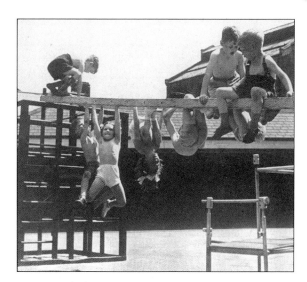

Fig. 25.9 Climbing apparatus in school.

task. At Halifax the individual disabilities of handicapped children led Miss Dudgeon to encourage individual interpretation of open tasks, where children were left to decide rhythm and timing and work at their own level. After the war, this novel approach attracted most of the progressive physical educationists in the country; they noticed that the levels of child involvement, enjoyment and personal skill achievement were unequalled elsewhere in the country.

The outcome of these progressive developments was the publication of *Moving and Growing*[6] and *Planning the Programme*.[7] These 'revolutionary' books replaced the formal training syllabuses by introducing a child-centred approach to primary physical education. Both these publications are still to be found in book shops. A small sample of the activities is shown in Figure 25.10 and it would be an excellent role-play experience to use these or others from *Planning the Programme* to show how free and individualised physical education had become, compared with the initial Model Course.

25.5 Summary of cultural influences in the 20th century

By the turn of the century, the population in the industrial towns had stabilised, with the working-class population continuing to be housed in back-to-back properties, but with skilled workers in particular benefiting from their union strength and the policy of

building council houses. Some of the worst inner-city slums were being cleared for commercial development in the town centres and the number of city parks increased as a result of the Open Spaces Act in 1906. Much of this progress should be put down to the

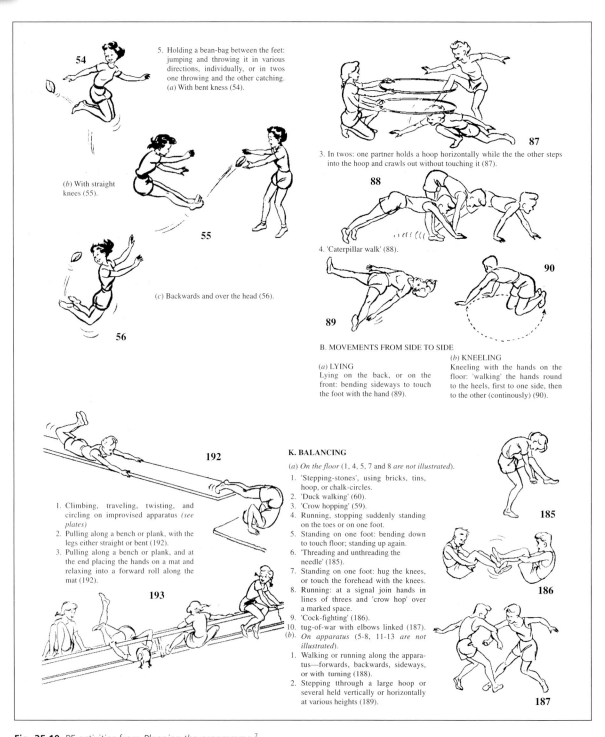

5. Holding a bean-bag between the feet: jumping and throwing it in various directions, individually, or in twos one throwing and the other catching. (*a*) With bent kness (54).

(*b*) With straight knees (55).

(*c*) Backwards and over the head (56).

3. In twos: one partner holds a hoop horizontally while the the other steps into the hoop and crawls out without touching it (87).

4. 'Caterpillar walk' (88).

B. MOVEMENTS FROM SIDE TO SIDE

(*a*) LYING
Lying on the back, or on the front: bending sideways to touch the foot with the hand (89).

(*b*) KNEELING
Kneeling with the hands on the floor: 'walking' the hands round to the heels, first to one side, then to the other (continously) (90).

1. Climbing, traveling, twisting, and circling on improvised apparatus (*see plates*)
2. Pulling along a bench or plank, with the legs either straight or bent (192).
3. Pulling along a bench or plank, and at the end placing the hands on a mat and relaxing into a forward roll along the mat (192).

K. BALANCING

(*a*) *On the floor* (1, 4, 5, 7 and 8 *are not illustrated*).
1. 'Stepping-stones', using bricks, tins, hoop, or chalk-circles.
2. 'Duck walking' (60).
3. 'Crow hopping' (59).
4. Running, stopping suddenly standing on the toes or on one foot.
5. Standing on one foot: bending down to touch floor; standing up again.
6. 'Threading and unthreading the needle' (185).
7. Standing on one foot: hug the knees, or touch the forehead with the knees.
8. Running: at a signal join hands in lines of threes and 'crow hop' over a marked space.
9. 'Cock-fighting' (186).
10. tug-of-war with elbows linked (187).
(*b*). *On apparatus* (5-8, 11-13 *are not illustrated*).
1. Walking or running along the apparatus—forwards, backwards, sideways, or with turning (188).
2. Stepping tthrough a large hoop or several held vertically or horizontally at various heights (189).

Fig. 25.10 PE activities from *Planning the programme*.[7]

Liberal governments of Lloyd George from 1906 to 1914 that marked the foundation of our welfare state and included the National Insurance Act.

The 1914–1918 war interrupted this progress but after the war there was a short period of revival. However, the expansion of the 'conveyor belt industry' led to overproduction and a decade of industrial slump and financial chaos between 1929 and 1939. It was during this period that fascism spread in Europe and the seeds were set for the Second World War.

The centre of this mass production was the car and this led to a reduction in the dominance of the railways and the introduction of 'independent' holidays for the middle classes, reflected in the growth of rambling, camping and cycling and the development of the Youth Hostel Association.

It was in this atmosphere of increased freedom, but economic instability, that women won the right to vote, to wear less inhibiting fashions and to achieve an increased opportunity to participate in sport. However, it took a second world war, the destruction of our cities from bombing and the fear of the atom bomb to prevent a third world war, leaving a divided Europe to establish greater economic stability based on two different political principles.

It is important to recognise that a synoptic dimension exists between what happened in the schools and the cultural influences in society, but also at a comparative level when these developments are compared with what happens in primary school PE today. Alternatively, these developments in primary physical education can be compared with the public school developments as they concerned different sectors of the community in the 19th and 20th centuries. In all this synoptic analysis it is important to recognise that values, objectives, content and teaching methods changed as society changed.

Review questions

1. Use Figure 25.11 to explain the major changes that occurred in junior schools between 1902 and 1954.

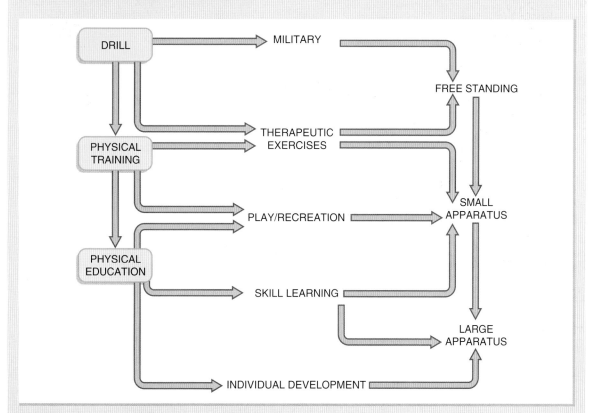

Fig. 25.11 Changes in PE in schools between 1902 and 1954.

▶ **2.** Compare the physical education envisaged for primary children in *Moving and Growing* with what is done in a secondary school today.

3. Use Figures 25.12 and 25.13 to explain the differences between drill and physical education.

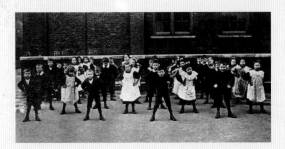

Fig. 25.12 Drill and PT from *Moving and growing*.[6]

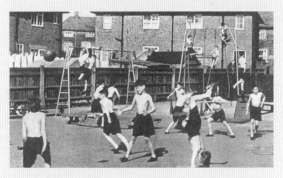

Fig. 25.13 Physical education from *Moving and growing*.[6]

Exam-style questions

Between 1902 and 1954 elementary school military drill changed to primary school physical education.

1. Describe the 1902 Model Course and explain why it was implemented. (*5 marks*)

2. Explain the transition to physical training and the form it took between 1904 and 1933. (*5 marks*)

3. How did the teacher and the teaching method change during this time? (*5 marks*)

4. Discuss the effects of the 1939–1945 war on physical education in the primary schools of Britain and the emergence of a broad physical education curriculum. (*10 marks*)

References

1. Board of Education 1902 *Model course.* HMSO, London
2. Board of Education 1904 *Syllabus.* HMSO, London
3. Board of Education 1909 *Syllabus.* HMSO, London
4. Board of Education 1919 *Syllabus.* HMSO, London
5. Board of Education 1933 *Syllabus.* HMSO, London
6. Ministry of Education 1952 *Moving and growing.* HMSO, London
7. Ministry of Education 1953 *Planning the programme.* HMSO, London

Further reading

McIntosh P C 1952 *Physical education in England since 1800.* Bell, London
Munden I 1947 *Suggestions for small apparatus in PE.* Ling, London
Roscoe D A, Roscoe J V, Honeybourne J, Davis R, Galligan F 2003 *Physical education and sport studies AS/A2 level student revision guide.* 3rd edn. Jan Roscoe Publications, Widnes
Smith W D 1974 *Stretching their bodies.* David and Charles, Newton Abbot

Glossary of terms

Chapters 22–25

agrarian revolution massive movement of people from rural to urban areas, largely as a result of the mechanisation of landwork and enclosure from the middle of the 18th century.

amateur initially gentleman amateur, identifying an elite land-owning group of men who played sport for the love of it. By the 1870s the 'gentleman' prefix was removed when middle-class and respectable working-class men were allowed to play a variety of organised sports as long as there was no financial gain involved. However, by the mid-20th century, the increased scope of amateur sport resulted in many participants needing expenses to cover travel and loss of earnings.

Arnold, Dr Thomas the liberal headmaster of Rugby School, 1814–1828, who is believed to have had a great influence on the development of athleticism in public schools.

athleticism the transition of popular recreations and pastimes to rationalised sport in public schools where they were invested with character-building qualities.

blood sports ancient sports where animals were killed as part of a sporting ritual. The most vicious, cock throwing and bull running, were the first to be banned but badger, bear and bull baiting, though banned in the middle of the 19th century, continued illegally for many years. Cock fighting, loved by peasantry and gentry alike, survived for most of the 19th century, often as part of race meetings.

Clarendon Report published in 1864, this reported on the standards in the nine most famous public schools in England: Eton, Charterhouse, Harrow, Rugby, Shrewsbury, Westminster, Winchester, Merchant Taylors and St Paul's. The statements on sport in these schools are the most valuable evidence available.

cottage industry before the Industrial Revolution and the introduction of factories, industry was controlled by families, often working from their own house. The whole family was often involved, but the hours of work were more loosely organised to meet the sale of products. As a result, there was the possibility of free time.

early closing movement shop assistants wanted a half-day off each week, but Saturdays and market days were very busy. If any shop selling a particular type of goods stayed open, others in the same trade did not dare close. Chemists' and drapers' shops were the first to organise this, but greengrocers with perishable goods would not cooperate. Sports teams grew up from groups of shop assistants, the best example being Sheffield Wednesday FC.

factory system this led to strictly regulated working hours, where the machines dictated free time. Starting with a 72-hour week, it was only when the machine operatives (fitters) won the 57-hour week that other workers had a chance of reducing their working hours.

fairs annual commercial fairs have an ancient history, with statutes which prevented them from being stopped. They were often linked with religious festivals, extending the merry making. Statute fairs or mops were linked with the employment of labour, male and female, as on that day occupations were settled for a year.

festivals normally an annual occasion in a community, where the whole area had a holiday and participated in a wide range of feasting, physical activities and fireworks.

field sports hunting coursing, angling and shooting belong to this group with killing selected wildlife as part of the presumed human right to kill for sport. They also involve such skills as marksmanship, horsemanship and bravery in the field.

girls public schools, though evident at an early date as academies (finishing schools) for young ladies, Victorian attitudes among the middle classes delayed private education for girls and particularly forms of athleticism in them. When the breakthrough was made, mainly in the 1880s, selected games like lawn tennis and hockey became widespread in the middle class high schools for girls.

holy days until the Industrial Revolution and factory production, there were as many as 44 holy days, which meant public holidays to allow worship and festivity (sacred and profane). Industrial employment and the rise of capitalism led to public holidays being reduced to three, Christmas, Easter and Whitsun, until the addition of August Bank Holiday late in the 19th century.

Hughes, Judge Thomas Old Boy of Rugby School who knew Thomas Arnold and wrote a best seller, *Tom Brown's school days* (1857) and later *Tom Brown at Oxford*. Though semi-fiction, it did as much to popularise Arnold and public school athleticism as the actual reforms.

Industrial Revolution claimed to cover the century 1750–1850, this marked the change of Britain from a feudal, rural society into an industrialised, capitalist country, dominated by coal, iron and steel and controlled by a powerful urban middle class.

lawn tennis supposedly the only game invented by the middle class. It gave them an alternative to the gentry game of real tennis; it reflected their status, requiring a large garden lawn; it was private and allowed young women to play sport; and in Wimbledon it had its festival occasion.

manliness originally based on masculine attributes of physical endeavour and prowess arising from militarism and developed as part of character building in boys' public schools, its function eventually overtook its original meaning as girls became part of this character-building experience, displacing masculinity with a commitment to living a noble, sporting life.

Merrie England no clear origin because it is wrapped up in myth, but centred on the Tudor period, 16th century, from Henry VIII to Elizabeth I. It marked the emergence of the 'Court' as a dynamic social element; the nation as an international power; the emergence of a high culture, illustrated by Shakespeare; and a rural peasantry who regularly celebrated religious and commercial festivals.

military drill exercise movements to increase military preparedness, which was associated with the physical training of young children. This was at the heart of all the European systems of gymnastics, but was particularly dominant in the 1902 Model Course, when the British War Department stipulated that all elementary children should receive drill from military instructors.

mob games occasional, violent festival games played in certain localities. They varied in each community, e.g. in Derby, it was football; in Lutterworth it was hockey; and in Haxey, it was the Haxey Hood. Attempts were made to curtail them but some in more remote areas have survived to the present day, e.g. the Ashbourne Game.

Model Course introduced in 1902 to compensate for an embarrassing Boer War in which the lack of fitness in the British Army was blamed for difficulties in defeating a small number of mobile Boer fighters. It was imposed on all elementary school children, treating them as little soldiers and controlled by regular soldiers.

moral integrity the second basic element of the public school athleticism ethic. It suggested that organised sport in school should lead to a sound sense of morality which would be retained as a lasting lifestyle quality.

muscular Christianity preceded by the Oxford Movement of Tractarians, the emphasis on athleticism in public school and at Oxbridge produced a cult where Christianity and athleticism were seen to be the finest interpretation of what the British Empire stood for. This movement owed much of its strength to such writers as Charles Kingsley, Thomas Hughes and Rudyard Kipling.

pedestrianism initially limited to a group of professional walkers who set themselves such impossible challenges as walking 1000 miles in 1000 hours for 1000 guineas. There was a great deal of wagering involved and huge crowds were attracted to these challenges.

physical endeavour this was the first element within the concept of public school athleticism, where physicality was part of the Spartan ethic and endeavour represented the significance of effort in terms of personal achievement.

physical training this followed on from military drill as teachers and the medical profession emphasised the need for young elementary children to experience a balanced set of therapeutic exercises. Largely drawn from the Swedish gymnastic system, they were free-standing exercises requiring minimal apparatus and designed to encourage the health and development of the body.

popular of the people; it does not so much mean popularity as popular with the lower classes.

popular recreation a basic term used to describe sports and pastimes which existed prior to the Industrial Revolution and had such characteristics as occasional, rural, local, violent, limited rules, festival and wagering.

prize ring the most popular combat in popular recreation, it started as a 'school' of fighters known as 'Masters of Defence' required to defend themselves against others using a wide range of weapons. Broughton later introduced rules which limited the prize ring to pugilism and out of this was born modern boxing.

professional the term initially referred to games players who earned their living from playing. They were largely cricketers in the first place, but the term spread to football and court games as the lower classes found employment performing for a crowd and teaching the game to children and amateur performers.

proprietary schools middle-class schools opened as business ventures, modelled on

the successful gentry public schools. Most of them were built in spa towns, designed to demonstrate a commitment to the games ethic, e.g. Cheltenham, Clifton and Malvern Colleges.

public schools independent schools, often of ancient origin, controlled by trustees rather than owned privately, e.g. Eton College, Charterhouse, etc.

rational recreation post-industrial development of sport, where respectability, regularity, stringent administration and codification were key characteristics. Though largely the product of public school athleticism, it was recognised as a social control vehicle when the lower classes were involved in the latter part of the 19th century.

real tennis taken from French high culture, this game became the elite game of the ruling class in England from the time of Henry VIII and was the fore-runner of rational recreation.

regularity a key feature of rational recreation, it was the possibility of regular play in gentry public schools which allowed prowess and rules to be developed and with them the birth of modern sport.

respectability a by-product of rational recreation in that it was the wealthy who had the opportunity to engage in sports regularly and through this, modern sport was invested with a set of respectable values epitomised by the code of amateurism.

ritual the religious connotations within the earliest sports and pastimes. Many sports date back to pagan times and as such were part of the worship ceremony. Christianity initially used this ritual component to expand the Church, but with the emergence of Puritanism, the attempt was made to separate the sacred from the profane.

sabbatharianism a highly influential Protestant movement that demanded that in keeping Sunday as a sacred day, it was essential that all sporting activities should be excluded from it because they distracted the population from prayer.

Saturday half-day the 72-hour week meant working all day Saturday, but in the 1870s skilled workers, mainly fitters, obtained a half-day on Saturday as a result of union action. Other workers had to wait several decades, depending on the strength of their unions. It allowed the typical British sporting Saturday afternoon to develop. Parallel to this development, the 12-hour day was gradually reduced to nine hours.

singlesticks called broadswords, but often with a smaller stick. Arising out of militaristic swordplay and duelling, this was the lower-class version of fencing, where combats were held during rural festivals. Many public schools also taught singlesticks as part of the gymnastic programme.

social control sometimes became a vehicle in public school sport. It involved the use of

sport to establish a code of behaviour and was intended to make use of social interaction at peer group, team and authority levels. The impact of this association of sport and education was such that many values were carried on into life and was reflected in the subsequent loyalty of old students.

spa movement part of the Regency fashion, where c.1800 the upper classes established elite watering places like Bath, Leamington and Cheltenham, where they 'took the water cure'. The fashion included hot and cold baths and was one of the sources of modern indoor bathing. The fashion later spread to seaside spas like Brighton.

steeplechasing originally an evening pastime for the gentry after a day's hunting, racing across open country guided by village steeples. It became professionalised and public schools developed footraces on the school fields as an athletics version.

stringent administration a feature of rational sport, where regular participation and the formation of clubs led to written rules. This was a major middle-class development given their management skills and level of literacy.

Swedish drill one of the European schools of gymnastics which had military, therapeutic, educational and sporting aspects. The Army, universities and public schools built gymnasia and developed all these aspects, but lack of facilities meant that until 1919, elementary schools tended to only use free-standing exercises.

syllabus, Board of Education there were four Board of Education syllabuses developed in the 20th century, in 1904, 1909, 1919 and 1933. They were basically concerned with physical training and centred on the health and development of generally undernourished young children. They consisted of systematic exercises, but progressively included gymnastic and minor games skills and gradually changed from a drill to a child-centred approach.

tournament a major festival occasion based on military prowess and chivalry, it was at its height from the Norman Conquest until its debasement in the 14th century. It reflected the social order of the day with the nobility and peasantry each demonstrating their own lifestyle through the activities they pursued, the knightly pursuits of jousting as compared with archery by the yeomen of England.

urban revolution this was the third social revolution and arose out of the massive expansion of the urban population as a result of industrialisation. From the 1850s the majority of the population lived in large towns and their status was reflected in the back-to-back terraces of the working class and the villas of the middle classes. Town councils, shopping centres, parks and urban sports were essential parts of the development of town life.

wakes these were rituals and festivals associated with the Church. At an individual level they were held at funerals, as is still the case in Ireland, but more generally they marked the veneration day of the parish church. They maintained a mixture of the sacred and profane, as after mass, there were general sporting festivities. Attempts were made to curtail them from Puritan times, because they were associated with excessive drinking, but it was only in the 1870s that rational recreation and garden fetes took their place.

watermen these were men who took an apprenticeship to work on the commercial rivers. Many of them worked on ferryboats and so were expert scullers, others owned small rowing boat firms and hired out gigs for the public and to rowing clubs. The Doggett Coat and Badge was the most famous waterman's race and this was very much a professional working-class event. In the older regattas there were always races for watermen as well as amateur rowers.

world wars the significance of the three 20th-century wars, Boer, World War I and World War II, cannot be over-estimated in terms of their effect on the development of physical education, but also on the development of sport in the UK.

YMCA a Christian organisation established to help young male clerical workers in the expanding towns. Many were away from home and liable to be corrupted. Accepting all Christians, except Roman Catholics, the movement embraced physical activity as a means of establishing moral integrity in an atmosphere of physical endeavour, but also recognised that sporting activities attracted membership. Though there was a wide range of sports clubs, the gymnasium was always the central facility. This was particularly the case in the USA where the strength of the YMCA led to the formation of such leading universities as Springfield, Mass. The YWCA grew as a parallel movement, but physical activities were delayed in line with the attitude to women and sport at the time.

Index

Page numbers in *italics* indicate glossary entries

Abduction, 15, 16, 17, *264*
Ability, 286–291, 386, 387, *431*
  testing, 290–291
Aboriginal Sport and Recreation Programme, 574
Aborigines, Australian, 496, 562, 564, 565
Academies, 482, *543*
Acceleration, 189, 192, 194, 195, 205, *264*
  angular, 247, *264*
  inertia and, 204
Acclimatisation, *264*
  altitude, 161–162
Acetyl coenzyme A (acetyl CoA), 96
Acetylcholine, 32, *264*
Acetylcholinesterase, 32–33
Achievement motivation, 382–385, *431*, 500
Acid—base balance, *264*
  respiratory system and, 74
Actin filaments, 41–42, *267*
Actin—myosin bonds, 42
Action potential, 32, 33, *264*
Action theory, sociology, 492, 493
Acupuncture, 163
Adaptation, 136–140, *264*
  reversal, 140–141
Adaption/maladaption, 357–358
Adaptive programme for special needs, 589, 593, *625*
Adduction, 15, 16, 17, *264*
Adenosine diphosphate (ADP), 95, *264*
Adenosine triphosphate (ATP), 94–99, 101, *264*
  replacement after exercise, 101
Adipose tissue, 114, 174
Adrenaline, 53, *264*
Advanced democracies, sport in, 498–500
Adventure, 465, 530, *543*
Advertising, 528
Aerobic, *264*
Aerobic adaptations, *264*
Aerobic capacity
  children, 170
  effect of altitude, 204
  effect of training, 136, 184
Aerobic energy system, 96–98, 137
  enhancement by training, 136
  weight training, 153

Aerobic power *see* V̇O₂max
Aerobic system, *264*
Aerobic tests, 107–109
Aerobic training/exercise
  children, 170
  effects, 136, 138–139, 184
  on obesity, 175–176
Africa, sport in, 498
Ageing, 181–186
Ageism, 525, *543*
Agencies, *543*
Aggression, 374–378, *431*, 512
  causes, 377
  definitions, 374–375
  elimination/prevention, 377
  hostile (reactive; angry), 374–375, *432*
  instrumental (channelled), 375, *432*, 512
  spectator, 377–378
  theories, 375–377
Aggressive cue hypothesis, 376–377, *431*
Agility, 120, *264*
  testing, 127
Agonist/antagonist muscles/response, 24, 35, 142, *264*
Agrarian revolution, 635–636, *693*
Air resistance, 193, 215, *264*
  flight and, 206
Alactacid oxygen debt component, 102–103, *264*
Alactic anaerobic (ATP-PC) energy system, 95–96, 136–137, *264*
  enhancement by training, 136
  weight training, 152–153
Alactic—lactic threshold, 95–96, 101
Alarm reaction, 423
All-or-none law, 33, 48, *264*
Altitude
  acclimatisation to, 161–162
  effect on aerobic capacity, 204
  effects on weight, 204
  training at, 161–162, 163, *264*
Alveolar ducts, 70, 71, *264*
Alveolar oxygen tension, *264*
Alveolar ventilation, 70, 82, *264*
Alveoli, 70, 71, 72, *264*
Amateur, *693*
Amateurism, *543*, 641
American Dream, 500
Amphetamines, 165
Anabolic androgenic steroids, 165
Anaerobic, *264*
Anaerobic adaptations, *264*

Anaerobic capacity, *264*
  children, 169–170
  effect of training, 136
  measurement, 110–111
Anaerobic energy systems
  alactic (ATP-PC), 95–96, 136–137, 152–153
  lactic acid system, 95, 96, 137, 153
  weight training, 152–153
Anaerobic power, 110, *264*
Anaerobic threshold, 74, *264*
Anaerobic training, effects, 137–138
Anatomical dead space, 82, *264*
Ancient cultures, 495–496
Angina, 178, *264*
Angles, 243, 244–245
Anglo-Saxons, 632
Angular acceleration, 247, 252, *264*
Angular displacement, 243–244, *264*
Angular momentum, 250–251, *264*
Angular velocity, 245, *264*
Anticipation, 313–314
Anticlockwise moment, 229, *265*
Anxiety, 419–424, *431*
  management, 424–426
    cognitive, 425–426, *431*
    somatic, 424–425, *434*
  measurement, 424
  multidimensional theory, 421, *433*
Aorta, 49, 61, *265*
Aponeurosis, 23, *265*
Archery, 645–646
Arnold, Dr Thomas, 656–658, *693*
Arousal, 417–419, 421, 424, *431*
Arteries, 60, 61, *265*
  narrowing/blockage, 178–179
Arterioles, 61, *265*
Arteriovenous oxygen difference (a-v̄O₂ diff), 61, 78, 81, 138, *265*
  children, 170
Articular surface, 3, *265*
Aspiration, groups, 512–513
Assertiveness, 374, 375, *431*
Assimilation, *543*
Association football, 672
Association theories of learning, 330–333, *431*
Asthma, 70, *265*
Atherosclerosis, 178, *265*
Athleticism in English public schools, 652, 656, 659–660, *693*
  character development and, 661–662
  influence on sport in society, 663–665

Athletics
  rational development, 671
  use of term in USA, 594, *625*
Atlas, 6
Atrioventricular (AV) node, 50, *265*
Atrioventricular valves, 49, 51, *265*
Atrium, 49, *265*
Atrophy, *265*
Attention, 312, 334, 398, *431*
  selective, 304–305, *434*
Attentional focus, 415–417, *431*
Attentional narrowing, 417, *431*
Attentional style, 416, *431*
Attitude(s), 369–373
  changing, 372–373
  components, 369–370
  definition, 369
  development, 370
  measurement, 371–372
  stereotypical, 371
  to sport and participation, 370–371
Attitude objects, 369
Attribution, 367, 385–389, 392, *431*
  errors, 387
  training/retraining, 388–389
Audience
  effects of, 410–412
  see also Crowd behaviour
Audition, 299, 300, *431*
Aussie Able Program, 566, 574, *625*
Aussie Sport, 568–569, *625*
Australia, physical education and sport
  administration of physical education, 566–571
  administration of sport, 571–577
  outdoor recreation and education, 577–581
  social setting, 559–566
Australian Athlete Scholarship Scheme (AASS), 573
Australian Coaching Council (ACC), 573
Australian College of Sports Education (ACSE), 570
Australian Institute of Sport (AIS), 571, 572–574
Australian Sports Commission (ASC), 571–572
Autocratic leadership, 406–407, *431*
Award schemes, 381–382, 479, 480
Axis
  frontal, 17, *268*
  sagittal, 17, *272*
  vertical, 17, *274*
Axis (vertebra), 6
Axis of rotation, 247, 249, *265*
Axons, 31, 32

Badminton, 675
Balance, 121, *265*, 287
  children, 170
  dynamic, *267*
  static, *273*, 290
  testing, 127
Balanced tension, 492, 493, 512
Ball and socket joint, 16, *265*
Ballistic skills, 317
Barometric pressure, *265*
Baroreceptors, 53, 63, *265*

Basal metabolic rate (BMR), 91, 93, 107, 115, 176, *265*
  gender differences, 130
Base of support, 239–240, *265*
Bathing, 671
Behaviourist theories of learning, 330–333
Bernoulli effect, 207, 217, *265*
Beta blockers, 165
Beta-hydroxy-betamethylbutyrate (HMB), 164
Bias, self-serving, 387
Bicarbonate ions, 79, *265*
Bicuspid valves, 49, 51
Biofeedback, 425, *431*
Biological ageing, 181, *265*
Biomechanics
  force, 199–242
  linear motion, 189–198
  rotating systems, 243–256
Bisham Abbey, 485
Blood
  acidity, 74, *265*
  cells, 58–59
  circulation, 59–62
  constituents, 58, *266*
  shunting, 64
  viscosity, 63
Blood doping, 163, 165, *265*
Blood flow, *265*
  effect of aerobic training, 138
  muscles, 63–69
  pulmonary circulatory system, 67
  resistance to, 63
Blood pressure, 64–67, *265*
  children, 170
  diastolic, *266*
  effect of ageing, 183
  effect of exercise, 179
  pulmonary, 77, *271*
  systolic, *273*
Blood sports, 639, *693*
Blood vessels, 60, 61–62
Blood volume, effect of aerobic training, 138
Body awareness, training and, 143
Body composition, 120, 176, *265*
  ageing and, 182
  evaluation, 125–126
  gender differences, 130
Body image, *431*
Body planes, 15, 16
Body types, 120
Böhr effect, 79
Bone(s), 9
  cancellous (spongy), 9, 12, *265*
  compact (hard), 9, 12, *266*
  development, 11–12
  flat, 4, 5, *267*
  irregular, 4, 5, *269*
  long, 4, 5, 10–11, *269*
  measurements, 7
  short, 4, 5, *272*
  structure, 10
  types, 4–5
Bony features, 5, *265*
Bowls, 674
Boycotts, international, 563–564, 586–587, 606

Bracketed morality, 377, *431*
Bradycardia, 138, *265*
Breathing, *265*
  effect of altitude, 162
  quiet, 82, 84–85, *272*
Breathing mechanism, 72–74
  regulators, 74–75
Breathing system, 70–71
  children, 170
Breaths, frequency, 84–85, *268*
Brevets, 551, *625*
British Olympic Committee (BOC), 485
British Sports Foundation (BSF), 485
Bronchi, 70, 71, *265*
Bronchioles, 70, *265*
  respiratory, 70, 71, *272*
Bull baiting, 639
Bull-running in Stamford, 633–634
Bundle of His, 50, *265*
Bursae, 14, *265*

Caffeine, 164
Calorimeter, 92
Camp schools/summer camps
  Soviet Union/Russia, 608, 619–621
  United States, 601
Canoeing, 676
Capillaries, 60, 61, *265*
Capillarisation, *265*
Carbaminohaemoglobin, 79, *265*
Carbohydrates, 114, 115, *266*
Carbo-loading, 115–116, 164, *266*
Carbon dioxide, *266*
  breathing regulation, 74
  tissue respiration, 78–79
Carbonic acid, 79, *266*
Cardiac, *266*
Cardiac arrest, 178, *266*
Cardiac cycle, 51–52, *266*
Cardiac impulse, 48, 50, *266*
Cardiac output (Q̇), 52, *266*
Cardiovascular disease, 178–181, *266*
Cardiovascular endurance, *266*
Cardiovascular system, 47
  children, 170
  effect of ageing, 183
  effect of obesity, 174
Carotid artery, *266*
Cartilage, 8–9, *266*
  hyaline (articular), 3, 8, 14, *268*
    effect of training, 139
  yellow elastic, 8, *275*
Cartilaginous joints, 5, 6, 13, *266*
Catastrophe theory, 421–422, 423–424, *431*
Catharsis, 376, *431*
Central Council of Physical Recreation (CCPR), 485
Central nervous system, 31, *266*, 299
  information processing, 296–297, 299
Centre of mass (gravity), 234–235, *266*
  jumper, 236–238
  stability and, 239–240
Centres de vacances, 556
Cerebellum, 36, *266*
Chaining, 332
Challenge, 510, *543*

Champion Coaching, 479–480
Chance, *543*
Cheltenham Ladies' College, 659
Chemoreceptors, *266*
    respiratory, 74, 75
Children
    overweight, 174
    physical activity and, 168–170
    see also Schools
Chins, 122
Cholesterol, blood, *266*
    effect of exercise, 179
Chunking of information, 307, *431*
Cilia, 70, 71
Circuit training, 153–155, *266*
Circulatory system, 59–62, *266*
    pulmonary, 60, *271*
    systemic, 60, *273*
Circumduction, 15, 16, *266*
Citric acid (Krebs) cycle, 96, 97
Civilisation, *543*
Clarendon Report, *693*
Classes Transplanteés, 556–557, *625*
Climbing, 677
Clockwise, *266*
Clockwise moment, 229
Closed loop theory, 317–318, 320, 321, *431*
Coaches
    role of, 517–518
    see also Leaders
Coactive skills/sports, 284, 410, *431*
Coccyx, 6
Cockfighting, 639
Cognitive dissonance theory, 373, *431*
Cognitive skill, 279, *431*
Cognitive state anxiety, 421, 421–422, 423, *431*
Cognitive theories of learning, 333
Cohesion
    groups/teams, 402–403, *431*, 510–511
    measurement, 402–403
Collagen, 9
Colonialism, 497, 498
Colonie de vacances, 556
Colostrum, 164
Combat, *543*
Combat activities/sports, 439–440, *543*, 633
Command style of teaching, 345, *431*
Commercialism, 457, 500, 506–507
Commitment, 414–415, *431*
Communication(s) and sport, 668
Communism, 500, 606–607
Communist Youth League, 619–620
Comparison in perceptual process, 302, 305
Competence, *431*
Competition, 510, *543*
Complexity, skills, 284–285
Computer analysis, 348
Concentration, 415–417, *431*
Conditioning
    classical, 330–331, *431*
    operant (instrumental), 331–332, *433*
Condyles, 5, 7
Condyloid joint, 16, *266*
Confidence, 390–392, *431*

Conflict, 511–512
Conflict theory, sociology, 492, 493
Connectionist theory *see* Association theories
Connective tissue, 24
    skeletal, 8–12
        see also Bone(s); Cartilage
Conquest activity, 440, *543*
Consistency, skill and, 281
Construct validation theory, 130, *266*
Contest, *543*
Control/controllability, 387, *431*
    emotional, 417–419
Cool-down (active recovery), 103, 104, 145, *273*
Cooper's 12-minute test, 131
Coordination, 121, *266*, 287, 289
    children, 169, 170
    gross body, 288
    groups, 401
    measurement, 290
    testing, 128
Coronary heart disease (CHD), 178–180
    exercise and, 179
Coronary thrombosis, 178, *266*
Corpuscles, 58, *266*
Cottage industry, *693*
Counter culture, United States, 592, 594, 600, *625*
Country parks, 488
Country sports, 636–638
Countryside Commission, 483, 488, 489
Couple, 228–229, 235, *266*
Coupled reaction, 95, *266*
Coursing, 636
Court(ly) games, 645–646, 675–676
Creatine, *266*
Creatine kinase, 95
Creatine supplementation, 116, 164
Crest (ridge), bone, 5, 7
Cricket, development, 640, 674
Cricket Academy, Australia, 572–573
Cross-bridges, 42, *266*
Cross-country running, 671
Crowd behaviour, 500, 504, 505, *543*
Crystal Palace sports centre, 485
Cues, 313, 314, 348
Culture, 494, *543*
    high, 445, 506–508, *543*
    low (mass), 445, 504–505, 508
    sport and, 494–508, 522, 524–525
        discrimination, 538
        outdoor sport, 532
    training approach and, 144
Cyclical loading, *266*
Cycling, 678

Deceleration, 192, *266*
    inertia and, 204
Decision making, 296, 308–314, *431*
Decreasing errors graph, 326, *431*
Defence mechanisms, 357–358
DEFRA, 483, 488
Degree (angle), 244
Delayed onset of muscle soreness (DOMS), 104, *266*
Democratic leadership, 407, *431*
Demonstration, 333, 344, 347

Dendrites, 31
Department of the Environment (DoE), 483, 488
Depolarisation, 32, 52, *266*
Depression, movement, 15, *266*
Depressions, bone, 6–7, *266*
Depth jumping (plyometrics), 27–28, *271*
Derby mob football game, 642
Detection in perceptual process, 302–303, 303
Development, children and adolescents, 168–169, *266*
Deviance, sociology, 492
Diaphragm, 73–74, *266*
Diaphysis, 11, *266*
Diastole, 51, *266*
Diet
    balanced, 113, 114, 175, *265*
    coronary heart disease and, 179
    glycogen-loaded, 115–116
    overeating, 174–175
Dietary supplements, 116, *266*
Dieting, 175
Diffusion, gaseous exchange, 76, 78, *267*
Disability, *543*
Disabled, activity/opportunities for, 525
    Australia, 566, 574
    Soviet Union/Russia, 609
    United Kingdom, 473
    United States, 589, 593
Discovery style of teaching, 345, *431*
Discrimination in sport, 524–525
    Australia, 564–566
    France, 548
    issue analysis, 534–538
    Soviet Union/Russia, 506, 535, 608–609
    United Kingdom, 470, 472–473, 525, 534–535
    United States, 535, 588–589
Displacement, 190, *267*
Display, input data, 298
Dissonance, cognitive, 373
Distance, 190, 196, *267*
Distraction-conflict theory, 411
Diuretics, 165
Doping, definition, 166
Dorsiflexion, 15, 17, *267*
Draft system, professional sport, 577, 598, *625*
Drag, 214, 216–217, *267*
Drill, 681–682
Drinks
    hypertonic, 116, 164
    isotonic, 116, 164
    sports, 116, 164
Drive theory, 335–336, 417–418, *431–432*
Drugs and sport, 527, 529, *543*, 574
Duke of Edinburgh's Award Scheme, 489
Dummy, 312–313

Early closing movement, *693*
Eco-sport, 595, *625*
Economy of effort, 281
Ectomorphs, 120, *272*

Education, *543*
    see also Schools; Public schools
Effector mechanism, information
        processing, 297, 298, 315, *432*
Efficiency of human body, 93, *267*
Effort, 228, 231–232, *267*
Ego/ego orientation, 357, 385, *432*
Egypt, Ancient, 495–496
Electrocardiogram (ECG), 52, *267*
Electromyography (EMG), 425
Electron transport chain, 98, *267*
Elevation, 15, *267*
Elitism, 497, 498, 522, 525, 527, *543*
Emergent countries, 497–498, *543*
Emotional arousal, 391
Emotional control, 417–419
Endocardium, 48, 49, *267*
Endochondral ossification, 11, *267*
Endomorphs, 120, *272*
Endomysium, 38, 39, *267*
Endothermic reactions, *267*
Endurance, 47, 120
    strength, 120, *273*
    testing, 122–123
Endurance training, 138, 139, 148
    fuel use and, 115
Energy, *267*
    chemical, 91–92, 94, *266*
    creation and release within muscle,
        94–100
    input, 114–116, *267*
    kinetic (motion), 189, 196, *269*
    measurement of energy usage, 91–92
        direct method, 91, *267*
        indirect method, 91–92, *268*
    metabolism, 114–116
    output/expenditure, 89–91, 93, *267*
    rotational, 250, *272*
Energy balance, 176
    negative, 175, *270*
    neutral, *270*
    positive, 174, *271*
Energy continuum, 98–99, *267*
Energy systems, 94, 95–100, 101
    aerobic, 96–98, 137
        weight training, 153
    alactic anaerobic (ATP-PC), 95–96,
        136–137, *264*
        enhancement by training, 136
        weight training, 152–153
    endothermic, 94
    enhancement by training, 136–137
    exothermic, 94
    lactic acid anaerobic, 95, 96, 137,
        139, *269*
        enhancement by training, 136
        weight training, 153
    metabolic effects of training, 136–137
    thresholds, 95, 136–137
England
    public schools, 651–666
    see also United Kingdom
English Institute of Sport (EIS), 471,
    483, 485
Enigma, *543*
Environment
    natural *see* Outdoor recreation/
        education
    skills classification, 283–284

EPI/EPQ, 363
Epicondyles, 7
Epiglottis, 70, 71, *267*
Epimysium, 24, 38, 39, *267*
Epiphyseal disc, 11
Epiphyseal plate, 11, *267*
Epiphysis, 11, *267*
Epithelium, respiratory system, 70, 71
Equilibrium, 200, 201, 229, 234–235,
    267, 300
    gross body, 288, 290
    neutral, 239, *270*
    stable, 239, *272*
    unstable, 239, *274*
Ergogenic aids, 163–165, *267*
Erythropoietin, rhesus (rEPO), 163, 165,
    267
Ethnic sport, 494, 500–501, *543*
Eustress, 423, *432*
Evaluation apprehension, 411, *432*
Eversion, 15, *267*
Excellence in sport, 458, *544*
    issue of, 522–530
Excess postexercise oxygen consumption
        (EPOC) *see* Oxygen debt
Executive programme, *432*
Exemplary schools, Australia, *625*
Exercise machines, 150
Exhaled air, 80, *267*
Exhaustion, 423
Exothermic reactions, *267*
Expectation, 389
    groups, 512–513
Expiration, 73–74, 76, *267*
Expiratory capacity (EC), 82, *267*
Expiratory reserve volume (ERV), 82, *267*
Extension, 15, 16, 17, *267*
Extrovert/extroversion, 359, *432*
Exultation, *543*
Eysenck Personality Inventory (or
        Questionnaire) (EPI; EPQ),
    363

Factory system, 669–670, *693*
Failure, attribution, 385–390
Fair play, 456, 457, *543*
Fairs, 637, *693*
    local, 501
Faking, 312–313
Falconry, 637–638
Fancy, The, 635
Far East, sport in, 498
Fartlek training, *267*
Fascia, 24, *267*
Fasciculi, 38, 39
Fat, pad of, 14, *270*
Fat, body, 176
    effect of exercise, 175
    evaluation/measurement, 125–126,
        176
Fatigue
    children, 169
    muscle, 105
    total body, 105
Fatigue index, 111, *267*
Fats, dietary, 114, 115, *267*
Fatty acids, 114, 174, *267*
Faulty processes, 404, *432*

Feedback, 296, 298, 336–339, *432*
    augmented (extrinsic), 320, 336–338
    delayed, *431*
    exteroceptive, 320
    functions, 336–338
    inherent (intrinsic), 300, 330, 336
    kinaesthetic, 317–318, 320, 321
    motor control, 320
    outcome, 317
    proprioceptive, 320
    terminal, 319, 337, *434*
Femur head, 10
Fencing, 645, 646
Festival wakes, 634–635
Festivals, 632–635, 637, *693*
    local, 500–501, 502
Fibre, dietary, 114
Fibrocartilage, white, 8–9, *275*
Fiedler's contingency model, 407–408,
    432
Field sports, 636–638, *693*
Fitness, *267*
    for life, 173–187
    measures, gender differences, 130
    motor, 119, 120–121, *270*
    physical, 119–120, *271*
Fitness testing, 119, 121–129
    maximal/submaximal tests, 129
    reliability, 130
    validity, 130
Fitness trail, 185–186
Flexibility, 120, *267*
    ageing and, 182
    children, 170
    dynamic, 287, 288
    extent, 288
    static, 287
    testing, 124
Flexion, 15, 16, 17, *268*
    plantar, 15, 17, *271*
    spinal lateral, 16
Flight/flight path, 205–208
    centre of mass and, 236–237
Fluency, skill and, 281
Fluid friction, 193, 214–216, *268*
Fluids
    supplementation, 116
    see also Water
Focus
    attentional, 415–417, *431*
    intensity of, 515
Folk games, 641–644
Foot, movement, 4
Footwear, surfaces and, 213–214
Force, 189, 192–195, 199–227, *268*
    components, 202
    friction, 194–195, 200, 201, 212–213,
        268
    internal, 227–242, *269*
    measurement, 202–203
    net (resultant), 200–202
    reaction, 195, 200, 201, 209–212, *272*
    as vector, 200–202
Force field, 203
Fossa, bone, 5
Fox hunting, 636, 638–639
France, physical education and sport
    administration of physical education,
        549–552

France, physical education and sport
administration of physical
education   (cont'd)
administration of sport, 553–555
outdoor recreation and education,
555–557
social setting, 545–548
Frequency of breaths, 84–85, *268*
Friction, fluid, 193, 214–216, *268*
Friction forces, 194–195, 200, 201,
212–213, *268*
Frontal axis, 17, *268*
Frontal plane, 16, *268*
Frontier spirit, United States, *625*
Frustration—aggression theory, 376, *432*
Fulcrum (pivot), 228, 231–232, *268*
Function, sociology, 492, 493
Functional residual capacity (FRC), 82,
268

Game occurrence, 451, *625*
Game simulation, 159
Game(s), 439
courtly, 645–646, 675–676
definition, 440, *543*
invasion, 672–673
target, 673–674
Gaseous exchange, *268*
capillaries, 60, 61, 67, 70
lungs, 76–82
Gender differences
adaptation to overload training, 140
body composition, 130
fitness measures, 130
reaction time, 310
sports opportunities, 473
strength, 130
training needs/responses, 145
General Adaptation Syndrome (GAS),
422–423
Gestalt theory, 333, *432*
Glandular malfunction, *268*
obesity and, 174
Gliding joint, 16, *268*
Glottis, 70, *268*
Gluconeogenesis, 104, *268*
Glucose, 114, *268*
Glutamine, *268*
supplementation, 116, 164
Glycerol, 114, 174
Glycogen, 96, 114, 115, *268*
replacement, 102
Glycogen sparing, 136, 139
Glycogen stores
children, 169
effect of training, 136
muscle, *270*
restoration, 105
Glycolysis, 96, 101, *268*
Goal setting, 338, 414–415, *432*
Goblet cells, 70, 71
Golf, 674
Golgi tendon organs, 35, *268*
Gravitational field strength, 203, *268*
Gravity, 203–204
centre of *see* Centre of mass
Gravity field, 203, 205, *268*
Great Britain *see* United Kingdom

Greece, Ancient, 496
Grip strength test, 121
Group, 399–404
leadership, 405–409
Group dynamics in sport, 508–515
Growth, 168, *268*
GTO award system, Soviet Union/
Russia, 612–615, *625*
Guidance, 346–349, *432*
manual/mechanical, 348, *432*
verbal, 348–349, *434*
visual, 347–348, *434*
Gymnastics, development, 671, 681–682
Gyration, radius of, 250, *272*

Habit, 332, 335
Haemoglobin, *268*
children, 170
effect of aerobic training, 138
effect of altitude, 161–162
oxygenation, 77–78
Haemoglobinic acid, 79, *268*
Haka, 497
Halifax Experiment, 689
Hallaton Bottle Game, 643
Haversian systems, 9, *268*
Haxey Hood Game, 643
Hearing, 299, 300
Heart
action, 50–53
children, 170
effect of aerobic training, 138
effect of obesity, 174
Starling's Law, 52, *273*
structure, 48–50
Heart attack (coronary thrombosis),
178
Heart rate, 51, *268*
effect of ageing, 183
effect of endurance training, 138
HRmax, *268*
measurement, 52, 54–55
regulation, 53
training, 149
Heart sounds, 52, *268*
Heart valves, 49, 51
semilunar, *272*
Hegemony, 525, 538, *543*
Height, 8
Herbal medicines, 163
Hering—Breuer reflex, 74, 75, *268*
Hick's Law, 311
High Performance (Training) Centres
(HPCs), 472, 483, 485–486,
543
Hinge joint, 16, *268*
Historical studies, 627–629
origins of sport, 630
popular recreation in Great Britain,
630–649
HMB, 164
Hockey, 673
Holme Pierrepont, 485
Holy Day festivals, 501
Holy days, *693*
Home advantage/disadvantage, 411, *432*
Homeostasis, 139
Hooligan behaviour, 505

Hors Limites, 557
Horse racing, 638–639
Hughes, Judge Thomas, *693*
Human growth hormone (HGH), 165
Humanist psychology, 361, 365
Hunting, 636, 638–639
Hyaline cartilage, 3, 8, 14, *268*
Hydrogen atoms, oxidation, 98
Hyperextension, 17
Hyperpolarisation, 32, *268*
Hypertension, 178, *268*
Hypertrophy, *268*
Hypnosis, 164

Illinois Agility Run, 127
Imagery, 425–426, *432*
relaxation, 424
Impact, impulse and, 218–224
Impulse, *268*
impact and, 218–224
Industrial Revolution, 635–636, *693*
Industry and recreation provision,
669–670
Inertia, 204
moment of, 247–255, *269*
Information processing, 295–323, *432*
perception in, 301–308
Schmidt's model, 296–297
sensory input, 299–301
Welford's model, 321
Whiting's model, 297
Inhaled air, 80, *268*
Inhibition
learning, 335
muscle, *268*
Injury, training, 143
Input, information processing, 296
Inspiration, 70, 73, 74, 76, *268*
Inspiratory capacity (IC), 82
Inspiratory reserve volume (IRV), 82,
268–269
Instinct theories, aggression, 376, *432*
Institut National de Sport et Education
Physique (INSEP), 551, 555
Institutes of sport, *543*
Institutions, definition, 494, *543*
Instruction, 344
verbal, 348–349
Interaction
between competitors, 284
groups/teams, 399–401
Interactionist (interactional) theory, 361,
406, *432*
Intercostal muscles, 72–73, 74
Intercostal nerves, 73, *269*
Interval, *269*
Interval training, 148–156, *269*
Intervertebral disc, 5, 6
Introversion, 359, *432*
Invasion games, 672–673
Inversion, 15, *269*
Inverted-U theory, 418, *432*
Isokinetic training/muscle contraction,
27, *269*
Isometric training/muscle contraction,
27, 35, 42, 155, *269*
Isotonic exercise/muscle contraction, 27,
269

Issues in physical education and sport, 521–541

Jackson Pollock Equation, 126
Jogging, 147
John Major Initiative, 480, 481
Joint capsule, 14, *269*
Joints, 3
   ageing, 182
   angle, effect on load force, 229, 234
   cartilaginous, 5, 6, 13, *266*
   fibrous (fixed), 5, 13, *267*
   movements, 3–4, 12–20
   synovial, 5, 13–16, *273*
Joule (J), 89, *269*
Jousting, 633
Juggling, 128
Jumper, motion of, 236–238

Karvonen method/principle, 149, *269*
Kenya, sport in, 498
Kinaesthesis, 300, 301, *432*
Kinetic energy (motion energy), 189, 196, *269*
   rotational, 250, *272*
Knee, 14
Knowledge of performance, 320, 336, 337, *432*
Knowledge of results, 320, 336, *432*
Kollectivs, 615–616
Komsomol, 619–620, *625*
Krebs (citric acid) cycle, 96, 97, *269*

Lactacid oxygen debt component, 103–105, *269*
Lactate, *269*
Lactate shuttle, 104, *269*
Lactate threshold (LT), 104, 139
Lactic acid, *269*
   removal following exercise, 103–104
Lactic acid energy system, 95, 96, 137, *269*
   effect of training, 136, 139
   weight training, 153
Laissez-faire leadership, 407, *431*
Laminar flow, 216, *269*
Larynx, 70, 71, *269*
Law of effect, 381, *432*
Law of exercise, *432*
Lawn tennis, 675, *693*
Leaders/leadership, 405–409
   qualities/styles, 406–408
   theories, 406
Learned helplessness, 387, *432*
Learning, 281, 325–326, *432*
   association theories, 330–333
   causes of plateaux, 326–327
   cognitive theories, 333
   information processing, 295–323
   phases, 329–330
   principles and theories, 328–334
   self-esteem and, 367–368
   social (observational) theory, 333–334, 397–398, *433*
   Thorndike's laws, 332
   transfer of, 340–343, *434*
   trial and error, 332

Learning curves, 326–327, *432*
Leisure
   as basis of self-realisation, 446
   concept of, 441–446, *543*
   as economic condition, 444–445
   as form of social control, 445
   purposeful, 445
   as spare time, 444
Levers, 228, 231–234, *269*
Lifetime sport, 594–595
Lift forces, 206
Ligaments, 14, *269*
   effect of training, 139
Lilleshall Hall, 485
Line (ridge), bone, 5, 7
Lipids, 175, *269*
Load, 228, 231–233, *269*
Loafing, 401–402
Local festivals, 500–501, 502
Locus of causality/control, 386–387, *432*
Lombardism, 457, 594
Lung stretch receptors, 74, 75
Lung volumes, 82–87
   children, 170
   effects of ageing, 183
   measurement, 83–84
Lungs
   gas exchange, 76–82
   structure, 70–71
Lymph, *269*
Lymph nodes, 68

Maclaren, Archibald, 671, 681
Macrocycles, 144, *269*
Macrophages, 70
Magnus effect, 207, 208, 217–218, *269*
Manliness, *693*
Marxism, 500
Masking agents, 165
Mass, 204, *269*
   centre of, 234–235, 236–238, *266*
Mass culture, 504–505, 508
Massovost, 451, 615, *625*
Masterstvo, 615, *625*
Mastery learning, 333
Mastery orientation, 358, 388
Materialism, 500
May Day festivals, 632–633
Media and sport, 528
Medulla oblongata, 73, 74, *269*
Memory, *433*
   long-term, 305, 306–308, *432*
   short-term, 304, 305–306, *434*
   for skills, 307
   strategies for improving retention, 307–308
Memory trace, 318
Menisci, 14, *269*
Mental imagery, 164
Mental preparation, 413–428
Mental rehearsal, 349–350, 425–426, *433*
Merrie England, *693*
Mesocycles, 144, 160, *269*
Mesomorphs, 120, *272*
Metabolic rate, *269*
   basal, 91, 93, 107, 115, 176, *265*
   effect of exercise, 175
   total, 115, 177, *273*

Metabolism, 94–95, *269*
   children, 170
   energy, 114–116
Microcycles, 144, 160, *269*
Military drill, 681, *693*
   1902 Model course, 682–684
Minerals, dietary, 113, *269*
Minoan Crete, 495
Minorities, *543*
Minute ventilation/volume ($\dot{V}I$ or $\dot{V}E$), 82, 84–85, *269*
Mitochondria, 38, 40, 94, 96, 98, *269*
Mitral valves, 49, 51, *269*
Mob games, 641–644, 656, *693*
Mobility
   active, 157, *264*
   kinetic (ballistic), 157–158, *269*
   passive, 157, 158, *271*
Mobility training, 156–158, *269*
Model course (1902), 682–684, *693–694*
Modelling, 333–334, 391, 398, *433*
Moment of force, 228–229, *269*
Moment of inertia, 247–255, *269*
Moments, principle of, *271*
Momentum, *269*
   angular, 250–251, *264*
   conservation in collisions, 224–225
   impact and, 218–219
Mop days, 501
Moral integrity, *694*
Morality, bracketed, 377, *431*
Motion
   energy, 189, 196
   equations of, 195
   general, *268*
   linear, 189–198, *269*
   Newton's Laws, 192, 193, 194–195
   rotational, *272*
Motivation, 335–336, 379–393, *433*
   achievement, 382–385
   attribution in, 385–389
   components, 379
   feedback as, 338
   group, 401
   measuring, 382
   self-motivation, 385
   types, 381
Motor abilities, 286–291
   gross, 288
   measurement, 290–291
Motor control
   closed loop theory, 317–318, 320, 321, *431*
   feedback, 321
   levels, 320–321
   open loop theory, 316–317, 320, *433*
   schema theory, 318–319
Motor end-plates, 31, 33, *269*
Motor fitness, 119, 120–121, *270*
Motor neurone, 31–33, *270*
Motor neurone pools, 33, *270*
Motor programmes, 315–316, *433*
Motor skills, 280, 307
   coordination, *270*
   fundamental, 316, *543*
   learning
      information processing, 315–319
      phases, 329–330
      theories, 330–335

Motor units, 31, 33–35, *270*
Mountaineering, 677
Movement
  axes of, 17
  coordinated, 31–37
    role of reflexes, 36
    sensory feedback in, 35
  voluntary, *274*
Movement education, 568, 590, 592
Movement patterns, synovial joints, 15
Movement time, 309, *433*
Muscle(s)
  action, 20–26
  agonist/antagonist, 24, 35, *264*
  agonist/antagonist response, 142
  atrophy, 182
  blood flow in, 63–69
  cardiac, 48
  effects of ageing, 182–183
  extensor, 24
  fatigue, 105, *270*
  fixator, 24, *267*
  flexor, 24
  force in, 228–231
  fusiform, 21, 22, *268*
  hypertrophy, 137–138, 155
  insertion, 24, *268*
  local endurance, *269*
  origin, 24, *271*
  pennate, 21–22, *271*
  red, 40, *272*
  relaxation, 425
    progressive, *433*
  respiratory, 72–73
  response to overload training,
    137–138, 139
  restoration of glycogen stores, 105
  shapes, 21–22
  skeletal (striated; striped; voluntary),
    38–40, 60, *272*
  smooth, 60, 61, 138, *272*
  soreness, 104, *270*
  spasms, 104
  synergistic, 224, *273*
  white, 40, *275*
Muscle contraction, 21
  concentric, 27, 42, 155, *266*
  dynamic, 27, *267*
  eccentric, 27–28, 42, 155, *267*
  effects on body shape/movement,
    227–228
  energy and, 95
  gradation, 34, *268*
  Huxley's sliding filament theory,
    41–42, *268*
  inhibition, 35
  nervous system and, 31
  reaction forces and, 211–212
  static (isometric), 27, 35, 42, 155, *269*
  tetanic, 34
  types, 26–30, 42
Muscle fibres, 38–40, *270*
  fast-twitch (type II), 21, 43, 44, 96,
    270
    effects of training, 136, 137–138
    weight training, 152–153
  single muscle fibre block, 31, *272*
  slow-twitch (type I), 21, 40, 43, 44,
    96, *270*

  effects of training, 136, 139
    weight training, 153
Muscle group, *270*
Muscle pump, 67, *270*
Muscle spindles, 35, *270*
Muscle twitch, 33, *270*
Muscular Christianity, 661–662, 668,
  671, *694*
Myelin sheath, 31, 32
Myelination, 168–169, *270*
Myocardium, 48, 49, *270*
  effect of aerobic training, 138
  striped tissue, *273*
Myofibrils, 39, 40, *270*
Myogenic, *270*
Myoglobin, 40, 78, *270*
  role in recovery, 103
Myosin filaments, 41, 42, *267*

Nasal cavity, 70, 71, *270*
Nasal strips, 164
National Coaching Foundation, United
  Kingdom, 483
National Institute of Sports and Physical
  Education (INSEP), France,
  551, 555
National Lottery, 472, 527
National parks
  Australia, 578
  England and Wales, 488
  United States, 599–600
National Trust, 489
Nationalism/national identity, sport and
  emergent countries, 497–498
  France, 547–548
  Soviet Union/Russia, 606
  United Kingdom, 470
  United States, 585–586
Native Americans, *625*
Nervous impulse, *270*
Nervous system, 31, 53, 63
Net force, 200–202, *270*
Net oxygen cost, 93, 109–110, *270*
Neuromuscular junction, impulse
  transmission at, 33
Neuromuscular system, effects of
  ageing, 183–184
Neurones
  effects of ageing, 182
  motor, 31–33, *270*
  sensory, 35, *272*
Neuroticism, 359, *433*
Newton's Laws of Motion, 192, 193,
  194–195
Newtons, 89, 202, *270*
Nodes of Ranvier, 32
Noise, information processing, 302,
  433
Noradrenaline, 53
Notch, bone, 5
Nutrition, 112–117
Nutritional aids, 164
Nutritional balance, *270*

Obesity, 173–176, *270*
Observational learning, 333–334,
  397–398

Olympian rural games, 501
Olympic Movement/Olympism, 456,
  494, 501, 503–504, *543*
One repetition maximum (1RM), *270*
Onset of blood lactate accumulation
  (OBLA), 104, *270*
  effect of endurance training, 139
Open loop theory, 316–317, 320, *433*
Operant conditioning, 331–332
Organisation, skills classification, 285
Origins of sport, 630
Ossification, 11–12
  intramembranous, 11–12, *269*
Osteoarthritis, 182, *270*
Osteoblasts, 11–12, *270*
Osteoclasts, 11, *270*
Osteocytes, 11, *270*
Osteoporosis, 181, *270*
Otter hunting, 636
Outcome orientation, 388
Outdoor pursuits, 486–487, *543*
Outdoor recreation/education, 451, 465
  Australia, 577–581
  definitions, 465, 486–487, *543*
  France, 555–557
  issue analysis, 530–534
  Soviet Union/Russia, 618–621
  United Kingdom, 486–489
  United States, 598–601
Output, information processing, 296
Outward Bound movement, *543*
  Australia, 581
  France, 557
  United Kingdom, 489
  United States, 600–601
Overeating, 174–175, *270*
Overload training, 133–135
  effects/adaptation, 136–140
    gender differences, 140
    reversibility, 140–141
Oxidation of hydrogen atoms, *270*
Oxygen, *270*
  arteriovenous oxygen difference
    (a-$\bar{v}O_2$ diff), 78, 81, 138, *265*
    children, 170
  consumption (uptake), 93, 107, *270*
    during recovery, 101–102
    maximum (aerobic power;
      $\dot{V}O_2$max), 107
    in measurement of energy costs,
      109–110
  net oxygen cost, 93, 109–110
  tissue respiration, 78
Oxygen debt, 102, *267*
  alactic (fast component), 102–103,
    264
  children, 169
  lactacid (slow component), 103–105,
    269
Oxygen deficit, 101, 102, *270*
Oxygen dissociation curve, 77, 80, *270*
Oxygen recovery *see* Oxygen debt
Oxygen transport system, effect of
  altitude, 162
Oxygenation, haemoglobin, 77–78
Oxyhaemoglobin, 78, *270*
Oxymyoglobin, 101, *270*
  function in purging oxygen debt,
    103

Pacemaker, cardiac (sinoatrial node), 48, 50, 51, *272*
Pacing, 282–283, *433*
Parasympathetic nervous system, 53, 63, 270–271
Parietal membrane, 70, 71, *271*
Partial pressure (p) of a gas, 76–77, 80, 81, *271*
Pedestrianism, 640–641, *694*
Perception, 296, 301–308
Perceptual abilities, 169, *271*, 289
Perceptual—motor skills, 280, *433*
Perceptual skill, 279, *433*
Perceptual trace, 318
Performance, 281, 325–326, *433*
Performance accomplishments, 391
Pericardium, 48, 49, *271*
Perimysium, 38, 39, *271*
Period, *271*
Periodisation, training, 143–144, *271*
Periosteum, 10, 24, *271*
Peripheral nervous system, *271*, 299, *433*
Peripheral resistance, 63, *271*
Personal development, 489, *544*
Personal performance programmes (PPP), 160
Personality, 356–369
    achievement motivation and, 383
    assessment, 361–363, 364
    definitions, 356
    self-concept/self-esteem, 365–368
    sport and, 363–365
    structure, 356–357
    theories, 357–361
Persuasive communication, 373, 391
16PF questionnaire/profile, 362
Pharynx, 70, 71, *271*
Phosphagen restoration, 102, 103, *271*
Phosphocreatine (PC), 95, *271*
    regeneration, 102
Phrenic nerves, 73, *271*
Physical Activity Readiness Questionnaire (PARQ), 121
Physical education
    Australia, 559–582
    definitions, 438, 462–463, *544*
    France, 545–558
    philosophical perspective, 437–441
    school curriculum in, 463, 474–476, 477–478, 482
    Soviet Union/Russia, 603–623
    United Kingdom, 469–490
    United States, 583–602
    value, 463–465
Physical endeavour, *544*, *694*
Physical fitness, 119–120, *271*
Physical performance
    categories of, 438–440
    social setting (extrinisic factors), 440–441
Physical prowess, *544*
Physical recreation, definition, 438
Physical training, *694*
Physiotherapy, 163
Pioneer movement, Soviet Union/ Russia, 605, 610, 620, *625*
Pivot *see* Fulcrum
Pivot joint, 16, *271*
Plan of action *see* Motor programmes

Planes, body, 15, 16
    frontal, 16, *268*
    sagittal (median), 16, *272*
    transverse (horizontal), 16, *274*
Plantar flexion, 15, 17, *271*
Plas y Brenin National Centre for Mountain Activities, 485
Plasma, 58, *271*
Platelets, *271*
Play, 438, 447–444
Pleura, pulmonary, 70, *271*
Pleural cavity, 70, *271*
Pleural fluid, 70, *271*
Pluralism, *544*, 585, *625*
Plyometric work, 27–28, *271*
Pneumotaxic centre, 74, *271*
Pocket valve, *271*
Politics and sport, 500
    Soviet Union, 606–607
    United Kingdom, 470–471
Polycythaemia, 162
Polynesia, 496
Popular, *694*
Popular recreation, *694*
    history in Great Britain, 630–649
    in public schools, 654–656
Position, 190, *271*
Posture, 19, *271*
Potassium/sodium exchange pump, 32, *271*
Power, 90–91, 121, 189, 196, *271*
    aerobic, 107, *264*
    anaerobic, 110, *264*
    decline, 111, *271*
    peak, 136, 137
Practice, 347
    distributed (spaced), 349, *431*
    fixed, 349
    learning and, 329, 332–333
    massed, 349, *432*
    part, 346
    types, 349–350
    variable, 349, *434*
    whole, 346
    whole-part-whole, 347
Practice style of teaching, 345, *433*
Preadolescence, *271*
Precapillary sphincter, *271*
Prejudice, 371
Pressure
    barometric, *265*
    footwear/surfaces, 214
Prize ring/prizefighting, 646–648, *694*
Productivity, teams, 401, 404, *433*
Professional, *694*
Professionalism, 457, 458, 527, *544*, 640–641
Profile of Mood States (POMS), 364
Pronation, 15, 17, *271*
Proprietary schools, 653, *694*
Proprioception, 299–300
Proprioceptive neuromuscular facilitation (PNF), 157, *271*
Proprioceptors, 74, 75, *271*
    feedback from, 320
Protein, dietary, 113, *271*
Protrusions, bone, 6–7, *271*
Psychoanalytic theory, 357–359
Psychodynamic theories, 357–359

Psychological needs, training, 144
Psychological refractory period, 312–313, *433*
Psychological stress, 423
Psychological testing, 361–363, 364
Psychology of sport, 353–429
    history, 354–355
Psychometry, personality assessment, 362, *433*
Psychomotor abilities, 286–291
    measurement, 290–291
Psychomotor skills, 280
Puberty, 169, *271*
Public schools (England), *694*
    athleticism in, 652, 656, 659–665
    background to development, 651
    girls schools, 659, 663, 665, *693*
    social control through physical activity, 659–660, *694*
    sport and character development, 661–662
    structural basis, 652–654
    technical development of sports, 654–661
    types, nineteenth century, 653–654
Pueblo baseball, 497
Pugilism, 647
Pulmonary arteries, 49, *271*
Pulmonary veins, 49, *271*
Pulmonary ventilation, 70, *271*
Pulse, 52, *271*
Punishment, 332, 337, *433*
Purkinje fibres, 50, *271*
PWC-170 test, 130, *272*
Pyruvic acid, 96, *272*

Queen's College Step Test, 108–109, 123
Quest, *544*

Racism, 473, 525, *544*
Rackets, 675
Radial artery, *272*
Radian, 243, 244, *272*
Radius of gyration, *272*
Rankings structure, 524–525
Ratchet mechanism, 42, *272*
Rational recreation, 659, 663, *694*
    19th century Britain, 667–680
Reaction forces, 195, 200, 201, 209–212, *272*
Reaction time, 121, *272*, 297, 309–312, *433*
    choice, 310, *431*
    measuring, 128, 311
    simple, 310
Readiness, 332
Real tennis, 644–645, *694*
Recall, 307
Recall schema, 319
Reciprocal innervation (inhibition), 36
Reciprocal style of teaching, 345, *433*
Recognition in perceptual process, 302, 306–308
Recognition schema, 319
Recovery after exercise, 101–106
    active recovery (cool-down), 103, 104, 145

Recovery after exercise (*cont'd*)
    effect of aerobic training, 139
    passive recovery, 103
Recreation
    concept of, 450, *544*
    physical, 450–452, *544*
    see also Outdoor recreation; Popular
        recreation; Rational
        recreation
Red blood cells, 58, *272*
Reflexes, 36, 330–331
Regularity, *694*
Rehearsal, mental, 349–350, 425–426,
    433
Reinforcement, 332, 335, 398, *433*
    feedback for, 338
Relationships, 492
    group dynamics, 508–515
Relaxation, differential, 287
Relaxation techniques, 424–425
Religion and sport
    19th century Britain, 668, 669
    tribal societies, 497
Repetitions, interval training, 148, *272*
Repolarisation, 32, 52, *272*
Residual volume (RV), 82, *272*
Respectability, *694*
Respiration
    aerobic, 96–98, 99, 137
    anaerobic, 95–96, 99, 136–137
    tissue, 70, 77, 78–79, 94
Respiratory centre, 74, 75, *272*
Respiratory exchange ratio (RER;
        respiratory quotient), 92–93,
        139, *272*
Respiratory pump, 67, *272*
Respiratory system, 70–88
    children, 170
    effect of aerobic training, 138
    effect of ageing, 183
    effect of obesity, 174
Response
    dominant, *431*
    programming, 297, 315
    selection, 296, 315
    to information processing, 296–297,
        298
    see also Stimulus—response
Response time, 309, *433*
    improving, 313
Rest relief, 148, 155, *272*
Resting potential, 31–32
Resultant force, 200–202, *272*
Retention, learning, 334
Reversal theory, 421
Rewards, extrinsic, 381–382
Ridge, bone, 5, 7
Ringelmann effect, 401–402, *433*
Risk, 465, *544*
Risk taking, 383–384
Ritual, 496, 497, 501, 630, *694*
Role models, emergent countries, 497
Role play, 515–518
Role theory, sociology, 492, 493
Roles, 366–367
    sport and physical education,
        515–518
    within group/team, 400–401
Roman Britain, 630–631

Rome, Ancient, 496
Rotating systems, 243–256, *272*
Rotation, 15, 16, 17, *272*
    external, *267*
    internal, *269*
Rotational energy, 250, *272*
Roughage, 114
Rowing, 676
Rugby football, 673
Rugby School, 656–658
Ruler drop test, 311
Rules, 397
Rural (rustic) simplicity, France, 556,
    557, *625*
Russia *see* Soviet Union/Russia

Sabbatarianism, *694*
Sacrum, 6
Saddle joint, 16, *272*
Sagittal axis, 17, *272*
Sagittal (median) plane, 16, *272*
Sailing, 676
Saltatory conduction, 32, *272*
Samoa, 497
Sarcolemma, 38, 39, *272*
Sarcomeres, 39, 40–41, *272*
Sarcoplasm, 38, 39, 94, 96, *272*
Saturday half-day, 669, *694*
Saxons, 632
Scalar, *272*
Scales, attitude, 371–372
SCCAMP goals, 415, *433*
Schema, *433*
Scholarships, United States, 596–597
Schools
    Australia, 566–570
    England and Wales, 474–478, 479,
        480–482
        early physical training syllabuses,
            684–687, 688, *694*
        transitions in English elementary
            schools, 681–692
    France, 549–552
    physical education in, 462, 463,
        474–478, 479, 480–482
    Soviet Union/Russia, 610–612
    sports, 480
    United States, 589–594
    see also Public schools
Self concept, 365–368, *434*
Self-confidence, 390–392, *434*
Self-efficacy, 390–392, *434*
Self-esteem, 365, 366, 367–368, *434*
Self-fulfilling prophecy, 390–392
Self-motivation, 385
Self-talk, 426, *434*
Sensory input systems, 299–301
Sensory neurones, 35, *272*
Sensory stores, short-term, 303–304,
    434
Separatism, *544*
Sets, interval training, 148, *272*
Sex discrimination, 534–538
    United Kingdom, 473
Shaping, 332
Sharpey's fibres, 24
Shivering, 93
Shooting, 638

Shop window, Soviet Union/Russian
    sport, 500, *625*
Shoulder joint, movements, 4
Singlesticks, 646, *694*
Sinoatrial node (cardiac pacemaker), 48,
    50, 51, *272*
Sit and reach test, 124
Sit-ups, 123
Skating, 676–677
Skeleton, *272*
    appendicular, 3, *265*
    axial, 3, *265*
    functions, 4
    movement and, 3–12
Skiing, 677
Skill(s)
    ability and, 286–291
    classification, 281–286
    closed, 283–284, *431*
    coactive, 284, 410, *431*
    continuous, 282, 307, *431*
    definition, 279–281
    discrete, 282, *431*
    fine, 282, *432*
    gross, 282, *432*
    individual, 284, *432*
    information processing and,
        295–323
    interactive, 284, *432*
    learning, 141–142, 281
    memory for, 307
    open, 283–284, 307, *433*
    pacing and, 282–283
    serial, 282
    training, 159
    transfer, 142
Skinfold measurements, 125–126, *272*
SMART goals, *434*
SMART(ER) goals, 414–415
Smooth muscle, 60, 61, *272*
    effect of aerobic training, 138
Social cohesion, 402, *434*
Social control through physical activity,
    public schools, 659–660, *694*
Social facilitation, 410–412, *434*
Social inhibition, 410, 411, *434*
Social learning theory, 333–334, 361,
    376, 397–398, 406, *434*
Social loafing, 401–402, *434*
Social setting of performance, 440–441
Socialisation, 397–398, 498, 513–514
Society, 494, *544*
    culture/sport and, 494–508, 522,
        524–525
Sociology
    definitions, 491
    sport/physical education and,
        491–519
    theories, 492–494
Sociometry, 403–404, *434*
Sodium/potassium exchange pump, 32
Somatic state anxiety, 421, *434*
Somatotypes, 120, *272*
South America, sport in, 498
Soviet Union/Russia, physical education
    and sport
    administration of physical education,
        610–614
    administration of sport, 614–618

Soviet Union/Russia, physical education
    and sport (*cont'd*)
    outdoor recreation (tourism),
        618–621
    social setting, 603–609
Spa movement, 671, *694*
Spartakiads, 605, 612, 615, *625*
Spatial summation, 34–35, *272*
Special needs *see* Disabled
Specific dynamic action (SDA), 177, *272*
Spectators *see* Audience; Crowd
Speed, 120, 189, 190, 191–192, 194, 195,
    272
    testing, 124
Sphygmomanometer, 65, *272*
Spin, flight and, 217–218
Spine, bone, 5, 7
Spinning *see* Rotating systems
Spirometer, 82, 83–84, *272*
Sport
    Australia, 559–582
    classification, 455–456
    concept of, 454–461, *544*
    culture and, 494–508, 522, 524–525
    definition, 438
    ethnic, 494, 500–501, *543*
    France, 545–558
    social setting, 440–441
    Soviet Union/Russia, 603–623
    structure, 523
    United Kingdom, 469–490
    United States, 583–602
Sport Aid Foundation (SAF), 485
Sport for All, 451, 458, *544*, 553
Sport Competition Anxiety Test (SCAT),
    420
Sport education, 533
Sport England, 483
Sport science, 570
Sports coach UK, 483
Sports colleges, 474–475, 482, *544*
Sports Council(s), 483
Sports drinks, 116, 164
SportsLEAP, 574
Sportsmanship, 456, 457, *544*
Stability, 239–240, *272*
    personality, 359, *434*
Stacking, 500, 588–589, *625*
Stage training, 153, 155, *273*
Stamford, bull-running, 633–634
Stamina, 288
Starling's Law of the Heart, 52, *273*
State anxiety, 420, *434*
State measures, 363, *434*
State Trait Anxiety Inventory (STAI),
    420
Steady state, *273*
Steeplechasing, 639, *694*
STEN score, 362, *434*
Step tests, 107–109, 123
Stereotyping, 371, 534–535
Steroids, anabolic androgenic, 165
Stick drop test, 128
Stimulus
    identification, 296, 303
    information processing, 302
    response to, 309–313
Stimulus—response (S-R) learning,
    330–333, 335, 361

Streamlining, 193, 216, *273*
Strength, 119–120, *273*
    dynamic, 120, *267*, 288
    effect of ageing, 182
    endurance, 120, *273*
    explosive/elastic, 120, *267*, 288
    gender differences, 130
    maximal, 120, *273*
    static, 120, *273*, 288
    testing, 121
    trunk, 288
    types, 120
Strength training, 133–134, 135–136
    children and adolescents, 169
Strength work, elastic/explosive *see*
        Plyometric work
Stress, 422–423, *434*
Stretch reflexes, 35
Stringent administration, *694*
Stroke volume, 52, *273*
    children, 170
    effect of exercise, 179
Structure, sociology, 492, 493
Supination, 15, 17, *273*
Sweating, 139–140
Swedish drill, 681–682, *694*
Swimming, 147, 148
    rational development, 671
Swordplay, 646
Sympathetic nervous system, 53, 63, *273*
Synapses, 32, *273*
Synovial fluid, 14, *273*
Synovial joints, 13–16, *273*
Synovial membrane, 14, *273*
Systems, society, *544*
Systole, 51, *273*

Tailteann Games, 630
Target games, 673–674
Target zone, *273*
Task analysis, 346
Task cohesion, 402, *434*
Task orientation, 358, 388
Teaching, 343–351
    forms of guidance, 346–349
    modes of presentation, 345–347
    process, 344
    styles, 344–345
Team, 399–404, 509
    leadership, 405–409
Team spirit, 509, 510
Tendons, 23–24, *273*
    effect of training, 139
    tension, 35
Tension, balanced, 492, 493, 512
Tetanic contraction, 34, *273*
Thermoregulation, 139
    children, 170
Thorndike's laws of learning, 332
Thought-stopping, 426, *434*
Thresholds, *273*
    alactic—lactic, 95–96, 101
    anaerobic, 74, *264*
    energy systems, 95, 136–137
    lactate, 104, 139
Tidal volume (TV), 82, 84–86, *273*
    effect of aerobic training, 138
Tiers-temps pedagogique, 549–550, *625*

Timbertop, 580, *625*
Tissue fluid, 67–68, *273*
Tissue respiration, 70, 77, 78–79, 94,
    273
Title IX, US Education Amendment Act
        of 1972, 535, 588, 593, *625*
Torque, 228–229, *273*
Total body fatigue, 105
Total lung capacity (TLC), 82
Total metabolic rate, 115, 177, *273*
Touch, 299
Tourism (outdoor recreation), Soviet
        Union/Russia, 618–621, *625*
Tournament, 633, *694*
Trabeculae, 9
Trachea, 70, 71, *273*
Traditional sports, 496–497, 501
Training, 132–170, 347
    altitude, 161–162, 163
    circuit, 153–155, *266*
    continuous, 147, *266*
    cyclical loading, 143
    duration, 133, *273*
    endurance, 115, 148
    fuel use and, 115
    individual response, 144–145, *273*
    interval, 148–156
    mobility, 156–158, *269*
    moderation in, 143, *273*
    overload, 133–135, *273*
        effects/adaptation, 136–140
    periodisation, 143–144
    regression after stopping, 140–141,
        274
    repetition in, 143, *274*
    specificity, 141, *274*
    stage, 153, 155
    variance in, 143–144, *274*
Training heart rate (THR), 149
Training principles, *273–274*
Training programmes, 160–161
    children, 169, 170
    coronary heart disease prevention,
        179–180
    health-related fitness, 184–185
Trait, 359, *434*
Trait anxiety, 420, *434*
Trait measures, 362–363
Trait theories, 359–361
Transfer (of learning), *274*, 340–343, *434*
Travel and sport, 668
Triad ('T') vesicles, 38, *274*
Tribal societies, 496–497, 498, *544*
Tricuspid valves, 49, 51, *274*
Triglycerides, 114, 174, *274*
    effect of exercise, 179
Tropomyosin, 41–42, *274*
Troponin, 41–42, *274*
Trunk strength, 288
Tubercle, 5, 7
Tuberosity, 5, 7

UK Sports Institute (UKSI), 485
Union National du Sport Scolaire
        (UNSS), 551, 552, *625*
United Kingdom
    history of popular recreation,
        630–649

United Kingdom (*cont'd*)
 physical education and sport
  administration of physical
   education, 474–482
  administration of sport, 483–486
  outdoor recreation/education,
   486–489
  rational recreation in 19th
   century, 667–680
  social setting, 469–473
 see also England
United Kingdom Sports Trust (UKST)
 see Youth Sports Trust
United States of America, physical
 education and sport
 administration of physical education,
  589–594
 administration of sport, 594–598
 outdoor recreation and education,
  598–601
 social setting, 583–589
Universities
 Australia, 570–571
 Soviet Union/Russia, 612, 614
 United States, 596–597
Urban revolution, 636, *694*
Urbanisation, 667–668
USSR *see* Soviet Union/Russia

Vascular shunt, 64, *274*
Vascular system, 47, 58–62
 children, 170
 effect of aerobic training, 138
Vasoconstriction, 61, 64, *274*
Vasodilation, 61, 64, *274*
Vasomotor centre, 63–64, *274*
Vasomotor control, 61, 63–64, *274*
Vectors, 200–202, *274*
 components, 202, *266*
Veins, 60, 61–62, *274*

Velocity, 190, 194, 195, *274*
 angular, 245, *264*
Venae cavae, 49, 62, *274*
Venoconstriction, *274*
Venomotor control, 64, *274*
Venomotor tone, *274*
Venous return, 52, 61–62, 67, *274*
Ventilation
 alveolar, 70, 82, *264*
 minute, 82, 84–85
 pulmonary, 70, *271*
Ventricle, 49, *274*
Venules, 60, 61–62, *274*
Vertebral column, 4, 6
Vertical axis, 17, *274*
Vertical jump test, 122
Vertigo, *544*
Victory ceremony, 496
Video, 348
Violence in sport, 377–378
 see also Aggression
Visceral membrane, 70, 71, *274*
Viscosity of fluid, 214
Vision, 299, 300
Visual aids, 347–348
Vital capacity (VC), 82, 84, *274*
Vitamin C, 164
Vitamin E, 164
Vitamins, 113, *274*
V̇O$_2$max, 107, *274*
 effect of ageing, 183, 184
 effects of exercise, 184
Voluntary movement, *274*

Wakes, 634–635, *695*
 local, 501
Warm-up, 145, *274*
Water intake, 113
Watermen, 640, *695*
Watt, 90, *274*

Wave summation, 34, *274*
Weighing, underwater, 176, *274*
Weight, body, 89–90
 reduction/control, 175–177
 see also Obesity
Weight (physics), 193, 203–204, *275*
 effects of altitude, 204
 mass and, 204–205
Weight training, 149–153
 choice of exercise, 153
 frequency and intensity, 152
 response to overload, 133–135
 safety, 152
West Indies, sport in, 498
White blood cells, 59, *275*
Wilderness areas, 578–579, 598–600,
 618, *625*
Wingate Anaerobic Cycling Test,
 110–111, *275*
Women in sport, 525
 Australia, 564–565, 574
 issue analysis, 534–540
 Moslem women, 470, 474
 Soviet Union/Russia, 608–609
 United Kingdom, 470
 United States, 588, 593, 595, 597
Work, 89, 196, *275*
World wars, effect on development of
 physical education and sport,
 686–689, *695*
Wrestling, 647

Yachting, 676
YMCA, 668, 669, 671, *695*
Youth Sports Trust, 474, 485

Zero-sum, *625*
Zone of optimal functioning, 421, *434*